A Clinical Guide to the Treatment of the Human Stress Response

Third Edition

George S. Everly, Jr. • Jeffrey M. Lating

A Clinical Guide to the Treatment of the Human Stress Response

Third Edition

With:

Chapter 13 contributed by Melvin A. Gravitz and Roger A. Page
Chapter 16 contributed by Jason M. Noel and Judy L. Curtis
Chapter 18 contributed by Rich Blake, Jeffrey M. Lating and George S. Everly, Jr.
Chapter 23 contributed by Paul J. Rosch

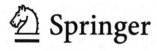 Springer

George S. Everly, Jr.
The Johns Hopkins University
    School of Medicine
The Johns Hopkins Bloomberg
    School of Public Health
Baltimore, MD, USA

Jeffrey M. Lating
Loyola University Maryland
Baltimore, MD, USA

ISBN 978-1-4614-5537-0   ISBN 978-1-4614-5538-7 (eBook)
DOI 10.1007/978-1-4614-5538-7
Springer New York Heidelberg Dordrecht London

Library of Congress Control Number: 2012946740

Printed on acid-free paper

Springer is part of Springer Science+Business Media (www.springer.com)

To George S. Everly, Sr. (1916–2011). A truly "good man" whose kindness, work ethic, and dedication to family personified the "greatest generation."

To Olivia Gayle Berhardt, may you know only health, kindness, and gentility.

To Marideth Everly Bernhardt, you make us all very proud.

To George, Carpe Diem!

To Andi, you are truly a blessing!

—GSE, Jr

To Dorothy Lating (1938–2011). Your determination and resolve are instilled life lessons that all of us who love you will always cherish.

To Austin, for allowing me to experience unmitigated pride and joy.

To Jenna, for making every day of my life special and more meaningful.

—JML

Preface to the Third Edition

The idea for our original volume first arose in 1979. At that time, the study of human stress was by no means new. More than four decades earlier, the brilliant endocrinologist Hans Selye had coined the term "stress" and along with Harvard's Walter Cannon had pioneered the study of its then perplexing physiology. John Mason, at Yale, had not only expanded the work of Selye and Cannon but also offered a heuristic formulation that made the physiology, especially the endocrinology, of stress accessible to even the non-physiologist. In 1939, the *Journal of Psychosomatic Medicine* was first published and offered explorations of the interrelationships between psychological and physiological processes, with the subsequent goal to integrate somatic and psychologically anchored therapies. Thus the basis for the science and practice of what some would later call "psychosomatic medicine" and later "stress medicine" was established. The late 1960s and early 1970s saw a virtual "epidemic" of stress-related physical and psychiatric disorders. Whether it was truly an increase in the incidence of such disorders or simply an increased acuity in the recognition of such disorders is unclear. Nevertheless, psychiatrists, psychologists, and non-psychiatric physicians were being challenged with patients who clearly presented with disorders of over arousal and disturbances in mind-body relationships. Traditional patterns of medical practice for stress-related illnesses typically focused upon treatment of the end-organ. While this is often useful and necessary, something seemed to be missing in the treatment mosaic.

One of the first groups to recognize this omission was the interdisciplinary group at Harvard Medical School headed by Herbert Benson. Benson, Joan Borysenko, David Eisenberg, and others who were predecessors or contemporaries of that group including Paul Rosch, Ernst Gellhorn, Gary Schwartz, and Edmund Jacobson, believed that in many instances the most effective treatment for stress-related disorders would be those interventions that served to mitigate pathogenic arousal, not just to mitigate the target organ disease or dysfunction. Sadly, there were no textbooks that attempted to edify and instruct the clinician in the *mosaic or continuum of treatments of the human stress response* itself, rather than just its somatic and psychological manifestations. The first addition of this book and its predecessor, a volume entitled *The Nature and Treatment of the Stress Response*, were clinical guides that endeavored to focus on the management and treatment of pathogenic arousal. As a result of its unique focus, earlier versions of this book found a receptive audience.

Thus 33 years later, this volume has once again been updated. Its purpose remains the same, that is, to serve as a useful introduction to the psychophysiologic nature of the human stress response, as well as a practical clinical resource for anyone interested in managing or treating excessive stress. This book is designed for students and practitioners in the fields of psychology, psychiatry, social work, education, and public health, as well as anyone else seeking a better understanding of the complexities of mind-body relationships and further seeking practical guidelines for intervention.

There seems little doubt that such a volume is still needed. The field of disaster mental health continues to grow, terrorism remains a constant concern internationally, volatile economic conditions as well as political unrest have set the foundation for a most anxiogenic world. While the need for a volume such as this seemed great 30 years ago, it seems even greater now as we realize we cannot just continue to solely treat the manifestation of excessive stress, we must treat the pathogenic processes, as well. This is especially true in an environment of rising healthcare costs.

Lastly, given the previous discussion, we must look to the final frontier…human resilience. In this volume we examine the notions of psychological immunity and human resilience as we attempt to complete the continuum of care in "stress medicine."

Baltimore, MD, USA   George S. Everly Jr., PhD, ABPP
                                                                                   Jeffrey M. Lating, PhD

Acknowledgments

George S. Everly, Jr. wishes to thank the following individuals for their contributions, either direct or indirect, to the creation of this volume: Theodore Millon, Ph.D., D.Sc., for his mentorship; Bertram Brown, M.D., M.P.H., for his support and guidance in international affairs; David C. McClelland, Ph.D., for his friendship and mentorship; Paul Rosch, M.D., for his support; Jeffrey T. Mitchell, Ph.D., for his friendship and support over the two decades, but most of all, he thanks his family.

Jeffrey M. Lating wishes to thank Stephen Bono, Ph.D., for his twenty years of mentoring and invaluable friendship, along with his thoughtful review of the chapter on nutrition and stress. He would also like to thank his colleague and friend Russ Hibler, Ph.D., ABPP, for his review of the biofeedback chapter. Thanks also to Lee McCabe, Ph.D., and Don Wilmes, Ph.D., for their continued mentorship, guidance, and friendship. He is particularly grateful to Ginny Jump, whose "undeniable" presence and support during the timing of this project will always be very much appreciated…UBU. Most importantly, he would like to thank his family for always providing grounding, special meaning, comfort, and laughter.

Both authors would like to thank Melvin Gravitz, Ph.D., Roger Page, Ph.D., Jason Noel, Pharm.D., BCPP, Judy Curtis, Pharm.D., Rich Blake, M.S., and Paul J. Rosch, M.D. for their scholarly contributions. They are indebted to Heather Roy, B.A., Rebecca Dean, M.S., Michelle Siegel, M.S., and Emily Shivo, B.A., for their assistance in locating and updating references and to David Essien, B.S., and Andrea N. Everly, for their artistic contributions. They would also like to thank Casey Hofmann, Phyllis Grupp, Nina Morrison, Megan Kerns, Hannah Rockwood, Molly Corry, and Connor Riegel for their production assistance in the development of this text, and Sylvana Ruggirello and Sharon Panulla from Springer for their patience, editorial guidance, and help during this project. Lastly, both authors are tremendously indebted to Traci Martino, M.S., whose organizational and technical skills allowed this work to be completed in a timely manner.

About the Authors

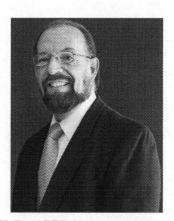

George S. Everly, Jr., Ph.D., ABPP is an Associate Professor of Psychiatry and Behavioral Sciences at The Johns Hopkins University School of Medicine and serves as a faculty member at The Johns Hopkins Bloomberg School of Public Health and the Johns Hopkins Public Health Preparedness Program. In addition, Dr. Everly serves as Professor of Psychology at Loyola University Maryland (core faculty) and as Chairman of the Board Emeritus of the International Critical Incident Stress Foundation, a United Nations-affiliated organization providing consultation and training in emergency, mental health, and disaster response. Formerly Chief Psychologist and Director of Behavioral Medicine at the Johns Hopkins Homewood Hospital Center, Dr. Everly has also held appointments at Harvard University and Harvard Medical School. He has authored or edited 20 other books, including *Secrets of Resilient Leadership, The Resilient Child, Mental Heath Aspects of Disaster* (with C. Parker), *Integrative Crisis Intervention and Disaster Mental Health* (with J. Mitchell), *Psychotraumatology: Key Papers and Core Concepts in Posttraumatic Stress* (with J. Lating), *Critical Incident Stress Management* (with J. Mitchell), and *Personality and Its Disorders* (with T. Millon). Dr. Everly has given invited lectures in 22 countries on six continents and has held visiting or honorary professorships in Argentina, Peru, and Hong Kong. He is a Fellow of the American Psychological Association and a Fellow of the Academy of Psychosomatic Medicine.

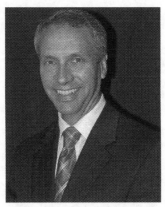

Jeffrey M. Lating, Ph.D., is a Professor of Psychology and Director of Clinical Training of the Doctor of Psychology Program at Loyola University Maryland. He also is a Senior Associate in the Department of Environmental Health Sciences in the Johns Hopkins Bloomberg School of Public Health and a faculty member of the International Critical Incident Stress Foundation. He was formerly the Director of Clinical Training and Chief Psychologist at The Union Memorial Hospital in Baltimore. He earned his B.A., in psychology at Swarthmore College, his Ph.D., in clinical psychology at the University of Georgia, and completed a postdoctoral fellowship in medical psychology at the Johns Hopkins Hospital. He has served as a consultant with the US Secret Service and currently serves as a consultant with the US Senate and the US Department of State. He has coedited or coauthored three other texts, including *Personality-Guided Therapy for Posttraumatic Stress Disorder* (with G.S. Everly, Jr).

Contents

Part III   Special Topics and the Human Stress Response

Part I
First Study the Science, Then Practice the Art

Leonardo da Vinci

Part I is the first of three parts that constitute this volume on the nature and treatment of the human stress response. This series of chapters is dedicated to providing the reader with a comprehensive introduction to stress phenomenology. The need to adhere to da Vinci's urgings to study the science before we practice the art is a virtual imperative in the case of human stress. The human stress response represents the ultimate intertwining of physiology and psychology. One cannot understand nor fully appreciate the stress response without a working knowledge of both. Thus we begin.

Chapter 1 is entitled "The Concept of Stress." It provides the reader with a working definition of the stress response and related term and concepts derived from the Selyean tradition.

Chapter 2, entitled "The Anatomy and Physiology of Human Stress" is a functional review of the core anatomical substrates and physiological mechanisms that constitute human stress. Contained in this chapter, the reader will also find a unique "systems' model" that will be used throughout the text to demonstrate the phenomenology, measurement, and treatment of human stress. In addition, the reader will find a "multi-axial" flow chart that should prove of value in better understanding various interacting physiological mechanisms.

Chapter 3 is entitled "The Link from Stress Arousal to Disease." It examines major models of target organ pathogenesis, i.e., the mechanisms that link stress arousal to disease.

Chapter 4 provides an introductory review of putative stress-related diseases. While the reviews are by no means comprehensive, they should serve as a useful introduction to core aspects of psychosomatic medicine.

Chapter 5 addresses the measurement of human stress. Though less enigmatic than in earlier years, the measurement of human stress remains a most challenging endeavor fraught with pitfalls than can bias or even cast serious epistemological doubt on the entire field.

Chapter 6 "Personologic Diathesis" introduces the somewhat novel idea that human personality can serve to buffer or accentuate exposure to psychosocial stressors. In this chapter, we introduce the work of Theodore Millon, one of the world's greatest personologists and apply his work to suggest that there may be value in understanding that various personality styles may actually have diatheses, or vulnerabilities, related to the manifestation of the stress response.

Finally, Chap. 7 introduces a rather new topic to the mainstream study of human stress, i.e., human resilience. Resilience is certainly timely and has attracted the interest of a wide variety of scholars and clinicians.

Chapter 1
The Concept of Stress

> To study medicine without reading is like sailing
> an uncharted sea.
>
> Sir William Osler, M.D.

Stress, Behavior, and Health

Scientists investigating human health and disease are now reformulating the basic tenets upon which disease theory is based. For generations, the delivery of health care services was built upon the "one-germ, one-disease, one-treatment" formulations that arose from the work of Louis Pasteur. Although clearly one of the great advances in medicine, yielding massive gains against the infectious diseases that plagued humanity, the "germ theory" of disease also represents an intellectual quagmire that threatens to entrap us in a unidimensional quest to improve human health.

The germ theory of disease ignores the fact that by the year 1960, the primary causes of death in the USA were no longer microbial in nature. Rather, other pathogenic factors had emerged. Even four decades ago, it was noted, "New knowledge... has increased the recognition that the etiology of poor health is multifactorial. The virulence of infection interacts with the particular susceptibility of the host" (American Psychological Association, 1976, p. 264). Thus, in addition to mere exposure to a pathogen, one's overall risk of ill health seems also to be greatly influenced by other factors. Recent evidence points toward health-related behavior patterns and overall lifestyle as important health determinants.

The significance of health-related behavior in the overall determination of health status is cogently discussed by Jonas Salk (1973) in his treatise *The Survival of the Wisest*. Salk argues that we are leaving the era in which the greatest threat to human health was microbial disease, only to enter an era in which the greatest threat to human health resides in humanity itself. He emphasizes that we must actively confront health-eroding practices such as pollution, sedentary lifestyles, diets void of nutrients, and practices that disregard the fundamentals of personal and interpersonal hygiene at the same time that we endeavor to treat disease.

G.S. Everly and J.M. Lating, *A Clinical Guide to the Treatment of the Human Stress Response*, DOI 10.1007/978-1-4614-5538-7_1,
© Springer Science+Business Media New York 2013

Stress! While this word is relatively new in the English lexicon, few words have had such far-reaching implications. Evidence of the adverse effects of stress is well documented in innumerable sources. Homer's *Iliad* describes the symptoms of post-traumatic stress as suffered by Achilles. In *The New Testament*, Acts, Chap. 5, describes what may be the sudden death syndrome as it befell Ananias and his wife Saphira, after being confronted by Peter the Apostle, for withholding money intended for missionary service.

Excessive stress has emerged as a significant challenge to public health. More than 30 years ago, the Office of the US Surgeon General declared that when stress reaches excessive proportions, psychological changes can be so dramatic as to have serious implications for both mental and physical health (US Public Health Service, 1979). More recently, the Global Burden of Disease Study (Lopez, Mathers, Ezzati, Jamison, & Murray, 2006) revealed that mental illnesses represent a significant contributor to the burden of global disease in high-income and low- and middle-income countries. The disability-adjusted life year (DALY) represents the number of years of life lost to premature death and disability; the disease burdens are listed by selected illnesses for high-income countries:

Ischemic heart disease	12.39 DALY
Cerebrovascular disease	9.35 DALY
Unipolar depressive disorders	8.41 DALY
Alzheimer's disease and other dementias	7.47 DALY
Trachea, bronchus, lung cancers	5.40 DALY
Hearing loss, adult onset	5.39 DALY
Chronic obstructive pulmonary disease	5.28 DALY
Diabetes mellitus	4.19 DALY
Alcohol use disorders	4.17 DALY
Osteoarthritis	3.79 DALY
Ten leading causes of burden of disease (DALYs) by high income group, 2001	

It should be noted that mental illnesses not only rank as the third most burdensome disease process but also consistent with the observations of Salk (1973) almost 40 years ago, infectious diseases represent significantly less of a global burden upon health compared to neuropsychiatric disorders and alcohol use. According to the US Surgeon General (U.S. Department of Health and Human Services, 1999), for persons ages 18–54 years, anxiety and stress-related diseases are the major contributors to the mental illness in the USA, with more than twice the prevalence (16.4%) of mood disorders (7.1%). Stress seems to have reached almost epidemic proportions. Table 1.1 underscores the role that stress may play as a public health challenge.

Finally, reviews by McEwen (2008), Marketon and Glaser (2008), Black and Garbutt (2002), Kubzansky and Adler (2010) and Brydon, Magid, & Steptoe (2006) point out the contribution that stress makes to a wide variety of physical diseases.

Contained within the Surgeon General's report, *Healthy People* (U.S. Public Health Service, 1979), was the most significant indication ever that stress and its potentially pathological effects are considered serious public health factors. The Surgeon General's report on mental health (U.S. Department of Health and Human

Table 1.1 Stress and trauma as public health challenge

- Recent evidence suggests that 82.8% of adults in the USA will be exposed to a traumatic event during their lifetime (Breslau, 2009)
- Suicide rates in the military seem to be increasing (Kang & Bullman, 2009)
- Twelve-month DSM-IV disorders are highly prevalent in the USA, with 14% experiencing moderate to severe cases (Kessler, Chiu, Demler, & Walters, 2005)
- Suicide was the tenth leading cause of death in the USA in 2007 and an estimated 11 attempted suicides occur per every suicide death
- An elevated rate of major depression was equal to the rate of PTSD in New York City residents several months after the attacks on the World Trade Center of September 11, 2001 (Galea et al., 2002)
- Rates of trauma occurrence related to violence, injury/shock trauma, trauma to others, and unexpected death peaked sharply at age 16–20 years (Breslau, 2009)
- The lifetime prevalence of criminal victimization was assessed among female health management organization patients and found to be about 57%
- In 2001, the terrorist attacks against the World Trade Center and the Pentagon focus terrorism against the USA
- Of 2050 American Airlines (AA) flight attendants, 18.2% reported symptoms consistent with probable posttraumatic stress disorder (PTSD) in the aftermath of the September 11 attacks (Lating, Sherman, Everly, Lowry, & Peragine, 2004)
- Clearly, trauma and stress are at epidemic proportions in the USA. It seems clear that such conditions represent a "clear and present danger" to the psychological health of American society
- Perhaps of greatest concern, from a public health perspective is the realization that veterans returning from military service in Iraq and Afghanistan are returning home with a high prevalence of PTSD and PTSD-like syndromes. A recent review of 29 published studies revealed varying estimates of PTSD. "Among previously deployed personnel not seeking treatment, most prevalence estimates range from 5 to 20%. Prevalence estimates are generally higher among those seeking treatment: As many as 50% of veterans seeking treatment screen positive for PTSD...Combat exposure is the only correlate consistently associated with PTSD" (Ramchand et al., 2010, p. 59)
- The Veterans Affairs (VA) estimate that about 26% of veterans seeking treatment at VA facilities meet criteria for PTSD (U.S. Department of Veteran Affairs, Veterans Health Administration, Office of Public Health and Environmental Hazards, 2010)

Services, 1999) extended those observations made 20 years earlier and even sought to quantify the burden that mental illnesses represent as a disease entity. If, indeed, the aforementioned appraisals are credible, then what has emerged is a powerful rationale for the study of the nature and treatment of the human stress response. To that end, this book is written.

Defining Stress

In this book written for clinicians, the focus is on the treatment of pathogenic stress. Yet it may be argued that effective treatment emerges from an understanding of the phenomenology of the pathognomonic entity itself. In this first chapter, the reader will encounter some of the basic foundations and definitions upon which the treatment of pathognomonic stress is inevitably based.

It seems appropriate to begin a text on stress with a basic definition of the stress response itself. The term *stress* was first introduced into the health sciences in 1926 by Hans Selye. As a second-year medical student at the University of Prague, he noted that individuals suffering from a wide range of physical ailments all seemed to have a common constellation of symptoms, including loss of appetite, decreased muscular strength, elevated blood pressure, and a loss of ambition (Selye, 1974). Wondering why these symptoms seemed to appear commonly, regardless of the nature of the somatic disorder, led Selye to label this condition as "the syndrome of just being sick" (Selye, 1956).

In his early writings, Selye used the term *stress* to describe the "sum of all nonspecific changes (within an organism) caused by function or damage" or, more simply, "the rate of wear and tear in the body." In a more recent definition, the Selyean concept of stress is "the nonspecific response of the body to any demand" (Selye, 1974, p. 14).

Paul Rosch (1986) provides an interesting anecdote. Recognizing that the term stress was originally borrowed from the science of physics, he relates how Selye's usage of the term did not conform to original intent:

> In 1676, Hooke's Law described the effect of external stresses, or loads, that produced various degrees of "strain," or distortion, on different materials. Selye once complained to me that had his knowledge of English been more precise, he might have labeled his hypothesis the "strain concept," and he did encounter all sorts of problems when his research had to be translated. (Rosch, 1986, p. ix)

Indeed, confusion concerning whether stress was a "stimulus," as used in physics, or a "response," as used by Selye, has plagued the stress literature. As Rosch (1986) describes:

> The problem was that some used stress to refer to disturbing emotional or physical stimuli, others to describe the body's biochemical and physiologic response … and still others to depict the pathologic consequences of such interactions. This led one confused British critic to complain, 35 years ago, that stress in addition to being itself was also the cause of itself and the result of itself, (p. ix)

To summarize the discussion so far, the term *stress* used in the Selyean tradition refers to a response, whereas in its original usage, within the science of physics, it referred to a stimulus, and the term *strain* referred to the response.

Using the term *stress* to denote a response left Selye without a term to describe the stimulus that engenders a stress response. Selye chose the term *stressor* to denote any stimulus that gives rise to a stress response.

In summary, drawing upon historical precedent, and consistent with Selye's original notion, the term *stress* is used within this volume to refer to a physiological reaction, or response, regardless of the source of the reaction. The term *stressor* refers to the stimulus that serves to engender the stress response.

With this fundamental introduction to the concept of stress, let us extend the conceptualization a bit further.

Ten Key Concepts in the Study of Stress

1. The stimulus that evokes a stress response is referred to a *stressor*. There are two primary forms of stressors (Girdano, Dusek, & Everly, 2009): (a) psychosocial stressors (including personality-based stressors) and (b) biogenic stressors.

2. *Psychosocial stressors* become stressors by virtue of the cognitive interpretation of the event, that is, the manner in which they are interpreted, the meanings they are assigned (Ellis, 1973; Lazarus, 1966, 1991, 1999; Lazarus & Folkman, 1984; Meichenbaum, 1977). Selye once noted, "It's not what happens to you that matters, but how you take it." Epictetus is credited with saying, "Men are disturbed, not by things, but the views which they take of them." For example, a traffic jam is really a neutral event; it only becomes a stressor by virtue of how the individual interprets the event (i.e., as threatening or otherwise undesirable). If the individual views the traffic jam as neutral or positive, no stress response ensues. Some stressors are inherently more stressful than others and leave less potential variation for cognitive interpretation (e.g., objective external threats to one's safety or well-being, grief, guilt, etc.). But even in these cases, cognitive interpretation will play a role in the adjustment to the stressor and serve to augment or mitigate the resultant stress response.

   Phenomenological research conducted by Smith, Everly, and Johns (1992, 1993) evaluated the credibility of this notion of a mediating role for psychological variables in the relation between stressor stimuli and the signs and symptoms of distress. Using structural mathematical modeling, exploratory and confirmatory factor analyses, they demonstrated that psychosocial environmental stressors exert their pathogenic effect upon the human organism primarily through cognitive processes. More specifically, evidence of cognitive–affective discord predicted signs and symptoms of physical ill health as well as maladaptive coping behaviors. This notion of a mediating role for cognitive–affective processes in the stressor-to-illness paradigm is explored in Chap. 2.

3. *Biogenic stressors,* on the other hand, require no cognitive appraisal in order to assume stressor qualities; rather, biogenic stimuli possess an inherent stimulant quality. This stimulant characteristic, commonly referred to as a sympathomimetic characteristic, is found in substances such as tea, coffee, ginseng, guarana, ginkgo biloba, yohimbine, amphetamines, and cocaine. Extremes of heat and cold and even physical exercise exert sympathomimetic effects. Biogenic stressors directly cause physiological arousal without the necessity of cognitive appraisal (Ganong, 1997; Widmaier, Raff, & Strang, 2004).

   The inclusion of the biogenic sympathomimetic category of stressors in no way contradicts the work of Lazarus and others who have studied the critical role that interpretation plays in the formation of psychosocial stressors. Such an inclusion merely extends the stressor concept to recognize that stimuli that alter the normal anatomical or physiological integrity of the individual are also capable of activating many of the same psychoendocrinological mechanisms that we refer to as the *stress response*. Thus, even if a patient convincingly reports that he or she really enjoys drinking 15 cups of caffeinated coffee per day, the clinician must be sensitive to the fact that those 15 "enjoyable" cups of coffee can serve as a powerful stressor activating an extraordinary systemic release of stress-response hormones such as epinephrine and norepinephrine, and in doing so can be a contributing factor in cardiac conduction abnormalities, for example. Similarly, individuals who belong to "Polar Bear" clubs and voluntarily immerse themselves in frigid waters during the winter undergo an extraordinary stress response characterized by massive sympathetic nervous system (SNS) arousal. Thus, even though the consumption of caffeine and the immersion of oneself into frigid bodies of water may truly be reinforcing, that person still experiences a form of physiological arousal that is accurately described as a stress response and may pose some risk to health, depending upon the intensity and chronicity of the exposure to the stressors. These issues are reiterated once again in Chap. 2.In general, it is important for the clinician to understand that by far the greater part of the excessive stress in the patient's life is self-initiated and self-propagated, owing to the fact that it is the patient who interprets many otherwise neutral stimuli as possessing stress-evoking characteristics. Kirtz and Moos (1974) suggest that social stimuli do not directly affect the individual. Rather, the individual reacts to the environment in accordance with his or her interpretations of the environmental stimuli. These interpretations are affected by such variables as personality components or status and social role behaviors. These cognitive–affective reactions are also subject to exacerbation through usually self-initiated exposures to sympathomimetic stimuli, such as excessive caffeine consumption and the like. Having the patient realize and accept reasonable responsibility for the cause and reduction of excessive stress can be a major crossroads in the therapeutic intervention. Therefore, we also discuss this issue in greater detail in Chap. 3.

4. Stress is a response, or reaction, to some stimulus. The stressor–stress response notion is illustrated in Fig. 1.1.

5. The stress response represents a physiological reaction, as defined in the Selyean tradition (Cannon, 1914; Selye, 1956) has extended this concept somewhat and conceptualizes the stress response as a "physiologic mechanism of mediation," that is, a medium to bring about a result or effect. More specifically, the stress response may be viewed as the physiological link between any given stressor and its target-organ effect. This then will be the working definition of stress used in this volume: *Stress is a physiological response that serves as a mechanism of mediation linking any given stressor to its target-organ effect or arousal.* This notion is captured in Fig. 1.2.

When communicating with patients or simply conceptualizing the clinical importance of the stress response, however, (Selye's 1974, 1976) notion that stress is the "sum total of wear and tear" on the individual seems useful.

6. The stress response, as a physiological mechanism of mediation, can be characterized by a widely diverse constellation of physiological mechanisms (Cannon, 1914; Godbout & Glaser, 2006; Gruenewald & Kemeny, 2007;

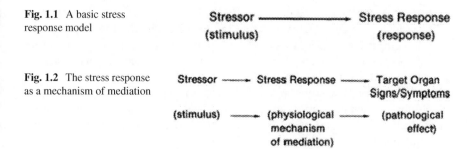

Fig. 1.1 A basic stress response model

Stressor ⎯⎯⎯⎯⎯⎯⎯→ Stress Response

(stimulus)   (response)

Fig. 1.2 The stress response as a mechanism of mediation

Stressor ⎯⎯→ Stress Response ⎯⎯→ Target Organ Signs/Symptoms

(stimulus) ⎯⎯→ (physiological ⎯⎯→ (pathological mechanism   effect) of mediation)

Kiecolt-Glaser, McGuire, Robles, & Glaser, 2002; Mason, 1972; Selye, 1976; Widmaier, Raff, & Strang, 2004) that may be categorized as (1) neurological response pathways, (2) neuroendocrine response mechanisms, and (3) endocrine response pathways. These potential response mechanisms will be reviewed in detail in Chap. 2.

Although the mechanisms of the stress response are processes of arousal, and the target-organ effects are usually indicative of arousal, the stress response has been noted as entailing such forms of arousal as to cause actual slowing, inhibition, or complete stoppage of target-organ systems (Engel, 1971; Gellhorn 1968, 1969; Gray, 1985; Selye, 1976; Widmaier, Raff, & Strang, 2004). These inhibiting or depressive effects are typically a result of the fact that, upon occasion, stress arousal constitutes the activation of inhibitory neurons, inhibitory hormones, or simply an acute hyperstimulation that results in a nonfunctional state (e.g., cardiac fibrillation). This seeming paradox is often a point of confusion for the clinician; hence, its mention here.

7. Selye (1956, 1976) has argued for the "nonspecificity" of the stress response. Other authors (Harris, 1991; Mason, 1971; Mason et al., 1976; Monroe, 2008) have argued that the psychophysiology of stress may be highly specific with various stressors and various individuals showing different degrees of stimulus or response specificity, respectively. Current evidence strongly supports the existence of highly specific neuroendocrine and endocrine efferent mechanisms. Whether there exists another way of collectively categorizing stress-response mechanisms may be as much a semantic as a physiological issue (Brosschot, Gerin, & Thayer, 2006; Everly, 1985a; Selye, 1980).

8. A vast literature argues that when stress arousal becomes excessively chronic or intense in amplitude, target-organ (the organ affected by the stress response) disease and/or dysfunction will result (Godbout & Glaser, 2006; Gruenwald & Kemeny, 2007; Selye, 1956). When stress results in *organic* biochemical and/or structural changes in the target organ, these results are referred to as a *psychophysiological disease* (American Psychiatric Association, 1968) or a *psychosomatic disease* (Lipowski, 1984). Psychosomatic diseases were first cogently described by Felix Deutsch in 1927. However, it was Helen Dunbar (1935) who published the first major treatise on psychosomatic phenomena. In 1968, in the *Diagnostic and Statistical Manual of Mental Disorders*, second

edition (American Psychiatric Association, 1968), the term *psychophysiological disorder* was used to define a "group of disorders characterized by physical symptoms that are caused by emotional factors" (p. 46). Thus, we see the terms *psychosomatic* and *psychophysiological* used interchangeably to refer to organically based physical conditions resulting from excessive stress.

Sometimes these terms are confused with the development of neurotic-like physical symptoms without any basis in organic pathology. The terms *conversion hysteria* or *somatoform disorders* are usually used to designate such nonorganic physical symptomatology.

The *Diagnostic and Statistical Manual of Mental Disorders,* fourth edition text revision, used the designation "Psychological Factors Affecting Medical Condition" to encompass stress-related physical disorders (American Psychiatric Association, 2000). By virtue of its multiaxial diagnostic schema, this nosological manual allowed clinicians to assess levels of stress and environmental support as they may affect not only physical symptoms but also psychiatric symptoms. Physical symptoms without a basis in or manifestation of organic pathology are subsumed under the somatoform category.

In the context of this volume, it is recognized that stress can be directed toward discrete anatomical or physiological target organs and therefore can lead to physical disorders characterized by organic pathology (i.e., psychophysiological or psychosomatic disorders); yet we must also recognize that the human mind can serve as a target organ. Thus, in addition to somatic stress-related disorders, it seems reasonable to include psychiatric-stress-related disorders as potential target-organ effects as well.

In summary, the terms *psychosomatic* and *psychophysiological* disorders are considered in this book as terms that refer to disorders characterized by physical alterations initiated or exacerbated by psychological processes. If tissue alterations are significant enough, and if the target organ is essential, then psychosomatic disorders could be life threatening. Neurotic-like somatoform disorders, on the other hand, involve only functional impairments of the sensory or motor systems and therefore cannot threaten life. Like the psychosomatic disorder, somatoform disorders are psychogenic; unlike psychosomatic processes, somatoform disorders entail no real tissue pathology. Confusion between the psychosomatic concept, on one hand, and the somatoform concept, on the other, is easily understandable. Yet, such confusion may lead to an underestimation of the potential severity of the disorder, thereby affecting treatment motivation and compliance.

9. Although recent reports emphasize the negative aspects of stress, there do exist positive aspects as well. Previous writers have viewed the stress response as an innate preservation mechanism, which in earlier periods of evolutionary development allowed us to endure the challenges to survival. Numerous researchers (Cannon, 1953; Chavat, Dell, & Folkow, 1964; Henry & Stephens, 1977; Widmaier, Raff, & Strang, 2004) have concluded, and we shall see in later chapters, that the nature of the psychophysiological stress response is that of apparent preparatory arousal–arousal in preparation for physical exertion.

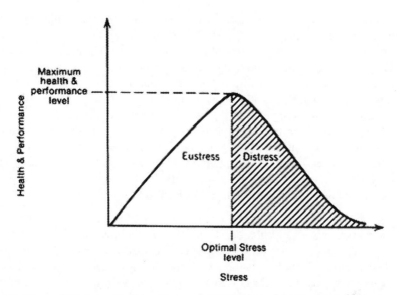

Fig. 1.3 The graphic relationship between stress arousal (*horizontal axis*) and performance (*vertical axis*). As stress increases, so does performance (eustress). At the optimal stress level, performance has reached its maximum level. If stress continues to increase into the "distress" region, performance quickly declines. Should stress levels remain excessive, health will begin to erode as well

When used in such a way, it is easy to see the adaptive utility of the stress response. Yet stress arousal in modern times under circumstances of strictly psychosocial stimulation might be viewed as inappropriate arousal of primitive survival mechanisms, in that the organism is aroused for physical activity but seldom is such activity truly warranted and, therefore, seldom does it follow (Benson, 1975; Widmaier, Raff, & Strang, 2004).

Selye (1956, 1974) further distinguishes constructive from destructive stress clearly pointing out that not all stress is deleterious. He argues that stress arousal can be a positive, motivating force that improves the quality of life. He calls such positive stress "eustress" (prefix *eu* from the Greek meaning "good") and debilitating, excessive stress "distress." Figure 1.3 depicts the relation between stress and health/performance. As stress increases, so does health/performance and general well being. However, as stress continues to increase, a point of maximal return is reached. This point may be called the *optimal stress level,* because it becomes deleterious to the organism should stress arousal increase. The point at which an individual's optimal stress level is reached, that is, the apex of one's tolerance for stress as a productive force, seems to be a function of genetic, biological, acquired physiological, and behavioral factors.

10. Last in this series of assumptions about what stress is and is not, is the point that confusion exists regarding the role of the nonmedical clinician in the treatment of the stress response. This is so primarily because the target-organ effects or

pathologies that result from excessive stress are mistakenly thought of as the psychophysiological stress response itself. It is important to remember the distinction that stress is a process of psychophysiological arousal (as detailed in Chap. 2), whereas the effects and pathologies (such as migraine headache, peptic ulcers, etc.) are the manifestations of chronically repeated and/or intense triggerings of the psychophysiological stress response (see Chap. 3). Treating the end-organ pathologies is clearly within the realm of the physician or nonmedical specialist in behavioral medicine. However, the traditional psychologist, counselor, physical therapist, social worker, or health educator can effectively intervene in the treatment of the stress arousal process itself. This includes treating the excessive stress/anxiety that accompanies, and often exacerbates, chronic infectious and degenerative diseases.

It is important to understand that this text addresses the clinical problem of excessive psychophysiological arousal—that is, the excessive stress-response process itself. It is not a detailed guide for psychotherapeutic intervention in the psychological trauma or conflict that may be at the root of the arousal (although such intervention can play a useful role). Nor does this text address the direct treatment of the target organ pathologies that might arise as a result of excessive stress. We shall limit ourselves to a discussion of the clinical treatment of the psychophysiological stress-response process itself.

Based on a review of the literature, we may conclude that treatment of the process of excessive psychophysiological stress arousal may take the form of three discrete interventions (see Girdano, Dusek, & Everly, 2009):

1. Helping the patient develop and implement strategies by which to avoid/minimize/modify exposure to stressors, thus reducing the patient's tendency to experience the stress response (Ellis, 1973; Lazarus, 1991, 2006; Meichenbaum, 2007).
2. Helping the patient develop and implement skills that reduce excessive psychophysiological functioning and reactivity (Girdano et al., 2009; Lazarus, 2006; Lehrer, Woolfolk, & Sime, 2007).
3. Helping the patient develop and implement techniques for the healthful expression, or utilization, of the stress response (see Girdano, Dusek, & Everly, 2009; Lehrer, Woolfolk, & Sime, 2007).

Finally, it has been suggested that the clinicians who are the most successful in treating the stress response have training not only in the psychology of human behavior but also medical physiology (Miller, 1978; Miller & Dworkin, 1977). Our own teaching and clinical observations support this conclusion. If indeed accurate, this conclusion may be due to the fact that stress represents the epitome of mind–body interaction. As Miller (1979) suggests, mere knowledge of therapeutic techniques is not enough. The clinician must understand the nature of the clinical problem as well. Therefore, the reader will find that the treatment section of this text is preceded by a basic discussion of the functional anatomy and physiology of the stress response.

Plan of the Book

The purpose of this text is to provide an up-to-date discourse on the phenomenology and treatment of pathogenic human stress arousal. As noted earlier, once target-organ signs and symptoms have been adequately stabilized, or ameliorated, the logical target for therapeutic intervention becomes the pathogenic process of stress arousal that caused the target-organ signs and symptoms in the first place. To treat the target-organ effects of stress arousal while ignoring their pathogenic, phenom-enological origins is palliative at best, and often predicts a subsequent relapse.

The unique interaction of psychological and physiological phenomena that embodies the stress response requires a unique therapeutic understanding, as Miller has noted. Therefore, this volume is divided into three sections: Part I addresses the anatomical and physiological nature of stress arousal. Also discussed are measurement and other phenomenological considerations. Part II offers a practical clinical guide for the actual treatment of the human stress response and addresses a multitude of various technologies. Finally, Part III discusses special topics in the treatment of the human stress response. Also included in this volume are appendices that provide a series of brief discussions on considerations and innovations relevant to clinical practice.

References

American Psychiatric Association. (1968). *Diagnostic and statistical manual of mental disorders* (2nd ed.). Washington, DC: Author

American Psychiatric Association. (2000). *Diagnostic and statistical manual of mental disorders* (4th ed. Text revision). Washington, DC: Author

American Psychological Association. (1976). Contributions of psychology to health research. *The American Psychologist, 31*, 263–273.

Benson, H. (1975). *The relaxation response*. New York, NY: Morrow.

Black, P. H., & Garbutt, L. D. (2002). Stress, inflammation and cardiovascular disease. *Journal of Psychosomatic Research, 52*(1), 1–23.

Breslau, N. (2009). The epidemiology of Trauma, PTSD, and other posttrauma disorders. *Trauma, Violence and Abuse: A Review Journal, 10*(3), 198–210.

Brosschot, J. F., Gerin, W., & Thayer, J. F. (2006). The preservative cognition hypothesis: A review of worry, prolonged stress-related physiological activation, and health. *Journal of Psychosomatic Research, 60*(2), 113–124.

Brydon, L., Magid, K., & Steptoe, A. (2006). Platelets, coronary heart disease, and stress. *Brain, Behavior, and Immunity, 20*(2), 113–119.

Cannon, W. B. (1914). The emergency function of the adrenal medulla in pain and in the major emotions. *American Journal of Physiology, 33*, 356–372.

Cannon, W. B. (1953). *Bodily changes in pain, hunger, fear, and rage*. Boston, MA: Branford.

Chavat, J., Dell, P., & Folkow, B. (1964). Mental factors and cardiovascular disorders. *Cardiologia, 44*, 124–141.

Dunbar, H. F. (1935). *Emotions and bodily changes*. New York, NY: Columbia University Press.

Ellis, A. (1973). *Humanistic psychology: The rational-emotive approach*. New York, NY: Julian.

Engel, G. L. (1971). Sudden and rapid death during psychological stress. *Annals of Internal Medicine, 74*, 771–782.

Everly, G. S., Jr. (1985). Occupational stress. In G. S. Everly & R. Feldman (Eds.), *Occupational health promotion* (pp. 49–73). New York, NY: Wiley.

Galea, S., Ahern, J., Resnick, H., Kilpatrick, D., Bucuvalas, M., Gold, J., & Vlahov, D. (2002). Psychological sequelae of the September 11 terrorist attacks in New York City. *New England Journal of Medicine, 346,* 982–987.

Ganong, W. F. (1997). *Review of medical physiology* (18th ed.). Stamford, CT: Appleton & Lange.

Gellhorn, E. (1968). Central nervous system tuning and its implications for neuropsychiatry. *Journal of Nervous and Mental Disease, 147,* 148–162.

Gellhorn, E. (1969). Further studies on the physiology and pathophysiology of the tuning of the central nervous system. *Psychosomatics, 10,* 94–104.

Girdano, D., Dusek, D., & Everly, G. S., Jr. (2009). *Controlling stress and tension*. San Francisco, CA: Pearson Benjamin Cummings.

Godbout, J. P., & Glaser, R. (2006). Stress-induced immune dysregulation: Implications for wound healing, infection disease and cancer. *Neuroimmune Pharmacology, 1*(4), 421–427.

Gray, J. (1985). Issues in the neuropsychology of anxiety. In A. Tuma & J. Maser (Eds.), *Anxiety and anxiety disorders* (pp. 5–26). Hillsdale, NJ: Erlbaum.

Gruenewald, T. L., & Kemeny, M. E. (2007). Aging and health: Psychoneuroimmunological processes. In C. M. Aldwin, C. L. Park, & A. Spiro III (Eds.), *Handbook of health psychology and aging* (pp. 97–118). New York, NY: Guilford Press.

Harris, T. (1991). Life stress and illness: The question of specificity. *Annals of Behavioral Medicine, 13,* 211–219.

Henry, J. P., & Stephens, P. (1977). *Stress, health, and the social environment*. New York, NY: Springer-Verlag.

Kang, H. K., & Bullman, T. A. (2009). Is there an epidemic of suicides among current and former military personnel? *Annals of Epidemiology, 19*(10), 757–760.

Kessler, R. C., Chiu, W. T., Demler, O., Merikangas, K. R., & Walters, E. E. (2005). Prevalence, severity, and comorbidity of 12-month DSM-IV disorders in the National Comorbidity Survey Replication. *Archives of General Psychiatry, 62,* 617–627.

Kiecolt-Glaser, J. K., McGuire, L., Robles, T. F., & Glaser, R. (2002). Emotions, morbidity, and mortality: new perspectives from psychoneuroimmunology. *Annual Review of Psychology, 53,* 83–107.

Kirtz, S., & Moos, R. H. (1974). Physiological effects of social environments. *Psychosomatic Medicine, 36,* 96–114.

Kubzansky, L. D., & Adler, G. K. (2010). Aldosterone: A forgotten mediator of the relationship between psychological stress and heart disease. *Neuroscience & Biobehavioral Reviews, 34*(1), 80–86.

Lating, J. M., Sherman, M. F., Everly, G. S., Lowry, J. L., & Peragine, T. F. (2004). PTSD reactions and functioning of American airlines flight attendants in the wake of September 11. *Journal of Nervous and Mental Disease, 192*(6), 435–441.

Lazarus, R. S. (1966). *Psychological stress and the coping process*. New York: McGraw-Hill.

Lazarus, R. S. (1991). *Emotion and adaptation*. New York: Oxford University Press.

Lazarus, R. S. (1999). *Stress and emotion: A new synthesis*. New York: Springer.

Lazarus, R. S. (2006). *Stress and Emotion: A new synthesis*. New York, NY: Springer.

Lazarus, R. S., & Folkman, S. (1984). *Stress, appraisal, and coping*. New York: Springer.

Lehrer, P. M., Woolfolk, R. L., & Sime, W. E. (2007). *Principles and Practice of Stress Management* (3rd ed.). New York, NY: The Guildford Press.

Lipowski, Z. J. (1984). What does the word "psychosomatic" really mean? *Psychosomatic Medicine, 46,* 153–171.

Lopez, A. D., Mathers, C. D., Ezzati, M., Jamison, D. T., & Murray, C. J. (2006). Global and regional burden of disease and risk factors, 2001: Systematic analysis of population health data. *The Lancet, 367*(9524), 1747–1757.

Marketon, J. W., & Glaser, R. (2008). Stress hormones and immune function. *Cellular Immunology,* *252*(1–2), 16–26.

Mason, J. W. (1971). A re-evaluation of the concept of "non-specificity" in stress theory. *Journal of Psychiatric Research, 8*(3–4), 323–333.

Mason, J. W. (1972). Organization of psychoendocrine mechanisms: A review and reconsideration of research. In N. Greenfield & R. Sternbach (Eds.), *Handbook of psychophysiology* (pp. 3–76). New York: Holt, Rinehart & Winston.

Mason, J. W., Maher, J., Hartley, L., Mougey, E., Perlow, M., & Jones, L. (1976). Selectivity of corticosteroid and catecholamine responses to various natural stimuli. In G. Servan (Ed.), *Psychopathology of human adaptation* (pp. 147–171). New York: Plenum Press.

McEwen, B. S. (2008). Central effects of stress hormones in health and disease: Understanding the protective and damaging effects of stress and stress mediators. *European Journal of Pharmacology, 583*(2–3), 174–185.

Meichenbaum, D. (1977). *Cognitive-behavior modification.* New York: Plenum Press.

Meichenbaum, D. (2007). Stress inoculation training. A preventative and treatment approach. In P. M. Lehrer, R. L. Woolfolk, & W. E. Sime (Eds.) *Principles and practice of stress mamangement* (3rd ed., pp. 497–516. New York: Guilford

Miller, N. E. (1978). Biofeedback and visceral learning. *Annual Review of Psychology, 29,* 373–404.

Miller, N. E. (1979). General discussion and a review of recent results with paralyzed patients. In R. Gatchel & K. Price (Eds.), *Clinical applications of biofeedback* (pp. 215–225). Oxford, UK: Pergamon Press.

Miller, N. E., & Dworkin, B. (1977). Critical issues in therapeutic applications of biofeedback. In G. Schwartz &J. Beatty (Eds.), *Biofeedback: Theory and research* (pp. 129–162). Chicago: Aldine.

Monroe, S. M. (2008). Modern approaches to conceptualizing and measuring human life stress. *Annual Review of Clinical Psychology, 4,* 33–52.

Ramchand, R., Schell, T. L., Karney, B. R., Osilla, K. C., Burns, R. M., & Caldarone, L. B. (2010). Disparate prevalence estimates of PTSD among service members who served in Iraq and Afghanistan: possible explanations. *Journal of Trauma and Stress, 23*(1), 59–68.

Rosch, P. (1986). Foreword. In J. Humphrey (Ed.), *Human stress* (pp. ix-xi). New York: American Management Systems Press.

Salk, J. (1973). *The survival of the wisest.* New York: Harper & Row.

Selye, H. (1956). *The stress of life.* New York: McGraw-Hill.

Selye, H. (1974). *Stress without distress.* Philadelphia: Lippincott.

Selye, H. (1976). *Stress in health and disease.* Boston: Butterworth.

Selye, H. (1980). *Selye's Guide to Stress Research.* New York: Van Nostrand Reinhold Co.

Smith, K. J., Everly, G. S., & Johns, T. (1992, December). A structural modeling analysis of the mediating role of cognitive-affective arousal in the relationship between job stressors and illness among accountants. Paper presented to the Second APA/NIOSH Conference on Occupational Stress, Washington, DC.

Smith, K. J., Everly, G. S., & Johns, T. (1993). The role of stress arousal in the dynamics of the stressor-to-illness process among accountants. *Contemporary Accounting Research, 9,* 432–449.

U. S. Department of Health and Human Services. (1999). *Mental health: Report of the surgeon general.* Rockville, MD: Author.

U. S. Public Health Service. (1979). *Healthy people.* Washington, DC: U.S. Government Printing Office.

U.S. Department of Veterans Affairs, Veterans Health Administration, Office of Public Health and Environmental Hazards. (2010). Analysis of VA health care utilization among U.S. Global War of Terrorism (GWOT) veterans. Unpublished quarterly report (cumulative through 4th quarter FY 2009). Washington, DC: Author.

Widmaier, E. P., Raff, H., & Strang, K. T. (2004). *Vander, Sherman, Luciano's Human Physiology: The Mechanisms of Body Function.* New York, NY: McGraw-Hill.

Chapter 2
The Anatomy and Physiology of the Human Stress Response

It is highly dishonorable for a Reasonable Soul to live in so Divinely built a Mansion as the Body she resides in, altogether unacquainted with the exquisite structure of it.

Robert Boyle

In the first chapter, we provided the following working definition of the stress response: "Stress is a physiological response that serves as a mechanism of mediation linking any given stressor to its target-organ effect." By viewing the phenomenology of stress within the context of a "linking" mechanism, we can answer one of the most critical questions in psychosomatic medicine, that is, through what mechanisms can stressor stimuli, such as life events, lead to disease and dysfunction? The response to that query will be addressed within the next two chapters.

This chapter describes, within the boundaries of historical reviews and foundations, current findings and speculation, the anatomical and physiological foundations of the human stress response by (1) addressing basic neuroanatomical structures and (2) tracing the psychophysiological effector mechanisms that actually represent the stress response, as currently defined. To assist in the pedagogical process, a basic model of the human stress response is constructed to serve as a unifying thread for better understanding of not only the phenomenology of human stress but also its measurement and treatment. Chapter 3 will pursue the logical extension by reviewing several models of pathogenesis, that is, the process by which stress arousal leads to disease.

Neurological Foundations

In order to understand the stress response, we must first understand its foundations, which reside in the structure and function of the human nervous systems.

The basic anatomical unit of the nervous systems is the *neuron* (see Fig. 2.1). Indeed the smallest functional unit of the nervous system, the neuron serves to

G.S. Everly and J.M. Lating, *A Clinical Guide to the Treatment of the Human Stress Response*, DOI 10.1007/978-1-4614-5538-7_2,
© Springer Science+Business Media New York 2013

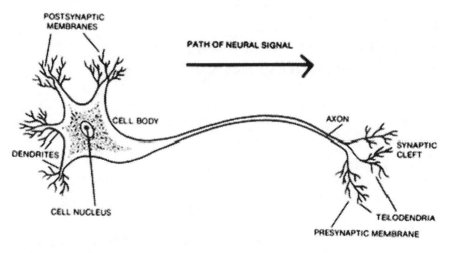

Fig. 2.1 A typical neuron

conduct sensory, motor, and regulatory signals throughout the body. The neuron consists of three basic units: (1) the *dendrites* and their outermost membranes—the postsynaptic dendritic membranes; (2) the *neural cell body*, which contains the nucleus of the cell; and (3) the *axon*, with its branching projections called the *telodendria* and their end points, the presynaptic membranes.

Neural Transmission

An incoming signal is first received by the postsynaptic membranes of the dendrites. Chemical (metabotropic) or electrical (ionotropic) processes are initiated upon stimulation of the postsynaptic dendritic membranes, which cause the neuron to conduct the incoming signal through the dendrites and the cell body. Finally, a neural impulse relayed to the axon travels down the axon until it reaches the telodendria and ultimately the presynaptic membranes. It is the task of the presynaptic membrane to relay the signal to the subsequent postsynaptic membrane of the next neuron. This is not easily achieved, however, because the neurons do not actually touch one another. Rather, there exists a space between neurons called the *synaptic cleft.*

In order for a signal to cross the synaptic cleft, chemical substances called *neurotransmitters* are required. Residing in storage vesicles in the telodendria, chemical neurotransmitters await the proper cues to migrate toward the presynaptic membrane. Once there, they are ultimately discharged into the synaptic cleft to stimulate (or inhibit) the postsynaptic membrane of the next neuron. Table 2.1 contains a list of major neurotransmitters and their anatomical loci.

Having completed a basic overview of the anatomy of neural transmission, it is necessary to return to a brief discussion of the dynamics of intraneuronal communication. For clinicians, this phenomenon is extremely important because it serves as

Table 2.1 Major neurotransmitters and their loci

Neurotransmitter	Neuronal pathways
Norepinephrine (NE) (a major excitatory neurotransmitter)	Locus ceruleus
	Limbic system, especially
	Amygdala
	Hippocampus
	Septum
	And interconnecting pathways
	Postganglionic sympathetic nervous system
	Cerebellum
Serotonin (5-HT)	Brain stem
	Limbic system
Acetylcholine (Ach)	Neuromuscular junctions
	Preganglionic sympathetic nervous system
	Preganglionic parasympathetic nervous system
	Postganglionic parasympathetic nervous system
	Septal–hippocampal system
Gamma amino butyric acid (GABA) (a major inhibitory neurotransmitter)	Hippocampus
	Substantia nigra
	Limbic system–general
Dopamine (DA)	Mesolimbic system
	Nigrostriatal system

the basis for electrophysiological events such as electromyography, electrocardiography, and electroencephalography.

Shortly after the incoming signal passes the postsynaptic dendritic membrane and moves away from the cell body toward the axon, it becomes a measurable electrical event that serves as the basis for electrophysiological techniques such as electrocardiography. The foundations of these electrical events are based upon the dynamics of ionic transport.

The neuron at rest has ions both within the boundaries of its membranes and outside, around its membranes. Sodium (Na^+) is the positively charged ion that makes up the majority of the ionic constituency outside the neuron. In addition to the sodium concentration outside the neuron (about 0.142 M) there resides another ion, chloride (Cl^-). Chloride is a negatively charged ion that makes up the second largest ionic constituency outside the neuron (about 0.103 M). Whereas Na^+ and Cl^- predominate in the extraneural space, negatively charged protein anions dominate the internal milieu of the neuron along with potassium (K^+). Thus, relatively speaking, the outside of the neuron possesses a positive charge and the inside, a negative charge. This resting status is called a polarized state (*polarization*). The relative intensity of the negatively charged intraneuronal constituency is about −70 mV and is called the *resting electrical potential.*

When a neuron is in the act of transmitting a neural signal, the resting status of the neuron is altered. Ionically, (Na^+) rushes across the membrane of the neuron and enters the intraneuronal space. This influx of Na^+ pushes the electrical gradient to

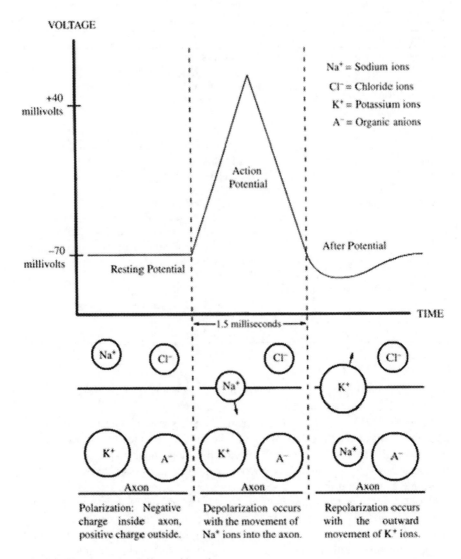

Fig. 2.2 The electrochemical neural impulse

about +50 mV (from the resting −70 mV). This process of sodium ion influx is called *depolarization* and represents the actual firing, or discharge, of the neuron. Depolarization lasts about 1.5 ms. Depolarization moves longitudinally along the axon as a wave of ionic influx. After 1.5 ms, however, the neuron begins to repolarize. *Repolarization* occurs as K+ and Na+ are pumped out of the neuron and any remaining Na+ is assimilated into the neuron itself. The result of repolarization is the return of the +50 mV to a resting −70 mV, ready for subsequent discharge. This process is shown in Fig. 2.2.

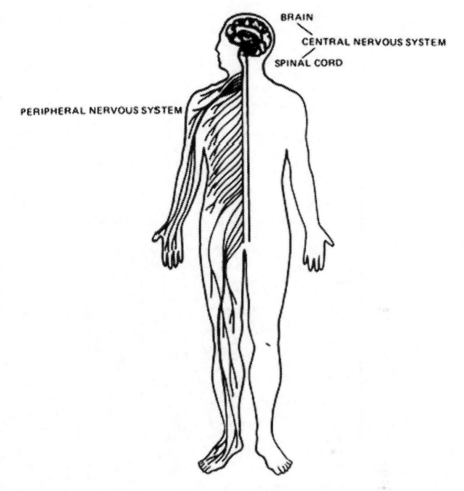

Fig. 2.3 Nervous systems (adapted from Lachman, 1972)

Basic Neuroanatomy

From the preceding discussion of basic neural transmission, the next step to be undertaken is an analysis of the fundamental anatomical structures involved in the human stress response.

The nervous systems, the functional structures within which millions upon millions of neurons reside, may be classified from either an anatomical or a functional perspective. For the sake of parsimony, we describe the nervous systems from an anatomical perspective.

From an anatomical perspective, there are two fundamental nervous systems: *the central nervous system* (CNS) and *the peripheral nervous system* (PNS) (see Fig. 2.3).

Table 2.2 The human nervous systems

The central nervous system (CNS)
   Brain
   Spinal cord
The peripheral nervous systems (PNS)
   The somatic branch
   The autonomic branches (ANS)
      Sympathetic (SNS)
      Parasympathetic (PSNS)

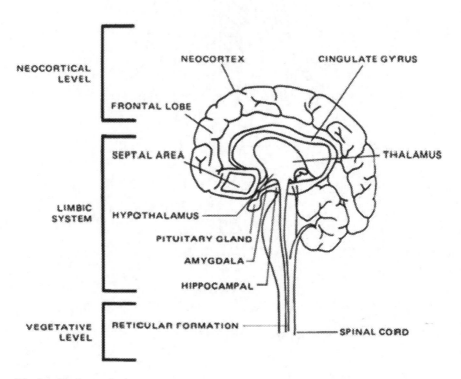

Fig. 2.4 The human brain

The CNS

The CNS consists of the brain and the spinal cord (see Table 2.2). MacLean (1975) has called the human brain the "triune brain" because it can be classified as having three functional levels (see Fig. 2.4). The *neocortex* represents the highest level of the triune brain and is the most sophisticated component of the human brain. Among other functions, such as the decoding and interpretation of sensory signals, communications, and gross control of motor (musculoskeletal) behaviors, the neocortex (primarily the *frontal lobe*) presides over imagination, logic, decision making, memory, problem solving, planning, and apprehension.

The *limbic system* represents the major component of the second level of the triune brain. The limbic brain is of interest in the discussion of stress because of its role as the emotional (affective) control center for the human brain. The limbic system is believed to be just that, that is, a *system*, consisting of numerous neural structures, for example, the *hypothalamus, hippocampus, septum, cingulate gyrus*, and *amygdala*. The *pituitary gland* plays a major functional role in this system in that *it is a major effector* endocrine gland. The limbic system is examined in greater detail in Chap. 9.

The *reticular formation* and the *brain stem* represent the lowest level of the triune brain. The major functions of this level are the maintenance of vegetative functions (heartbeat, respiration, vasomotor activity) and the conduction of impulses through the reticular formation and relay centers of the *thalamus* en route to the higher levels of the triune brain.

The spinal cord represents the central pathway for neurons as they conduct signals to and from the brain. It is also involved in some autonomically regulated reflexes.

The PNS

The PNS consists of all neurons exclusive of the CNS. Anatomically, the PNS may be thought of as an extension of the CNS in that the functional control centers for the PNS lie in the CNS. The PNS may be divided into two networks: the *somatic* (SNS) and the *autonomic nervous systems* (ANS).

The somatic branch of the PNS carries sensory and motor signals to and from the CNS. Thus, it innervates sensory organs as well as the striate musculature (skeletal musculature).

The autonomic branches carry impulses that are concerned with the regulation of the body's internal environment and the maintenance of the homeostasis (balance). The autonomic network, therefore, innervates the heart, the smooth muscles, and the glands.

The ANS can be further subdivided into two branches, the *sympathetic* and the *parasympathetic* (see Fig. 2.5 for details of autonomic innervation). The sympathetic branch of the ANS is concerned with preparing the body for action. Its effect on the organs it innervates is that of generalized arousal. The parasympathetic branch of the ANS is concerned with restorative functions and the relaxation of the body. Its general effects are those of slowing and maintenance of basic bodily requirements. The specific effects of sympathetic and parasympathetic activation on end organs are summarized later in this chapter (see Table 2.3).

To this point, we have briefly described the most basic anatomical and functional aspects of the human nervous system. We are now ready to see how these elements become interrelated as constituents of the human stress-response process.

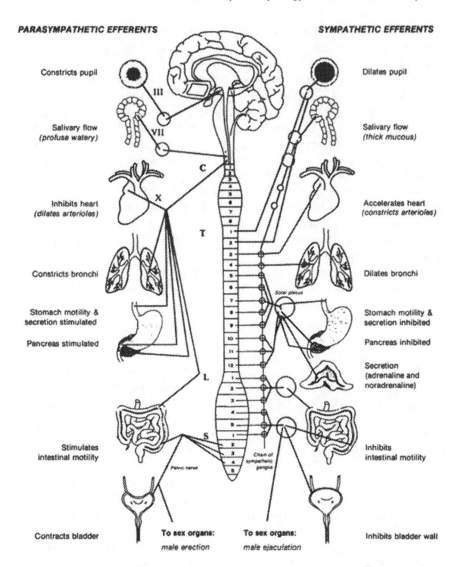

Fig. 2.5 Efferent autonomic pathways

A Systems Model of the Human Stress Response

The human stress response is perhaps best described within the context of the dynamic "process" it represents. This process may then be delineated from a "systems" perspective, that is, one of interrelated multidimensionality. Figure 2.6 details a systems perspective brought to bear upon the phenomenology of the human stress response.

Table 2.3 Responses of effector organs to autonomic nervous system impulses

	SNS	PNS
Function	Ergotropic; catabolism	Trophotropic; anabolism
Activity	Diffuse	Discrete
Anatomy		
Emerges from spinal cord	Thoracolumbar	Craniosacral
Location of ganglia	Close to spinal cord	Close to target organ
Postganglionic neurotransmitter	Noradrenalin[a] (adrenergic)	Acetylcholine (cholinergic)
Specific actions		
Pupil of eye	Dilates	Constricts
Lacrimal gland	–	Stimulates secretion
Salivary glands	Scanty, thick secretion	Profuse, water secretion
Heart	Increases heart rate	Decreases heart rate
	Increases contractility	Decreases metabolism
	Increases rate of idiopathic pacemakers in ventricles	
Blood vessels		
Skin and mucosa	Constricts	–
Skeletal muscles	Dilates	–
Cerebral	Constricts	Dilates
Renal	Constricts	–
Abdominal viscera	Mostly constricts	–
Lungs: bronchial tubes	Dilates	Constricts
Sweat glands	Stimulates[a]	Constricts
Liver	Glycogenolysis for release of glucose	Expels bile
Spleen	Contracts to release blood high in erythrocytes	–
Adrenal medulla	Secretes adrenaline (epinephrine) and noradrenaline (norepinephrine)[a]	–
Gastrointestinal tract	Inhibits digestion	Increases digestion
	Decreases peristalsis and tone	Increases peristalsis and tone
Kidney	Decreases output of urine	?
Hair follicles	Piloerection	–
Male sex organ	Ejaculation	Erection

[a]Postganglionic SNS neurotransmitter is acetylcholine for most sweat glands and some blood vessels in skeletal muscles. Adrenal medulla is innervated by cholinergic sympathetic neurons. Partially adapted from Hassett (1978)

This model, which has evolved significantly in recent years, will serve as a unifying theme to assist in gaining a better understanding of not only the phenomenology of human stress but also its measurement and treatment. These latter themes will be expanded upon later in the text.

An analysis of Fig. 2.6 reveals the epiphenomenology of the human stress response to be that of a multidimensional, interactive process possessing several key elements:

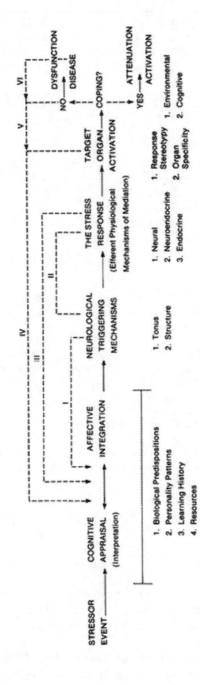

Fig. 2.6 A systems model of the human stress response

1. Stressor events (real or imagined).
2. Cognitive appraisal and affective integration.
3. Neurological triggering mechanisms (e.g., locus ceruleus, limbic nuclei, hypo-thalamic nuclei).
4. The stress response (a physiological mechanism of mediation).
5. Target-organ activation.
6. Coping behavior.

A detailed analysis of each of these elements is appropriate at this point.

Stressor Events

Because Selye used the term *stress* to refer to a "response," it was necessary to employ a word to delineate the stimulus for the stress response—that word is *stressor.* Stressor events, as noted earlier, fall in one of the two categories: (1) psychosocial stressors and (2) biogenic stressors (Girdano, Dusek, & Everly, 2009).

Psychosocial stressors are either real or imagined environmental events that "set the stage" for the elicitation of the stress response. They cannot directly "cause" the stress response but must work through cognitive appraisal mechanics. Most stressors are, indeed, psychosocial stressors. For this reason, one may argue that "stressors, like beauty, reside in the eye of the beholder."

Biogenic stressors, however, actually "cause" the elicitation of the stress response. Such stimuli bypass the higher cognitive appraisal mechanisms and work directly on affective and neurological triggering nuclei. Thus, by virtue of their biochemical properties, they directly initiate the stress response without the usual requisite cognitive–affective processing. Examples of such stimuli include the following:

- Ginseng
- Ginkgo biloba
- Amphetamine
- Phenylpropanolamine
- Caffeine
- Theobromine
- Theophylline
- Nicotine
- Certain physical factors such as pain-evoking stimuli, extreme heat, and extreme cold
- Guarana
- Yohimbine

As just mentioned, however, most stressors are not biogenic stressors. Therefore, in clinical practice, therapists will most likely be treating patients who are plagued by environmental events—real, imagined, anticipated, or recalled—that are perceived in such a manner as to lead to activation of the stress response. To better understand this process we move now to the second step in the model: the cognitive–affective integration stage.

Cognitive–Affective Domain

Practically speaking, there is simply no such thing as "reality" without considering the human perspective that might be brought to bear upon it. The cognitive–affective domain is delineated within this model in order to capture that notion.

Cognitive appraisal refers to the process of cognitive interpretation, that is, the meanings that we assign to the world as it unfolds before us. *Affective integration* refers to the blending and coloring of felt emotion into the cognitive interpretation. The resultant cognitive–affective complex represents how the stressors are ultimately perceived. In effect, this critical integrated perception represents the determination of whether psychosocial *stimuli* become psychosocial *stressors* or not. Such a perceptual process, however, is uniquely individualized and vulnerable to biological predispositions (Millon & Everly, 1985), personality patterns (Millon, Grossman, Millon, Meagher, & Ramnath, 2004), learning history (Lachman, 1972), and available resources for coping (Lazarus, 2006; Lazarus & Folkman, 1984).

Although Fig. 2.6 portrays a reciprocity between cognitive and affective mechanisms, it should be noted that there exists substantial evidence supporting the cognitive primacy hypothesis (see Chap. 8); that is, cognition determines affect (felt emotion) and thus assumes a superordinate role in the process of restructuring human behavior patterns. Let us explore this important notion further.

Perhaps the earliest recognition that cognition is superordinate to affect has been credited by Albert Ellis to the fifth-century Greco-Roman philosopher Epictetus, who reportedly said, "Men are disturbed not by things, but by the views which they take of them." The science of physiology follows in kind. Hans Selye, also known as the father of modern endocrinology, has summarized over 50 years of research into human stress with the conclusion, "It is not what happens to you that matters, but how you take it," Similarly, the noted neurophysiologist Ernest Gellhorn (Gellhorn & Loofbourrow, 1963) recognized the preeminent role of the prefrontal lobe cognitive processes in felt and expressed emotion in his research spanning the 1950s, 1960s, and 1970s. Influential authors such as Arnold (1970, 1984), Cassel (1974), Lazarus (1966, 1982, 1991), Meichenbaum (1985), Meichenbaum and Jaremko (1983), and Selye (1976) strongly support the cognitive primacy position as it relates to human stress.

More recently, Everly, Davy, Smith, Lating, and Nucifora (2011) [also see Everly, Smith, and Lating (2009) and Smith, Everly, and Johns (1992, 1993)] assessed the role of cognitive processes in the determination of stress-related illness. "Stressors, like beauty, lie in the eye of the beholder," is the assertion. Using a sample of 1,618 adults, Smith, Everly, and Johns (1993) employed structural modeling, exploratory, and confirmatory factor analyses to investigate the relative roles of environmental stressors compared to cognitive processes as predictors of physiological symptoms of stress-related illness or dysfunction. The role of coping mechanisms was also investigated. The results of this investigation indicated that, consistent with the speculations of Epictetus and even Selye, environmental stressors exert their pathogenic effect only indirectly. Rather, environmental stressors act "through their ability to cause psychological discord. In fact, psychological discord had the strongest influence on maladaptive coping behaviors and stress-related illness" (Smith et al., 1993, p. 445). Psychological discord, as assessed by these authors, reflects the cognitive interpretations of the environmental events.

An extended physiological perspective may be of value at this point. If a given, nonsympathomimetic stimulus is to engender a stress response, it must first be received by the receptors of the PNS. Once stimulated, these receptors send their impulses along the PNS toward the brain. According to Penfield (1975), once in the CNS, collateral neurons diverge from the main ascending pathways to the neocortical targets and innervate the reticular formation. These collaterals diverge and pass through limbic constituents, but seldom are such afferent diversions sufficient to generate full-blown emotional reactions. Rather, such diversions may account for nonspecific arousal (startle or defense reflexes) or subtle affective coloration ("gut reactions"). Cognitive theorists do not regard these momentary acute, ontogenetically primitive events as emotions (Lazarus, 1982).

These divergent pathways ultimately reunite with the main ascending pathways and innervate the primary sensory and appraisal loci. Arnold (1984) has written that "the sheer experience of things around us cannot lead to action unless they are appraised for their effect on us" (p. 125). She has hypothesized the anatomical locus of such appraisal to be the cingulate gyrus and the limbic–prefrontal neocortical interface (see Aggleton, 1992).

Arnold (1984) notes that the granular cells of the limbic–prefrontal interface contain relay centers that connect all sensory, motor, and association areas. She states:

> These connections would enable the individual to appraise information from every modality: smells, via relays from the posterior orbital cortex; movement and movement impulses, via relays from frontal and prefrontal cortex; somatic sensations can provide data via relays from parietal association areas; and things seen could be appraised over relays from occipital association areas. Finally, something heard can be appraised as soon as relays from the auditory association area reach the hippocampal gyrus. (pp. 128–129)

As noted in Fig. 2.6, appraisal is a function of any existing biological predispositions, personality patterns, learning history, and available coping resources. Once appraisal is made, efferent impulses project so as to potentiate the stimulation of two major effector systems:

1. Impulses project back to the highly sensitive emotional anatomy in the limbic system (Arnold, 1984; Cullinan, Herman, Helmreich, & Watson, 1995; Gellhorn & Loufbourrow, 1963; Gevarter, 1978; Nauta, 1979), especially the hippocampus (Reiman et al., 1986), for the experience of stimulus-specific felt emotion and the potential to trigger visceral effector mechanisms.
2. Impulses similarly project to the areas of the neocortex concerned with neuromuscular behavior where, through pyramidal and extrapyramidal systems, muscle tone (tension) is increased and the intention to act can be potentially translated to actual overt motor activity (Gellhorn, 1964a, 1964b).

Thus far, we have seen that psychosocial stimuli, once perceived, excite nonspecific arousal and cognitive appraisal mechanisms. If the appraisal of the stimulus is ultimately one of threat, challenge, or aversion, then emotional arousal will likely result.

In most individuals, activation of the limbic centers for emotional arousal leads to expression of the felt emotion in the form of visceral activation and neuromuscular activity. Such visceral and neuromuscular activation represents the multiaxial physiological mechanisms of mediation Selye called the "stress response." Thus, in the final analysis, it can be seen that physiological reactions to psychosocial stimuli result from the cognitive interpretations and emotional reactions to those stimuli, *not* the stimuli themselves. Stressors are, indeed, in the eye of the beholder!

Before turning to a discussion of the multiaxial nature of the stress response, we must first discuss a mechanism that prefaces activation of the stress response axes. Research in the last several years has necessitated specific consideration of mechanisms that serve to "trigger" the elicitation of the multiaxial stress response. These mechanisms are referred to as *neurological triggering mechanisms.*

Neurological Triggering Mechanisms

The next step in the model depicted in Fig. 2.6 is the neurological triggering mechanisms consisting of the locus ceruleus (LC), limbic system, and hypothalamic efferent triggering complex. Linked through ventral and dorsal adrenergic as well as serotonergic projections (among others), this complex appears to consist of the LC, the hippocampus, the septal–hippocampal–amygdaloid complexes, and the anterior and posterior hypothalamic nuclei (Nauta & Domesick, 1982; Reiman et al., 1986). These structures appear to be the anatomical epicenters for the visceral and somatic efferent discharges in response to emotional arousal (Aggleton, 1992; Gellhorn, 1964a, 1964b, 1965, 1967; MacLean, 1949; Nauta, 1979; Redmond, 1979); that is, these structures appear to give rise to the multiaxial stress response. Indeed, these centers even seem capable of establishing an endogenously determined neurological tone that is potentially self-perpetuating (Gellhorn, 1967; Weil, 1974). This notion of a positive feedback loop is initially depicted in Fig. 2.6 by the dotted line labeled I. Subsequent dotted lines are labeled with Roman numerals to show other feedback mechanisms that maintain what Gellhorn (1957) has called a state of "egotropic tuning," what Everly (Everly & Benson, 1989) calls "limbic hypersensitivity" (discussed in Chap. 3), and what Weil (1974) has called a "charged arousal system." Each of these terms is indicative of a predisposition for physiological arousal.

More specifically, these terms describe a preferential pattern of SNS (and related arousal mechanism) responsiveness. Such a chronic tonic status may, over time, serve as the basis for a host of psychiatric and psychophysiological disorders (Gellhorn, 1967). The mechanisms by which such neurological tone can exert an effect upon a given target organ is the subject of the next phase of the system's model: the stress response—a physiological mechanism of mediation.

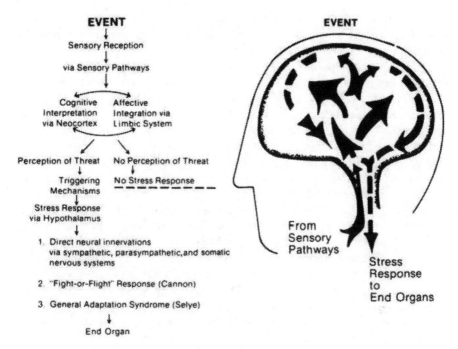

Fig. 2.7 The stress response

The Stress Response

Recall the question that has plagued psychosomatic research: Through what mechanisms of pathogenic mediation can a stressor and its subsequent appraisal ultimately affect a target organ to such a degree as to result in dysfunction and disease? Although a definitive answer on *all* levels has yet to be found, research in applied physiology has yielded considerable insight into the mechanisms of pathogenesis by which stressors cause disease. This section details three such physiological pathways known to demonstrate extraordinary responsiveness with respect to psychosocial stimuli: (1) the neural axes, (2) the neuroendocrine axis, and (3) the endocrine axes (see Fig. 2.7).

The Neural Axes: Stress Response Via Neural Innervation of Target Organs

Three neural axes comprise the neural stress response: (1) the sympathetic nervous system, (2) the parasympathetic nervous system, and, (3) the neuromuscular nervous system. These neural pathways are the first of all stress response axes to become activated during stress arousal. This phenomenon is based upon the fact that the structure of these pathways, from origination to target-organ innervation, is completely neural, and therefore quickest.

It is clear that ANS activation occurs during states of emotional arousal in human beings (Widmaier, Raff, & Strang, 2004). These neural axes are the most direct of all stress pathways. Following the complex neocortical and limbic integrations that occur in the interpretation of a stimulus as "threatening," neural impulses descend to the posterior hypothalamus (in the case of a sympathetic activation) and the anterior hypothalamus (in the case of a parasympathetic activation). From here, sympathetic neural pathways descend from the anterior hypothalamus through the cranial and sacral spinal cord regions. Parasympathetic nerves then innervate the end organs.

Generally speaking, the release of the neurotransmitter norepinephrine from the sympathetic telodendria is responsible for changes in most end-organ activity. Acetylcholine is the neurotransmitter in the remaining cases and in parasympathetic postganglionic transmissions as well (see McCorry, 2007).

The effects of neural activation via the sympathetic system are those of generalized arousal within the end organs—what Hess (1957) referred to as an "ergotropic" response. The effects of activation via the parasympathetic system are inhibition, slowing, and "restorative" functions—what Hess called a "trophotropic" response. The specific end-organ effects of the sympathetic and the parasympathetic nervous systems are summarized in Table 2.3 (see Ganong, 1997).

Although the most common form of neural autonomic stress responsiveness in human beings is in the form of the ergotropic response (Johnson & Spalding, 1974), simultaneous trophotropic responses have been observed in human beings as well (Gellhorn, 1969). The trophotropic stress response may be perceived by some clinicians as paradoxical, owing to the expectation of manifestations of somation "arousal." However, the important work of Gellhorn (1968, 1969) and Williams (1986), in addition to the clinical observations of Carruthers and Taggart (1973), has demonstrated that sympathetic stress arousal can be accompanied by parasympathetic trophotropic activation.

Finally, there is evidence (Gellhorn, 1958a, 1958b, 1964b, 1967; Malmo, 1975; Williams, 1986) that the skeletal muscular is also a prime target for immediate activation during stress and emotional arousal. Such activation, if excessive, may lead to a host of neuromuscular dysfunctions as well as increased limbic excitation (Gellhorn, 1958b; Malmo, 1975; Weil, 1974) and therefore heightened emotional arousal.

Although neuromuscular activation may last virtually indefinitely—hence, the proliferation of various neuromuscular dysfunction syndromes—the major effects of autonomic neural activation on target organs are immediate but not potentially chronic. This is because of the limited ability of the sympathetic telodendria to continue to constantly release neurotransmitting substances under chronically high stimulation (LeBlanc, 1976). Therefore, in order to maintain high levels of stress arousal for prolonged periods, an additional physiological stress axis must be activated. This axis is the neuroendocrine "fight-or-flight" response axis.

The "Fight-or-Flight" Response: The Neuroendocrine Axis

In 1926, the same year that Selye first described the "syndrome of just being sick," physiologist Walter Cannon first wrote about a phenomenon that he termed *homeostasis*, described as the effort of the physiological systems within the body to actively maintain a level of functioning, within the limits of tolerance of the systems, in the face of ever-changing conditions. Homeostasis was the adaptational effort of the body to stay in balance. From his early efforts, it was clear that the work of Cannon was to parallel and augment that of Selye in terms of understanding the psychophysiological stress response.

Cannon wrote extensively on one particular aspect of the ANS's role in the stress response—the neuroendocrine process. He researched what he termed the "fight-or-flight" response. The pivotal organ in this response is the adrenal medulla—thus giving this response both neural ANS and endocrine characteristics (Cannon, 1914, 1953; Cannon & Paz, 1911).

The "fight-or-flight" response is thought to be a mobilization of the body to prepare for muscular activity in response to a perceived threat. This mechanism allows the organism either to fight or to flee from the perceived threat (Cannon, 1953).

Research has demonstrated that the homeostatic, neuroendocrine "fight-or-flight" response can be activated in human beings by numerous and diverse psychological influences, including varied psychosocial stimuli (Levi, 1972; Mason, 1968a, 1972).

The dorsomedial amygdalar complex appears to represent the highest point of origination for the "fight-or-flight" response as a functionally discrete psychophysiological axis (Lang, 1975; Roldan, Alvarez-Palaez, & de Molina, 1974). From that point, the downward flow of neural impulses passes to the lateral and posterior hypothalamic regions (Roldan et al., 1974). From here, neural impulses continue to descend through the thoracic spinal cord, converging at the celiac ganglion, then innervating the adrenal gland, or more specifically, the adrenal medulla.

The adrenal gland in mammals consists of two functionally and histologically discrete constituents: the adrenal medulla and the adrenal cortex. The adrenal medulla consists of chromaffin cells (pheochromoblasts) that lie at the core, or center, of the adrenal gland (*medulla* means stalk). Chromaffin cells are responsible for the creation and secretion of adrenal medullary catecholamines. This process is referred to as *catecholaminogenesis*.

The hormonal output of the neuroendocrine stress-response axis is the secretion of the adrenal medullary catecholamines. There are two adrenal medullary catecholamines: norepinephrine (noradrenaline) and epinephrine (adrenaline). These two hormones are collectively referred to as adrenal medullary catecholamines because of their origin and the chemical nature; that is, these hormones are secreted by the two adrenal medullae that lie at the superior poles of the kidneys. Furthermore, the biochemical structure of these hormones is related to a group of organic compounds referred to as *catechols* (or pyrocatechols).

The adrenal medullary cells are divided into two types: A cells, which secrete epinephrine, and N cells, which secrete norepinephrine. About 80% of the

Table 2.4 Effects of adrenal medullary axis stimulation

Increased arterial blood pressure

Increase blood supply to brain (moderate)

Increased heart rate and cardiac output

Increased stimulation of skeletal muscles

Increase plasma free fatty acids, triglycerides, cholesterol

Increased release of endogenous opioids

Decreased blood flow to kidneys

Decreased blood flow to gastrointestinal system

Decreased blood flow to skin

Increased risk of hypertension

Increased risk of thrombosis formation

Increased risk of angina pectoris attacks in persons so prone

Increased risk of arrhythmias

Increased risk of sudden death from lethal arrhythmia, myocardial ischemia, myocardial fibrillation, myocardial infarction

See Henry and Stephens (1977), Axelrod and Reisine (1984), McCabe and Schneiderman (1984), Guyenet (2006), Mazeh, Paldor, and Chen (2012), Florian and Pawelczyk (2010), Heim and Nemeroff (2009) Ray and Carter (2010), Lomax, Sharkey, and Furness (2010), Surges, Thijs, Tan, and Sander (2009), Hall (2011) for reviews

medullary catecholamine activity in humans is accounted for by epinephrine (Harper, 1975; Mazeh, Paldor, & Chen, 2012). It is critical to note at this juncture that norepinephrine is secreted by not only the adrenal medulla but also the adrenergic neurons of the CNS and the SNS. The biosynthesis and actions are the same regardless of whether the norepinephrine originates in the medulla or in the adrenergic neurons of the CNS or SNS.

Upon neural stimulation, the adrenal medulla releases the medullary catecholamines as just described. The effect of these medullary catecholamines is an increase in generalized adrenergic somatic activity in human beings (Folkow & Neil, 1971; Maranon, 1924; Wenger et al., 1960). The effect, therefore, is functionally identical to that of direct sympathetic innervation (see Table 2.3), except that the medullary catecholamines require a 20 to 30 second delay of onset for measurable effects and display a tenfold increase in effect duration (Usdin, Kretnansky, & Kopin, 1976). Also, the catecholamines only prolong the adrenergic sympathetic response. Cholinergic responses, such as increased electrodermal activity and bronchiole effects, are unaffected by medullary catecholamine release (Usdin et al).

The "fight-or-flight" response has been somewhat reformulated by writers such as Schneiderman (McCabe & Schneiderman, 1984), who view this system as an "active coping" system. This active coping system has been referred to as the "sympathoadrenomedullary system" (SAM).

Specific somatic effects that have been suggested or observed in humans as a result of activation of this axis in response to psychosocial stressor exposure are summarized in Table 2.4.

This brings us to a discussion of the third and final stress response mechanism — the endocrine axes.

Endocrine Axes

The most chronic and prolonged somatic responses to stress are the result of the endocrine axes (Mason, 1968b). Four well-established endocrine axes have been associated with the stress response:

1. The adrenal cortical axis.
2. The somatotropic axis.
3. The thyroid axis.
4. The posterior pituitary axis.

These axes not only represent the most chronic aspects of the stress response but also require greater intensity stimulation to activate (Levi, 1972).

Reviews by Axelrod and Reisine (1984), Levi (1972), Mason (1968c, 1972), Mason et al. (1995), Selye (1976), Yehuda, Giller, Levengood, Southwick, and Siever (1995), and more recently by, Entringer, Kumsta, Hellhammer, Wadhwa, and Wust (2009), and Foley and Kirschbaum (2010), demonstrate that these axes can be activated in humans by numerous and diverse psychological stimuli, including varied psychosocial stimuli.

The Adrenal Cortical Axis

The septal–hippocampal complex appears to represent the highest point of origination for the adrenal cortical axis as a physiologically discrete mechanism (Henry & Ely, 1976; Henry & Stephens, 1977). From these points, neural impulses descend to the median eminence of the hypothalamus. The neurosecretory cells in the median eminence release corticotropin-releasing factor (CRF) into the hypothalamic–hypophyseal portal system (Rochefort, Rosenberger, & Saffran, 1959). The CRF descends the infundibular stalk to the cells of the anterior pituitary. The chemophobes of the anterior pituitary are sensitive to the presence of CRF and respond by releasing adrenocorticotropic hormone (ACTH) in the systemic circulation. At the same time, the precursor to the various endogenous analgesic opioids (endorphins) is released. This precursor substance, beta lipotropin, yields the proliferation of endogenous opioids during human stress (Rossier, Bloom, & Guillemin, 1980).

ACTH is carried through the systemic circulation until it reaches its primary target organ: an endocrine gland, the adrenal cortex. The two adrenal cortices are wrapped around the two adrenal medullae (neuroendocrine axis) and sit at the superior poles of the kidneys.

ACTH appears to act upon three discrete layers, or zona, of the adrenal cortex. It stimulates the cells of the zona reticularis and zona fasciculata to release the glucocorticoids cortisol and corticosterone into the systemic circulation. The effects of the glucocorticoids in apparent response to stressful stimuli are summarized in Table 2.5.

Table 2.5 The effects of the glucocorticoid hormones and HPAC activation

Increased glucose production (gluconeogenesis)

Exacerbation of gastric irritation

Increased urea production

Increased release of free fatty acids into systemic circulation

Increased susceptibility arteherosclerotic processes

Increased susceptibility to nonthrombotic myocardial necrosis

Thymicolymphatic atrophy (demonstrated in animals only)

Suppression of immune mechanisms

Exacerbation of herpes simplex

Increased ketone body production

Appetite suppression

Associated feeling of depression, hopelessness, helplessness, and loss of control

See Henry and Stephens (1977), Selye (1976), Yuwiler (1976), McCabe and Schneiderman (1984), Makara, Palkovitzm, and Szentagothal (1980), van Raalte, Ouwens, and Diamant (2009), Macfarlane, Forbes, and Walker (2008), Schwarz et al. (2011), and Krishnan and Nestler (2008), Hall (2011)

Similarly, ACTH allows the zona glomerulosa to secrete the mineralocorticoids aldosterone and deoxycorticosterone into the systemic circulation. The primary effects of aldosterone release are an increase in the absorption of sodium and chloride by the renal tubules and a decrease in their excretion by the salivary glands, sweat glands, and gastrointestinal tract. Subsequent fluid retention is noted as a corollary of this process. Although cortisol does exhibit some of these properties, aldosterone is about 1,000 times more potent as an electrolyte effector. As the prepotent mineralocorticoid, aldosterone may affect other physiological outcomes, among them increasing glycogen deposits in the liver and decreasing circulating eosinophils.

Excessive activation of mineralocorticoid secretion in human beings has been implicated in the development of Cushing's syndrome (hyperadrenocorticism) by Gifford and Gunderson (1970) and in high blood pressure and myocardial necrosis by Selye (1976).

As a tropic hormone, the main function of ACTH is to stimulate the synthesis and secretion of the glucocorticoid hormones from the adrenal cortex, yet ACTH is known to cause the release of cortical adrenal androgenic hormones such as testosterone as well. Finally, there is evidence that ACTH affects the release of the catecholamines described earlier in this chapter. Its effect on the catecholamines epinephrine and norepinephrine appears to be through a modulation of tyrosine hydroxylase, which is the "rate-limiting" step in catecholamine synthesis. This effect is a minor one, however, compared with other influences on tyrosine hydroxylase. Thus, adrenal medullary and cortical activities can be highly separate, even inversely related, at times (Kopin, 1976; Lundberg & Forsman, 1978). See Axelrod and Reisine (1984) for an excellent review of hormonal interaction and regulation.

The adrenal cortical response axis has been referred to by various authors (e.g., McCabe & Schneiderman, 1984) as the hypothalamic–pituitary–adrenal cortical system (HPAC). Activation of this system in the aggregate has been associated with the helplessness/hopelessness depression syndrome, passivity, the perception of no control, immunosuppression, and gastrointestinal symptomatology. Behaviorally, the HPAC system appears to be activated when active coping is not possible; thus, it has been called the "passive coping" system. Considering the HPAC system with respect to the SAM, Frankenhauser (1980) has concluded:

1. Effort without distress → activation of the SAM response system.
2. Distress without effort → activation of the HPAC response system.
3. Effort with distress → activation of both SAM and HPAC.

The most extreme variation of the human stress response is, arguably, posttraumatic stress. The codified variant of this response is posttraumatic stress disorder (PTSD), the subject of a specialized review in Chap. 21. Nevertheless, we believe it warrants mention in this discussion of physiological mechanisms because of complex and often contradictory findings. In PTSD, both the adrenal medullary catecholamine axis and the HPAC pathways are implicated in PTSD. Given the aforementioned discussion, one would expect increased glucocorticoid secretion in PTSD given the intensity, chronicity, and overall severity of PTSD as a clinical syndrome. While enhanced cortisol secretion is, indeed, evidenced in PTSD patients, there is also evidence of decreased cortisol secretion. Yehuda et al. (1995) provide a useful review and reformulation of this issue. PTSD patients evidence enhanced CRF activity but lower overall cortisol levels in many instances. These authors summarize as follows:

> The study of PTSD, whose definition rests on being the sequelae of stress, represents an opportunity to express the effects of extreme stress... from a unique perspective. The findings suggest that... individuals who suffer from PTSD show evidence of a highly sensitized HPA axis characterized by decreased basal cortisol levels, increased number of lymphocyte glucocorticoid receptors, a greater suppression of cortisol to dexamethasone, and a more sensitized pituitary gland. (p. 362)

Thus, in summary, in addition to the more "classic" Selyean observation of increased cortisol as a constituent of extreme stress, PTSD may represent an extension of the Selyean formulation characterized by an increase in CRF, a hypersensitized pituitary, and a resultant down-regulation of the HPAC system via an enhanced negative feedback system. As Yehuda et al. (1995) note, "The findings challenge us to regard the stress response as diversified and varied, rather than as conforming to a simple, unidirectional pattern" (pp. 362–363).

The Somatotropic Axis

The somatotropic axis appears to share the same basic physiological mechanisms from the septal–hippocampal complex through the hypothalamic–hypophyseal portal system as the previous axis, with the exception that somatotropin-releasing factor (SRF) stimulates the anterior pituitary within this axis. The anterior pituitary responds to the SRF by releasing growth hormone (somatotropic hormone) into the systemic circulation (see Makara, Palkovitzm, & Szentagothal, 1980; Selye, 1976).

The role of growth hormone in stress is somewhat less clearly understood than that of the adrenal cortical axis. However, research has documented its release in response to psychological stimuli in human beings (Selye, 1976), and certain effects are suspected. Selye (1956) has stated that growth hormone stimulates the release of the mineralocorticoids. Yuwiler (1976), in his review of stress and endocrine function, suggests that growth hormone produces a diabetic-like insulin-resistant effect, as well as mobilization of fats stored in the body. The effect is an increase in the concentration of free fatty acids and glucose in the blood.

The Thyroid Axis

The thyroid axis is now a well-established stress response mechanism. From the median eminence of the hypothalamus is released thyrotropin-releasing factor (TRF). The infundibular stalk carries the TRF to its target—the anterior pituitary. From here, the tropic thyroid-stimulating hormone (TSH) is released into the systemic circulation. TSH ultimately stimulates the thyroid gland to release two thyroid hormones: triiodothyronine (T3) and thyroxine (T4). Once secreted into the systemic circulation system, these hormones are bound to specific plasma protein carriers, primarily thyroxin-binding globulin (TBG). A small amount of the thyroid hormones remains as "free" unbound hormones. About 0.4% of T4 and about 0.4% of T3 remain unbound. Proper evaluation of thyroid function is best based upon an assessment of free thyroid hormones. At the level of target-cell tissue, only free hormone is metabolically active. The T3 and T4 hormones serve to participate in a negative feedback loop, thus suppressing their own subsequent secretion.

In humans, psychosocial stimuli have generally led to an increase in thyroidal activity (Levi, 1972; Makara et al., 1980; Yuwiler, 1976). Levi has stated that the thyroid hormones have been shown to increase general metabolism, heart rate, heart contractility, peripheral vascular resistance (thereby increasing blood pressure), and the sensitivity of some tissues to catecholamines. Hypothyroidism has been linked to depressive episodes. Levi therefore concludes that the thyroid axis could play a significant role as a response axis in human stress. See Mason et al. (1995) for a comprehensive review.

The Posterior Pituitary Axis and Other Phenomena

Since the early 1930s, there has been speculation on the role of the posterior pituitary in the stress response. The posterior pituitary (neurohypophysis) receives neural impulses from the supraoptic nuclei of the hypothalamus. Stimulation from these nuclei results in the release of the hormones vasopressin (antidiuretic hormone, or ADH) and oxytocin into the systemic circulation.

ADH affects the human organism by increasing the permeability of the collecting ducts that lie subsequent to the distal ascending tubules within the glomerular struc-tures of the kidneys. The end result is water retention.

Corson and Corson (1971), in their review of psychosocial influences on renal function, note several studies that report significant amounts of water retention in apparent response to psychological influences in human beings. Although there seems to be agreement that water retention can be psychogenically induced, there is little agreement on the specific mechanism. Corson and Corson (1971) report studies that point to the release of elevated amounts of ADH in response to stressful episodes. On the other hand, some studies conclude that the antidiuretic effect is due to decreased renal blood flow. Some human participants even responded with a diuretic response to psychosocial stimuli.

Nevertheless, Makara et al. (1980), in their review of 25 years of research, found ample evidence for the increased responsiveness of ADH during the stress response. ADH is now seen as one of the wide range of diverse, stress-responsive hormones.

Oxytocin, the other major hormone found in the posterior pituitary axis, is syn-thesized in the same nuclei as ADH, but in different cells. Its role in the human stress response is currently unclear but may be involved in psychogenic labor con-tractions (Omer & Everly, 1988) and premature birth, as well as the stress response, particularly for women (Taylor, 2006).

Various investigations have shown that both interstitial cell-stimulating hormone (Sowers, Carlson, Brautbar, & Hershman, 1977), also known as luteinizing hor-mone, and testosterone (Williams, 1986) have been shown to be responsive to the presentation of various stressors.

Finally, the hormone prolactin has clearly shown responsiveness to psychosocial stimulation as well (see Makara et al., 1980, and more recently, Zimmermann et al., 2009). The role of prolactin in disease or dysfunction phenomena, however, has not been well established. Attempts to link prolactin with premenstrual dysfunction have yet to yield a clear line of evidence. The specific role of prolactin in stress-related disease needs further elucidation.

The "General Adaptation Syndrome"

As a means of integrating his psychoendocrinological research, Hans Seyle (1956) proposed an integrative model for the stress response, known as the "General Adaptation Syndrome" (GAS).

The GAS is a tri-phasic phenomenon. The first phase Selye refers to as the "alarm" phase, representing a generalized somatic shock, or "call to arms" of the body's defense mechanisms. The second phase is called the "stage of resistance," in which there is a dramatic reduction in most alarm stage processes and the body fights to reestablish and maintain homeostasis. Stages 1 and 2 can be repeated throughout one's life. Should the stressor persist, however, eventually the "adap-tive energy," that is, the adaptive mechanisms in the second stage, may become depleted. At this point, the body enters the third and final stage, the "stage of exhaustion," which, when applied to a target organ, is indicative of the exhaustion of that organ, and the symptoms of disease and dysfunction become manifest. When the final stage is applied to the entire body, life itself may be in jeopardy. The three stages of the GAS are detailed in Table 2.6.

The Stress Response: A Summary

In this section, we have presented a unifying perspective from which to view the complex psychophysiological processes that have come to be known as the stress response. The intention was to provide clinicians with an understandable interpretation of the complexities of the stress-response process that they often find themselves treating. Because effective treatment of the stress phenomenon is related to comprehension of the nature of the problem (Miller, 1978, 1979), it is our hope that this discussion will prove useful for the clinician.

The unifying thread throughout this discussion has been the temporal sequencing of the stress-response process. We have shown that the most immediate response to a stressful stimulus occurs via the direct neural innervations of end organs. The intermediate stress effects are due to the neuroendocrine "fight-or-flight" axis. The reaction time of this axis is reduced by its utilization of systemic circulation as a transport mechanism. However, its effects range from intermediate to chronic in duration and may overlap with the last stress-response system to respond to a stimulus—the endocrine axes. The endocrine axes are the final pathways to react to stressful stimuli, owing primarily to the almost total reliance on the circulatory system for transportation, as well as the fact that a higher intensity stimulus is needed to activate this axis. The GAS provides an additional schema to extend the endocrine response axis in the adaptation of the organism to the presence of a chronic stressor [see Selye (1956), for a discussion of diseases of adaptation]. Figure 2.8 summarizes the sequential activation of the stress-response axes.

It is important to understand that there is a potential for the activation of each of these axes to overlap. The most common axes to be simultaneously active are the neuroendocrine and endocrine axes—both of which have potential for chronic responsivity (Mason, 1968a, 1968c).

On the other hand, it is clear that all mechanisms and axes detailed cannot possibly discharge each and every time a person is faced with a stressor. Perhaps clearest of all is the fact that each sympathetic and parasympathetic effect is not manifest to all stressors. Therefore, what determines which stress-response mechanisms will be activated by which stressors in which individuals? The answer to this question is currently unknown. However, some evidence suggests the existence of a psychophysiological predisposition for some individuals to undergo stress-response pattern specificity (see Sternbach, 1966). We expand on this topic in Chap. 3.

These, then, are the stress-response axes and the various mechanisms that work within each. They represent the potential response patterns result each time the human organism is exposed to a stressor. As to when each responds and why, we are unsure at this time. Current speculations are reviewed in Chap. 3. Despite this

Table 2.6 The general adaptation syndrome

Alarm stage
  Sympathetic nervous system arousal
  Adrenal medullary stimulation
  ACTH release
  Cortisol release
  Growth hormone release
  Increased thyroid activity
  Gonadotropin activity increased
  Anxiety
Resistance stage
  Reduction in adrenal cortical activity
  Reduction in sympathetic nervous system activity
  Homeostatic mechanisms engaged
Exhaustion stage
  Enlargement of lymphatic structures
  Target organ disease/dysfunction manifest
  Increased vulnerability to opportunistic disease
  Psychological exhaustion: depression
  Physiological exhaustion: disease → death?

uncertainty, the clinician should gain useful insight into the treatment of the stress response by understanding the psychophysiological processes involved once the stress response becomes activated. To assist the reader in putting the picture together, Fig. 2.9 provides a unique "global" perspective into the multiaxial nature of psychophysiological stress.

As a final note, returning to Fig. 2.6, feedback loops II and III simply indicate the ability of the physiological stress response to further stimulate the cognitive–affective domain as well as the neurological triggering mechanisms, so as to further promulgate the stress response. Such a feedback mechanism may provide the potential for a psychophysiologically self-sustaining response. This, then, is the physiology of human stress as currently understood.

Target-Organ Activation

The term *target-organ activation* as used in the present model refers to the phenomenon in which the neural, neuroendocrine, and endocrine constituents of the stress response just described (1) activate, (2) increase or (3) inhibit normal activation, or (4) catabolize some organ system in the human body. Potential target-organ systems for the stress response include the cardiovascular system, the gastrointestinal system, the skin, the immune system, and even the brain and its mental status, to mention only a few. It is from activation of the target organs and the subsequent emergence of various clinical signs and symptoms that we often deduce the presence of excessive stress arousal.

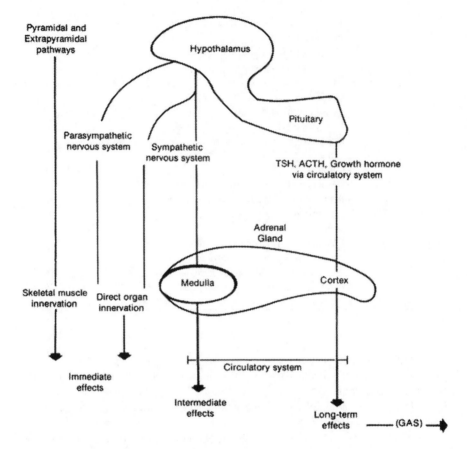

Fig. 2.8 Temporal relationship between primary stress axes

As for which target organs are most likely to manifest stress-related disease or dysfunction, it appears that two major biogenic factors assist in that determination: response mechanism stereotypy (Sternbach, 1966) and target-organ specificity (Everly, 1978). *Response mechanism stereotypy* refers to a preferential pattern of stress-related neural, neuroendocrine, or endocrine activation. Target-organ specificity refers to a predisposing vulnerability of the target organ to experience pathogenic arousal (Everly, 1986). Genetic, prenatal, neonatal, and traumatic stimuli may all play a role in such a determination.

Finally, feedback loop IV (in Fig. 2.6) indicates that target-organ activation and subsequent signs and symptoms of disease may affect the patient's cognitive–affective behavior and, therefore, further neurological triggering and continued stress-response activity. In some cases (e.g., agoraphobic patients, obsessive patients, and hysteria-prone patients), a hypersensitive awareness to target-organ symptoms can create a self-sustaining pathogenic feedback loop.

We elaborate upon the issue of target-organ disease in the next chapter.

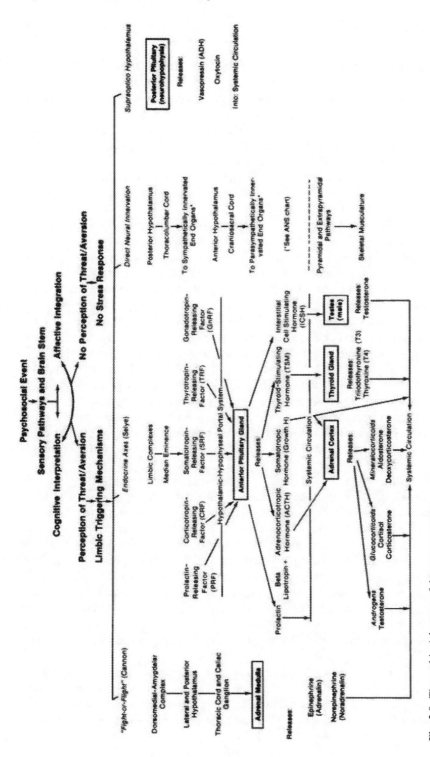

Fig. 2.9 The multiaxial nature of the stress response

Coping

The preceding two sections went into great detail in an attempt to describe what many phenomenologists have called the "missing link" in psychosomatic phenomena, that is, the physiological mechanisms of mediation by which cognitive–affective discord could result in physical disease and dysfunction. It is an understanding of these physiological mechanisms of mediation that allows us to see stress-related disorders as the quintessential intertwining of "mind and body" as opposed to some anomaly of hysteria. Yet we know that the manifestations of human stress are highly varied and individualistic. Whereas biological predisposition certainly plays a role in this process, a major factor in determining the impact of stress on the patient is his or her perceived ability to cope.

Coping is defined as: efforts, both action-oriented and intrapsychic, to manage (that is, master, tolerate, reduce, minimize) environmental and internal demands, and conflicts among them, which tax or exceed a person's resources. Coping can occur prior to a stressful confrontation, in which case it is called anticipatory coping, as well as in reaction to a present or past confrontation with harm. (Cohen & Lazarus, 1979, p. 219)

More recently, coping has been defined as "constantly changing cognitive and behavioral efforts to manage specific … demands that are appraised as taxing or exceeding the resources of the person" (Lazarus & Folkman, 1984, p. 141).

From the perspective of the current model (Fig. 2.6), coping may be thought of as environmental or cognitive tactics designed to attenuate the stress response. The present model views coping as residing subsequent to the physiological stress response and target-organ activation. Thus, coping is seen as an attempt to reestablish homeostasis. Anticipatory coping, as mentioned by Lazarus and other theorists, is subsumed, in the present model, in the complex interactions of the cognitive–affective domain.

To further refine the notion of coping, we suggest that coping strategies can be either adaptive or maladaptive (Girdano et al., 2009). Adaptive coping strategies reduce stress while at the same time promoting long-term health (e.g., exercise, relaxation, proper nutrition). Maladaptive coping strategies, on the other hand, do indeed reduce stress in the short term but serve to erode health in the long term (alcohol/drug abuse, cigarette smoking, interpersonal withdrawal) (see Everly, 1979a).

Figure 2.6 reflects the belief that when coping is successful, extraordinary target-organ activation is reduced or eliminated and homeostasis is reestablished. If coping strategies are unsuccessful, target-organ activation is maintained and the chances of target-organ disease are increased.

Feedback loops V and VI once again reflect the interrelatedness of all components included in Fig. 2.6.

The model depicted in Fig. 2.6 reflects an integration of recent research and critical thought concerning human stress. It is presented as nothing more than a pedagogical tool designed to facilitate the clinician's understanding of the phenomenology of the stress response. If it has sensitized the clinician to the major components of the stress response and shown their interrelatedness, it has served its purpose. This phenomenological model is used as a common reference in subsequent chapters to facilitate better understanding of the topics of measurement and treatment of the human stress response.

Summary

Our purpose has been to provide a somewhat detailed analysis of the psychophysiological nature of the human stress response. Let us review the main points of this chapter.

1. The nervous systems serve as the foundation of the stress response. The neuron is the smallest functional unit within any given nervous system. Communications between neurons, and therefore within nervous systems, are based upon electrical (ionic transport) and chemical (neurotransmitter mobilization) processes.
   Nervous systems are anatomically arranged in the following schema:

   (a) Central nervous system
       • Brain
       • Spinal cord

   (b) Peripheral nervous systems
       • Somatic (to skeletal musculature)
       • Autonomic (to glands, organs, viscera)
           – Sympathetic
           – Parasympathetic

2. Figure 2.6, which represents an integrative epiphenomenological model of the stress response, is reproduced once again here as Fig. 2.10 for review purposes. Let us summarize its components.
3. Environmental events (stressors) may either "cause" the activation of the stress response (as in the case of sympathomimetic stressors) or, as is usually the case, simply "set the stage" for the mobilization of the stress response.
4. The cognitive–affective domain is the critical "causal" phase in most stress reactions. Stress, like beauty, appears to be in the eye of the beholder. One's interpretation of the environmental event is what creates most stressors and subsequent stress responses.
5. The locus ceruleus, limbic complexes, and the hypothalamic nuclei trigger efferent neurological, neuroendocrine, and endocrine reactions in response to higher cognitive–affective interactions.
6. The actual stress response itself is the next step in the system's analysis. Possessing at least three major efferent axes—neurological, neuroendocrine, and endocrine—this "physiological mechanism of mediation" represents numerous combinations and permutations of efferent activity directed toward numerous and diverse target organs (see Fig. 2.9).

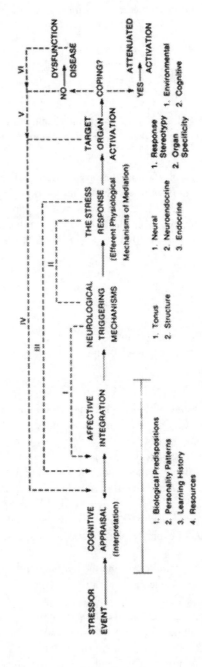

Fig. 2.10 A systems model of the human stress response

The most rapid of the physiological stress axes are the neurological axes. They consist of mobilization of the sympathetic, parasympathetic, and neuromuscular nervous systems. The neuroendocrine axis, sometimes called the sympathoadrenomedullary system (SAM), but better known as Cannon's "fight-or-flight" response, is next to be mobilized. Activation leads to the extraordinary release of epinephrine and norepinephrine. Finally, the endocrine axes, researched primarily by Hans Selye, are potential response mechanisms. Consisting of the adrenal cortical axis (HPAC system), the somatotropic axis, the thyroid axis, and the posterior pituitary axis, these axes play a major role in chronic disease and dysfunction. Selye's notion of the General Adaptation Syndrome is an attempt to unify these axes (see Table 2.6).

7. As a result of the stress response axes being extraordinarily mobilized, target-organ activation is realized.

8. The final step before pathogenic target-organ activation is coping. Here, the patient has the opportunity to act environmentally or cognitively, or both, so as to reduce or mitigate the overall amplitude and level of activation that reaches the target organs.

9. Should stress arousal be excessive in either acute intensity or chronicity, target-organ dysfunction and/or pathology will result.

10. As a final note, remember that the aforementioned axes are always activated at some level of functioning. Inclusion in this chapter simply reflects their potential for pathogenic arousal in response to stressor stimuli and thus their aggregate designation as the physiological mechanisms of the stress response.

11. In summary, this chapter was designed to provide the reader with a reasonable approximation of the mechanisms that serve to link the stressor stimulus with target-organ activation. Chapter 3 extends this examination into the link between stress arousal and subsequent disease.

References

Aggleton, J. P. (Ed.). (1992). *The Amygdala*. New York, NY: Wiley-Liss.

Arnold, M. (1970). *Feelings and emotions*. New York, NY: Academic.

Arnold, M. (1984). *Memory and the brain*. Hillsdale, NJ: Erlbaum.

Axelrod, J., & Reisine, T. (1984). Stress hormones. *Science, 224*, 452–459.

Cannon, W. B. (1914). The emergency function of the adrenal medulla in pain and in the major emotions. *American Journal of Physiology, 33*, 356–372.

Cannon, W. B. (1953). *Bodily changes in pain, hunger, fear, and rage*. Boston, MA: Branford.

Cannon, W. B., & Paz, D. (1911). Emotional stimulation of adrenal secretion. *American Journal of Physiology, 28*, 64–70.

Carruthers, M., & Taggart, P. (1973). Vagotonicity of violence. *British Medical Journal, 3*, 384–389.

Cassel, J. (1974). *Psychosocial processes and stress: The behavioral sciences and preventive medicine*. Washington, DC: Public Health Service.

Cohen, F., & Lazarus, R. S. (1979). Coping with the stresses of illness. In G. Stone, F. Cohen, & N. Adler (Eds.), *Health psychology* (pp. 217–254). San Francisco, CA: Jossey-Bass.

Corson, S., & Corson, E. (1971). Psychosocial influences on renal function: Implications for human pathophysiology. In L. Levi (Ed.), *Society, stress, and disease* (Vol. 1, pp. 338–351). New York, NY: Oxford University Press.

Cullinan, W., Herman, J. P., Helmreich, D., & Watson, S. (1995). A neuroanatomy of stress. In M. J. Friedman, D. Charney, & A. Deutch (Eds.), *Neurobiological and clinical consequences of stress* (pp. 3–26). Philadelphia, PA: Lippincott-Raven.

Entringer, S., Kumsta, R., Hellhammer, D. H., Wadhwa, P. D., & Wust, S. (2009). Prenatal exposure to maternal psychosocial stress and HPA axis regulation in young adults. *Hormones and Behavior, 55*, 292–298.

Everly, G. S., Jr. (1978). *The Organ Specificity Score as a measure of psychophysiological stress reactivity.* Unpublished doctoral dissertation, University of Maryland, College Park.

Everly, G. S., Jr. (1979a). *Strategies for coping with stress: An assessment scale.* Washington, DC: Office of Health Promotion, Department of Health and Human Services.

Everly, G. S., Jr. (1986). A "biopsychosocial analysis" of psychosomatic disease. In T. Millon & G. Kierman (Eds.), *Contemporary directions in psychopathology* (pp. 535–551). New York, NY: Guilford.

Everly, G. S., Jr., & Benson, H. (1989). Disorders of arousal and the relaxation response. *International Journal of Psychosomatics, 36*, 15–21.

Everly, G. S., Jr., Davy, J. A., Smith, K. J., Lating, J. M., & Nucifora, F. C., Jr. (2011). A defining aspect of human resilience in the workplace: A structural modeling approach. *Disaster Medicine and Public Health Preparedness, 5*(2), 98–105.

Everly, G. S., Jr., Smith, K. J., & Lating, J. M. (2009). A rationale for cognitively-based resilience and psychological first aid (PFA) training: A structural modeling analysis. *International Journal of Emergency Mental Health, 11*(4), 249–262.

Florian, J. P., & Pawelczyk, J. A. (2010). Non-esterified fatty acids increase arterial pressure via central sympathetic activation in humans. *Clinical Science, 118*, 61–69.

Foley, P., & Kirschbaum, C. (2010). Human hypothalamus-pituitary-adrenal axis responses to acute psychosocial stress in laboratory settings. *Neuroscience and Biobehavioral Reviews, 35*, 91–96.

Folkow, B., & Neil, E. (1971). *Circulation.* London: Oxford University Press.

Frankenhaeuser, M. (1980). Psychoneuroendocrine approaches to the study of stressful person-environment transactions. In H. Selye (Ed.), *Selye's guide to stress research* (pp. 46–70). New York, NY: Van Nostrand Reinhold.

Ganong, W. F. (1997). *Review of medical physiology* (18th ed.). Stamford, CT: Appleton & Lange.

Gellhorn, E. (1957). *Autonomic imbalance and the hypothalamus.* Minneapolis, MN: University of Minnesota Press.

Gellhorn, E. (1958a). The physiological basis of neuromuscular relaxation. *Archives of Internal Medicine, 102*, 392–399.

Gellhorn, E. (1958b). The influence of curare on hypothalamic excitability and the electroencephalogram. *Electroencephalography and Clinical Neurophysiology, 10*, 697–703.

Gellhorn, E. (1964a). Motion and emotion. *Psychological Review, 71*, 457–472.

Gellhorn, E. (1964b). Sympathetic reactivity in hypertension. *Acta Neurovegetative, 26*, 35–44.

Gellhorn, E. (1965). The neurophysiological basis of anxiety. *Perspectives in Biology and Medicine, 8*, 488–515.

Gellhorn, E. (1967). *Principles of autonomic-somatic integrations.* Minneapolis, MN: University of Minnesota Press.

Gellhorn, E. (1968). Central nervous system tuning and its implications for neuropsychiatry. *Journal of Nervous and Mental Disease, 147*, 148–162.

Gellhorn, E. (1969). Further studies on the physiology and pathophysiology of the tuning of the central nervous system. *Psychosomatics, 10*, 94–104.

Gellhorn, E., & Loofburrow, G. (1963). *Emotions and emotional disorders.* New York, NY: Harper & Row.

Gevarter, W. (1978).*Psychotherapy and the brain.* Unpublished paper, NASA, Washington, DC.

Gifford, S., & Gunderson, J. G. (1970). Cushing's disease as a psychosomatic disorder: A selective review. *Perspectives in Biology and Medicine, 13*, 169–221.

Girdano, D., Dusek, D., & Everly, G. (2009). *Controlling stress and tension.* San Francisco, CA: Pearson Benjamin Cummings.

Guyenet, P. G. (2006). The sympathetic control of blood pressure. *Nature Reviews/Neuroscience, 7*, 335–346.

Hall, J. E. (2011). *Guyton and Hall Textbook of Medical Physiology* (12th ed.). Philadelphia, PA: Saunders Elsevier.

Harper, H. A. (1975). *Review of physiological chemistry.* Los Altos, CA: Lange.

Hassett, J. (1978). *A primer of psychophysiology.* San Francisco, CA: W. H. Freeman.

Heim, C. & Nemeroff, C. B. (2009). Neurobiology of posttraumatic stress disorder. *CNS Spectrum, 14(1) (Suppl 1)*, 13–24.

Henry, J. P., & Ely, D. (1976). Biologic correlates of psychosomatic illness. In R. Grenen & S. Galay (Eds.), *Biological foundations of psychiatry* (pp. 945–986). New York, NY: Raven Press.

Henry, J. P., & Stephens, P. (1977). *Stress, health, and the social environment.* New York, NY: Springer-Verlag.

Hess, W. (1957). *The functional organization of the diencephalon.* New York, NY: Grune &Stratton.

Johnson, R. H., & Spalding, J. M. (1974). *Disorders of the autonomic nervous system.* Philadelphia: Davis.

Kopin, L. (1976). Catecholamines, adrenal hormones, and stress. *Hospital Practice, 11*, 49–55.

Krishnan, V., & Nestler, E. J. (2008). The molecular neurobiology of depression. *Nature, 455*(16), 894–902.

Lachman, S. (1972). *Psychosomatic disorders: A behavioristic interpretation.* New York: Wiley.

Lang, I. M. (1975). *Limbic involvement in the vagosympathetic arterial pressor response of the rat.* Unpublished master's thesis, Temple University, Philadelphia.

Lazarus, R. S. (1966). *Psychological stress and the coping process.* New York: McGraw-Hill.

Lazarus, R. S. (1982). Thoughts on the relations between emotions and cognition. *American Psychologist, 37*, 1019–1024.

Lazarus, R. S. (1991). *Emotion and adaptation.* New York: Oxford University Press.

Lazarus, R. S. (2006). *Stress and Emotion: A New Synthesis.* New York, NY: Springer Publishing Company, Inc.

Lazarus, R. S., & Folkman, S. (1984). *Stress, appraisal, and coping.* New York: Springer.

Le Blanc, J. (1976, July). *The role of catecholamines in adaptation to chronic and acute stress.* Paper presented at the proceedings of the International Symposium on Catecholamines and Stress, Bratislava, Czechoslovakia.

Levi, L. (1972). Psychosocial stimuli, psychophysiological reactions and disease. *Acta Medico Scandinavica (entire Suppl. 528).*

Lomax, A. E., Sharkey, K. A., & Furness, J. B. (2010). The participation of the sympathetic innervation of the gastrointestinal tract in disease states. *Neurogastroenterology & Motility, 22*, 7–18.

Lundberg, U., & Forsman, L. (1978). *Adrenal medullary and adrenal cortical responses to understimulation and overstimulation* (Report No. 541). Stockholm: Department of Psychology, University of Stockholm.

Macfarlane, D. P., Forbes, S., & Walker, B. R. (2008). Glucocoticoids and fatty acid metabolism in humans: fuelling fat redistribution in the metabolic syndrome. *Journal of Endocrinology, 197*, 189–204.

MacLean, P. D. (1949). Psychosomatic disease and the "visceral brain. *Psychosomatic Medicine, 11*, 338–353.

MacLean, P. D. (1975). On the evolution of three mentalities. *Man-Environment System, 5*, 213–994.

Makara, G., Palkovits, M., & Szentagothal, J. (1980). The endocrine hypothalamus and the hormonal response to stress. In H. Selye (Ed.), *Selye's guide to stress research* (pp. 280–337). New York: Van Nostrand Reinhold.

Malmo, R. B. (1975). *On emotions, needs, and our archaic brain*. New York: Holt, Rinehart & Winston.

Maranon, G. (1924). Contribution a l'etude de l'action emotive de l'ademaline. *Revue Francais d'Endrocrinologie, 2*, 301–325.

Mason, J. W. (1968a). A review of psychendocrine research on the sympathetic–adrenal medullary system. *Psychosomatic Medicine, 30*, 631–653.

Mason, J. W. (1968b). Organization of psychoendocrine mechanisms. *Psychosomatic Medicine, 30* (entire P. 2).

Mason, J. W. (1968c). A review of psychoendocrine research on the pituitary–adrenal–cortical system. *Psychosomatic Medicine, 30*, 576–607.

Mason, J. W. (1972). Organization of psychoendocrine mechanisms: A review and reconsideration of research. In N. Greenfield & R. Sternbach (Eds.), *Handbook of psychophysiology* (pp. 3–76). New York: Holt, Rinehart & Winston.

Mason, J. W., Wang, S., Yehuda, R., Bremner, J. D., Riney, S., Lubin, H., & Charney, D. (1995). Some approaches to the study of clinical implications of thyroid alterations in post-traumatic stress disorder. In M. J. Friedman, D. Charney, & A. Deutch (Eds.), *Neurobiological, and clinical consequences of stress,* (pp. 367–380). Philadelphia: Lippincott-Raven.

Mazeh, H., Paldor, I., & Chen, H. (2012). The endocrine system: Pituitary and adrenal glands. *ACS Surgery: Principles and Practice*, 1–13

McCabe, P., & Schneiderman, N. (1984). Psychophysiologic reactions to stress. In N. Schneiderman & J. Tapp (Eds.), *Behavioral medicine* (pp. 3–32). Hillsdale, NJ: Erlbaum.

McCorry, L. K., PhD. (2007). Physiology of the autonomic nervous system. *American Journal of Pharmaceutical Education, 71*(4), 1–78.

Meichenbaum, D. (1985). *Stress innoculation training*. New York: Plenum Press.

Meichenbaum, D., & Jaremko, M. (1983). *Stress reduction and prevention*. New York: Plenum Press.

Miller, N. E. (1978). Biofeedback and visceral learning. *Annual Review of Psychology, 29*, 373–404.

Miller, N. E. (1979). General discussion and a review of recent results with paralyzed patients. In R. Gatchel & K. Price (Eds.), *Clinical applications of biofeedback* (pp. 215–225). Oxford, UK: Pergamon Press.

Millon, T., & Everly, G. S., Jr. (1985). *Personality and its disorders*. New York: Wiley.

Millon, T., Grossman, S., Millon, C., Meagher, S., & Ramnath, R. (2004). *Personality disorders in modern life*. Hoboken, NJ: John Wiley & Sons, Inc.

Nauta, W. (1979). Expanding borders of the limbic system concept. In T. Rasmussen & R. Marino (Eds.), *Functional neurosurgery* (pp. 7–23). New York: Raven Press.

Nauta, W., & Domcsick, V. (1982). Neural associations of the limbic system. In A. Beckman (Ed.), *Neural substrates of behavior* (pp. 3–29). New York: Spectrum.

Omer, H., & Everly, G. S., Jr. (1988). Psychological influences on pre-term labor. *American Journal of Psychiatry, 145*(12), 1507–1513.

Penfield, W. (1975). *The mystery of the mind*. Princeton, NJ: Princeton University Press.

Ray, C. A. & Carter, J. R. (2010). Effects of aerobic exercise training on sympathetic and renal responses to mental stress in humans. *American Journal of Physiology – Heart and Circulatory Physiology, 298*, H229–H234.

Redmond, D. E. (1979). New and old evidence for the involvement of a brain norepinephrine system in anxiety. In W. Fann, I. Karacan, A. Pikomey, & R. Williams (Eds.), *Phenomenology and treatment of anxiety* (pp. 153–204). New York: Spectrum.

Reiman, E., Raichle, M. E., Robins, E., Butler, F. K., Herscovitch, P., Fox, P., & Perlmutter, J. (1986). The application of positron emission tomography to the study of panic disorder. *American Journal of Psychiatry, 143*, 469–477.

Rochefort, G. J., Rosenberger, J., & Saffran, M. (1959). Depletion of pituitary corticotropin by various stresses and by neurohypophyseal preparations. *Journal of Physiology, 146*, 105–116.

Roldan, E., Alvarez-Pelaez, P., & de Molina, F. (1974). Electrographic study of the amygdaloid defense response. *Physiology and Behavior, 13*, 779–787.

Rossier, J., Bloom, F., & Guillemin, R. (1980). In H. Selye (Ed.), *Selye's guide to stress research* (pp. 187–207). New York: Van Nostrand Reinhold.

Schwarz, N. A., Rigby, B. R., La Bounty, P., Shelmadine, B., & Bowden, R. G. (2011). A review of weight control strategies and their effects on the regulation of hormonal balance. *Journal of Nutrition and Metabolism, 2011*, 1–15.

Selye, H. (1956). *The stress of life*. New York: McGraw-Hill.

Selye, H. (1976). *Stress in health and disease*. Boston: Butterworth.

Smith, K. J., Everly, G. S., & Johns, T. (1992, December). A structural modeling analysis of the mediating role of cognitive-affective arousal in the relationship between job stressors and illness among accountants. Paper presented to the Second APA/NIOSH Conference on Occupational Stress, Washington, DC.

Smith, K. J., Everly, G. S., & Johns, T. (1993). The role of stress arousal in the dynamics of the stressor-to-illness process among accountants. *Contemporary Accounting Research, 9*, 432–449.

Sowers, J. R., Carlson, H. E., Brautbar, N., & Hershman, J. M. (1977). Effect of dexamethasone on prolactin and TSH responses to TRH and metoclopramide in man. *The Journal of Clinical Ednocrinology and Metabolism, 44*(2), 237–241.

Sternbach, R. (1966). *Principles of psychophysiology: An introductory text and readings*. Oxford, England: Academic Press.

Surges, R., Thijs, R. D., Tan, H. L., & Sander, J. W. (2009). Sudden unexpected death in epilepsy: risk factors and potential pathomechanisms. *Nature Reviews/Neurology, 5*, 492–504.

Taylor, S. E. (2006). Tend and befriend: Biobehavioral bases of affiliation under stress. *Current Directions in Psychological Science, 15*(6), 273–277.

Usdin, E., Kretnansky, R., & Kopin, L. (1976). *Catecholamines and stress*. Oxford, UK: Pergamon Press.

van Raalte, D. H., Ouwens, D. M., & Diamant, M. (2009). Novel insights into glucocorticoid-mediated diabetogenic effects: towards expansion of therapeutic options? *European Journal of Clinical Investigation, 39*(2), 81–93.

Weil, J. (1974). *A neurophysiological model of emotional and intentional behavior*. Springfield, IL: Charles C. Thomas.

Wenger, M. A., Clemens, T., Darsie, M. L., Engel, B. T., Estess, F. M., & Sonnenschien, R. R. (1960). Autonomic response patterns during intravenous infusion of epinephrme and norepinephrine. *Psychosomatic Medicine, 22*, 294–307.

Widmaier, E. P., Raff, H., & Strang, K. T. (2004). *Vander, Sherman, Luciano's Human Physiology: The Mechanisms of Body Function*. New York, NY: McGraw-Hill.

Williams, R. B. (1986). Patterns of reactivity and stress. In K. Matthews, R. R. Williams, S. B. Manuck, B. Faulkner, T. Dembroski, T. Detre, & S. M. Weiss (Eds.), *Handbook of stress, reactivity, and cardiovascular disease* (pp. 109–125). New York: Wiley.

Yehuda, R., Giller, E., Levengood, R., Southwick, S., & Siever, L. (1995). Hypothalamic–pituitary–adrenal-functioning in post-traumatic stress disorder. In M. J. Friedman, D. Charney, & A. Deutch (Eds.), *Neurobiological, and clinical consequences of stress* (pp. 351–366). Philadelphia: Lippincott-Raven.

Yuwiler, A. (1976). Stress, anxiety and endocrine function. In R. Grenell & S. Gabay (Eds.), *Biological foundations of psychiatry* (pp. 889–943). New York: Raven Press.

Zimmermann, U. S., Buchmann, A. F., Spring, C., Uhr, M., Holsboer, F., & Wittchen, H.-U. (2009). Ethanol administration dampens the prolactin response to psychosocial stress exposure in sons of alcohol-dependent fathers. *Psychoneuroendocrinology, 34*, 996–1003.

Chapter 3
The Link from Stress Arousal to Disease

The notion that one's psychosocial environment, lifestyle, and attitudes are linked to disease is by no means a new idea, as discussed in Chap. 1. In a scholarly meta-analysis, Tower (1984) reviewed 523 published reports investigating the relationship between psychosocial factors and disease. Ultimately selecting 60 of those studies on the basis of design considerations, she then submitted the data to a meta-analysis. The results supported the conclusion that there exists a strong relationship between psychosocial factors and illness. She notes, "Psychological well-being appeared to be most strongly associated with coronary heart disease and infectious processes ... although it was significantly associated with all diseases [investigated] except complications of pregnancy" (p. 51). To assess the power of her findings, Tower calculated the number of fugitive studies required to reject the findings of her meta-analysis. The results of this analysis of outcome tolerance revealed that over 28,000 fugitive studies would be required to reject the conclusion that psychosocial factors are related to disease. More recently, researchers have studied the link between psychosocial factors and heart disease (Low, Thurston, & Matthews, 2010), depression (Bonde, 2008) and even musculoskeletal pain (Macfarlane et al., 2009).

In the tradition of Pasteur, however, in order for a stimulus to be recognized as being a credible cause or contributor to disease, the pathophysiological processes that culminate in target-organ disease and dysfunction (sometimes called *mechanisms of mediation*) must be understood. Chapter 2 reviewed a model by which a *stressor* may activate *stress-response mechanisms*. That chapter further detailed potential stress-response effector mechanisms that might undergird such pathogenic relationships as confirmed by Tower (1984). The chapter offered evidence that an aggregation of neural, neuroendocrine, and endocrine response axes, collectively referred to as the *stress response*, were indeed vulnerable to extraordinary activation upon exposure to psychosocial stimuli. This chapter examines the logical extension of stress physiology by reviewing several noteworthy models of target-organ pathogenesis, that is, those proposed factors that link *stress arousal* mechanisms, once they are activated, to *target-organ disease.*

G.S. Everly and J.M. Lating, *A Clinical Guide to the Treatment*
of the Human Stress Response, DOI 10.1007/978-1-4614-5538-7_3,
© Springer Science+Business Media New York 2013

Although the literature in psychosomatic phenomenology as a global concept is voluminous, relatively few models exist that concern themselves more directly with the link between extraordinary arousal of the stress axes and the ultimate manifestations of stress-related disease. Let us take this opportunity to review several of those models.

Selye's "General Adaptation Syndrome"

In Chap. 2, Selye's General Adaptation Syndrome (GAS) was introduced as a means of integrating the manifestations of the stress response as a sequential series of physiological events. Its triphasic constituency was described at that point: (1) the alarm stage, (2) the stage of resistance (adaptation), and (3) the exhaustion stage. The GAS is mentioned in the present chapter because, not only does it serve to integrate, from a temporal perspective, many of the stress axes described earlier, but it also serves to explain the link from stress arousal to disease. As described by Selye (1956), Stage 1 of the GAS involves a somatic "shock" and initial "alarm reaction" for biological sources within the body following exposure to a stressor. The insult to the bodily tissues during this acute alarm phase could be so great as to deprive the target organ of its ability to compensate. If this happens, as might occur in cases of burns, electrical shock, or acute psychological trauma, the target organ may simply cease to function (e.g., in the case of cardiac fibrillation). Thus, the target organ will have been traumatically exhausted and rendered incapable of further functioning. Serious illness or death may then result.

If, however, the resources of the body are not completely compromised as a result of the "alarm" phase, then the stage of resistance is entered. Here the body's resources are mobilized to reestablish homeostasis. This is what usually occurs in most stress-related conditions. Yet, in order to maintain homeostasis in the face of a persistent stressor, there is a chronic drain of "adaptive energy," that is, physiological resources. Should the stressor persist indefinitely (even in the form of cognitive rumination) or should Stages 1 and 2 recycle themselves too frequently, eventual exhaustion of the target organ is predicted. This is the third and final stage in Selye's schema, the exhaustion phase. Thus, stress-related disease manifestation would occur as a result of a depletion of adaptive physiological resources and the subsequent target-organ exhaustion would be considered a result of excessive "wear and tear" (Selye, 1974). This then is the GAS as it attempts to define the stress-to-disease process. The GAS has been criticized for its global generality and lack of sensitivity for physiological response specificity (Mason, 1971).

In Selye's original exposition, he states, "It seems to us that more or less pronounced forms of this three-stage reaction represent the usual response of the organism to stimuli such as temperature changes, drugs, muscular exercise, etc., to which habituation or inurement can occur" (1936, p. 32). Yet subsequent researchers such as Mason (1971) argued that the stress response and subsequent target-organ pathology may indeed be rather specific, rather than generalized, pathogenic processes. This was a point with which Selye would have to contend for the rest of his career.

Given that Selye's important formulations were from the perspective of an endocrinologist more interested in pathogenic mechanisms than target-organ pathology per se, later writers in the emerging field of psychosomatic medicine would greatly elaborate upon the link from stress arousal to stress-related disease. Those mechanisms we consider most important are summarized below.

Lachman's Model

In a "behavioral interpretation" of psychosomatic disease, Lachman (1972) proposes an "autonomic learning theory" that emphasizes:

> ... the role of learning in the development of psychosomatic aberrations without minimizing the role of genetic factors or of nongenetic predisposing factors. The essence of the theory proposed is that psychosomatic manifestations result from frequent or prolonged or intense ... reactions elicited via stimulation of receptors. (pp. 62–63)

Lachman argues that a major source of frequent, prolonged, or intense emotional and physiological reactions is a *learned* pattern of emotional and autonomic responsiveness. More specifically, he notes with regard to the stress-to-disease phenomenon, "In order for emotional reactions to assume pathological significance such reactions must be intense or chronic or both" (p. 70). He goes on to state that which end-organ structure will be affected pathologically depends on the following:

1. Genetic factors that biologically predispose the organ to harm from psychophysiological arousal.
2. Environmental factors that predispose the organ to harm from psychophysiological arousal, including such things as nutritional influences, infectious disease influences, physical trauma influences, and so on.
3. The specific structures involved in the physiological reactivity.
4. The magnitude of involvement during the physiological response, which he has defined in terms of intensity, frequency, and duration of involvement of the organ.

Lachman (1972) concludes that the determination of which structure is ultimately affected in the psychosomatic reaction depends on "the biological condition of the structure" (whether a function of genetic or environmental influences), "on the initial reactivity threshold of the organ, and on ... learning factors" that affect the activation of the organ. He goes on to note that the "magnitude of the psychosomatic phenomenon" appears to be a function of the frequency, intensity, and chronicity of the organ's activation.

Sternbach's Model

In a somewhat more psychophysiologically oriented model, Sternbach (1966) provides another perspective on the stress-to-disease issue, which is considered a variation on the diathesis–stress model of Levi and Andersson (1975).

The first step in Sternbach's model is *response stereotypy*. This term generally refers to the tendency of an individual to exhibit characteristically similar patterns of psychophysiological reactivity to a variety of stressful stimuli. Sternbach views it as a "predisposed response set." That such a response stereotypy phenomenon does indeed exist has been clearly demonstrated in patient and normal populations (Lacey & Lacey, 1958, 1962; Malmo & Shagass, 1949; Moos & Engel, 1962; Schnore, 1959).

Response stereotypy may be generally thought of as a form of the "weak-link" or "weak-organ" theory of psychosomatic disease. Whether the weak organ is genetically determined, a function of conditioning, or acquired through disease or physical trauma is unclear.

The second step in the Sternbach model entails the frequent activation of the psychophysiological stress response within the stereotypical organ. The mere existence of response stereotypy is not enough to cause disease. It is obvious that the organ must be involved in frequent activation in order to be adversely affected.

Finally, Sternbach's model includes the requirement that homeostatic mechanisms fail; that is, once the stereotypical organ has undergone psychophysiological arousal, that stress-responsive organ must now evidence slow return to baseline level of activity. Such homeostatic failure has been implicated in the onset of disease since the work of Freeman (1939). Freeman advanced the theory that autonomic excitation that is slow to deactivate from an organ system does increase the strain on that system. Malmo, Shagass, and Davis (1950) empirically demonstrated that such a phenomenon exists. Lader's (1969) review on this issue implicates it as a potential precursor to disease.

Sternbach (1966) has then put forward these conditions as prerequisites for the development of a stress-related disorder. The reader is referred to the work of Stoyva for further commentary on the Sternbach model, as well as other theories of psychosomatic illness (Stoyva, 1976, Stoyva & Budzynski, 1974).

Kraus and Raab's "Hypokinetic Disease" Model

In their treatise on exercise and health, Kraus and Raab (1961) argue that many stress-related diseases are induced not so much by the direct physiology of the stress response, but by the lack of subsequent somatomotor expression of that physiology. They argue that a little over 100 years ago, vigorous physical labor was a way of life that actually served as a protective mechanism against diseases commonly referred to today as "diseases of civilization." These authors suggest that modern sedentary lifestyles have put that protective mechanism "all but out of commission." Kraus and Raab (1961) conclude:

> The system that has been put all but out of commission, the striated musculature … has an important role which exceeds the mere function of locomotion. Action of the striated muscle influences directly and indirectly circulation, metabolism, and endocrine balance. … Last but not least the striated muscle serves as an outlet for our emotions and nervous responses …. Obliteration of [this] important safety valve … might well upset the original balance to which the bodies of primitive man have been adapted. (p. 4)

Therefore, Kraus and Raab coined the term "hypokinetic disease" (*hypo* = under; *kinetic* = motion/exercise) to refer to a wide array of diseases that as a result of the lack of healthful expression/utilization of the physiological mechanisms of the stress response. The notion of the lack of physical activity serving as a risk factor for disease and dysfunction has been supported by the World Health Organization (Chavat et al., 1964), which concludes that suppression of somatomotor activity in response to stress arousal is likely to lead to increased cardiovascular strain.

Schwartz's "Disregulation" Model

Gary Schwartz, working at Yale University (1977, 1979), devised a general systems model of stress-related pathogenesis that revolves around homeostatic disregulation as its pathogenic core (see Fig. 3.1). He notes, "It follows directly from cybernetic and systems theory that a normally self-regulatory system can become disordered when communication … between specific parts of the system is … disrupted" (1979, p. 563).

> Schwartz (1977) describes his model:When the environment (Stage 1) places demands on a person, the brain (Stage 2) performs the regulatory functions necessary to meet the specific demands. Depending on the nature of the environmental demand on stress, certain bodily systems (Stage 3) will be activated, while others may be simultaneously inhibited. However,

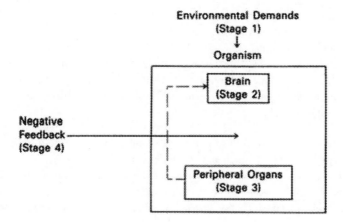

Fig. 3.1 Schwartz's model

if this process is sustained to the point where the tissue suffers deterioration or injury, the
negative feedback loops (Stage 4) of the homeostatic mechanism will normally come into
play, forcing the brain to modify its directives to aid the afflicted organ. (p. 76)

Thus, the negative feedback loops described by Schwartz dominate the normal
physiological milieu and are necessary to effective, adaptive functioning. Yet
Schwartz argues that it is a *disregulation* in Stage 4 homeostatic mechanisms that
may lead to a host of stress-related diseases through target-organ overstimulation.
Overstimulation may occur by the creation of positive, self-sustaining feedback
mechanisms or the blockage of natural inhibitory processes. Schwartz argues that
disconnection of any feedback mechanism, from a systems view, is capable of leading to disregulation and thus to disease.

Congruent with the aforementioned model, therapeutic interventions would
entail reestablishing homeostasis (homeostatic regulation). Consistent with this is
Greengard's (1978) perspective based on the observation of physiological systems:
"It seems probable that derangements of homeostatic processes are responsible for
many disease states. Conversely, it seems likely that the effects of many therapeutic
… agents are exerted on such homeostatic systems" (p. 146). Therefore, as one
might expect, Schwartz sees biofeedback and other auto-regulatory therapies as
useful agents for the treatment of stress-related disorders.

Conflict Theory of Psychosomatic Disease

Spawned in the formulative years of psychosomatic medicine, Alexander (1950)
postulated that specific types of conflicts lead to specific types of physical illnesses.
More specifically, specific psychical conflicts engendered specific mechanisms of
physiological pathogenesis. The result was a specific target-organ illness. Several
specific conflict–illness relationships were suggested:

Guilt → vomiting

Alienation → constipation

Repressed hostility → migraine headaches

Dependence → asthma

More recently, Harris (1991), using a specially designed psychometric instrument, the Life Events and Difficulties Schedule (LEDS), empirically investigated
the relation between life events and illness. The following relations emerged:

Long-term threat and loss → depression

Danger → anxiety

Goal frustration → gastrointestinal disorders and Coronary artery disease

Major challenge → amenorrhea or dysmenorrhea

With the possible exception of Rosenman and Friedman's (1974) Type A behavior
pattern and its predictive relationship with premature coronary artery disease, the
specific conflict approach to psychosomatic illness has not proven very predictive
of any specific physical or psychological disorder.

Everly and Benson's "Disorders of Arousal" Model

The "disorders of arousal" model of pathogenesis (Everly & Benson, 1989) is a direct result of an integration of efforts from Harvard University to understand the mechanisms of pathogenesis in psychosomatic disorders (Everly, 1986) and the mechanisms active in the amelioration of such psychosomatic disorders (Benson, 1975, 1987, 1996).

It has been observed for over five decades that various technologies that could be used to induce a hypoarousal relaxation response were able to ameliorate, or at least diminish, the severity of a wide and diverse variety of diseases. Despite data supporting specific clinical and experimental effects for various stress-management methods (Lehrer, Carr, Sargunaraj, & Woolfolk, 1994; Lehrer, Woolfolk, & Sime, 2007), it also seems that the initiation of what Herbert Benson (1975) has called the "relaxation response" has virtually a generic applicability across a wide spectrum of stress-related, psychosomatic diseases. That observation led to an investigation of the source of the broad-spectrum therapeutic effect of the relaxation response as a way of understanding the disorders it was useful in treating. The investigation culminated in an analysis of common phenomenological mechanisms, that is, common denominators (latent), occurring across anxiety and stress-related diseases that would serve to homogenize such disorders.

Based upon an integration of the work of Goddard on "kindling" (Goddard & Douglas, 1976), Post on "sensitization" (Post & Ballenger, 1981), Gellhorn on "ergotropic tuning" (1967), and Gray (1982) on the limbic system, it has been proposed by Everly that the phenomenology of many chronic anxiety- and stress-related diseases is undergirded by the existence of a latent, yet common denominator, existing in the form of a neurological hypersensitivity for excitation (or arousal) residing within the subcortical limbic circuitry (Everly, 1985b). This limbic hypersensitivity phenomenon (LHP) may be understood as an unusually high propensity for neurological arousal/excitation with the potential to lead to, or exist as, a pathognomonic state of excessive arousal within the limbic system. "Hyperstartle reaction," "autonomic hyperfunction," and "autonomic lability" are diagnostic terms commonly used to capture such a notion. The LHP is believed to develop as a result of either acutely traumatic or repeated extraordinary limbic excitation and is credited with the potential to ignite a cascade of extraordinary arousal of numerous and varied neurological, neuroendocrine, and endocrine efferent mechanisms (as discussed in Chap. 2) and, therefore, the potential to give rise to a host of varied psychiatric and somatic disorders. The subsequent disorders are then referred to as "disorders of arousal." This concept is captured in Fig. 3.2.

Figure 3.2 depicts the notion that, responsive to a host of widely disparate etiological factors (stressors) including environmental events, cognitive–affective dynamics, personologic predispositions, and the like, there exists a subtle, latent mechanism of pathogenesis: a neurological hypersensitivity for pathogenic arousal located within the limbic circuitry. Such arousal is believed to be capable of triggering a subsequent variety of physiological effector mechanisms (stress-response axes)

Fig. 3.2 Limbic
hypersensitivity
phenomenon: the latent taxon
in stress-related "disorders of
arousal"

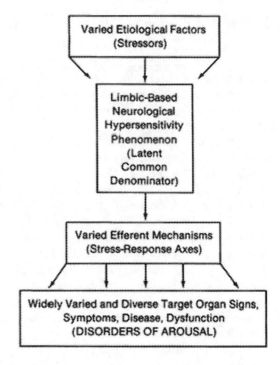

within existing patterns of response predisposition (response stereotypy), so as to ultimately give rise to a wide and diverse spectrum of target-organ disorders (disorders of arousal). Included in the disorders of arousal taxonomy would be most anxiety and adjustment disorders, including some forms of depression, as well as virtually any and all stress-related physical disorders. The disorders of arousal will be enumerated in greater detail later in this volume. The reader may also refer to Everly and Benson (1989), Doane (1986), and Post (1986).

The natural corollary of the disorders of arousal model of pathogenesis is the notion that effective treatment of such disorders is highly related to reducing the subcortical hypersensitivity through the use of some "antiarousal" therapy. In addition to various pharmacological interventions, Benson's concept of the relaxation response represents a natural antiarousal phenomenon that appears antithetical to the mechanisms that undergird the disorders of arousal. Thus, it may well be that a major source of the broad-spectrum therapeutic effect exhibited by the relaxation response resides in the homeostasis-seeking, antiarousal phenomenology of the relaxation response, which serves to inhibit the mechanism of limbic hypersensitivity believed to exist as a common denominator among the various disorders of arousal.

In summary, the disorders of arousal model of stress-induced pathology recognizes the influences of environmental factors, cognitive–affective dynamics, patterns of previous learning, and patterns of preferential psychophysiological excitation as described in previous models and summarized elsewhere (Everly, 1986). Yet it focuses upon the limbic system proper, its efferent influences on cognitive processes, and its effector mechanisms through the hypothalamus. More specifically, it focuses upon a proposed LHP, developed as a result of extraordinary limbic excitation, as key constituents in linking the stress response to stress-related disease formation, especially chronic manifestations of such diseases.

Several different theories have been enumerated here to explain how psychophysiological arousal can be channeled to affect target organs adversely. Despite the disparity between the theories mentioned, there does appear to be one element, either directly stated or implied, that is common to all. That commonality pertains to how the target organs ultimately become dysfunctional or pathological—simply stated, if any given target organ is subjected to psychophysiological overload (overstimulation) for a long enough period, that organ will eventually manifest symptoms of dysfunction or pathology due to excessive "wear and tear," be it biochemically induced trauma or toxicity, or actual visceromotor fatigue or exhaustion. According to Stoyva (1976) in his review of stress-related disorders, "A number of investigators have hypothesized that if the stress response is evoked too often, or sustained for too long, then disorders are likely to develop" (p. 370). In a "behavioristic interpretation" of psychosomatic disorders, Lachman (1972) states, "The longer a given structure is involved in an ongoing emotional reaction pattern, the greater is the likelihood of it being involved in a psychosomatic disorder" (pp. 69–70). Lachman concludes, "Theoretically, any bodily structure or function can become the end focus of psychosomatic phenomena—but especially those directly innervated and regulated by the autonomic nervous system" (p. 71).

Perhaps of greater interest to the clinician than the theory concerning what causes a target-organ symptom to be overloaded is the widely accepted conclusion that target-organ stress-related diseases result from excessively frequent, intense, and/or prolonged activation, that is, overstimulation (see Everly, 1986; Everly & Benson, 1989; Kraus & Raab, 1961; Lachman, 1972; Sternbach, 1966; Stoyva, 1976; Stoyva & Budzynski, 1974). See Table 3.1.

Summary

Chapter 2 described a mechanism by which psychosocial factors could serve to ignite extraordinary arousal of the physiological stress-response axes through cognitive–affective integrations and limbic–hypothalamic neurological mechanisms. This chapter pursued the logical extension of stress–axis arousal by reviewing the pathogenic mechanisms that are postulated to link the stress response to subsequent target-organ disease. Let us review the main points covered in this review.

1. All major theories agree that target-organ pathology ultimately results when the specific target organ is overstimulated. Overstimulation may occur as a result of excessively frequent, chronic, or intense stimulation. Pathological states emerge from excessive "wear and tear" on the target organ and can be caused by

Table 3.1 From stress to disease: theories of psychosomatic pathogenesis

Theory	Pathogenic mechanisms	Result
Selye's "General Adaptation Syndrome"	Triphasic fluctuation of neuroendocrine and endocrine mechanisms, especially ACTH. The chronic maintenance of the stage of resistance yields a depletion of adaptive energy	Depletion of adaptive physiological energy → exhaustion → disease, due to excessive wear and tear
Lachman's "behavioral" model	Biological and learned factors interact to establish predisposing patterns of target-organ arousal and disease from excessively frequent stress arousal. Emotional and autonomic learning play a major role in repeated target-organ excitation	Excessively intense or excessively chronic activation of target organs → stress-related disease (excessive wear and tear)
Sternbach's model	Response stereotypy. Frequent stress arousal. Homeostatic recovery failure	Frequent target-organ activation → organ fatigue and pathology
Kraus and Raab's "hypokinetic disease" model	Suppression of somatomotor behavior. Failure to ventilate and utilize the stress response once activated. Increased pathogenic risk	Target-organ overload and pathology
Schwartz's "disregulation" model	Failure in homeostatic feedback mechanisms following stressor exposure	Target-organ overload and pathology
Conflict theory	Specific psychic conflicts lead to specific physical illnesses	Target-organ overload and pathology
Everly and Benson's "disorders of arousal" model	Limbic hypersensitivity phenomenon causing extraordinary arousal of stress response axes	Excessively intense and/or excessively frequent or chronic activation of stress response axes → target-organ overstimulation and pathology

biochemical toxicity or trauma (e.g., necrosis) as well as structural alteration and visceromotor fatigue or exhaustion.

2. The GAS of Selye presents a triphasic model by which acute "shock" or chronic excitation could ultimately deplete the physiological constituents that normally allow target organs to continue to function in the face of stress arousals. The results would be target-organ exhaustion and perhaps even death.

3. Lachman's behavioral model emphasizes the point that emotional and autonomic responses could be learned. Interacting with other biological factors that are not learned, emotional and autonomic learning can cause repeated target-organ excitation. Excessively prolonged, frequent, or intense target-organ stimulation may then lead to disease.

4. Sternbach's psychophysiological model cites response stereotypy, frequent arousal of stress-response axes, and homeostatic recovery delay as factors that

serve to exhaust target organs and lead to disease. Once again, the theme of overutilization emerges as the key pathogenic constituent.

5. Kraus and Raab's model emphasizes the role of suppressed somatomotor expression in the etiology of stress-related pathology. Such suppression leads to target-organ overstimulation, exhaustion, and ultimately disease.
6. Schwartz's "disregulation" model also accepts the overload/overstimulation concept, but emphasizes the role of faulty negative feedback mechanisms in the pathological etiology.
7. The conflict theory postulates that specific psychological conflicts lead to specific physical and/or psychological disorders. This is clearly the weakest of the major psychosomatic theories.
8. Finally, Everly and Benson propose a model that serves to unite stress-related illnesses on the basis of a LHP, that is, a sensitization (increased propensity for activation) of cognitive, affective, and stress-response efferents in the formulation of stress-related disease. It is proposed that excessively frequent, chronic, or intense activation of target organs based upon the limbic hypersensitivity could ultimately exhaust the target organ and lead to a stress-related disease.
9. Thus, we see that all theories of pathogenesis, while emphasizing different phenomenological aspects as to why target-organ overstimulation occurs, agree that, indeed, overstimulation and excessive wear of target organs lead to stress-related dysfunction and disease. Chapter 4 will review specific stress-related diseases commonly encountered in clinical practice.

References

Alexander, F. (1950). *Psychosomatic medium*. New York, NY: Norton.

Benson, H. (1975). *The relaxation response*. New York, NY: Morrow.

Benson, H. (1987). *Your maximum mind*. New York, NY: Times Books.

Benson, H. (1996). *Timeless healing: The power and biology of belief*. New York, NY: Scribner.

Bonde, J. P. E. (2008). Psychosocial factors at work and risk of depression: A systematic review of the epidemiological evidence. *Occupational and Environmental Medicine, 65*(7), 438–445.

Chavat, J., Dell, P., & Folkow, B. (1964). Mental factors and cardiovascular disorders. *Cardiologia, 44*, 124–141.

Doane, B. (1986). Clinical psychiatry and the physiodynamics of the limbic system. In B. Doane & K. Livingston (Eds.), *The limbic system* (pp. 285–315). New York, NY: Raven Press.

Everly, G. S., Jr. (1985b, November). *Biological foundations of psychiatric sequelae in trauma and stress-related "disorders of arousal."* Paper presented to the 8th National Trauma Symposium, Baltimore, MD.

Everly, G. S., Jr. (1986). A "biopsychosocial analysis" of psychosomatic disease. In T. Millon & G. Kierman (Eds.), *Contemporary directions in psychopathology* (pp. 535–551). New York, NY: Guilford.

Everly, G. S., Jr., & Benson, H. (1989). Disorders of arousal and the relaxation response. *International Journal of Psychosomatics, 36*, 15–21.

Everly, G. S., Jr., Welzant, V., Machado, P. & Miller, K. (1989). *The correlation between frontalis muscle tension and sympathetic nervous system activity*. Unpublished research report.

Freeman, G. L. (1939). Toward a psychiatric Plimsoll Mark. *Journal of Psychology, 8*, 247–252.

Gellhorn, E. (1967). *Principles of autonomic-somatic integrations*. Minneapolis, MN: University of Minnesota Press.

Goddard, G., & Douglas, R. (1976). Does the engram of kindling model the engram of normal long-term memory? In J. Wads (Ed.), *Kindling* (pp. 1–18). New York, NY: Raven Press.

Gray, J. (1982). *The neuropsychology of anxiety*. New York, NY: Oxford University Press.

Greengard, P. (1978). Phosphorylated proteins and physiological affectors. *Science, 199*, 146–152.

Harris, T. (1991). Life stress and illness: The question of specificity. *Annals of Behavioral Medicine, 13*, 211–219.

Kraus, H., & Raab, W. (1961). *Hypokinetic disease*. Springfield, IL: Charles C. Thomas.

Lacey, J., & Lacey, B. (1958). Verification and extension of the principle of autonomic response-stereotype. *American Journal of Psychology, 71*, 50–73.

Lacey, J., & Lacey, B. (1962). The law of initial value in the longitudinal study of autonomic constitution. *Annals of the New York Academy of Sciences, 98*, 1257–1290.

Lachman, S. (1972). *Psychosomatic disorders: A behavioristic interpretation*. New York: Wiley.

Lader, M. H. (1969). Psychophysiological aspects of anxiety. In M. H. Lader (Ed.), *Studies of anxiety* (pp. 53–61). Ashford, Kent, UK: Headly Brothers.

Lehrer, P. M., Carr, R., Sargunaraj, D., & Woolfolk, R. L. (1994). Stress management techniques: Are they all equivalent, or do they have specific effects? *Biofeedback and Self-Regulation, 19*(4), 353–401.

Lehrer, P. M., Woolfolk, R. L., & Sime, W. E. (2007). *Principles and practice of stress management* (3rd ed.). New York, NY: The Guildford Press.

Levi, L., & Andersson, L. (1975). *Psychosocial stress*. New York: Wiley.

Low, C. A., Thurston, R. C., & Matthews, K. A. (2010). Psychosocial factors in the development of heart disease in women: current research and future directions. *Psychosomatic Medicine, 72*(9), 842–854.

Macfarlane, G. J., Pallewatte, N., Paudyal, P., Blyth, F. M., Coggon, D., Crombez, G., … van der Windt, D. (2009). Evaluation of work-related psychosocial factors and regional musculoskeletal pain: results from a EULAR Task Force. *Annals of Rheumatoid Disorders, 68*, 885–891.

Malmo, R. B., & Shagass, C. (1949). Physiologic study of symptom mechanisms in psychiatric patients under stress. *Psychosomatic Medicine, 11*, 25–29.

Malmo, R. B., Shagass, C., & Davis, J. (1950). A method for the investigation of somatic response mechanisms in psychoneurosis. *Science, 112*, 325–328.

Mason, J. W. (1971). A re-evaluation of the concept of "non-specificity" in stress theory. *Journal of Psychiatric Research, 8*(3–4), 323–333.

Moos, R., & Engel, B. (1962). Psychophysiological reactions in hypertensive and arthritic patients. *Journal of Psychosomatic Research, 6*, 222–241.

Post, R. (1986). Does limbic system dysfunction play a role in affective illness? In B. Doane & K. Livingston (Eds.), *The limbic system* (pp. 229–249). New York: Raven Press.

Post, R., & Ballenger, J. (1981). Kindling models for the progressive development of psychopathology. In H. van Pragg (Ed.), *Handbook of biological psychiatry* (pp. 609–651). New York: Marcel Dekker.

Rosenman, R., & Friedman, M. (1974). *Type A behavior and your heart*. New York: Knopf.

Schnore, M. M. (1959). Individual patterns of physiological activity as a function of task differences and degree of arousal. *Journal of Experimental Psychology, 58*, 117–128.

Schwartz, G. (1977). Psychosomatic disorders and biofeedback: A psychobiological model of disregulation. In J. Maser & M. Seligman (Eds.), *Psychopathology: Experimental models* (pp. 270–307). San Francisco: Freeman.

Schwartz, G. (1979). The brain as a health care system. In C. Stone, F. Cohen, & N. Adler (Eds.), *Health psychology* (pp. 549–573). San Francisco: Jossey-Bass.

Selye, H. (1936). A syndrome produced by diverse noxious agents. *Nature, 138*, 32–33.

Selye, H. (1956). *The stress of life*. New York: McGraw-Hill.

Selye, H. (1974). *Stress without distress*. Philadelphia: Lippincott.

Sternbach, R. (1966). *Principles of psychophysiology: An introductory text and readings*. Oxford, England: Academic Press.

Stoyva, J. M. (1976). Self-regulation and stress-related disorders: A perspective on biofeedback. In D. I. Mostofsky (Ed.), *Behavior control and modification of physiological activity*. Englewood Cliffs, NJ: Prentice-Hall.

Stoyva, J. M., & Budzynski, T. H. (1974). Cultivated low-arousal: An anti-stress response? In L. DiCara (Ed.), *Recent advances in limbic and autonomic nervous systems research* (pp. 369–394). New York: Plenum Press.

Tower, J. F. (1984). A meta-analysis of the relationships among stress, social supports, and illness and their implications for health professions education. Unpublished doctoral dissertation, University of Pennsylvania, Philadelphia.

Chapter 4
Stress-Related Disease: A Review

I'm at the mercy of any rogue who cares to annoy and tease me.

John Hunter, eighteenth-century physician

There has been skepticism that emotions aroused in a social context can so seriously affect the body as to lead to long-term disease or death. But the work, such as that of Wolf, shows that machinery of the human body is very much at the disposal of the higher centers of the brain.... Given the right circumstances, these higher controls can drive it mercilessly, often without awareness on the part of the individual of how close he is to the fine edge.

(Henry & Stephens, 1977, p. 11)

To review what we have covered so far, Chap. 2 proposed a model of how psychosocial factors can activate a complex myriad of neurological, neuroendocrine, and endocrine response axes. Similarly, Chap. 2 reviewed the physiological constituents of these stress axes in considerable detail. Chapter 3 reviewed the link from stress arousal to disease by summarizing several noteworthy models constructed to elucidate how stress arousal can lead to disease and dysfunction, that is, mechanisms of pathogenesis that link causally stress arousal to target-organ pathology. The goal of this chapter is to review some of the most common clinical manifestations of excessive stress, and more specifically, to familiarize the reader with some of the most frequently encountered target-organ disorders believed to be related to excessive stress arousal.

Gastrointestinal Disorders

Excessive stress and the diseases of the gastrointestinal (GI) system have been thought to be related for decades. The most commonly encountered stress-related GI disorders are peptic ulcers, ulcerative colitis, irritable bowel syndrome, and esophageal reflux.

G.S. Everly and J.M. Lating, *A Clinical Guide to the Treatment of the Human Stress Response*, DOI 10.1007/978-1-4614-5538-7_4,
© Springer Science+Business Media New York 2013

Gastrointestinal Physiology

Before reviewing specific disorders, let us briefly review the basic physiology of the GI system. As described by Weinstock and Clouse (1987), the GI system involves a series of sequentially arranged tubular organs separated by sphincters. This system includes the esophagus, the stomach, the duodenum, the small intestine, and the large intestine (colon). See Fig. 4.1.

The esophagus provides a tubular canal for the connection of the mouth and the stomach. The activity of the esophagus is primarily under vagal control and neural mechanisms are primarily responsible for esophageal motility. The upper border of the esophagus is the cricopharyngeus (upper esophageal sphincter). The lower border is the lower esophageal sphincter, the gateway to the stomach.

The basic functions of the stomach are to receive, pulverize, nutritionally regulate, and temporarily store the food one consumes. The stomach is lined with a mucosal tissue that serves to protect it from its own digestive processes. Under the influence of factors such as gastrin, histamine, and vagal and sympathetic stimulation, intragastric dynamics involving the release of hydrochloric acid, pepsin, and mucus, as well as muscular contractions, act upon food that has been delivered to the stomach from the esophagus.

From the stomach, the food passes through the pyloric sphincter to the duodenum. The gallbladder is responsible for releasing bile into the duodenum.

The small intestine and its specialized mucosal lining serves as the primary location for digestion and nutrient absorption. Finally, the large intestine is designed for the absorption and orderly evacuation of concentrated waste products (Weinstock & Clouse, 1987). Let us now review several common stress-related GI disorders.

Peptic Ulcers

Peptic ulcers are usually further classified by their location in the GI system: gastric or stomach ulcers and duodenal ulcers. The incidence of peptic ulcer disease is about 18 in 10,000, with duodendal ulcers accounting for about 75% of those cases.

It was demonstrated many years ago that emotions of anger and rage are related to increased secretion of acid and pepsin by the stomach and that this secretion decreased with depression (Mahl & Brody, 1954; Mittelman & Wolff, 1942; Wolf & Glass, 1950). Although it might be concluded that what one sees in gastric ulcers, that is, an erosion of the wall of the stomach by the acid and enzyme it produces, is simply an exaggeration of a normal physiological response; actually it is not quite so simple. Certainly, emotions can raise gastric acid secretion and exacerbate an already existing ulcer, but normally the stomach wall is protected from the acid within it by a lining of mucus secreted by other cells in its wall. How this protective system breaks down and what predisposes a person to such an event remains elusive.

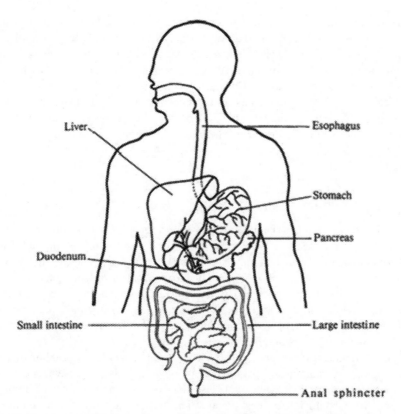

Fig. 4.1 The gastrointestinal system. (*Source*: Daniel A. Girdano and George S. Everly, Jr. (1986). *Controlling Stress and Tension: A Holistic Approach*, 2nd ed., pp. 36, 39. Reprinted by permission of Prentice-Hall, Inc., Englewood Cliffs, NJ)

There seems to be a combination of emotional and genetic factors involved in the pathogenesis of gastric ulcers, and such studies as that of Weiner, Thaler, Reiser, and Mirsky (1957) have demonstrated this quite well. These investigators were able to predict which individuals in a group of recruits in basic training in the army would develop gastric ulcers on the basis of serum pepsinogen levels—a genetic trait that is apparently a necessary but not sufficient factor in the formation of gastric ulcers. Gastric ulcers were also of interest to Selye (1951), who described ulcers apparently in response to chronic arousal of the endocrine stress axes in the general adaptation syndrome. One could thus conceive of a mechanism whereby stress, through the intermediation of neural or hormonal mechanisms, could result in significant irritation. In individuals who are so predisposed, ulceration of the stomach would occur given sufficient time and continued exposure to the stress. The picture is less clear-cut, however, in that it has been suggested that the duodenal ulcer results from changes in the mucosal wall "associated with sustained activation and a feeling of being deprived" (Backus & Dudley, 1977, p. 199).

Therefore, strongly implicated in the stress response, the specific causal mechanisms involved in peptic ulcer formation are probably multifactorial. Vagus-stimulated gastric hypersecretion as well as glucocorticoid anti-inflammatory activity on the mucous lining has been implicated. Yet conclusive data are lacking at present with regard to the selective activation of each mechanism. Bacteriological infections have most recently been implicated in ulcer formation, but a primary main effect seems doubtful. Rather, some complex interaction effect between arousal and bacteria seems more likely in instances where bacteria are, indeed, implicated.

Ulcerative Colitis

Ulcerative colitis is an inflammation and ulceration of the lining of the colon. Research by Grace, Seton, Wolf, and Wolff (1949) and Almy, Kern, and Tulin (1949) produced evidence that the colon becomes hyperactive and hyperemic with an increase in lysozyme levels (a proteolytic enzyme that can dissolve mucus) under stress. The emotions of anger and resentment are reported to create observable ulcerations of the bowel (Grace et al.). "Sustained feelings of this sort might be sufficient to produce enough reduction in bowel wall defenses to the point that the condition becomes self-sustaining" (Backus & Dudley, 1977, p. 199).

The predominant symptom of ulcerative colitis is rectal bleeding, although diarrhea, abdominal cramping and pain, and weight loss may also be present. Ulcerative colitis is sometimes associated with disorders of the spine, liver, and immune system. Rosenbaum (1985) has stated, "The frequency with which emotional precipitating-factors are identified varies, being as high as 74% in adults and 95% in children" (p. 79). Personologic investigations of colitis patients commonly find them to possess an immature personality structure often demonstrating extreme compulsive traits.

Irritable Bowel Syndrome

Mitchell and Drossman (1987) refer to irritable bowel syndrome (IBS) as the most common of the functional disorders. It is viewed as a syndrome of dysfunctional colonic motility; that is, the colon proves to be overreactive to psychological as well as physiological stimuli.

The diagnostic criteria for IBS include atypical abdominal pain, altered bowel habits, symptomatic duration of 3 months or more, and disruption of normal lifestyle (Latimer, 1985). Abdominal distention, mucus in the stools, fecal urgency, nausea, loss of appetite, and even vomiting are other IBS symptoms.

The pathophysiology of IBS is clearly multifactorial, with abnormal myoelectric phenomena, altered gut opiate receptors, abnormal calcium channel activity, and increased alpha-adrenergic activity. Personality characteristics of IBS patients often

Table 4.1 Psychological stimuli and gastrointestinal responses

Psychological state	GI response
Anxiety	Increased esophageal motility
	Increased colonic contractions
	Increased intraluminal pressure of the colon
Hostility, resentment, aggression (without somatomotor expression)	Increased colonic contractions
	Increased gastric acid
	Increased contractile activity of stomach
Depression	Decreased gastric acid
	Decreased colonic contractions
Wish to be rid of trouble	Rapid colonic transit with diarrhea

include compulsiveness, overly conscientious behavior, interpersonal sensitivity, and nonassertiveness (Latimer, 1985). Whitehead (1992) found stress to be related to acute IBS exacerbation and disability.

Esophageal Reflux

Before leaving this section on GI disorders it would be prudent to mention gastroesophageal reflux and its frequent corollary, esophagitis. Dotevall (1985) has indicated that these syndromes are common stress-related disorders. According to Young, Richter, Bradley, and Anderson (1987):

> Heartburn, a common GI symptom, generally is experienced as a painful substernal burning sensation. However, sensations can radiate into the arms or jaw and mimic pain associated with coronary artery disease. Heartburn [esophageal reflux] symptoms typically occur after eating, when lying down, or during bending or straining. The symptoms result from frequent irritation of the sensitive mucosal lining of the esophagus by the usually acidic gastric contents. (p. 8)

Although the primary physiological cause of esophageal reflux and esophagitis is a weakened lower esophageal sphincter, psychological factors are known to contribute to the reflux phenomenon (Dotevall, 1985).

In his superb review of GI physiology and stress, Dotevall (1985) listed the known effects of varied emotional reactions on GI activity. These are summarized in Table 4.1.

Cardiovascular Disorders

The cardiovascular system is thought by many researchers and clinicians to be the prime-target end organ for the stress response. The cardiovascular disorders most often associated with excessive stress are essential hypertension, migraine headache, and Raynaud's disease.

Cardiovascular Physiology

Before reviewing those specific disorders, a brief review of cardiovascular physiology is appropriate. Figure 4.2 details the cardiovascular system.

The heart is the key component in the cardiovascular system. It pumps nutrient-rich, oxygenated arterial blood to the cells of the body while at the same time pumping venous blood, which carries the various metabolic waste products.

The heart is divided into two halves: a right heart and a left heart. The circulatory cycle begins with blood entering the right heart. This blood supply is waste-filled venous blood. It has traveled throughout the venules and veins once it left the capillary beds, where the nutrient and gaseous exchanges initially took place within the body. The venous blood enters the resting heart and fills a small feeder chamber called the right atrium. Blood then passively moves through the tricuspid valve into the pumping chamber of the right heart, the right ventricle. Once the right ventricle is almost completely filled, an electrical impulse begins in the sinoatrial conducting node so as to contract the right atrium. This action forces any remaining blood into the right ventricle.

More specifically, the electrical impulse transverses the atrium until it reaches the atrioventricular node, where there is a fraction-of-a-second delay completing the filling of the right ventricle. Then the electrical impulse is sent through the ventricle, forcing it to contract and pump the venous blood through the pulmonary valve toward the lungs via the pulmonary artery. Once the blood arrives in the lungs, waste products such as carbon dioxide are exchanged for oxygen and the blood is returned to the heart.

The left heart receives the fresh, oxygenated blood from the lungs via the pulmonary vein. This blood enters the left heart at the point of the left atrium. From here the blood is moved through the mitral valve into the left heart's pumping chamber, the left ventricle. Once again, when the heart beats, it sends the electrical impulse from the sinoatrial node through the left atrium to the atrioventricular node, ultimately culminating in the contraction of the left ventricle. Blood pumped from the left ventricle passes through the aortic valve through the aorta into the arterial system, including the coronary arteries. The arteries narrow into arterioles, which feed the capillary beds where the cells exchange gases and nutrients. Then the capillaries feed the venules, which feed the veins, and the cycle is repeated.

Both the right and left hearts pump simultaneously; therefore, blood is being pumped to the lungs at the same time it is being pumped out to the body.

The cardiovascular system is a closed-loop system. As such, pressure within the system is a necessary driving force. The arterial system, including the left heart, is a high-pressure system driven by the contraction of the left ventricle. The venous system, including the right heart, is a low-pressure system, assisted in venous return by the contraction of the skeletal muscles during movement. Blood pressure, as it is typically measured and expressed, relates to the arterial system pressures. Blood pressure is measured in millimeters of mercury (mmHg) and is expressed in terms equivalent to the amount of pressure required to raise a column of mercury so many

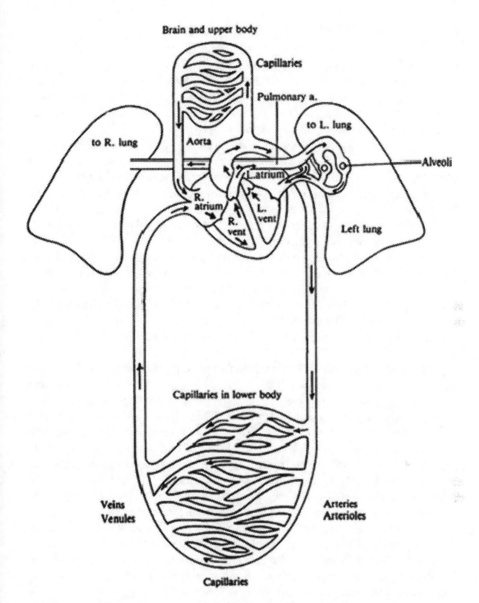

Fig. 4.2 The cardiovascular system. (*Source*: Daniel A. Girdano and George S. Everly, Jr. (1986). *Controlling Stress and Tension: A Holistic Approach*, 2nd ed., pp. 36, 39. Reprinted by permission of Prentice-Hall, Inc., Englewood Cliffs, NJ.)

millimeters. Blood pressure is expressed in terms of the systolic pressure (the pressure within the arteries during the contraction of the ventricles—called *systole*) and the diastolic pressure (the pressure within the arteries when the ventricles are filling at rest—called *diastole*).

Essential Hypertension

According to current estimates, 33% of adult Americans suffer from "the silent killer," cardiovascular hypertension. Cardiovascular hypertension is usually defined as arterial pressures over 140 mmHg systolic pressure and/or 80 mmHg diastolic pressure, although many authorities will adjust these figures upward (especially the systolic pressure) if the patient is advanced in age.

There are basically two types of cardiovascular hypertension: secondary and essential. Secondary cardiovascular hypertension represents a status of elevated blood pressure due to some organic dysfunction, for example, a pheochromocytoma (tumor of the adrenal gland). Essential hypertension has been loosely interpreted as being related to stress and such factors as diet. The term "essential" reflects the once-held notion that with advancing age one always acquired elevated blood pressure. This notion has been refuted (Henry & Stephens, 1977).

In a review of the pathophysiology of hypertension, Eliot (1979) states that in less than 10% of the cases, organic disorders explain hypertension. However, he suggests that both the SAM and the anterior pituitary–adrenocortical stress axes are capable of increasing blood pressure in response to psychosocial factors alone. This may occur through a wide range of diverse mechanisms (see also Selye, 1976). With chronic activation, he concludes, the deterioration of the cardiovascular system may be irreversible.

Henry and Stephens (1977), in a useful review of psychosocial stimulation and hypertension, present evidence similar to that of Eliot. In their review of animal and human studies, they point to the ability of the psychophysiological stress mechanisms to effect an increase in blood pressure. They point to the role of medullary norepinephrine as a vasoconstrictive force capable of increasing blood pressure. In addition, they point to the notion that increased sympathetic tonus (apparently regardless of origin) will lead to further increased sympathetic discharge. The end result may well be the tendency for the carotid sinus and aortic baroreceptors to "reset" themselves at a higher level of blood pressure. The normal effect of the baroreceptors is to act to moderate blood pressure elevations. However, if they are reset at higher levels, they will tolerate greater blood pressure before intervening. Therefore, resting blood pressure may be allowed to rise slowly over time. Finally, these authors point to the role of the adrenocortical response in the elevation of blood pressure, perhaps through some arterial narrowing or sodium-retaining mechanism. They suggest that psychosocial disturbance can play a major role in blood pressure elevations that could become chronic in nature (see Steptoe, 1981).

Weiner (1977), however, states that "psychosocial factors do not by themselves "cause" essential hypertension" (p. 183). They do, however, "interact with other predispositions" to produce high blood pressure (p. 185). He concludes that the available data point toward the conclusion that hypertension essentially can be caused by a wide variety of influences and that psychological and sociological factors "may play a different etiological, pathogenetic, and sustaining role in its different forms" (p. 185).

Vasospastic Phenomena

Stress-related vasospastic phenomena include migraine headaches and Raynaud's disease. These disorders involve vascular spasms; more specifically, their phenomenology involves spasms of the arterial vasculature induced by excessive neurological tone (usually SNS activity) (see Ganong, 1997).

Migraine headaches may affect as many as 29 million Americans. There are two basic subtypes: classical migraine and common migraine. Although both are characterized by vasomotor spasms, the classical migraine is accompanied by a prodrome. The prodrome often manifests in the form of visual disturbances, hearing dysfunction, expressive aphasia, and/or GI dysfunction. The most common form of prodrome is the visual prodrome, for example, the development of an acute visual scotoma. The prodrome is a symptom of severe arterial vasoconstriction. The pain that accompanies migraine headaches occurs on the "rebound," that is, the point at which the arterial vasculature vasodilates in response to the original vasoconstriction. It is unclear whether the pain actually results from the physical dystension of the arterial vasculature or from associated biochemical processes (see Raskin, 1985; Wolff, 1963).

Raynaud's disease is another vasospastic disorder characterized by episodic pallor and cyanosis of the fingers and/or toes. Upon rebound vasodilation, there can be extreme pain characterized by sensations of aching and throbbing. Both exposures to cold and psychosocially induced stress can induce an attack of Raynaud's (Taub & Stroebel, 1978) (see Appendices C and D).

Myocardial Ischemia and Coronary Artery Disease

Myocardial ischemia is a condition wherein the heart muscle endures a state of significantly reduced blood flow. "Myocardial ischemia occurs frequently in patients with coronary artery disease (CAD) and is a significant predictor of future cardiac events" (Gullette et al., 1997, p. 1521). Using a case-crossover design, Gullette and her colleagues demonstrated that mental stress can induce myocardial ischemia. Electrocardiogram (ECG) data were gathered with specific foci upon the emotions of negative tension, sadness, and frustration. Results of this investigation indicated that these negative emotions during daily life can more than double the risk of myocardial ischemia in the subsequent hour. Such ischemic findings were not in evidence subsequent to the states of happiness and feeling in control.

Previous studies have shown a significant correlation between myocardial episodes and the emotion of anger (Mittleman et al., 1995). Other studies have shown a significant relationship between the stress associated with mass disasters (Leor, Poole, & Kloner, 1996) and even missile attacks (Kark, Goldman, & Epstein, 1995), and subsequent cardiac death. Yet the Gullette et al. (1997) study is important in that the mechanisms of pathogenesis were observed rather than inferred.

Finally, the relationship between stress and CAD has been vigorously debated. In a review of investigations, Niaura and Goldstein (1995) conclude, "Our review of sociocultural and interpersonal factors … has identified evidence for a positive association among the following factors and CAD: occupational factors (e.g., job strain, low control, few possibilities for growth, low social support, life stress, and social isolation" (pp. 45–46). An important paper by Manuck, Marsland, Kaplan, and Williams (1995) that reviewed animal research concluded that psychosocial variables and social stress are associated with the promotion of coronary atherogenesis, impaired vasomotor responses of the coronary arteries, coronary lesions, and specific injury to arterial endothelium.

While more research is clearly needed, the argument in support of a significant role for stress in the etiology of CAD appears to be growing.

Respiratory Disorders

Allergy

An allergy is a hypersensitivity that some people develop to a particular agent. The patient's body reacts with an exaggerated immune-defensive response when it encounters the agent (antigen).

One of the most familiar forms of allergy is hay fever. In this condition, the individual is sensitive to some forms of plant pollen, and when these are inhaled from the air, mucous membranes swell, nasal secretion becomes excessive, and nasal obstruction can occur. Because other particles in the air do not seem to elicit such a response, this is clearly an overreaction to a stimulus. However, hay fever has been generally thought to be a phenomenon related only to the body, as opposed to the mind. Yet the mind–body dualism is once again questioned by the finding that some subject with hay fever may respond minimally, if at all, when challenged with the allergenic substance in an environment in which he or she feels secure and comfortable, whereas in other, more stressful situations, the same challenge is met with the usual nasal hypersecretion, congestion, and the like (Holmes, Trenting, & Wolff, 1951).

Bronchial Asthma

Although sharing some similarities with allergy, asthma is a more complex and potentially serious disorder. In asthmatic patients, bronchial secretions increase, mucosal swelling takes place and, finally, smooth muscle surrounding the bronchioles contracts, leading to a great difficulty in expiring air from the lungs. This "inability to breath" is, of course, anxiety producing, and this stress itself leads to a need for more oxygen, thus exacerbating the stress response caused by the original stimulus no matter what its nature. That bronchial asthmatic attacks can be caused by or at least exacerbated by psychosocial stimulation is no longer in question. Research reviewed by Lachman (1972) warrants such a conclusion, as does the work of Knapp (1982). Stress-related asthma appears to be related to activation of the parasympathetic nervous system (Moran, 1995).

Hyperventilation

Hyperventilation may be considered an example of an acute stress response. However, episodic hyperventilation can become a long-standing problem that goes undiagnosed for long periods of time in patients presenting vague problems that do not fit any particular pattern, such as vague aches and pains, nausea, vomiting, chest pains, and the like. The clinician must be on guard for this particular manifestation of the stress response, in order to protect the individual from unnecessary suffering and expense while searching for the cause. This, again, is a part of the fight-or-flight response in which the body is readied for action by increasing O_2 and decreasing CO_2; however, no action takes place. It has been suggested that any time a patient presents such vague problems that seem elusive, the clinician should maintain a high degree of suspicion regarding hyperventilation. Consideration may then be given to asking the patient to hyperventilate in the office. If the symptoms are reproduced, much time and effort of both physician and patient may be saved. For methods and cautions, refer to articles by Campernolle, Kees, and Leen (1979) and Lum (1975); see also Knapp (1982).

Musculoskeletal Disorders

This system comprises, as its name implies, all the body's muscles and bony support. It is thus the system that is responsible for the body's mobility and therefore plays one of the more obvious roles in a fight-or-flight type of response. At such a time, the muscles tense, blood flow is increased to them, and the very word "tension" associated with emotions such as anger or anxiety relates to this state of the musculoskeletal system (Tomita, 1975).

The stress-related disorders here are quite predictable. Low back pain may often be produced in a situation in which there is contraction of the back muscles as if to keep the body erect for fleeing a situation. If the contraction continues but there is no associated action (and therefore the stress situation remains), blood flow to the muscles decreases, metabolites increase, and pain is produced (Dorpat & Holmes, 1955; Holmes & Wolff, 1952).

Tension headache is a similar situation. The muscles of the head and neck are kept in prolonged contraction, resulting in pain by the same mechanism. This is to be differentiated from the pain of vascular headaches, which seems to begin in periods *following* tension.

There have even been some studies that indicate a possible role for stress in the development or influence of the course of the inflammatory joint disease, rheumatoid arthritis (Amkraut & Solomon, 1974; Heisel, 1972; Selye, 1956).

Skin Disorders

The skin is thought to be a common target end organ for excessive arousal (Musaph, 1977). Common stress-related disorders include eczema, acne, urticaria, psoriasis, and alopecia areata (patchy hair loss) (Engels, 1985; Lachman, 1972). According to Medansky (1971), 80% of dermatological patients have a psychological overlay. Supporting such a conclusion is empirical evidence that various neurodermatological syndromes have either been initiated or exacerbated through the controlled manipulation of psychosocial variables (Engels, Lachman). The specific mechanisms of pathogenesis have yet to be satisfactorily detailed in most instances, however. Folks and Kinney (1995) provide a useful review of the role of psychological factors and various dermatological conditions.

Immune System

Perhaps the most intriguing and complex somatic target organ in the human body is the immune system. The implications for health and disease are literally profound. Imagine if psychological process can affect the immune system then virtually every cell in the human body can be a target of excessive stress and both noncommunicable and even communicable diseases then have the potential to be "stress-related" diseases. Let us explore the fascinating target organ in greater depth.

The immune system basically serves to protect the body from invading toxins and microorganisms that may damage organs and tissues. Some of the protective functions of the immune system are to eliminate bacteria and to reject foreign substances, known as antigens, that have entered the body. In addition, the immune system possesses a "memory" for encounters with foreign substances, such that a subsequent encounter induces a more rapid and potent response (Borysenko, 1987; Guyton & Hall, 2006). The immune system is often conceptually divided into innate or nonspecific immunity, which provides a general defense, and specific or acquired immunity, which acts against particular threatening antigens.

Innate Immunity

As the term implies, *innate immunity* refers to processes that are apparent from birth and provide a general or nonspecific defense by acting against anything identified as foreign or *not self* (Thibodeau & Patton, 1993). There are many variations of innate immunity. For example, species-resistant, innate immunity makes the human body unsuitable to some potentially lethal animal diseases such as distemper. Conversely, dogs and cats are resistant to human diseases such as mumps or measles. Other nonspecific types of immunity include physical barriers, such as the skin's outer keratin layer, which limits entry into the body, and biochemical substances, such as tears, saliva, and perspiration, which contain enzymes that digest or weaken the walls surrounding bacterial cells (Parslow, 1994). These anatomical and chemical barriers serve as the body's *first line of defense* against invading toxins (Abbas & Lichtman, 2011; Guyton & Hall, 2006; Thibodeau & Patton, 1993).

If bacteria or other microorganisms penetrate this first line of defense, the body has a second, nonspecific or general line of innate protection that incorporates phagocytosis, natural killer (NK) cells, interferon, and inflammation. Phagocytosis, which involves the destruction and absorption of microorganisms, utilizes cells known as phagocytes to eliminate pathogens (any organism causing disease). Nearly all tissues and organs possess inhabitant phagocytes. There are a variety of phagocytic cells, including (1) neutrophils, the most numerous type, accounting for one-half to two-thirds of circulating white blood cells (which are primarily involved in destroying pathogens); (2) monocytes, which are relatively large cells produced in the bone marrow and released into the blood for about 1 day before settling in a selective tissue; and (3) macrophages, the settled or mature monocytic cells, which are large, avid eliminators of foreign particles and debris (Abbas & Lichtman, 2011; Guyton & Hall, 2006).

In addition to phagocytes, the body possesses natural killer (NK) cells, which are lymphocytes (one type of white blood cell) that kill various tumor cells and cells infected by viruses. One of the common ways NK cells function is by breaking down or lysing cells by damaging their plasma membrane. NK cells are currently considered to be an initial or frontline protective response that is utilized before a more specific response can be exhibited (Imboden, 1994). Therefore, although probably related to cytotoxic T lymphocytes (see acquired immunity below), NK cells serve a broad surveillance-like function that, unlike T cells, do not require prior antigen interaction (McDaniel, 1992). Therefore, NK cells are often included as part of the nonspecific immune functions.

About 40 years ago, it was discovered that some cells exposed to viruses produce a secretory protein known as interferon, which, as the name implies, "interferes" with the ability of viruses to produce diseases. Basically, interferon works by producing an antiviral state within the host that prevents viruses from replicating in cells. Interferon has also been associated with the modulation of immune responses.

Inflammation, or the inflammatory response, is also considered part of the body's second line of defense and characterizes the complex manner in which tissues and cells react to an insult or microbial invasion. Immediately after an injury, there is a brief constriction, followed by dilation, of blood vessels. Injured tissues then release a number of chemical mediators, such as histamine, kinins, and prostaglandins (Abbas & Lichtman, 2011; Thibodeau & Patton, 1993). The factors involved in the inflammatory response characteristically results in redness, warmth, swelling, and pain. Although the inflammatory response is considered beneficial, it can be detrimental if it permanently injures the host tissues and/or impedes normal functioning.

Acquired Immunity

Contrary to nonspecific immunity described earlier, acquired or specific immune mechanisms attack certain agents that the body recognizes as *not self*. Therefore, specific immunity may be considered the body's *third line of defense* (Thibodeau & Patton, 1993). Acquired immunity develops in late fetal and neonatal life and is part of the body's lymphatic system. The lymphatic system, a part of the circulatory system, consists of a vast network of vessels and organs that drains excess fluid and provides a defense for the body (Moore, 1992). Lymphocytes, which circulate in the body's fluids, are the major cells controlling the immune response. They are found most extensively in the lymph nodes, which are glands composed of composites of lymphoid tissues, but are also located in special lymphoid tissues such as the spleen, bone marrow, and gastrointestinal tract (Moore). Lymphoid tissue is strategically disseminated throughout the body and allows for rapid interception and filtering of invading organisms and toxins. Two major types of lymphocytes involved in acquired immunity are T (thymus-derived) cells that form activated lymphocytes and are primarily involved in the slower acting cell-mediated immunity, and B (bone-marrow derived) cells that form circulating antibodies and are primarily involved in the more rapidly responding humoral immunity. Although these two types of lymphocytes are structurally similar, T and B cells are functionally distinct in their reaction to antigens (Abbas & Lichtman, 2011).

Cell-Mediated Processes

In cell-mediated immunity, each T lymphocyte, or T cell, operates by having a precisely distinctive surface receptor that allows it to recognize and bind to only one invading antigen. Thus, a T cell may have numerous receptor sites; however, all of them will be specific for only a certain antigen. T cells, which account for 70–80% of disseminated lymphocytes, circulate in the blood in an inactive form and are incapable of recognizing antigens without assistance. Therefore, when an antigen invades the body, it is typically first identified and then ingested by macrophages, which initiate the process of digestion. The T cells, whose surface receptors match the antigens, then travel to the now inflamed tissues and bind to the antigen.

Once in contact with the antigen, the sensitized T cell begins to divide repeatedly to form a clone of identical, activated T cells (Abbas & Lichtman, 2011; Guyton & Hall, 2006; Thibodeau & Patton, 1993). The antigen-bound, sensitized T cells then release lymphocyte-derived chemical messengers, commonly called cytokines, into the inflamed tissue to facilitate the immune response (Dunn, 1989). Several variations of T lymphocytes, or T cells, include, for example, helper cells (T-4). The T-helper cell, once activated by the cytokine interleukin-1 (IL-1), releases interleukin-2 (IL-2), which fosters the maturation and marshals the subsequent immune response, including the promotion and multiplication of cytotoxic cells used to combat the invading antigen. There are also suppressor cells (T-8), which inhibit the immune response in order to regulate it, memory T cells, which initiate a rapid response if the antigen is encountered again, and cytotoxic or killer cells, which release a powerfully destructive cytokine called lymphotoxin (Borysenko, 1987).

A distinguishing characteristic of cell-mediated immunity is that specifically sensitized or activated lymphocytes are employed to pursue and contact the invading antigen. Typically, these antigen cells are foreign to the body, malignant, or have been transplanted into the tissue. Therefore, cell-mediated immunity, which requires a localized response that may require several days to detect the invader and to employ the necessary cells to battle it, not only defends us from viruses and cancer but also is directly involved in the rejection of organ and tissue transplants.

Humoral Responses

Comparable to T lymphocytes, B lymphocytes, or B cells, are also initiated by macrophage stimulation. In humoral immunity, an encounter with an antigen activates the B lymphocytes, which, after being released from the bone marrow, circulate to the lymph nodes, spleen, and other lymphoid tissues. Whereas cytotoxic T cells, as described earlier, exit lymphoid tissue to encounter an antigen directly, B cells produce their effects indirectly (McDaniel, 1992). When an antigen binds to antigen receptors on the B cell, the activated B cell divides to form a clone or group of identical B cells. Some of the offspring of these B cells become differentiated to form plasma cells known as antibodies that circulate in the lymph and the blood, and combine selectively with the triggering antigen (Abbas & Lichtman, 2011; Guyton & Hall, 2006). Thus, antibodies are produced within a species to fit part of the antigen (Abbas & Lichtman; Guyton & Hall; Kendall, 1998). The binding of the antigen to the antibodies forms a complex that may (1) render the toxic antigens innocuous, (2) facilitate a bundling of antigens that allows phagocytes and macrophages to dispose of them rapidly, or (3) slightly alter the contour of the antibody, allowing the destruction of the foreign cells.

Antibodies belong to a group of proteins called globulins and are, therefore, referred to as immunoglobulins. The five different classes of antibodies or immunoglobulins known to exist in humans are designated as IgG, IgA, IgM, IgD, and IgE. Each immunoglobulin has a unique structure and function, and as mentioned earlier, generally defends the host by neutralizing toxins, blocking attachment of viruses to cells, or inducing phagocytosis of bacteria or other microorganisms. IgG is the most common immunoglobulin, accounting for around 70% of the circulating antibodies (Goldsby, Kindt, & Osborne, 2000). Therefore, immunoglobulins "not only serve as surface receptors for foreign substances but also can be released to search out and bind their targets at a considerable distance from the cell" (Parslow, 1994, p. 26).

Activated B cells that do not differentiate into plasma cells are known as memory B cells. Memory B cells do not produce or secrete antibodies. However, if they are exposed at some later time to the antigen responsible for their initial formation, then memory B cells convert into plasma cells that secrete antibodies (Guyton & Hall, 2006). Because there are many more memory cells than the initial B lymphocyte that was cloned, subsequent exposure to the same antigen will produce a more rapid and formidable antibody response (Abbas & Lichtman, 2011; Guyton & Hall).

Different antigens stimulate distinct B cells to develop into plasma cells and memory B cells. Most antigens activate both T and B lymphocytes concurrently, and there is in fact a cooperative relationship between the two (Guyton & Hall, 2006). The primary difference between the T and B cells is that B cells release antibodies, whereas whole T cells are activated and released into the lymph. Therefore, these latter cells may last for months to years in the body fluid (Abbas & Lichtman, 2011; Guyton & Hall).

Also of note, the effects of circulating antibodies and cellular immunity are influenced by a component of blood plasma enzymes known as the complement system, which entails different protein compounds. This system can be initiated by specific or nonspecific immune mechanisms and is closely involved in destroying various foreign tissues in a process known as cytolysis.

Because there is no easy access to the organs containing immune cells, and given that components of the immune system circulate in blood, it is not surprising that psychoneuroimmunological research often involves assessing the immune processes occurring in circulating peripheral blood. However, although peripheral blood is a key factor in immune responses and relatively easy to access (Herbert & Cohen, 1993), some researchers have questioned whether quantifying the typically variable and minute changes in the number or percentages of various white blood cells (neutrophils, monocytes, and lymphocytes) allows for a consistently reliable and completely valid detection of altered immune functioning (Cohen & Herbert, 1996).

Immune functioning has also been assessed by stimulating lymphocytes through incubation with mitogens, which produce nonspecific divergence of T or B cells. In this type of research, greater propagation of cells is usually equated with more effectiveness. Phytohemagglutinin (PHA), pokeweed mitogen (PWM), and concanavalin A (ConA) are the most commonly investigated mitogens. The procedures just described utilize what are known as in vitro tests, in which cells are removed from an organism and their function is then studied in a lab. There are also in vivo tests that study cellular function in living organisms. The quantification of antibodies to herpes viruses is an in vivo test frequently used in psychoneuroimmunology research. Basically, herpes viruses are common viruses that we have all been exposed to at some time in our lives. What makes them unique, however, is that after exposure, they usually remain present yet inactive in the body. When the immune system is threatened or challenged, this inactive virus may begin to replicate. Therefore, assessing and quantifying the level of antibodies to the herpes viruses provides evidence of immune function. More specifically, greater levels of herpes virus antibodies indicate suppressed cellular immune function (Herbert & Cohen, 1993).

Stress and Immune Functioning: Animal Studies

There has been an evolution from animal and human research investigating the link between biogenic and psychosocial stressors, immune functioning, and disease processes. The effects of humoral and cell-mediated immunity, as well as tumor growth and survival, have been used as outcome variables (Bohus & Koolhaas, 1991). In the animal literature, myriad stressors have been used to investigate the impact on immunological functioning. For example, Hans Selye's original description of the GAS was in response to exposing laboratory rats to diverse, nocuous agents, such as cold temperatures, severed spinal cords, excessive exercise, or drug injections. Following exposure to these stimuli, Selye (1936) documented decreased circulating lymphocytes; rapid decreased size of the thymus, spleen, lymph glands, and liver; formation of erosions in the stomach; and loss of muscle tone. He further noted that the animals often developed "resistance" with continued exposure to the stressors that mimicked normal functioning; however, with additional exposure of 1–3 months, the animals became "exhausted" and developed the symptoms described earlier.

The impact of environmental stressors on infectious disease processes has been reviewed extensively in the literature (Glaser & Kiecolt-Glaser, 2005; Segerstrom & Miller, 2004). Laboratory animals have been exposed to electric foot shocks, cold temperatures, loud noises, restraints, crowding, handling, and isolation. For example, restraint models that place rats or mice in narrow tubes or use adhesive substances placed on boards to maintain immobilization often prohibit their movement. These types of studies have often resulted in cellular and humoral suppression, as well as impaired NK-cell activity (Koolhaas & Bohus, 1995; Steplewski & Vogel, 1986). Studies examining the effects of handling, picking up, and holding laboratory animals for various lengths of time have shown a decrease in IgG antibody production and decreased T-cell function (Moynihan et al., 1994). However, additional data have shown that adding another stressor, such as an intraperitoneal injection, resulted in attenuated corticosterone and catecholamine responses in previously handled mice compared to unhandled mice. Thus, Moynihan and colleagues suggested that the psychosocial stressor of handling may result in habituation to the effects of the stress response.

The general immune responses of decreased IgG-antibody production, NK-cell activity, and lymphocyte generation have been fairly well established in response to electric shocks (Cunnick, Lysle, Armfield, & Rabin, 1988; Laudenslager et al., 1988). Other researchers have expanded these findings to include an investigation of psychosocial stressors such as decreased predictability and control. Despite equivocal data, evidence suggests that laboratory rats provided an opportunity to perform a response to avoid or eliminate electric shock developed less severe gastric ulceration and less rapid tumor growth formation than those exposed to the same amount of electric shocks without controllability (Sklar & Anisman, 1979; Weiss, 1968). Foot shock as a physical stressor causes release of pheromones that are an important aspect of rodent communication. Moynihan and colleagues (1994) reported on the results of an investigation in which pheromones produced by foot-shocked mice changed immune functioning in those mice receiving the odor.

Interestingly, they reported suppression in cell-mediated responses and enhanced humoral responses in the odor-exposed mice. Other data have suggested that learning and memory circuits may be conditioned at the CNS level following acute exposure to electric shock, and that these conditioned responses may have both immunosuppressive and immunoenhancement effects (Koolhaas & Bohus, 1995).

Psychosocial stressors induced by crowding and isolation have also been widely studied for their modulating effects on immunity. The results of numerous studies of high-density crowding have generally demonstrated increased disease susceptibility and decreased survival. In one of the original studies of this phenomenon, Vessey (1964) reported that placing typically isolated male mice in a group setting for 4 h a day resulted in lower antibody responses to a mitogen. Of particular interest, the dominant male mouse in the group had the highest antibody production. Other studies have shown that physically dominant or aggressive male rats in a social colony have higher antibody generation, whereas submissive or defeated rats and mice have demonstrated increased immunosuppression (Bohus & Koolhaas, 1991; Koolhaas & Bohus, 1989). Fleshner, Laudenslager, Simons, and Maier (1989) have also shown that engaging in submissive behaviors, as compared to continuing to react aggressively and receiving multiple bites, correlated with reduced antibody formation to an injected antigen. These data suggest that animals may evidence individual differences in coping styles to given stressors. The active coping style has been associated with high SNS reactivity, whereas passive coping has been considered to be affiliated with increased reactivity of the pituitary–adrenocortical axis. As noted by Koolhaas and Bohus (1995), "This interaction between environment and individual is… crucial to understanding the relationship between stress and immunity" (p. 78).

Stress and Immune Function: Human Studies

While the bulk of early empirical data on the effects of "psychological factors" on the immune system was derived from animal studies, in the past 35 years there has been a proliferation of studies conducted with human participants. Since human research is more focused on whether psychological factors or mood states alter immunity and health outcomes, we will briefly review some of the more salient findings that have recently occurred. This in no way is meant to minimize the relevance or impact of animal research, but for sake of space, and consistent with the purpose of this text, we will focus briefly on human studies.

In preface, we should note that investigators need to consider the subtle, selective, multifaceted nature of the precipitants (e.g., age, gender, emotional status, and genetic factors) and physical consequences of stress, in addition to the complex and often lengthy duration of immune responses before generating broadly conclusive causal statements about how stress directly alters immune function (Zeller, McCain, McCann, Swanson, & Colletti, 1996; see Maier et al., 1994, for a detailed discussion on this topic). As the eminent Paul Rosch (1995) noted, "These and other caveats must be considered when evaluating sweeping statements and conclusions about the effect of "stress" on "immune function" or therapeutic triumphs based on psychoneuroimmunological approaches" (p. 214).

These precautionary notes are not intended to diminish the outstanding advancements and notable influence of stress-induced immunomodulation research or the unequivocal impact that emotions such as stress have on immunity. Instead, they are intended to inform the reader that exploring, uncovering, and externally validating generally accepted tenets between psychological variables such as stress and immunity involve a complex process that continues to evolve. For example, it is worth considering that many of the proposed relations between psychosocial stressors (e.g., loss of a spouse) and disease (e.g., depression) that are often credited to immune changes may be strongly affected by behavioral health changes such as alcohol or drug consumption, noncompliance with medications, decreased sleep, and poorer diets that occur following the stressor (Cohen & Herbert, 1996). That having been said, let us briefly review the putative impact of selected "psychological factors" upon the immune system.

Bereavement

The preponderance of early evidence relating psychological components of human health and disease has been anecdotal, and, of course, ethical considerations have usually precluded the type of controlled experimental research conducted on animals. Correlational designs have primarily been used to examine the impact of stressors such as negative life events on illness and immune function. For example, bereavement studies have consistently demonstrated differences between unmarried and married individuals in terms of physical health. Immune functioning in the form of lymphocyte production was shown to be decreased in several prospective studies of bereaved and nonbereaved men and women who had lost a spouse due to illnesses such as breast and lung cancer (Bartrop, Luckhurst, Lazarus, Kiloh, & Penny, 1977; Irwin, Daniels, Smith, Bloom, & Weiner, 1987; Schleifer, Keller, Camerino, Thornton, & Stein, 1983). In a separate but related study, Linn, Linn, and Jensen, (1984) suggested that reduction in lymphocytes was more influenced by level of depression than by bereavement. A meta-analysis demonstrated that clinically depressed individuals have a poorer response to mitogens PHA, ConA, and PWM, and lowered NK- and helper T-cell activity (Herbert & Cohen, 1993). Irwin, Lacher, and Caldwell (1992) have provided longitudinal data suggesting that with successful treatment of depression, decreased NK activity is abrogated. However, the data on immune correlates of depression are not universally supportive (Ravindran, Griffiths, Merali, & Anisman, 1995), and discrepant findings have led researchers to suggest that compromised immune functioning may be more evident in elderly, severely depressed, and hospitalized patients (Houldin, Lev, Prystowsky, Redei, & Lowery, 1991). In a 10-year follow-up of the long-term impact of bereavement on spousal health in a sample of 152 participants, Jones, Bartrop, Forcier, and Penny (2010) reported an overall increase in morbidity of 10–20% compared with a control sample. The information in this chapter is limited to bereavement and immune function. For a comprehensive overview of grief, loss, and stress, see Chap. 20.

Depression

Major depressive disorder (MDD) has been associated with various changes in levels of the neurotransmitters serotonin, norepinephrine, and dopamine, There has been growing theoretical and empirical evidence to suggest, however, that the inflammatory response of the immune system (which is thought to affect neuroendocrine and central nervous system neurotransmitter processes synergistically), more specifically the release of cytokines (substances secreted by specific cells of the immune system that serve to foster communication or cross-talk between the CNS and immune system) might be associated with how neurochemical changes induced by stressors may contribute to MDD (Anisman, 2009). It is thought that the current or past stressful experiences may impact the neurochemical actions of the inflammatory immune system and lead to a MDD diathesis. Human studies, both correlational and case control, have shown an association between elevated levels of circulating proinflammatory cytokines (which indicate a disruption of cell replication and function and are associated with earlier onset and faster progression of disease) and MDD. In addition, several studies have demonstrated how the use of immunotherapy, such as interferon-α to treat certain types of cancer and hepatitis C may result in depressive symptoms (Bonaccorso et al., 2002; Capuron, Ravaud, & Dantzer, 2000; Capuron et al., 2002; Maes & Bonaccorso, 2004; Scalori et al., 2005). Interferon-α also alters levels of serotonin (5-HT), which is involved in depression, but as Anisman (2009) notes, interferon-α is also associated with other nonspecific symptoms not related to depression.

Schizophrenia

With regard to another major psychiatric disorder, researchers have also long noted the heterogenous pathophysiology of schizophrenia. Although not conclusive, studies examining immunoglobulin (IgG) (the most common of the antibodies produced by the body to fight bacterial and viral infections) in cerebrospinal fluid (CSF) in some patients have shown raised levels that may be due to impaired permeability of the blood–brain barrier (Muller & Ackenheil, 1995). Other studies in a subgroup of schizophrenic patients have revealed additional immunological abnormalities such as increased occurrence of autoimmune diseases and decreased lymphocyte (IL-2) production, a cytokine released by T-helper cells to combat an invading antigen, among other immune changes. Muller and Ackenheil have proposed that schizophrenic patients should be classified as those with and without immune alterations. Moreover, preliminary epidemiological evidence utilizing maternal recall has demonstrated an association between second-trimester gestational influenza infections, obstetrical complications (e.g., anemia, emergency cesarean section, breech presentation), and low birth weights in newborns who later developed schizophrenia (Wright, Takei, Rifkin, & Murray, 1995). A meta-analysis of 62 in vivo and in vitro studies with a total sample size of 2,298 schizophrenic and 1,858 healthy participants showed significant increases in certain cytokines in vivo (circulating cytokine levels with plasma samples) (IL-1RA, sIL-2R, and IL-6), and a decrease in vitro (secretion by peripheral white blood cells (leukocytes) stimulated or not by mitogens (potent stimulators of T cell activation), which collectively provides evidence of an ongoing inflammatory process (Potvin et al., 2008).

Personal Relationships

Studies examining the link between personal relationships (e.g., marital conflict, divorce, and separation) and immune function have provided some notable findings. In a study of 32 women, the 16 women who had been separated 1 year or less showed poorer immune function on immunological blood assays compared to matched controls (Kiecolt-Glaser et al., 1987). In a recent study of 1,211 sexual minority male patients in a community-based health center in Massachusetts 12 months after the legalization of same-sex marriage, participants had decreased medical and mental health care visits and mental health care costs compared to the 12 months before the law change (Hatzenbuehler et al., 2011). Of note, these results were similar for partnered as well as nonpartnered men.

In a study of 64 men, Kiecolt-Glaser and associates (1988) found that the 32 men who had been separated or divorced reported feeling more lonely and described more recent illnesses. Evidence suggests, however, that participants who initiate the separation and those who have less preoccupation with their ex-spouse may experience less distress and have better immune functioning (Keicolt-Glaser et al; Weiss, 1975). In a study of 42 married couples, Kiecolt-Glaser and colleagues (2005) found that those who evinced hostile behavioral exchanges or interactions during a monitored conflict resolution task in a laboratory setting showed poorer wound healing and higher levels of circulating proinflammatory cytokines levels (including interleukin-6 (IL-6) 24 h after a baseline observation, when compared to low-hostile couples.

In general, however, there has been data to suggest that there may be some benefits of emotional disclosure, particularly if expressing negative emotions about stressful experiences occurs in writing (Pennebaker & Beall, 1986; Pennebaker, Kiecolt-Glaser, & Glaser, 1988; Petrie, Fontanilla, Thomas, Booth, & Pennebaker, 2004). There is some suggestion that the benefits may be induced by alterations in cognitive processing, or how participants think about and then express their negative emotions. A method used to assess cognitive processing is the amount of words used related to expressions of insight (e.g., realize, see, understand) and causation (e.g., because, infer, thus), and the use of these words has been shown to predict greater total circulating lymphocyte counts over 3 days of writing in a sample of 65 first-year medical students (Pennebaker, Mayne, & Francis, 1997; Pennebaker, Mehl, & Niederhoffer, 2003; Petrie, Booth, & Pennebaker, 1998)

Graham and colleagues (2009) in a study of 42 married couples involved first in a "nonconflictive" and then in a "conflictive" discussion task, showed that individuals who engaged in the greater use of cognitive processing [words indicative of causal reasoning (e.g., because), insight (e.g., understand), and thinking (e.g., ought)], showed less increases in cytokine production over 24 h when in the conflictive task. This attenuation, even when cognitive processing words were used, did not occur in the nonconflicted discussion task.

Academic Stress

Keicolt-Glaser and her colleagues have also been responsible for some of the most methodologically sound, large-scale human stress studies investigating the immunological effects of the predictable acute stressor of academic examinations on medical students (Kiecolt-Glaser et al., 1984). These data have shown a decay in NK-cell activity when compared to baseline blood samples obtained 1 month prior to the exams. Additionally, in main effects noted for stressful life events in self-report inventories of the Holmes–Rahe Social Readjustment Scale and the UCLA Loneliness Scale, high scorers had lower NK activity than low scorers. The use of protein markers ruled out the possibility that the differences in NK-cell response were due to nutritional deficiencies. Also of note, there was no difference in received grades between students who did and did not participate. Other data (Glaser et al., 1992) have suggested that academic stress could negatively impact the ability of hepatitis vaccines to evoke antibody responses in a sample of medical students. Kang, Coe, and McCarthy (1996) recently expanded this line of research when they investigated whether differences in immune responses between healthy and asthmatic adolescents in response to academic examinations. Results revealed alterations in immune functioning, for example, decreased NK-cytolytic activity in both groups, without concurrent changes in lung function for the well-managing asthmatics.

Chronic Stress

Researchers have also investigated the effects of chronic stressors on immune functioning, and Glaser and Kiecolt-Glaser (2005) note, "chronic stressors might accelerate the risk of developing many age-related diseases by "premature ageing" of the immune response" (p. 249). Specifically, the health of family members who provide long-term care of loved ones with Alzheimer's disease, often considered a form of living bereavement, has been examined over time. Results suggest that caregiving may produce more depression in family members (Crook & Miller, 1985; Kiecolt-Glaser et al., 2003), in addition to impaired immune responses compared to a matched-control sample when exposed to ConA, PHA, and latent Epstein–Barr virus (Kiecolt-Glaser, Dura, Speicher, Trask, & Glaser, 1991). Moreover, caregivers experienced significantly more days ill from upper respiratory tract infections, and the poorest immune functioning was observed in caregivers who had institutionalized their spouse within the previous year after caring for them for an average of 5 years. Esterling, Kiecolt-Glaser, Bodnar, and Glaser (1994) expanded these findings by including a group of former Alzheimer's disease caregivers (those whose spouse had died at least 2 years earlier) along with current caregivers and a control group. Results revealed no difference in symptoms of depression or perceived distress between the continuing and former caregivers, and both groups were significantly more depressed than the control group. Similarly, the continuing and former caregivers did not differ in the functional responsiveness of NK-cell cytotoxicity to cytokine incubation, and both groups had a significantly poorer immune response than controls. A study has manipulated NK-cell composition at a cellular level to investigate the mechanisms of immune effects on caregivers (Esterling, Kiecolt-Glaser, & Glaser, 1996). Considering how the population is aging, this area of research will be increasingly valuable in the future.

Psychological Factors and HIV/AIDS

First recognized in the early 1980s, human immunodeficiency virus (HIV) is the virus that causes acquired immune deficiency syndrome (AIDS). The virus weakens an infected person's ability to fight infections and cancer, and AIDS is the final stage of HIV infection. The myriad implications associated with the course of HIV and AIDS) have provided a prototypical illness to study from a psychoneuroimmuno-logical perspective (McCain & Zeller, 1996). For example, Kemeny and her colleagues (1995), who reported that HIV-positive men who recently lost an intimate partner to AIDS evidence decreased immune functioning, have also suggested that grief and depression may have different immunological correlates in HIV.

The hallmark of AIDS is a quantitative pattern of depletion of a subset of T-lymphocyte cells, the T-helper or CD4 cells (CD=cluster designation) to a level below 200 (a healthy person's CD4 count can vary from 500 to more than 100) (McCain & Zeller, 1996; US Department of Health and Human Services, 2009). This is the result of HIV disease leading to CD4 cells becoming continually infected, destroyed, and regenerated, and the decline in CD4 cell number is the result of the proportional rate of cell destruction exceeding cell regeneration (Ho et al., 1995; Wei et al., 1995). As the aggregate of CD4 cells continues to decline, the signaling required for normal cellular and humoral responsivity is negatively impacted, leading to the development of opportunistic infections and various diseases that are pathognomonic of AIDS (Kemeny, 1994). The steady immunological decline noted in the beginning stages of HIV-seropositive individuals suggests that early psycho-social interventions may be particularly beneficial in helping patients to enhance their functioning (Antoni et al., 1990).

Estimates are that rates of depression may range from 21% to as high as 42% in HIV+ patients (Gaynes, Pence, Eron, & Miller, 2008; Horberg et al., 2008). Intervention studies of individuals with HIV have often involved exercise training and cognitive-behavioral approaches such as guided imagery and active neuromus-cular relaxation (see Chaps. 10, 12, 15, and Appendix B for detailed discussions of these topics). Compared to a group of HIV-seropositive men who improved their aerobic capacity by riding a stationary bicycle for 45 min, three times per week, HIV-seropositive men who did not exercise demonstrated significant increases in anxiety and depression, and decreases in immune functioning (LaPerriere et al., 1990, 1991). In a randomized control study of 60 HIV-infected adults, those who participated in a 12-week supervised aerobic exercise training program for 3 h per week, consisting of treadmill use, stationary biking, and walking, showed improvements in depressive mood and depressive symptoms compared to the control group (Neidig, Smith, & Brashers, 2003). In a randomized control trial testing whether the effectiveness of three different 10-week stress management approaches (i.e., cognitive-behavioral relaxation training, focused tai chi training, and spiritual growth groups) would improve and then sustain improvements 6 months later in areas of psychosocial functioning, quality of life, and physical health in a sample of 252 individuals with HIV infection, McCain and her colleagues (2008) reported that, in comparison to the control group, both the cognitive-behavioral relaxation training and tai chi training groups showed an enhancement in coping strategies (less emotion focused) and all three intervention groups had higher lymphocyte proliferation function. Guided imagery as a therapeutic intervention gained notoriety in the area of psychoneuroimmunology when researchers claimed that cancer patients who used the technique to most likely envision their body attacking and destroying invading infections were able almost to double their mean survival time (Hall & O'Grady, 1991; Hall, Anderson, & O'Grady, 1994; Holland & Tross, 1987; Simonton, Matthews-Simonton, & Sparks, 1980). Eller (1996) reported that 6 weeks of training in guided imagery and progressive relaxation training (PRT) were associated with less depression and fatigue and increased CD4 cells in a group of individuals with HIV.

Humor

Norman Cousins, the noted essayist and editor of the *Saturday Review*, addressed the potential therapeutic impact of humor on the immune system when he described in detail his use of laughter during his treatment for ankylosing spondylitis, a very uncomfortable inflammation of the vertebrae. Cousins dedicated more than a decade to amassing empirical evidence for his postulate that "laughter is the best medicine," and established the Humor Research Task Force (Wooten, 1996). Controlled studies have shown that laughter lowers cortisol levels and increases lymphocytes, NK cells, and concentration of salivary IgA (Berk, 1989a, b; Dillon & Baker, 1985; McClelland & Cheriff, 1997). Therefore, through the use of what may be considered cathartic liberation, humor and laughter seem to serve a protective immune function. Some hospitals have recognized the positive emotions engendered by humor and have introduced "Laugh Mobiles" that sell humorous novelties (Erdman, 1993).

Traumas

Investigators have also focused on acute and chronic immune system alterations following natural and man-made traumas, as well as technological disasters. One of the first instances of this type of exploration occurred following the nuclear accident at Three Mile Island (Hatch, Wallenstein, Beyea, Nieves, & Susser, 1991). Compared to control participants, residents near the event had greater numbers of neutrophils (a type of white blood cell that is the first to arrive at an infection site), and fewer B, T, and NK cells (types of lymphocytes or small white blood cells that realize antibodies as part of the immune response) 6 years later, suggesting chronic immune changes. In the Canadian Community Health Survey Cycle ($n = 36,984$), participants with a diagnosis of PTSD had significantly higher rates of cancer, chronic pain, cardiovascular diseases, gastrointestinal illnesses, and respiratory diseases, and after adjusting for the effects of other mental disorders and medical morbidity, PTSD was also associated with suicide attempts, poor quality of life, and disability (Sareen et al., 2007). In a longitudinal study of 896 participants following a fireworks depot explosion in a residential area in the Netherlands that killed 23 people and injured about 1,000 others, Dirkzwager, van der Velden, Grievink, and Yzermans (2007) reported that after adjusting for smoking, demographics, and previous health problems, a diagnosis of PTSD was associated with increased vascular (e.g., peripheral vascular disease, artherosclerosis, varicose veins, and edema), musculoskeletal, and dermatological difficulties. In comparison of 14 patients with PTSD, who were otherwise healthy, and 14 matched controls (age and gender) without PTSD, von Kanel and colleagues (2006) reported that more severe PTSD, as assessed by the German version of the Clinician-Administered PTSD Scale (CAPS) was associated with higher levels of plasma clotting factors (e.g., fibrinogen, which is a soluble protein that aids in clotting and high levels are associated with CVD and FVIII:C, a coagulant that is deficient in hemophilia). The authors concluded that even at subthreshold levels PTSD might produce hypercoagulability that may increase the risk of cardiovascular disease by speeding up platelet aggregation and thrombus formation.

Studies have also examined immune effects following the North Ridge earthquake in Southern California and Hurricane Andrew in South Florida (Ironson et al., 1997; Solomon, Segerstrom, Grohr, Kemeny, & Fahey, 1997). In both studies, NK cell cytotoxicity (NKCC) was lower over time. In the latter study, severity of symptoms (particularly perceived loss and intrusive thoughts) was negatively related to NKCC and positively related to white blood cell counts. Of special interest for therapeutic interventions was the evidence of new-onset sleep difficulties as possibly mediating the PTSD symptom–NKCC relationship.

Psychological Manifestations of the Stress Response

The final category of disease to be discussed in this chapter is the diverse psychological manifestations of the stress response. Although we have noted implications for depression, bereavement, trauma, and schizophrenia above; and we shall be examining trauma in far greater detail later in the text, here we shall briefly review the "psyche" as a target organ.

Acute and chronic stress episodes are implicated in the development of both diffuse anxiety and manic behavior patterns that are without defined direction or purpose.

Gellhorn (1969) argues that high levels of sympathetic activity can result in anxiety reactions. This anxiety may occur as a result of SNS and proprioceptive discharges at the cerebral cortical level. Thus, generalized ergotropic tone may then lead to conditions of chronic and diffuse anxiety. Guyton (1982), in apparent agreement with Gellhorn, notes that general sympathetic discharge and proprioceptive feedback may contribute to arousal states such as mania, anxiety, and insomnia. Greden (1974) and Stephenson (1977) have both found that the consumption of methylated xanthines (primarily caffeine) can create signs of diffuse anxiety as well as insomnia and may lead to a diagnosis of anxiety neurosis. The action of the methylated xanthines rests on their ability to stimulate a psychophysiological stress response primarily through sympathetic activation. Finally, Jacobson (1938, 1978) has argued that proprioceptive impulses as such would be found in conditions of high musculoskeletal tension and can contribute to anxiety reactions (see also Everly, 1985b).

Physiologically, in each of the cases just cited, it may be suggested that an ascending neural overload via the reticular activating system to the limbic and neocortical areas may be responsible for creating unorganized and dysfunctional discharges of neural activity that are manifested in clients' presenting symptoms of insomnia, undefined anxiety, and in some cases manic behavior patterns lacking direction or apparent purpose (see Everly, 1985b; Guyton & Hall, 2006).

In each of the three examples, activation of the psychophysiological stress response preceded the manifestation of diffuse, undefined anxiety, often diagnosed as generalized anxiety disorder or atypical anxiety disorder.

It is interesting to note that one link between anxiety and sympathetic stress arousal, specifically, striate muscle tension (Gellhorn, 1969; Jacobson, 1938, 1978), has prompted the development of techniques designed to reduce anxiety through the reduction of muscle tension. We review such techniques later in this text.

Another psychological manifestation of excessive stress is thought to be depressive reactions. Stressor events that lead the patient to the interpretation that his or her efforts are useless, that is, that he or she is in a helpless situation, are clearly associated with arousal of the psychophysiological stress response (Henry & Stephens, 1977). The affective manifestation that typically follows is depression. Henry and Stephens have compiled an impressive review that points to the reactivity of the anterior pituitary–adrenocortical axes during depressive episodes.

In addition to physiological evidence, there is psychological evidence to support the notion that excessive stress can precipitate a depressive reaction. Sociobehavioral research with depressed patients (see Brown, 1972; Paykel et al., 1969) produced somewhat similar evidence that social stressors can lead to major affective syndromes. Rabkin (1982), in her review of stress and affective disorders, states, "Overall, it seems justifiable to conclude that life events do play a role in the genesis of depressive disorders" (p. 578). Indeed, depressed patients report more stressful life events than do normal controls. This was especially true for a 3-week period immediately preceding the onset of the depression (Rabkin).

As noted, evidence supports a link between stress and schizophrenia as well. One behavioral interpretation of schizophrenia views the illness as a maladaptive avoidance

Table 4.2 Psychological disorders
and excessive stress
Brief reactive psychosis
Posttraumatic stress disorder
Adjustment disorders
Various anxiety disorders
Various affective disorders
Some forms of schizophrenia

mechanism in the face of an anxiety-producing environment (Epstein & Coleman, 1970). Serban (1975) found in a study of 125 acute and 516 chronic schizophrenics that excessive stress did play a role in the precipitation of hospital readmission. A more far-reaching view of psychopathology and stress is presented by Eisler and Polak (1971). In a study of 172 psychiatric patients, they concluded that excessive stress could contribute to a wide range of psychiatric disorders, including depression and schizophrenia, as well as personality disturbance—depending on the predisposing characteristics of the individual (see Millon & Everly, 1985). Rabkin (1982) concludes that stress may well be associated with schizophrenic relapse and subsequent hospitalization.

Most important, however, with the advent of the multiaxial DSM, came the identification of psychiatric disorders that were, by definition, a result of stressful life events. Thus, for such categories, mental status, that is, the mind, need no longer be seen as a viable target organ only by inference. Both the diagnoses of *brief reactive psychosis* and *posttraumatic stress disorder* are viewed diagnostically as being a *direct* consequence of a "recognizable stressor." So, too, would be the diagnostic categories of *adjustment disorders*. Diagnoses such as adjustment disorder with anxious mood, adjustment disorder with depressed mood, and adjustment disorder with mixed emotional features demonstrate an official nosological acceptance of the wide spectrum of psychiatric manifestations that can result directly from stress (Everly & Lating, 2004).

Thus, we see that in the last several years, the "mind" has been officially recognized as a potential target organ for pathogenic stress arousal. Table 4.2 summarizes diagnostic categories that serve as psychological target-organ manifestations of excessive stress.

Summary

The purpose of this chapter has been to briefly review some of the more common disorders seen in clinical practice that potentially possess a significant stress-related component. Let us review some of the main points addressed in this chapter:

1. There is a well-established literature linking the GI system to the stress response. The most commonly encountered stress-related GI disorders are peptic ulcers (gastric and duodenal), ulcerative colitis, irritable bowel syndrome, and esophageal

reflux. There appear to be two major pathogenic mechanisms in these disorders: vagus-induced hypersecretion of digestive acids and glucocorticoid (cortisol)-induced diminution of the protective mucosal lining of the GI system. Gastric acid hypersecretion has been shown to be related to anger and rage (Wolfe & Glass, 1950), whereas alterations in mucosal integrity have been shown to be related to depression and feelings of deprivation (Backus & Dudley, 1977).

2. The cardiovascular system is believed by many to be the prime target organ of the stress response, especially in males (Humphrey & Everly, 1980). The cardio-vascular disorders most commonly associated with excessive stress are essential hypertension, migraine headaches, and Raynaud's disease. Essential hyperten-sion is clearly a multifactorial phenomenon. Although stress may not be the soli-tary etiological factor in the majority of cases of essential hypertension, it appears to be a contributory factor in the majority of cases in a nonobese popula-tion. Mechanisms within the stress response that may contribute to the acute and chronic elevation of blood pressure include SNS activity and adrenomedullary activity, as well as cortisol and aldosterone hyperactivity (refer to Chap. 2).

3. Vasospastic phenomena such as migraine headaches and Raynaud's disease seem to be primarily a function of excessive SNS activity, as are myocardial ischemia and coronary endothelial injury.

4. There is evidence that the respiratory system can also be a target organ for the stress response. Bronchial asthma, hyperventilation syndrome, and even some forms of allergies may be stress related. Mechanisms of mediation may include excessive parasympathetic activation, excessive sympathetic activation, and extraordinary adrenomedullary activity, respectively.

5. According to Jacobson (1938, 1970), Gellhorn (1967), and Tomita (1975), the striated neuromuscular system is an underestimated yet prime target for exces-sive stress arousal. Stress-response efferent mechanisms of mediation include alpha-motoneuron innervation, adrenomedullary activity, and perhaps even SNS activity.

6. The skin serves as a target for excessive stress. Disorders such as eczema, acne, psoriasis, and alopecia areata have been implicated as stress-related disorders. Specific mechanisms of mediation are unclear.

7. Animal studies have demonstrated the connection between biogenic and psy-chosocial stressors and immune function. Hans Selye's seminal work investi-gating the General Adaptation Syndrome (GAS) is an early example of how biogenic stressors adversely affect immune function.

8. The impact of stress on immune function in humans has explored areas such as bereavement, marital conflict, and effects of taking exams, and providing long-term care to loved ones with Alzheimer's disease and AIDS. It is important to keep in mind, however, that individual variables and modifying factors need to be considered before coming to general conclusions about stress and immune function.

9. The impact of humor on immune function, most often credited to Norman Cousins, is an example of a positive and potential therapeutic intervention that may enhance immune functioning.

10. A final yet important target organ for the stress response must be the "mind," that is, psychological status. Mental disorders such as brief reactive psychosis, posttraumatic stress disorder, adjustment disorders, certain anxiety and affective disorders, and even some forms of schizophrenia may possess significant stress-related components.

11. In summary, this rather ambitious chapter has attempted to review the vast field of psychosomatics. There would appear to be considerable professional opinion and scientific data to support the widely held view that disease is a multifactorial, biopsychosocial phenomenon in terms of onset, course, and intervention. That is certainly the view supported by the volume, in general.

12. In closing this chapter, it should be noted that the concept of stress-related psychosomatic diseases has been far broadened with the advent of the multiaxial DSM. Now, via such diagnostic perspectives, the clinician can indicate the degree to which stress may have contributed to the primary Axis I diagnosis through the use of Axis III, Axis IV, and Axis V. Finally, data from the field of psychosomatics cogently suggest that even infectious and degenerative diseases may have significant stress-related components in their initiation or exacerbation.

References

Abbas, A. K., & Lichtman, A. H. (2011). *Basic Immunology updated edition: Functions and disorders of the immune system*. Philadelphia, PA: Elsevier Saunders.

Almy, T. P., Kern, F., & Tulin, M. (1949). Alterations in colonic function in man under stress. *Gastroenterology, 12*, 425–436.

Amkraut, A., & Solomon, G. (1974). From symbolic stimulus to the pathophysiologic response: Immune mechanisms. *International Journal of Psychiatry in Medicine, 5*, 541–563.

Anisman, H. (2009). Cascading effects of stressors and inflammatory immune system activation: Implications for major depressive disorder. *Journal of Psychiatry & Neuroscience, 34*(1), 4–20.

Antoni, M. H., Schneiderman, N., Fletcher, M. A., Goldstein, D. A., Ironson, G., & Laperriere, A. (1990). Psychoneuroimmunology and HIV-1. *Journal of Consulting and Clinical Psychology, 58*(1), 38–49.

Backus, F., & Dudley, D. (1977). Observations of psychosocial factors and their relationship to organic disease. In Z. J. Lipowski, D. Lipsitt, & P. Whybrow (Eds.), *Psychosomatic medicine* (pp. 187–205). New York, NY: Oxford University Press.

Bartrop, R. W., Luckhurst, E., Lazarus, L., Kiloh, L. G., & Penny, R. (1977). Depressed lymphocyte function after bereavement. *Lancet, 1*, 834–836.

Berk, L. (1989a). Eustress of mirthful laughter modifies natural killer cell activity. *Clinical Research, 37*, 115.

Berk, L. (1989b). Neuroendocrine and stress hormone changes during mirthful laughter. *American Journal of Medical Science, 298*, 390–396.

Bohus, B., & Koolhaas, J. M. (1991). Psychoimmunology of social factors in rodents and other subprimate vertebrates. In R. Ader, D. L. Felten, & N. Cohen (Eds.), *Psychoneuroimmunology* (2nd ed., pp. 807–830). New York, NY: Academic Press.

Bonaccorso, S., Marino, V., Puzella, A., Pasquini, M., Biondi, M., Artini, M., & Maes, M. (2002). Increased depressive ratings in patients with hepatitis C receiving interferon-[alpha]-based immunotherapy are related to interferon-[alpha]-induced changes in the serotonergic system. *Journal of Clinical Psychopharmacology, 22(1),* 86–90.

Borysenko, M. (1987). The immune system. *Annals of Behavioral Medicine, 9,* 3–10.

Brown, G. W. (1972). Life events and psychiatric illness. *Journal of Psychosomatic Research, 16,* 311–320.

Campernolle, T., Kees, H., & Leen, J. (1979). Diagnosis and treatment of the hyperventilation syndrome. *Psychosomalics, 20,* 612–625.

Capuron, L., Gumnick, J. F., Musselman, D. L., Lawson, D. H., Reedmsnyder, A., Nemeroff, C. B., & Miller, A. H. (2002). Neurobehavioral effects of interferon-α in cancer patients: phenomenology and paroxetine responsiveness of symptom dimensions. *Neuropsychopharmacology, 26*(5), 643–652.

Capuron, L., Ravaud, A., & Dantzer, R. (2000). Early depressive symptoms in cancer patients receiving interleukin 2 and/or interferon-alfa-2b therapy. *Journal of Clinical Oncology, 18*(10), 2143–2151.

Cohen, S., & Herbert, T. B. (1996). Health psychology: Psychological factors and physical disease from the perspective of human psychoneuroimmunology. *Annual Review of Psychology, 47,* 113–142.

Crook, T. H., & Miller, N. E. (1985). The challenge of Alzheimer's disease. *American Psychologist, 40*(11), 1245–1250.

Cunnick, J. E., Lysle, D. T., Armfield, A., & Rabin, B. S. (1988). Shock induced modulation of lymphocyte responsiveness and natural killer cell activity: Differential mechanisms of induction. *Brain, Behavior, and Immunity, 2,* 102–112.

Dillon, K., & Baker, K. (1985). Positive emotional states and enhancement of the immune system. *International Journal of Psychiatric Medicine, 5,* 13–18.

Dirkzwager, A. J. E., van der Velden, P. G., Grievink, L., & Yzermans, J. (2007). Disaster-related posttraumatic stress disorder and physical health. *Psychosomatic Medicine, 69,* 435–440.

Dorpat, T. L., & Holmes, T. H. (1955). Mechanisms of skeletal muscle pain and fatigue. *Archives of Neurology and Psychiatry, 74,* 628–640.

Dotevall, G. (1985). *Stress and the common gastrointestinal disorders.* New York, NY: Praeger.

Dunn, A. J. (1989). Psychoneuroimmunology for the psychoneuroendocrinologist: A review of animal studies of nervous-immune system interactions. *Psychoneuroendocrinology, 14,* 251–274.

Eisler, R., & Polak, P. (1971). Social stress and psychiatric disorder. *Journal of Nervous and Mental Disease, 153,* 227–233.

Eliot, R. (1979). *Stress and the major cardiovascular diseases.* Mt. Kisco, NY: Futura.

Eller, L. S. (1996). Effects of two cognitive-behavioral interventions on immunity and symptoms in persons with HIV. *Annals of Behavioral Medicine, 17,* 339–348.

Engels, W. (1985). Dermatological disorders. In W. Dorftnan & L. Cristofar (Eds.), *Psychosomatic illness review* (pp. 146–161). New York, NY: Macmillan.

Epstein, S., & Coleman, M. (1970). Drive theories of schizophrenia. *Psychosomatic Medicine, 32,* 114–141.

Erdman, L. (1993). Laughter therapy for patients with cancer. *Journal of Psychosocial Oncology, 11*(4), 55–67.

Esterling, B. A., Kiecolt-Glaser, J. K., Bodnar, J. C., & Glaser, R. (1994). Chronic stress, social support, and persistent alterations in the natural killer cell response to cytokines in older adults. *Health Psychology, 13*(4), 291–298.

Esterling, B. A., Kiecolt-Glaser, J. K., & Glaser, R. (1996). Psychosocial modulation of cytokine-induced natural killer cell activity in older adults. *Psychosomatic Medicine, 58,* 264–272.

Everly, G. S., Jr. (1985b, November). *Biological foundations of psychiatric sequelae in trauma and stress-related "disorders of arousal."* Paper presented to the 8th National Trauma Symposium, Baltimore, MD.

Everly, G. S., Jr., & Lating, J. M. (2004). *Personality guided therapy of posttraumatic stress disorder.* Washington, DC: American Psychological Association.

Fleshner, M., Laudenslager, M. L., Simons, L., & Maier, S. F. (1989). Reduced serum antibodies associated with social defeat in rats. *Physiology and Behavior, 42*, 485–489.

Folks, D. G., & Kinney, F. C. (1995). Dermatologic conditions. In A. Stoudemire (Ed.), *Psychological factors affecting medical conditions* (pp. 123–140). Washington, DC: American Psychiatric Press.

Ganong, W. F. (1997). *Review of medical physiology* (18th ed.). Stamford, CT: Appleton & Lange.

Gaynes, B. N., Pence, B. W., Eron, J. J., Jr., & Miller, W. C. (2008). Prevalence and comorbidity of psychiatric diagnoses based on reference standard in and HIV+ patient population. *Psychosomatic Medicine, 70*(4), 505–511.

Gellhorn, E. (1967). *Principles of autonomic-somatic integrations*. Minneapolis, MN: University of Minnesota Press.

Gellhorn, E. (1969). Further studies on the physiology and pathophysiology of the tuning of the central nervous system. *Psychosomatics, 10*, 94–104.

Girdano, D. A., & Everly, G. S., Jr. (1986). *Controlling stress and tension* (2nd ed.). Englewood Cliffs, NJ: Prentice-Hall.

Glaser, R., & Kiecolt-Glaser, J. K. (2005). Stress-induced immune dysfunction: Implications for health. *Nature Reviews Immunology, 5*, 243–251.

Glaser, R., Kiecolt-Glaser, J. K., Bonneau, R. H., Malarkey, W., Kennedy, S., & Hughes, J. (1992). Stress-induced modulation of the immune response to recombinant hepatitis B vaccine. *Psychosomatic Medicine, 54*, 22–29.

Goldsby, R. A., Kindt, T. J., & Osborne, B. A. (2000). *Kuby immunology*. New York, NY: W. H. Freeman.

Grace, W., Seton, P., Wolf, S., & Wolff, H. G. (1949). Studies of the human colon: 1. *American Journal of Medical Science, 217*, 241–251.

Graham, J. E., Glaser, R., Loving, T. J., Malarkey, W. B., Stowell, J. R., & Kiecolt-Glaser, J. K. (2009). Cognitive word use during marital conflict and increases in proinflammatory cytokines. *Health Psychology, 28*(5), 621–630.

Greden, J. F. (1974). Anxiety or caffeinism: A diagnostic dilemma. *American Journal of Psychiatry, 131*, 1089–1092.

Gullette, E. C., Blumenthal, J. A., Babyak, M., Jiang, W., Waugh, R. A., Frid, D. J., & Krantz, D. S. (1997). Effects of mental stress on myocardial ischemia during daily life. *Journal of the American Medical Association, 277*(19), 1521–1526.

Guyton, A. C. (1982). *Textbook of medical physiology*. Philadelphia, PA: Saunders.

Guyton, A. C., & Hall, J. E. (2006). *Guyton and hall textbook of medical physiology with student consult online access* (11th ed.). Philadelphia, PA: Elsevier Saunders.

Hall, N. R. S., Anderson, J. A., & O'Grady, M. P. (1994). Stress and immunity in humans: Modifying variables. In R. Glaser & J. K. Kiecolt-Glaser (Eds.), *Handbook of human stress and immunity* (pp. 183–215). San Diego: Academic Press.

Hall, N. R. S., & O'Grady, M. P. (1991). Psychosocial interventions and immune function. In R. Ader, D. L. Felten, & N. Cohen (Eds.), *Psychoneuroimmunology* (2nd ed., pp. 1067–1080). New York, NY: Academic Press.

Hatch, M. C., Wallenstein, S., Beyea, J., Nieves, J. W., & Susser, M. (1991). Cancer raters after the Three Mile Island nuclear accident and proximity of residence to the plant. *American Journal of Public Health, 81*(6), 719–724.

Hatzenbuehler, M. L., O'Cleirigh, C., Grasso, C., Mayer, K., Safren, S., & Bradford, J. (2011). Effect of same-sex marriage laws on health use and expenditures in sexual minority men: A quasi-natural experiment. *American Journal of Public Health, 102*(2), 285–291.

Heisel, J. S. (1972). Life changes as etiologic factors in juvenile rheumatoid arthritis. *Journal of Psychosomatic Research, 17*, 411–420.

Henry, J. P., & Stephens, P. (1977). *Stress, health, and the social environment*. New York, NY: Springer-Verlag.

Herbert, T. B., & Cohen, S. (1993). Stress and immunity in humans: A meta-analytic review. *Psychosomatic Medicine, 55*, 364–379.

Ho, D. D., Neumann, A. U., Perelson, A. S., Chen, W., Leonard, J. M., & Markowitz, M. (1995). Rapid turnover of plasma virions and CD4 lymphocytes in HIV-1 infection. *Nature, 373*, 123–126.

Holland, J. C., & Tross, S. (1987). Psychosocial considerations in the therapy of epidemic Kaposi's sarcoma. *Seminars in Oncology, 14*, 48–53.

Holmes, T. H., Trenting, T., & Wolff, H. (1951). Lift situations, emotions, and nasal disease. *Psychosomatic Medicine, 13*, 71–82.

Holmes, T. H., & Wolff, H. G. (1952). Lift situations, emotions and backache. *Psychosomatic Medicine, 14*, 18–33.

Horberg, M. A., Silverberg, M. J., Hurley, L. B., Townder, W. J., Klein, D. B., Bersoff-Matcha, S., & Dovach, D. A. (2008). *Journal of Acquired Immune Deficiency Syndrome, 47*, 384–390.

Houldin, A. D., Lev, E., Prystowsky, M. B., Redei, E., & Lowery, B. J. (1991). Psychoneuroimmunology: A review of literature. *Holistic Nursing Practice, 5*(4), 10–21.

Humphrey, J., & Everly, G. S., Jr. (1980). Factor dimensions of stress responsiveness in male and female students. *Health Education, 11*, 38–39.

Imboden, B. (1994). T lymphocytes and natural killer cells. In D. Stites, A. I. Terr, & T. G. Parslow (Eds.), *Basic and clinical immunology* (8th ed., pp. 94–104). Norwalk, CT: Appleton & Lange.

Ironson, G., Wynings, C., Schneiderman, N., Baum, A., Rodriguez, M., & Greenwood, D., Fletcher, M. A. (1997). Posttraumatic stress symptoms, intrusive thoughts, loss, and immune function after Hurricane Andrew. *Psychosomatic Medicine, 59*, 128–141.

Irwin, M., Daniels, M., Smith, T. L., Bloom, E., & Weiner, H. (1987). Life events, depressive symptoms, and immune function. *American Journal of Psychiatry, 144*, 437–441.

Irwin, M., Lacher, U., & Caldwell, C. (1992). Depression and reduced natural killer cytotoxicity: A longitudinal study of depressed patients and control subjects. *Psychological Medicine, 22*, 1045–1050.

Jacobson, E. (1938). *Progressive relaxation*. Chicago: University of Chicago Press.

Jacobson, E. (1970). *Modern treatment of tense patients*. Springfield, IL: Charles C. Thomas.

Jacobson, E. (1978). *You must relax*. New York, NY: McGraw-Hill.

Jones, M. P., Bartrop, R. W., Forcier, L., & Penny, R. (2010). The long-term impact of bereavement upon spouse health: A 10-year follow-up. *Acta Neuropsychiatrica, 22*, 212–217.

Kang, D. H., Coe, C. L., & McCarthy, D. O. (1996). Academic examinations significantly impact immune responses, but not lung function, in healthy and well-managed asthmatic adolescents. *Brain, Behavior, and Immunity, 10*, 164–181.

Kark, J. D., Goldman, S., & Epstein, L. (1995). Iraqi missle attachs on Israel. The association of mortality with a life-threatening stressor. *Journal of the American Medical Association, 273*(15), 1208–1210.

Kemeny, M. E. (1994). Psychoneuroimmunology of HIV infection. *Psychiatric Clinics of North America, 17*(1), 55–68.

Kemeny, M. E., Weiner, H., Duran, R., Taylor, S. E., Visscher, B., & Fahey, J. L. (1995). Immune system changes after the death of a partner in HIV-positive gay men. *Psychosomatic Medicine, 57*, 547–554.

Kendall, M. D. (1998). *Dying to live: How our bodies fight disease*. Cambridge, UK: Cambridge University Press.

Kiecolt-Glaser, J. K., Dura, J. R., Speicher, C. E., Trask, O. J., & Glaser, R. (1991). Spousal caregivers of dementia victims: Longitudinal changes in immunity and health. *Psychosomatic Medicine, S3*, 345–362.

Kiecolt-Glaser, J. K., Fisher, L., Ogrocki, P., Stout, J. C., Speicher, C. E., & Glaser, R. (1987). Marital quality, marital disruption, and immune function. *Psychosomatic Medicine, 49*, 13–34.

Kiecolt-Glaser, J. K., Garner, W., Speicher, C., Penn, G. M., Holliday, J., & Glaser, R. (1984). Psychosocial modifiers of immunocompetence in medical students. *Psychosomatic Medicine, 46*, 7–13.

Kiecolt-Glaser, J. K., Kennedy, S., Malkoff, S., Fisher, L., Speicher, C. E., & Glaser, R. (1988). Marital discord and immunity in males. *Psychosomatic Medicine, 50*, 213–229.

Kiecolt-Glaser, J. K., Loving, T. J., Stowell, J. R., Malarkey, W. B., Lemeshow, S., Dickinson, S. L, & Glaser, R. (2005) Hostile marital interactions, proinflammatory cytokine production, and wound healing. *Archives of General Psychiatry, 62*, 1377–1384.

Kiecolt-Glaser, J. K., Preacher, K. J., MacCallum, R. C., Atkinson, C., Malarkey, W. B., & Glaser, R. (2003). Chronic stress and age-related increases in the proinflammatory cytokine IL-6. *Proccedings of the National Academy of Sciences of the United States, 100*(15), 9090–9095.

Knapp, P. (1982). Pulmonary disorders and psychosocial stress. In W. Farm, I. Karacan, A. Pakorny, & R. Williams (Eds.), *Phenomenology and treatment of psychophysiological disorders* (pp. 15–34). New York: Spectrum.

Koolhaas, J. M., & Bohus, B. (1989). Social control in relation to neuroendocrine and immunological responses. In A. Steptoe & A. Appels (Eds.), *Stress, personal control and health* (pp. 295–304). Chichester, UK: Wiley.

Koolhaas, J. M. & Bohus, B. (1995). Animal models of stress and immunity. In B. E, Leonard & K. Miller (Eds.), *Stress, the immune system and psychiatry* (pp. 69–83). Chichester, UK: Wiley.

Lachman, S. (1972). *Psychosomatic disorders: A behavioristic interpretation*. New York: Wiley.

LaPerriere, A. R., Antoni, M. H., Schneiderman, N., Ironson, G., Klimas, N., Caralis, P., & Fletcher, M. A. (1990). Exercise intervention attenuates emotional distress and natural killer cell decrements following notification of positive serologic status for HIV-1. *Biofeedback and Self-Regulation, 15*, 229–242.

LaPerriere, A. R., Fletcher, M. A., Antoni, M. H., Klimas, N. G., Ironson, G., & Schneiderman, N. (1991). Aerobic exercise training in an AIDS risk group. *International Journal of Sports Medicine, 12*(Suppl. 1), S53–S57.

Latimer, P. (1985). Irritable bowel syndrome. In W. Dorfman & L. Cristofar (Eds.), *Psychosomatic illness review* (pp. 61–75). New York: Macmillan.

Laudenslager, M. L., Fleshner, M., Hofstadter, P., Held, P. E., Simons, L., & Maier, S. F. (1988). Suppression of specific antibody production by inescapable shock: Stability under varying conditions. *Brain, Behavior, and Immunity, 2*, 92–101.

Leor, J., Poole, W. K., & Kloner, R. A. (1996). Sudden cardiac death triggered by an earthquake. *New England Journal of Medicine, 334*(7), 413–419.

Linn, M. W., Linn, B. S., & Jensen, J. (1984). Stressful events, dysphoric mood, and iuume responsiveness. *Psychological Reports, 54*, 219–222.

Lum, L. C. (1975). Hyperventilation: The tip of the iceberg. *Journal of Psychosomatic Research, 19*, 375–383.

Maes, M., & Bonaccorso, S. (2004). Lower activities of serum peptidases predict higher depressive and anxiety levels following interferon-alpha-based immunotherapy in patients with hepatitis c. *Acta Psychiatrca Scandinavica, 109*(2), 126–131.

Mahl, C. F., & Brody, E. (1954). Chronic anxiety symptomatology, experimental stress and HCL secretion. *Archives of Neurological Psychiatry, 71*, 314–325.

Maier, S. F., Watkins, L. R., & Fleshner, M. (1994). Psychoneuroimmunology: The interface between behavior, brain, and immunity. *American Psychologist, 49*(12), 1004–1017.

Manuck, S. B., Marsland, A. L., Kaplan, J. R., & Williams, J. K. (1995). The pathogenicity of behavior and its neuroendocrine mediation: An example from coronary artery disease. *Psychosomatic Medicine, 57*(3), 275–283.

McCain, N. L., Gray, D. P., Elswick, R. K., Jr., Robins, J. W., Tuck, I., Walter, J. M., Ketchum, J. M. (2008). A randomized clinical trial of alternative tress management interventions in persons with HIV infection. *Journal of Consulting and Clinical Psychology, 76*(3), 431–441

McCain, N. L., & Zeller, J. M. (1996). Psychoneuroimmunological studies in HIV disease. *Annual Review of Nursing Research, 14*, 23–55.

McClelland, D. C., & Cheriff, A. D. (1997). The immunoenhancing effects of humor on secretory IgA and resistance to respiratory infections. *Psychology and Health, 12*(3), 329–344.

McDaniel, J. S. (1992). Psychoimmunology: Implications for future research. *Southern Medical Journal, 85*(4), 388–396.

Medansky, R. S. (1971). Emotion and the skin. *Psychosomatics, 12*, 326–329.

Millon, T., & Everly, G. S., Jr. (1985). *Personality and its disorders*. New York: Wiley.

Mitchell, C. M., & Drossman, D. (1987). The irritable bowel syndrome. *Annals of Behavioral Medicine, 9*, 13–18.

Mittelman, B., & Wolff, H. G. (1942). Emotions and gastroduodenal function. *Psychosomatic Medicine, 4*, 5–19.

Mittleman, M. A., Maclure, M., Sherwood, J. B., Mulry, R. P., Tofler, G. H., Jacobs, S. C., & Muller, J. E. (1995). Triggering of acute myocardial infarction onset by episodes of anger. *Determinants of myocardial infarction onset study investigators. Circulation, 92*(7), 1720–1725.

Moore, J. I. (1992). *Pharmacology*. New York: Springer-Verlag.

Moran, M. G. (1995). Pulmonary and rheumatologic diseases. In A. Stoudemire (Ed.), *Psychological factors affecting medical conditions* (pp. 141–158). Washington, DC: American Psychiatric Press.

Moynihan, J. A., Brenner, G. J., Cocke, R., Karp, J. D., Breneman, S. M., Dopp, J. M., Ader, R., Cohen, N., Grota, L. J., & Felten, S. Y. (1994). Stress-induced modulation of immune function in mice. In R. Glaser & J. K. Kiecolt-Glaser (Eds.), *Handbook of human stress and immunity* (pp. 1–22). New York: Academic Press.

Muller, N., & Ackenheil, M. (1995). The immune system and schizophrenia. In B. Leonard & K. Miller (Eds.), *Stress, the immune system and psychiatry* (pp. 137–164). Chichester, UK: Wiley.

Musaph, H. (1977). Itching and other dermatoses. In E. Wittower & H. Wames (Eds.), *Psychosomatic medicine* (pp. 307–316). New York: Harper & Row.

Neidig, J. L., Smith, B. A., & Brashers, D. E. (2003). Aerorbic exercise training for depressive symptoms management in adults living with HIV infection. *Journal of the Association of Nurses in AIDS care, 14*(2), 30–40.

Niaura, R., & Goldstein, M. G. (1995). Cardiovascular disease, Part II: Coronary artery disease and sudden death and hypertension. In A. Stoudemire (Ed.), *Psychological factors affecting medical conditions* (pp. 39–56). Washington, DC: American Psychiatric Press.

Parslow, T. G. (1994). Lymphocytes and lymphoid tissues. In D. Stites, A. I. Terr, & T. G. Parslow (Eds.), *Basic and clinical immunology* (8th ed., pp. 22–39). Norwalk, CT: Appleton & Lange.

Paykel, E., Myers, J., Dienelt, M., Klerman, G., Lindenthal, J., & Pepper, J. (1969). Life events and depression: A controlled study. *Archives of General Psychiatry, 21*, 753–760.

Pennebaker, J. W., & Beall, S. K. (1986). Confronting a traumatic event: Toward an understanding of inhibition and disease. *Journal of Abnormal Psychology, 95*, 274–281.

Pennebaker, J. W., Kiecolt-Glaser, J. K., & Glaser, R. (1988). Disclosure of traumas and immune function: Health implications for psychotherapy. *Journal of Consulting and Clinical Psychology, 56*(2), 239–245.

Pennebaker, J. W., Mayne, T. J., & Francis, M. E. (1997). Linguistic predictors of adaptive bereavement. *Journal of Personality and Social Psychology, 72*(4), 863–871.

Pennebaker, J. W., Mehl, M. R., & Niederhoffer, K. G. (2003). Psychological aspects of natural language use: Our words, our selves. *Annual Review of Psychology, 54*, 547–577.

Petrie, K. J., Booth, R. J., & Pennebaker, J. W. (1998). The immunological effects of thought suppression. *Journal of Personality and Social Psychology, 75*(5), 1264–1272.

Petrie, K. J., Fontanilla, I., Thomas, M. G., Booth, R. J., & Pennebaker, J. W. (2004). Effect of written emotional expression on immune function in patients with human immunodeficiency virus infection: A randomized trial. *Psychosomatic Medicine, 66*(2), 272–275.

Potvin, S., Stip, E., Sepehry, A. A., Gendron, A., Bah, R., & Kouassi, E. (2008). Inflammatory cytokine alterations in schizophrenia: A systematic quantitative review. *Biological Psychiatry, 63*, 801–808.

Rabkin, J. G. (1982). Stress and psychiatric disorders. In L. Goldberger & S. Brenitz (Eds.), *Handbook of stress* (pp. 566–584). New York: Free Press.

Raskin, N. (1985). Migraine. In W. Dorfinan & L. Cristofar (Eds.), *Psychosomatic illness review* (pp. 11–22). New York: Macmillan.

Ravindran, A. V., Griffiths, J., Merali, Z., & Anisman, H. (1995). Lymphocyte subsets associated with major depression and dysthymia: Modification by antidepressant treatment. *Psychosomatic Medicine, 57*, 555–563.

Rosch, P. J. (1995). Future directions in psychoneuroimmunology: Psychoelectroneuroimmunology? In B. Leonard & K. Miller (Eds.), *Stress, the immune system and psychiatry* (pp. 206–231). Chichester, UK: Wiley.

Rosenbaum, M. (1985). Ulcerative colitis. In W. Dorfman & L. Cristofar (Eds.), *Psychosomatic illness review* (pp. 61–75). New York: Macmillan.

Sareen, J., Cox, B. J., Stein, M. B., Afifi, T. O., Fleet, C., & Asmundson, G. J. G. (2007). Physical and mental comorbidity, disability, and suicidal behavior associated with Posttraumatic Stress Disorder in a large community sample. *Psychosomatic Medicine, 69*, 242–248.

Scalori, A., Pozzi, M., Bellia, V., Apale, P., Santamaria, G., Bordoni, T., , Roffi, L. (2005). Interferon-induced depression: prevalence and management. *Digestive and Liver Disease, 37(2)*, 102–107.

Schleifer, S. J., Keller, S. E., Camerino, M., Thornton, J. C., & Stein, M. (1983). Suppression of lymphocyte stimulation following bereavement. *Journal of the American Medical Association, 250*, 374–377.

Segerstrom, S. C., & Miller, G. E. (2004). Psychological stress and the human immune system: A meta-analytic study of 30 years of inquiry. *Psychological Bulletin, 130*(4), 601–630.

Selye, H. (1936). A syndrome produced by diverse noxious agents. *Nature, 138*, 32–33.

Selye, H. (1951). The General Adaptation Syndrome and the gastrointestinal diseases of adaptation. *American Journal of Proctology, 2*, 167–184.

Selye, H. (1956). *The stress of life*. New York: McGraw-Hill.

Selye, H. (1976). *Stress in health and disease*. Boston: Butterworth.

Serban, G. (1975). Stress in schizophrenics and normals. *British Journal of Psychiatry, 126*, 397–407.

Simonton, C., Matthews-Simonton, S., & Sparks, T. (1980). Psychological intervention in the treatment of cancer. *Psychosomatics, 21*, 226–233.

Sklar, L. S., & Anisman, H. (1979). Stress and coping factors influence tumor growth. *Science, 205*, 513–515.

Solomon, G. F., Segerstrom, S. C., Grohr, P., Kemeny, M., & Fahey, J. (1997). Shaking up immunity: Psychological and immunologic changes after a natural disaster. *Psychosomatic Medicine, 59*, 114–127.

Stephenson, P. (1977). Physiologic and psychotropic effects of caffeine on man. *Journal of the American Dietetic Association, 71*, 240–247.

Steplewski, Z., & Vogel, W. H. (1986). Total leukocytes, T cell subpopulation, and natural killer (NK) cell activity in rats exposed to resistant stress. *Life Science, 38*, 2419–2427.

Steptoe, A. (1981). *Psychological factors in cardiovascular disorders*. New York: Academic Press.

Taub, E., & Stroebel, C. (1978). Biofeedback in the treatment of vasonconstrictive syndromes. *Biofeedback and Self-Regulation, 3*, 363–374.

Thibodeau, G. A., & Patton, K. T. (1993). *Anatomy and physiology* (2nd ed.). St. Louis: Mosby.

Tomita, T. (1975). Action of catecholamines on skeletal muscles. In S. Geigor (Ed.), *Handbook of physiology* (Vol. 6, pp. 537–552). Washington, DC: American Physiological Society.

U.S. Department of Health and Human Services. (2009). Guidelines for the use of antiretroviral agents in HIV-1-infected adults and adolescents. Retrieved from: http://www.aidsinfo.nih.gov/contentfiles/AdultandAdolescentGL.pdf

Vessey, S. H. (1964). Effects of grouping on levels of circulating antibodies in mice. *Proceedings of Social and Experimental Biological Medicine, 115*, 252–255.

von Känel, R., Hepp, U., Buddeberg, C., Keel, M., Mica, L., Aschbacher, K., & Schnyder, U. (2006). Altered blood coagulation in patients with posttraumatic stress disorder. *Psychosomatic Medicine, 68*, 598–604.

Wei, X., Ghosh, S. K., Taylor, M. E., Johnson, V. A., Emini, E. A., Deutsch, P., Lifson, J. D., Bonhoeffer, S., Nowak, M. A., Hahn, B. H., Saag, M. S., & Shaw, G. M. (1995). Viral dynamics in human immunodeficiency virus type 1 infection. *Nature, 373*, 117–122.

Weiner, H. (1977). *Psychobiology and human disease*. New York: Elsevier.

Weiner, H., Thaler, M., Reiser, M., & Mirsky, L. (1957). Etiology of duodenal ulcer. *Psychosomatic Medicine, 19*, 1–10.

Weinstock, L., & Cluse, R. (1987). A focused overview of gastrointestinal physiology. *Annals of Behavioral Medicine, 9*, 3–6.

Weiss, J. M. (1968). Effects of coping responses on stress. *Journal of Comparative Physiological Psychology, 65*, 251–260.

Weiss, R. S. (1975). *Marital separation*. New York: Basic Books.

Whitehead, W. E. (1992). Biofeedback treatment of gastrointestinal disorders. *Biofeedback and Self Regulation, 77*(1), 59–76.

Wolf, S., & Glass, G. B. (1950). Correlation of conscious and unconscious conflicts with changes in gastric function and structure. In H. G. Wolff & S. Wolf (Eds.), *Life stress and bodily disease* (pp. 17–35). Baltimore: Williams & Wilkins.

Wolff, H. G. (1963). *Headache and other head pain*. New York: Oxford University Press.

Wooten, P. (1996). Humor: An antidote for stress. *Holistic Nursing Practice, 10*(2), 49–56.

Wright, P., Takei, N., Rifkin, L., & Murray, R. M. (1995). Maternal influenza, obstetric complications, and schizophrenia. *American Journal of Psychiatry, 152*(12), 1714–1720.

Young, L., Richter, J., Bradley, L., & Anderson, K. (1987). Disorders of the upper gastrointestinal system. *Annals of Behavioral Medicine, 9*, 7–12.

Zeller, J. M., McCain, N. L., McCann, J. J., Swanson, B., & Colletti, M. A. (1996). Methodological issues in psychoneuroimmunology research. *Nursing Research, 45*(5), 314–318.

Chapter 5
Measurement of the Human Stress Response

In the final analysis, the empirical foundation of epistemology is measurement.

When an unexplained phenomenon, such as a stress-related disease, is first observed, it is common to search for possible etiological factors. This search often culminates in a phenomenological theory; in this case, perhaps a theory of stress arousal and subsequent pathogenesis. On the basis of the formulated theory, for example, of stress arousal, it is then a useful next step to design an experiment in order to test the theory and any proposed relationships critical to the theory. Inherent in the design of the experiment is the designation of key variables and some means of measuring, recording, or otherwise quantifying those relevant variables. Relevant to the present discussion, this would typically involve a means of measuring the stress response and perhaps its pathological effects.

As we review the literature concerning human stress, it is obvious that in addition to the lack of a universal definition of stress, the field has also been plagued by a plethora of inconsistencies and potential phenomenological errors in the measurement of the human stress response. If we cannot reliably and validly measure the human stress response, what degree of credibility do we place upon investigations into its phenomenology? Indeed, meta-analytic research has suggested that the measurement of independent and dependent variables may be the single most important aspect of research design—even more important than the structure of the research design itself (Cohen, 1984; Fiske, 1983; Smith, Glass, & Miller, 1980). With regard to stress research, it may be argued that the confounded or inappropriate measurement process has the greatest ability to limit the generation of useful data regarding this important public health phenomenon (Cattell & Scheier, 1961; Everly & Sobelman, 1987; Stamm, 1996). Thus, the purpose of this chapter is to discuss the measurement of the human stress response.

In Chap. 2, a systems model of the nature of the human stress response was constructed (Fig. 2.6). As a means of integrating the following measurement-based discussions, that basic model is reproduced here, with key measurement technologies having been superimposed (see Fig. 5.1). Let us take this opportunity to examine more closely the measurement of the human stress response.

G.S. Everly and J.M. Lating, *A Clinical Guide to the Treatment*   103
of the Human Stress Response, DOI 10.1007/978-1-4614-5538-7_5,
© Springer Science+Business Media New York 2013

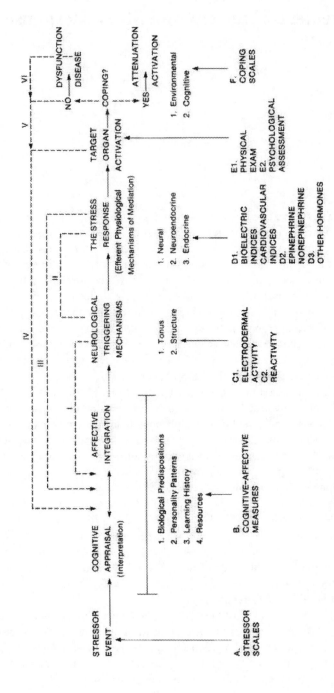

Fig. 5.1 Measurement of the human stress response

Stressor Scales

Historically, one of the most widely used measurement tool for the assessment of human stress, in reality, does not measure stress at all—it measures stressors. The Social Readjustment Rating Scale (SRRS), the "grandfather" of attempts at measuring stress, was developed by Thomas Holmes and Richard Rahe (1967), based upon the theory that "life change" is causally associated with subsequent illness. This notion was by no means a new idea. Adolph Meyer pioneered empirical investigations into the relationship between psychosocial events and illness with the advent of his "life chart" as a means of creating a medical history.

The SRRS contains 43 items consisting of commonly experienced "life events." Each life event is weighted with a life change unit score (LCU). Respondents are simply asked to check each of the items they have experienced within the last 12 months. The arithmetic summation of LCUs represents the total LCU score, which can then be converted to a relative health risk statement, that is, the risk of becoming ill within a stipulated time period. The association between high LCU scores and risk of subsequent illness is assumed to be a function of the fact that organisms must adapt to novel stimuli and otherwise new life events. The physiology of adaptation has long been known to be the same physiology as the stress response. Thus, stress may be seen as the linchpin between life events and illness as conceived of and measured by the SRRS.

The SRRS is not without its critics, however. Two major issues have been raised:

1. Life events scales should be modified so as to assess the perceived desirability of the life event. It has been suggested that negative life events are potentially more pathogenic than positive life events (Sarason, Johnson, & Siegel, 1978).
2. It has also been suggested that "minor hassles" are more important predictors of illness than major life events (Kanner, Coyne, Schaefer, & Lazarus, 1981).

Other noteworthy efforts in the assessment of stressor stimuli should be mentioned. In an attempt to improve the SRRS with regard to the issue of event desirability, Sarason and his colleagues (1978) created the Life Experiences Survey (LES), which not only lists a series of life events but also inquires into the desirability of each of the events. In a far more ingenious approach to the life events issue, Lazarus and his colleagues investigated the daily hassles versus major life events issue as it pertains to the prediction of subsequent illness (Kanner et al., 1981). The Hassles Scale lists a series of minor daily hassles, that is, sources of frustration that commonly recur to many individuals. The scale also includes an "uplifts" assessment that theoretically serves to mitigate the adverse impact of negative life events.

The LES and the Hassles Scale are creative and alternative approaches to the assessment of stressors. Another entry into the genre of stressor scales is the Stressful Life Experiences Screening (SLES; Stamm, 1996). This instrument consists of 20 items that inquire as to (1) the presence of a stressful life experience, and (2) the degree of "stressfulness" of that experience. The long form (SLES-L) takes 5–10 min to complete.

The Life Stressor Checklist—Revised (Wolfe & Kimerling, 1998) consists of 30 "events" that satisfy the DSM-IV definition of traumatic. The self-report scale takes 15–30 min to complete and is designed for use with adults. The scale is not only an indicator of traumatic events, but it also serves as an assessment of the events' current impact upon the individual.

Most recently, the Stress and Adversity Inventory (STRAIN) was created by the University of Los Angeles's Laboratory for Stress Assessment and Research. This is a computerized self-report inventory that consists of 96 questions that cover moderate to severe stressors that are typically experienced by the adult population. The strain is designed for use with adults and takes approximately 30–45 min to complete (UCLA Laboratory for Stress Assessment and Research: http://www.uclastresslab.org/products/strain–stress-and-adversity-inventory).

As for the genre of stressor scales, Monroe (1983) notes, "Although findings of event—illness associations appear to be consistent in that increased life events predict dysfunction in both retrospective and prospective studies, the magnitude of the association reported typically has been low" (p. 190). The recognized consistency in the life events research combined with its low-effect size leads one to believe that life events scales such as the SRRS do indeed tap some domain that has meaning in stress phenomenology; however, there appear to be other mediating variables that need to be better understood. From the view of the present model, life events scales tap the stressor domain and therefore cannot be said to assess either the stress response itself or the causal mechanisms that undergird stress arousal. Nevertheless, scales such as the SRRS can be of value, especially in stress research when the researcher wishes to obtain valid and reliable assessments of the "background noise," that is, intervening or other otherwise confounding variables in psychosocial stressor research (see Everly & Sobelman, 1987).

Cognitive–Affective Correlate Scales

Whereas in the preceding section we discussed the assessment of stressor stimuli, the reader will recall from Chap. 2 the agreement among most stress researchers that in order for psychosocial life events to engender a stress response and subsequent illness, they must first be processed via cognitive–affective mechanisms. It seems theoretically viable, therefore, that one might assess the cognitive–affective domain of respondents as an indirect assessment of the human stress response (Everly & Sobelman, 1987). Derogatis (1977) has argued that such a "self-report mode of psychological measurement contains much to recommend it" (p. 2). Furthermore, Everly has argued that assessment of this domain may be the most practical, efficient, and cost-effective way of measuring the human stress response (Everly & Sobelman, 1987; Everly, Davy, Smith, Lating, & Nucifora, 2011; Nucifora, Hall, & Everly, 2011).

The World Assumption Scale (WAS; Janoff-Bulman, 1996) assesses three core assumptions, or beliefs, about life: the benevolence of the world, the inherent meaningfulness of the world, and self-worth. This self-report scale requires 5–10 min to complete and consists of 32 items scored according to a 6-point Likert scale.

Neurological Triggering Mechanisms

The assessment of the sensitivity of neurological triggering mechanisms is by no means an easy task. Aberrant evoked potentials emerging from the subcortical limbic system would be one indication of an existing hypersensitivity phenomenon within the limbic system. The accurate assessment of subcortical activity via electroencephalography (EEG) is very difficult and may be considered a gross assessment at best, however. False-negative findings are a common problem with such assessment and EEGs in general. Electrodermal responsiveness as assessed via galvanic skin response (GSR) would be another way of assessing the reactivity of neurological triggering mechanisms (Peek, 2003).

Finally, the general assessment of psychophysiological reactivity is believed to be a viable process for assessing the efferent-discharge propensity of the limbic system (Everly & Sobelman, 1987). The phenomenology of this process is based upon the theories of Lacey, Malmo, and Sternbach discussed in Chap. 3.

Measuring the Physiology of the Stress Response

It will be recalled from Chap. 2 that the stress response can be divided into three broad categories: (1) the neural axes, (2) the neuroendocrine axis, and (3) the endocrine axes. Let us briefly review several of the more common assessment technologies used to tap these phenomenological domains.

Assessment of the Neural Axes

Assessment of the neural axes of the human stress response is for the most part an attempt to capture a transitory state measurement phenomenon, as opposed to a more consistent trait. Technologies used for such assessment include (1) electrodermal techniques, (2) electromyographic techniques, and (3) cardiovascular measures.

Electrodermal Measures

The physiological basis of the electrodermal assessment of the stress response is the eccrine sweat gland. Located primarily in the soles of the feet and the palms of the hands, these sweat glands respond to psychological stimuli rather than heat and emerge on the terminal efferent ends of sympathetic neurons. Although the neurotransmitter at the sweat gland itself is Ach, as opposed to NE, the assessment of this activity provides useful insight into the activity of the sympathetic nervous system.

Electrodermal activity may be assessed via active GSR techniques or through passive techniques such as skin potentials (SP), according to Edelberg (1972). Andreassi (1980) has stated that electrodermal techniques are useful indices of somatic arousal.

Electromyographic Measurement

The physiological basis of electromyographic measurement of the stress response is the neurological innervation of the striated skeletal muscles. Electromyography, although an indirect measure of muscle "tension," is a direct measure of the action potentials originating from the neurons that innervate the muscles.

Skeletal muscles receive their neural innervation primarily as a result of alpha motoneuron presence, on the efferent limb, and secondarily as a result of gamma motoneuron activity as well. From the afferent perspective, proprioceptive neurons arising from the muscle spindles contribute to the overall electrical activity that originates from the skeletal musculature. In a relaxed state, skeletal muscle tone serves as a very useful general index of arousal (Gellhorn, 1964a; Gellhorn & Loofburrow, 1963; Jacobson, 1929, 1970; Malmo, 1975; Weil, 1974), yet in a contracted state this utility appears to disappear. Thus, when using skeletal muscles as general indices of arousal and stress responsiveness, it becomes of critical importance to teach patients to first relax those muscles (Everly, Welzant, Machado, & Miller, 1989).

There has been debate on the utility of a particular set of muscles as an index of arousal. That set of muscles is the group known as the *frontalis*. Jacobson (1970) and Shagass and Malmo (1954) first recognized that the frontalis and related facial muscles were prime targets of the stress-arousal process. Budzynski and Stoyva (1969) and Stoyva (1979) explored and refined the clinical utility of these muscles in the treatment of stress-related disorders. Similar work was undertaken by Schwartz et al. (1978), who found the corrugator muscles of similar utility in relation to depression.

It may be argued that the frontalis muscles of the forehead provide a useful site for the assessment of stress arousal. These muscles have been termed "quasi-voluntary" muscles because their autonomic-like properties manifest during emotional states. In support of such a view are the studies indicating that when simple facial expressions are mimicked, an alteration in heart rate and skin temperature can be observed, even when the subjects were simply asked to mimic the expression without any consideration for the cognitive or affective state that might be associated with it. Similarly, Rubin (1977) suggests that the frontalis muscles, in particular, may possess properties of dual innervation: skeletal alpha motoneuron and ANS innervation.

Although, clearly, the frontalis musculature is predominately striated in nature (thus receiving efferent innervation from the alpha motoneuron assemblies), Rubin (1977) has argued that the frontalis also possesses thin nonstriated layers of musculature. These nonstriated muscles apparently receive their innervation (directly or indirectly) from the SNS (Miehlke, 1973). Thus, assessment of the frontalis muscles through electromyographic procedures may well provide insight into alpha motoneuron activity, sympathetic neural activity, as well as neuroendocrine activity (Everly & Sobelman, 1987). Although there is not total agreement on the utility of the frontalis musculature (Alexander, 1975), Stoyva (1979) provides useful guidelines for the use of that measurement variable.

Clinical biofeedback experience shows the frontalis muscles are useful in the treatment of a wide range of stress-related disorders, including essential hypertension and disorders of the GI system. Most clinicians, over the years, have reported use of the frontalis muscle in electromyographic assessment; however, the trapezius, brachioradialis, and sternocleidomastoid muscle groups have also been utilized.

In summary, most evidence suggests that the electromyographic assessment yields insight into the activity of other major muscle groups (Freedman & Papsdorf, 1976; Glaus & Kotses, 1977, 1978) as well as the generalized activity of the SNS (Arnarson & Sheffield, 1980; Budzynski, 1979; Donaldson, Donaldson, & Snelling, 2003; Field, 2009; Jacobson, 1970; Malmo, 1966; Rubin, 1977; Schwartz & Andrasik, 2003).

Cardiovascular Measurement

Cardiovascular measurement of the stress response entails the assessment of effects of the stress response upon the heart and vascular systems. Common cardiovascular measures include heart rate, peripheral blood flow, and blood pressure.

Heart rate activity as a function of the stress response is a result of direct neural innervation as well as neuroendocrine activity of epinephrine and norepinephrine. During psychosocially induced stress, epinephrine is preferentially released from the adrenal medullae. The ventricles of the heart are maximally responsive to circulating epinephrine and will respond with increased speed and force of ventricular contraction. Of course, direct sympathetic neural activation increases heart rate as well. The measurement of heart rate is most commonly achieved through the use of audio-metric or oscillometric techniques during the normal assessment of blood pressure. Occasionally, heart rate will be measured from ECG techniques via the use of passive electrodes or even through plethysmography.

Plethysmography focuses upon the volume of blood in a selected anatomical site. The most common areas for such assessment of the stress response are the fingers, toes, calves, and forearms. During the stress response, most patients will suffer a reduction of blood flow from these areas. This vasoconstrictive effect is a result of direct sympathetic activity to the arteries and arterioles, as well as of circulating norepinephrine (Hall, 2011). A decline of blood flow to these areas will also result in a reduction of skin temperature. Therefore, skin temperature is also sometimes utilized, although it is not as reliable as plethysmography. So we see that the assessment of peripheral blood flow can be accomplished via the use of plethysmography as well as skin temperature.

Finally, blood pressure is sometimes used as an *acute* index of the stress response. The assessment of blood pressure is generally achieved through the quantification of systolic and diastolic blood pressure, and may be considered highly state dependent.

Systolic blood pressure is the hemodynamic pressure exerted within the arterial system during systole (the ventricular contraction phase). Diastolic blood pressure is the hemodynamic pressure exerted within the arterial system during diastole (relaxation and filling of the ventricular chambers).

Blood pressure is a function of several variables revealed in the following equation:

$$BP = CO \times TPR$$

where
  BP = blood pressure
  CO = cardiac output = stroke volume × heart rate
  TPR = total hemodynamic peripheral resistance

Blood pressure can be measured noninvasively through auscultation, audiometry, or oscillometry. In noninvasive paradigms, a sampled artery (usually the brachial) is compressed through the use of an inflatable rubber tube or bladder. The bladder is inflated until it totally blocks the passage of blood through the artery. Air pressure, measured in millimeters of mercury (mm Hg) is slowly released from the bladder until a sound is heard or a distension sensed. This sound and distension (called a Korotkoff sound) is indicative of blood being allowed to pass through the once blocked artery. Korotkoff sounds continue until the artery is fully opened and returned back to its natural status. The first Korotkoff sound is indicative of the systolic blood pressure. The passing of the last Korotkoff sound is indicative of the diastolic blood pressure. The technique of audiometry measures blood pressure by the use of a microphone to sense the Korotkoff sounds. Oscillometry detects the Korotkoff phenomenon via a pressure-sensitive device placed on the outside of the artery. Finally, auscultation is the sensing of the Korotkoff sound via stethoscope. Audiometric and oscillometric techniques are far more reliable than is manual auscultation.

In summary, the measurement of cardiovascular phenomena can be seen to tap both neural and neuroendocrine domains; thus, there is an overlap in phenomenology. Also, when using the cardiovascular domain to measure stress arousal, the clinician is interested only in the *acute* fluctuations, as opposed to chronic levels. This is due to the fact that stress exerts its most measurable effect upon the acute status of the cardiovascular system. A multitude of other factors enter into, and otherwise confound, the measurement process when examining cardiovascular indices such as chronic blood pressure and peripheral blood flow, for example.

Assessment of the Neuroendocrine Axis

Assessment of the neuroendocrine axis of the stress response entails measurement of the adrenal medullary catecholamines: epinephrine (adrenaline) and norepinephrine (noradrenaline).

Aggregated medullary catecholamines may be sampled from blood or urine and assayed via fluorometric methods. Reference values range for random sampling up to 18 µg/100 ml urine, for a 24-h urine sample up to 135 µg, and for timed samples, 1.4–7.3 µg/h during daylight hours (Bio-Science, 1982). For aggregated catecholamines sampled from plasma, values range from 140 to 165 pg/ml via radioenzymatic procedures (Bio-Science).

Various fluorometric (Anderson, Hovmoller, Karlsson, & Svensson, 1974; Euler & Lishajko, 1961; Jacobs et al., 1994), chromatographic (Jacobs et al.; Lake, Ziegler, & Kopin, 1976; Mason, 1972), and radioimmunoassay (Jacobs et al.; Mason) methods are available for the assessment of catecholamines. The most useful of all methods may be the high pressure liquid chromatography (HPLC) with electrochemical detection as described in Hegstrand and Eichelman (1981) and McClelland, Ross, and Patel (1985). HPLC allows multiple catecholamines to be derived from sampled plasma, urine, and saliva with superior ease and sensitivity.

Epinephrine can be sampled from urine, plasma, or saliva. When sampled from urine a typical distribution is as follows: (see Jacobs et al., 1994; Katzung, 1992):

Unchanged epinephrine	6%
Metanephrine	40%
Vanillylmandelic acid	41%
4-Hydroxy-3-methoxy-phenylglycol	7%
3, 4-Dihydroxymandelic acid	2%
Other	4%
	100%

Norepinephrine can also be sampled from urine, plasma, and saliva. Table 5.1 provides a range of epinephrine and norepinephrine values when sampled from urine.

Despite the availability of methods such as HPLC, some researchers prefer the assessment of catecholamines by indirect routes, for example, through the assessment of urinary metabolites. Metanephrines and vanillylmandelic acid (VMA) are two popular choices.

In the case of the metanephrines, one of the major deactivating substances acting upon epinephrine and norepinephrine is the enzyme catecholamine-O-methyltransferase (COMT). Metabolites of this deactivation process are metanephrine and normetanephine. Aggregated metanephrines range from 0.3 to 0.9 mg/day in urine. VMA levels range from 0.7 to 6.8 mg/day. VMA is the urinary metabolite of COMT and monoamine oxidase.

Assessment of the Endocrine Axes

According to Hans Selye (1976), the most direct way of measuring the stress response is via ACTH, the corticosteroids, and the catecholamines. The catecholamines have already been discussed. The most commonly used index of ACTH

Table 5.1 Value ranges for urinary epinephrine and norepinephrine

	Epinephrine	Norepinephrine
Basal levels	4–5 μg/day	28–30 μg/day
Aroused	10–15 μg/day	50–70 μg/day
Significant stress	>15 μg/day	>70 μg/day

and corticosteroid activity is the measurement of the hormone cortisol. Cortisol is secreted by the adrenal cortices, activated by ACTH, at a rate of about 25–30 mg/ day and accounts for about 90% of glucocorticoid activity.

Cortisol may be sampled from either plasma or urine. Radioimmunoassay plasma levels for a normal adult may range from 5 to 20 μg/100 ml plasma (8 A.M. sample). The normal diurnal decline may result in a level of plasma cortisol at 4 P.M. about one half of the 8 A.M. level. Normal urinary-free cortisol may range from 20 to 90 μg/24 h (see Bio-Science, 1982). It has been suggested that urinary-free cortisol is the most sensitive and reliable indicator of adrenal cortical hyperfunction, followed by plasma cortisol and finally 17-hydroxycorticosteroid (17-OHCS), a cortisol metabolite (Damon, 1981). Normal values for 17-OHCS measured from urine typically range from 2.5 to 10 mg/24 h in the female to 4.5 to 12 mg/24 h in the male adult (Porter–Silber method). Slight increases in 17-OHCS are evidenced in the first trimester of pregnancy and in severe hypertension. Moderate increases can be observed in the third trimester of pregnancy and as a result of infectious disease, burns, surgery, and stress (Bio-Science). In conditions of extreme stress, urinary 17-OHCS may exceed 15 mg/24 h. Plasma assessments of 17-OHCS range from 10 to 14 μg% at 8 A.M. basal levels to 18 to 24 μg% under moderate stress, to an excess of 24 μg% in extremely stressful situations (Mason, 1972).

This section has discussed the assessment of the physiological constituents of the stress response. It should be noted that the assessment of this domain represents a challenging and potentially frustrating exercise. One major factor that confounds the assessment of most physiological variables is the fact that most physiological phenomena used to assess stress arousal are state-dependent variables that wax and wane throughout the course of a day as well as with acute situational demands. Normal diurnal fluctuations as well as acute situational variability can serve to yield false-positive or false-negative findings in the absence of meaningful baseline data. There has even been some question as to the predictive validity of acute physiological indices. Another issue that confounds the overall utility of many physiological measures is that such measures usually require special training, special equipment, or both. The difficulties associated with physiological assessment of the human stress response have been summarized by Everly and Sobelman (1987). Other issues, such as response specificity and organ reactivity, are also reviewed.

Assessment of Target-Organ Effects

Once the stress response has been activated to pathogenic proportions, there emerges another possible assessment strategy for measuring human stress—the assessment of the target-organ effects of the stress response. The assessment of target-organ effects can consist of measuring physical as well as psychological variables.

Physical Diagnosis

The assessment of the physical effects of stress would involve the use of standard diagnostic techniques common to the practice of physical medicine. The goal of such assessments is to measure the integrity of the target organ's structural and functional status. An in-depth discussion of such procedures is far beyond the scope of this volume, however.

It should be mentioned that such assessments are never clearly assessments of stress. One never really knows to what degree pathogenic stress arousal has contributed to the manifestation of target-organ pathology. For this reason, the diagnosis of stress-related target-organ disease is typically a diagnosis by exclusion; that is, one systematically excludes non-stress-related etiological factors while at the same time looking for evidence of pathogenic stress arousal through the assessment of other measurement domains as well. The stress-related diagnosis then emerges from a convergence of these data sets. There are also self-report scales that have shown to be valid and reliable indices of experienced physical illness. The Seriousness of Illness Rating Scale (SIRS; Wyler, Masuda, & Holmes, 1968; see also Rosenberg, Hayes, & Peterson, 1987) is one useful self-report tool for measuring illness and weighting its impact. The Stress Audit Questionnaire (Miller & Smith, 1982) is another. It is important to keep in mind that there is still no certainty as to the extent of the role of stress arousal in the formation of the emergent illnesses/reactions.

Finally, the Family Disruption from Illness Scale (Ide, 1996) extends the assessment of physical symptoms somewhat by assessing the degree of disruption that 53 health-related symptoms impose upon daily functioning. Most items represent physical illnesses. This scale, while more recent than the SIRS, is not as comprehensive, nor have its psychometric properties been adequately assessed.

Psychological Diagnosis

The psychological diagnosis of the stress response refers to the measurement of the "psychological" effects of the stress response. There currently exist numerous and diverse methods for the measurement of psychological states and traits. To cover this topic fully would require a volume of its own. Therefore, what we shall do in this section is merely highlight the paper-and-pencil questionnaires that a clinician might find most useful in measuring the psychological effects of the stress response.

Minnesota Multiphasic Personality Inventory—2

The Minnesota Multiphasic Personality Inventory—2 (MMPI-2) (Butcher, Dahlstrom, Graham, Tellegren & Kraemmer, 1989) is a revision of perhaps one of the most valid and reliable inventories for the assessment of long-term stress on the personality structure of the patient. The numerous clinical and content scales of the MMPI-2 yield a wealth of valuable information. These scales sample a wide range of "abnormal" or maladjusted personality traits (a personality trait is a rather chronic and consistent pattern of thinking and behavior).

The MMPI-2 consists of ten basic clinical scales developed on the basis of actuarial data:

1. Hs: Hypochondriasis
2. D: Depression
3. Hy: Conversion Hysteria
4. Pd: Psychopathic Deviate
5. Mf: Masculinity–Femininity
6. Pa: Paranoia
7. Pt: Psychasthenia (trait anxiety)
8. Sc: Schizophrenia
9. Ma: Hypomania (manifest energy)
10. Si: Social Introversion (preference for being alone)

In addition to the highly researched clinical scales, the MMPI-2 has validity scales that give the clinician a general idea of how valid any given set of test scores is for the patient. This unique feature of the MMPI-2 increases its desirability to many clinicians.

The MMPI-2 offers a virtual wealth of information to the trained clinician; its only major drawback appears to be its length of over 560 items.

The Sixteen Personality Factor Questionnaire (16-PF)

The 16-PF (Cattell, 1972), much the same as the MMPI, assesses a wide range of personality traits. It measures 16 "functionally independent and psychologically meaningful dimensions isolated and replicated in more than 30 years of factor-analytic research on normal and clinical groups" (p. 5).

The 16-PF consists of 187 items distributed across the following scales:

• Reserved–Outgoing

- Less Intelligent–More Intelligent
- Affected by Feelings–Emotionally Stable
- Humble–Assertive
- Sober–Happy-Go-Lucky
- Conservative–Experimenting
- Group-Dependent–Self-Sufficient
- Expedient-Conscientious
- Shy-Venturesome
- Tough-minded-Tender-minded
- Trusting-Suspicious
- Practical-Imaginative
- Forthright-Astute
- Self-Assured-Apprehensive
- Undisciplined Self-Conflict-Controlled
- Relaxed-Tense

Millon Clinical Multiaxial Inventory—II

The Millon Clinical Multiaxial Inventory (MCMI) (Millon, 1983) is a 175-item self-report, true–false questionnaire. The MCMI-II, although not as widely utilized as the MMPI in the diagnosis of major psychiatric disorders, is clearly the instrument of choice when the clinician is primarily interested in personologic variables and their relationship to excessive stress. Furthermore, the MCMI-II offers valuable insight into treatment planning. Another major advantage of the MCMI-II over the MMPI and 16-PF is that it consists of only 175 items. The MCMI-II includes 22 clinical scales broken down into three broad categories; ten basic personality scales reflective of the personality theory of Theodore Millon (1981); three pathological personality syndromes; and nine major clinical psychiatric syndromes (Millon, 1983). From a psychometric perspective, the MCMI-II offers the best of both worlds: an inventory founded in a practical, clinically useful theory as well as rigorous empirical development. The clinical scales of the MCMI-II are listed below:

Schizoid; Avoidant; Antisocial; Narcissism; Passive–aggressive; Compulsive; Dependent; Histrionic; Schizotypal; Borderline; Sadistic; Paranoid; Anxiety; Somatoform; Hypomania; Dysthymia; Alcohol abuse; Drug abuse; Psychotic thinking; Psychotic depression; Psychotic delusions.

Millon Clinical Multiaxial Inventory—III

While the MCMI-II is still in use, Millon has published an even more current version of the MCMI, the Millon Clinical Multiaxial Inventory—III (MCMI-III) (Millon, Millon, Davis, & Grossman, 2009). The MCMI-III still contains 175 items but 95 were changed or reworded from the MCMI-II. The MCMI-III has been updated into a 4th edition. The updated MCMI-III scales are as follows:

There exist *14 Personality Disorder Scales* that are coordinated with the *DSM-IV* Axis II disorders:

1—Schizoid
2A—Avoidant
2B—Depressive
3—Dependent
4—Histrionic
5—Narcissistic
6A—Antisocial
6B—Sadistic (Aggressive)
7—Compulsive
8A—Negativistic (Passive-Aggressive)
8B—Masochistic (Self-Defeating)
S—Schizotypal
C—Borderline
P—Paranoid

In addition there are ten Clinical Syndrome Scales:

A—Anxiety
H—Somatoform
N—Bipolar: Manic
D—Dysthymia
B—Alcohol Dependence
T—Drug Dependence
R—Posttraumatic Stress Disorder
SS—Thought Disorder
CC—Major Depression
PP—Delusional Disorder

There are also five scales that serve to detect response patterns that might call into question the test results:
Modifying Indices

X—Disclosure
Y—Desirability
Z—Debasement

Random Response Indicators

V—Invalidity
W—Inconsistency

Lastly, there are 42 subscales that serve to give the clinician insight into the psychological processes that undergird clinically significant elevations. These are the Grossman Facet Scales.

Common Grief Response Questionnaire

The Common Grief Response Questionnaire (CGQ) (McNeil, 1996) consists of 86 self-report items using a 7-point Likert response scale. The purpose of the CGQ is to assess the frequency of occurrence of numerous grief reactions to the death of a loved one.

Impact of Events Scale—Revised

The Impact of Events Scale—Revised (IES-R) (Weiss & Marmar, 1993) is a revision of the original IES. The IES-R consists of 22 self-report items purported to assess posttraumatic stress. Three response dimensions are tapped: intrusive ideation, avoidance and numbing, as well as hyper-arousal. The IES-R takes about 10 min to complete and is a widely used research tool.

Penn Inventory for Posttraumatic Stress Disorder (PENN)

Similar to the IES-R, the PENN (Hammarberg, 1992) is a measure of posttraumatic symptoms. It is, however, is a more global measure, consisting of 26 self-report items.

Stanford Acute Stress Reaction Questionnaire

The Stanford Acute Stress Reaction Questionnaire (SASRQ) (Cardena & Spiegel, 1993; Shalev, Peri, Canetti, & Schreiber, 1996) consists of 30 self-report items that assess acute stress disorder. The scale takes 5–10 min to complete and appears to be useful in predicting PTSD.

Taylor Manifest Anxiety Scale

The Taylor Manifest Anxiety Scale (TAS) (Taylor, 1953), unlike the inventories previously described, measures only one trait—anxiety. Its 50 items are derived from the MMPI. The TAS measures how generally anxious the patient is and has little ability to reflect situational fluctuations in anxiety.

State–Trait Anxiety Inventory

The State–Trait Anxiety Inventory (STAI) (Spielberger, Gorsuch, & Luchene, 1970) is a highly unique inventory in that it is two scales in one. The first 20 items measure state anxiety (a psychological state is an acute, usually situationally dependent condition of psychological functioning). The second 20 items measure trait anxiety. This is the same basic phenomenon as that measured by the TAS. The STAI can be administered in full form (40 items) or be used to measure only state or trait anxiety.

Affect Adjective Checklist

Another unusual measuring device is the Affect Adjective Checklist (AACL) (Zuckerman, 1960). Like the STAI, the AACL can be used to measure a psychological state or trait by using the same items (21 adjectives) and merely changing the instructions. The client may use the checklist of adjectives to describe how he or she feels in general or under a specific set of conditions—"now" for instance. Zuckerman and Lubin (1965) later expanded the AACL by adding specific items to assess hostility and depression. The more recent (1985) scale is called the Multiple Affect Adjective Checklist (MAACL).

Subjective Stress Scale

The Subjective Stress Scale (SSS) (Berkun, 1962) is designed to measure situational (state) effects of stress on the individual. The scale consists of 14 descriptors that the patient can use to identify his or her subjective reactions during a stressful situation. Each of these descriptors comes with an empirically derived numerical weight, which the clinician then uses to generate a subjective stress score.

Profile of Mood States

The Profile of Mood States (POMS) (McNair, Lorr, & Droppleman, 1971) is a factor-analytically derived self-report inventory that measures six identifiable mood or affective states (p. 5):

> Tension–Anxiety Depression–Dejection Anger–Hostility Vigor–Activity Fatigue–Inertia Confusion–Bewilderment

The POMS consists of 65 adjectives, each followed by a 5-point rating scale that the patient uses to indicate the subjective presence of that condition. The instructions ask the patient to use the 65 adjectives to indicate "How you have been feeling during the past week including today." Other time states have been used, for example: "right now," "today," and for "the past three minutes."

The POMS offers a broader range of state measures for the subjective assessment of stress when compared with the STAI, the AACL-MAACL, and the SSS.

Connor Davidson Resilience Measure

The Connor Davidson Resilience Measure (CD-RISC) (Connor & Davidson, 2003) is a rating scale that assesses resilience. It is composed of 25 items that are rated on a scale of 1–4. Higher scores indicate greater resilience.

Inventory of Complicated Grief Scale

The Inventory of Complicated Grief Scale (Prigerson et al., 1995) is a scale designed to assess symptoms of complicated grief. This scale is designed to assess the complicated bereavement symptoms of depression and anxiety that predict long-term functional impairments. The scale consists of 22 items corresponding to the cognitive, emotional, and behavioral states that are associated with complicated grief. Each of the items is rated on a scale of 1–4, depending on how frequently they experience each of the states.

Generalized Anxiety Disorder Questionnaire

The Generalized Anxiety Disorder Questionnaire (GADQ-IV) (Newman et al., 2002) is a self-report questionnaire that has items that are reflective of the DSM-IV's criteria for Generalized Anxiety Disorder. Most of the items are dichotomous and ask the respondent to give yes/no answers, one item is left open ended and two items utilize a rating scale from one (meaning no distress) to eight (meaning severe distress) to assess distress and impairment.

Beck Anxiety Inventory

The Beck Anxiety Inventory (BAI) (Beck & Steer, 1990) is a widely used 21 item self-report symptom inventory that is used to assess anxiety in adolescents and adults. The items reflect symptoms of anxiety and the respondents are asked to rate them on a scale of 0 (not experiencing symptoms at all) to 3 (severe symptoms). This can be used as a screening or diagnostic tool for Generalized Anxiety Disorder. It can also be used to assess treatment progress.

Symptom Checklist-90 Revised

The Symptoms Checklist 90 (SCL-90-R) (Derogatis, 1994) is a self-report measure assessing symptoms of psychopathology on nine different dimensions and three global indices. The dimensions include anxiety, obsessive-compulsive disorder, phobic anxiety, and paranoid ideation. The SCL-90 consists of 90 items and takes approximately 12–15 min to administer. There is also a shorter form called the Brief Symptom Inventory (BSI; Derogatis, 1993) that is composed of 53 items and provides scores on the same dimensions and global indices as the SCL-90. These tools can both be used to determine treatment progress or treatment outcome.

Screen for Posttraumatic Stress Symptoms

The Screen for Posttraumatic Stress Symptoms (SPTSS) (Carlson, 2001) is a 17-item self-report inventory that assesses the symptoms of PTSD listed in the DSM-IV. Respondents rate each of the items on an 11-point scale indicating frequency of symptoms from 0 (never) to 10 (always). This is recommended for screening of PTSD in both research and clinical settings.

Inventory of Psychosocial Functioning

The Inventory of Psychosocial Functioning is an 87-item self-report measure that assesses functional impairment experienced by active-duty service members and veterans over the past 30 days on a 7-point scale ranging from 1 ("never") to 7 ("always"). The IPF provides a total score for each of seven subscales (romantic relationships with a spouse or partner, family relationships, work, friendships and socializing, parenting, education, and day-today functioning), and an overall functional impairment score is computed by calculating the mean of the scores for each completed subscale. In a sample of veterans meeting diagnostic criteria for PTSD, their overall mean score on the IPF was 3.86 (SD = 1.06) (Castro, Hayes, & Keane, 2011).

The Assessment of Coping

The Millon Behavioral Health Inventory (MBHI) (Millon, Green, & Meagher, 1982) assesses the patient's characterological coping style. The Hassles Scale measures an indirect form of coping within its "uplifts" subscale. Everly created a simple coping inventory for use in conjunction with the National Health Fair (Everly, 1979a; Girdano & Everly, 1986). This checklist can be found in Appendix H.

Finally, perhaps the most popular of the coping indices is the Ways of Coping Checklist developed by Lazarus and Folkman (1984). This 67-item checklist that assesses an individual's preference for various styles of coping patterns (e.g., defensive coping, information seeking, problem solving) enjoys a considerable empirical foundation and can be found in their 1984 textbook on stress, appraisal, and coping.

In the broadest sense, coping may be viewed as any effort to reduce or mitigate the aversive effects of stress. These efforts may be psychological or behavioral. The scales mentioned sample both domains.

Law of Initial Values

A final point should be made regarding the role of individual differences in the process of measurement. No two patients are exactly alike in their manifestations of the stress response. When measuring psychophysiological reactivity, or any physiological index, the clinician must understand that the patient's baseline level of functioning on any physiological variable affects any subsequent degree of activity or reactivity in that same physiological parameter. This is Wilder's Law of Initial Values (Wilder, 1950). In order to compare an individual's stress reactivity (assuming variant baselines), a statistical correction must be made in order to assure that the correlation between baseline activity and stressful reactivity is equal to zero. Such a correction must be made in order to compare groups as well. Benjamin (1963) has written a very useful paper that addresses the necessary statistical corrections that must be made. She concludes that a covariance model must be adopted in order to correct for the law of initial values, though specific calculations will differ when comparing groups or individuals.[1] It must be remembered that the Law of Initial Values will affect not only the measurement of stress arousal but also stress reduction.

Summary

In this chapter we have described briefly some of the most commonly used methods of measuring the effects of the stress response. The methods described have included physiological and psychological criteria.

---

[1] One useful formula for correcting for the Law of Initial Values when comparing individuals is the Autonomic Lability Score (ALS; Lacey & Lacey, 1962). The ALS, a form of covariance and therefore consistent with Benjamin's recommendation, is expressed as

$$ALS = 50 + 10 \left[\frac{y_z - x_{z r_{xy}}}{\left(1 - r^{2xy^{0.5}}\right)} \right]$$

where X_z = client's standardized prestressor autonomic level, Y_z = client's standardized poststressor autonomic level, and r_{xy} = correlation for sample between pre- and poststressor levels.

The most important question surrounding the measurement of the stress response is "How do you select the most appropriate measurement criterion?" The answer to this question is in no way clear-cut. Generally speaking, to begin with you should consider the state versus trait measurement criterion issue. Basically, state criteria should be used to measure immediate and/or short-lived phenomena. Trait criteria should be used to measure phenomena that take a longer term to manifest themselves and/or have greater stability and duration. The psychological criteria discussed in this chapter are fairly straightforward as to their state or trait nature. The physiological criteria are somewhat less clear. Some physiological criteria possess both state and trait characteristics. Furthermore, normal values for blood and urinary stress indicators may vary somewhat from lab to lab. Therefore, the clinician should familiarize him- or herself with the lab's standard values. Before using physiological measurement criteria in the assessment of the stress response, the reader who has no background in physiology would benefit from consulting any useful physiology or psychophysiology text (see, e.g., Everly & Sobelman, 1987; Greenfield & Sternbach, 1972; Levi, 1975; Selye, 1976; Stern, Ray, & Davis, 1980). Finally, because no two patients are alike in their response to stressors, the clinician might consider measuring multiple and diverse response mechanisms (or stress axes) in order to increase the sensitivity of any given assessment procedure designed to measure the stress response (see Fig. 5.1).

Having provided these closing points, let us review the major issues discussed within this chapter:

1. It has been argued that the single most important aspect of empirical investigation is the process of the *measurement* of relevant variables. This is true of investigations into the nature of human stress as well.
2. The Social Readjustment Rating Scale (Holmes & Rahe, 1967), the Life Experiences Survey (Sarason et al., 1978), and the Hassles Scale (Kanner et al., 1981) are all self-report inventories that assess the patient's exposure to critical "life events." Collectively, these scales do not measure stress; rather, they assess the patient's exposure to stressors. Stressor scales are correlated with stress arousal because the physiology of adaptation to novel or challenging stimuli is also the physiology of the stress response.
3. The Derogatis Stress Scale (Derogatis, 1980) and the Millon Behavioral Health Inventory (Millon, et al., 1982) represent scales designed to assess the patient's cognitive–affective status. The stress response is thus assessed indirectly through the measurement of cognitive–affective states known to be highly associated with stress arousal. It has been argued that such assessments may well be the most efficient, practical, and cost-effective way of assessing stress arousal. All of these scales also include symptom indices.
4. Albeit an important clinical phenomenon, the assessment of propensities for limbic efferent discharge (limbic hypersensitivity phenomenon) is extremely difficult. Subcortical electroencephalography is a crude measure at best. Electrodermal and general psychophysiological reactivity may be the best options currently available for the assessment of neurological triggering mechanisms of the human stress response.

5. Numerous measurement options exist for the assessment of the physiological stress response itself (if deemed appropriate).

   (a) The neural stress axes may be assessed via electrodermal measures, electromyographic measures, as well as cardiovascular measures (heart rate, peripheral blood flow, blood pressures).
   (b) The neuroendocrine stress axis can be measured via the assessment adrenal medullary catecholamines.
   (c) The assessment of the endocrine stress axes is most commonly conducted via the assessment of cortisol.

6. The assessment of target-organ effects of pathogenic stress arousal can be conducted via standard physical medicine examination or the use of self-report inventories such as the Seriousness of Illness Rating Scale (Wyler et al., 1968) to measure *physical effects. Psychological effects* may be assessed via self-report scales such as the MMPI, the MCMI, the 16-PF, IES-R, PENN, SASRQ, CGO, the TAS, the STAI, the AACL, the SSS, and the POMS.

7. Coping is an important potential mediating variable. It may be assessed via the MBHI; the Hassles Scale, a coping scale developed by Everly (1979a) for the US Public Health Service; or the Ways of Coping Checklist (Lazarus & Folkman, 1984).

References

Alexander, A. B. (1975). An experimental test of the assumptions relating to the use of EMG: biofeedback as a general relaxation training technique. *Psychophysiology, 12,* 656–662.

Anderson, B., Hovmoller, S., Karlsson, C., & Svensson, S. (1974). Analysis of urinary catecholarnines. *Clinica Chimica Acta, 51,* 13–28.

Andreassi, J. (1980). Psychophysiology. New York: Oxford University Press.

Arnarson, E., & Sheffield, B. (1980, March). *The generalization of the effects of EMG and temperature biofeedback.* Paper presented at the Annual Meeting of the Biofeedback Society of America, Colorado Springs, CO.

Beck, A. T., & Steer, R. A. (1990). Manual for the Beck anxiety inventory. San Antonio, TX: Psychological Corporation.

Benjamin, L. (1963). Statistical treatment of the law of the initial values in autonomic research. *Psychosomatic Medicine, 25,* 556–566.

Berkun, M. (1962). Experimental studies of psychological stress in man. *Psychological Monographs, 76* (Whole No. 534).

Bio-Science. (1982). *Bio-Science handbook.* Van Nuys, CA: Author.

Budzynski, T. (1979, November). *Biofeedback and stress management.* Paper presented at the Johns Hopkins Conference on Clinical Biofeedback, Baltimore, MD.

Budzynski, T., & Stoyva, J. (1969). An instrument for producing deep muscle relaxation by means of analog information feedback. *Journal of Applied Behavioral Analysis, 2,* 231–237.

Butcher, J. N., Dahlstrom, W. G., Graham, J. R., Tellegren, A., & Kaemmer, B. (1989). *Manual for the restandardized Minnesota Multiphasic Personality Inventory: MMPI-2. An administrative and interpretive guide.* Minneapolis: University of Minnesota Press.

Cardena, E., & Spiegel, D. (1993). Dissociative reactions to the Bay Area Earthquake. *The American Journal of Psychiatry, 150,* 474–478.

Carlson, E. B. (2001). Psychometric study of a brief screen for PTSD: Assessing the impact of multiple traumatic events. *Assessment, 8*(4), 431–441.

Castro, F., Hayes, J. P., & Keane, T. M. (2011). Issues in assessment of PTSD within the military culture. In B. A. Moore & W. E. Penk (Eds.), *Treating PTSD in military personnel. A clinical handbook* (pp. 23–41). New York, NY: Guilford.

Cattell, R. B. (1972). *The sixteen personality factor.* Champaign, IL: Institute for Personality and Ability Testing.

Cattell, R. B., & Scheier, I. (1961). *The meaning and measurement of neuroticism and anxiety.* New York, NY: Ronald Press.

Cohen, J. (1984). The benefits of meta-analysis. In J. Williams & R. Spitzer (Eds.), *Psychotherapy research* (pp. 332–339). New York, NY: Guilford.

Connor, K. M., & Davidson, J. R. T. (2003). Development of a new resilience scale: The Connor-Davidson Resilience Scale (DC-RISC). *Depression and Anxiety, 18*(2), 76–82.

Damon Corporation. (1981). *Evaluation of adrenocortical function.* Needham Heights, MA: Author.

Derogatis, L. (1977). *The SCL-90-R: Administration, scoring and procedures manual 1.* Baltimore, MA: Clinical Psychometric Research.

Derogatis, L. (1980). *The Derogatis stress profile.* Baltimore, MA: Clinical Psychometric Research.

Derogatis, L. R. (1993). *Brief Symptom Inventory (BSI): Administration, scoring, and procedures manual.* Minneapolis, MN: National Computer Systems.

Derogatis, L. R. (1994). *SCL-90-R: Symptom Checklist-90-R: Administration, Scoring & Procedures Manual* (3rd ed.). Minneapolis, MN: National Computer Systems.

Donaldson, S., Donaldson, M., & Snelling, L. (2003). SEMG Evaluations: An overview. *Applied Psychophysiology and Biofeedback, 28*(2), 121–127.

Edelberg, R. (1972). Electrical activity of the skin. In N. Greenfield & R. Sternbach (Eds.), Handbook of Psychophysiology (pp. 367–418). New York: Holt, Rinehart & Winston.

Euler, U. S. V., & Lishajko, F. (1961). Improved techniques for the fluorimetric estimation of catecholamines. *Acta Physiologica Scandinavia, 51,* 348–355.

Everly, G. S., Jr. (1979a). *Strategies for coping with stress: An assessment scale.* Washington, DC: Office of Health Promotion, Department of Health and Human Services.

Everly, G. S., Jr., Davy, J. A., Smith, K. J., Lating, J. M., & Nucifora, F. C., Jr. (2011). A defining aspect of human resilience in the workplace: A structural modeling approach. *Disaster Medicine and Public Health Preparedness, 5*(2), 98–105.

Everly, G. S., Jr., & Sobelman, S. H. (1987). *The assessment of the human stress response: Neurological, biochemical, and psychological foundations.* New York, NY: American Management Systems Press.

Everly, G. S., Jr., Welzant, V., Machado, P. & Miller, K. (1989). *The correlation between frontalis muscle tension and sympathetic nervous system activity.* Unpublished research report.

Field, T. (2009). *Complementary and alternative therapies research.* Washington, DC: American Psychological Association.

Fiske, D. W. (1983). The meta-analysis revolution in outcome research. *Journal of Consulting and Clinical Psychology, 51,* 65–70.

Freedman, R., & Papsdorf, J. (1976). *Generalization of frontal EMG biofeedback training to other muscles.* Paper presented to the 7th Annual Meeting of the Biofeedback Society, Colorado Springs.

Gellhorn, E. (1964a). Motion and emotion. *Psychological Review, 71,* 457–472.

Gellhorn, E., & Loofburrow, G. (1963). *Emotions and emotional disorders.* New York, NY: Harper & Row.

Girdano, D. A., & Everly, G. S., Jr. (1986). *Controlling stress and tension* (2nd ed.). Englewood Cliffs, NJ: Prentice-Hall.

Glaus, K., & Kotses, H. (1977). *Generalization of conditioned frontalis tension.* Paper presented to the 8th Annual Meeting of the Biofeedback Society. Orlando, FL.

Glaus, K., & Kotses, H. (1978). *Generalization of conditioned frontalis tension: a closer look.* Paper presented to the 9th Annual Meeting of the Biofeedback Society. Albuquerque, NM.

Greenfield, N., & Sternbach, R. (1972). *Handbook of psychophysiology.* New York, NY: Holt, Rinehart & Winston.

Hall, J. E. (2011). *Guyton and Hall Textbook of Medical Physiology* (12th ed.). Philadelphia, PA: Saunders Elsevier.

Hammarberg, M. (1992). Penn Inventory for posttraumatic stress disorder: Psychometric properties. *Psychological Assessment, 4,* 67–76.

Hegstrand, L. R., & Eichelman, B. (1981). Determination of rat brain tissue catecholamines using liquid chromatography with electrochemical detection. *Journal of Chromatography, 22,* 107–111.

Holmes, T. H., & Rahe, R. (1967). The social readjustment rating scale. *Journal of Psychosomatic Research, 11,* 213–218.

Ide, B. A. (1996). Psychometric review of family disruption from Illness Scale. In B. H. Stamm (Ed.), *Measurement of stress trauma, and adaptation.* Lutherville, MD: Sidran Press.

Jacobs, D. S., Demott, W., Finly, P., Horvat, R., Kasten, B., & Tilzer, L. (1994). *Laboratory test handbook* (3rd ed.). Cleveland: Lexi-Comp.

Jacobson, E. (1929). *Progressive relaxation.* Chicago, IL: University of Chicago Press.

Jacobson, E. (1970). *Modern treatment of tense patients.* Springfield, IL: Charles C. Thomas.

Janoff-Bulman, R. (1996). Psychometric review of World Assumption Scale. In B. H. Stamm (Ed.), *Measurement of stress, trauma, and adaptation.* Lutherville, MD: Sidran Press.

Kanner, A. D., Coyne, J. C., Schaefer, C., & Lazarus, R. S. (1981). Comparison of two modes of stress measurement: Daily hassles and uplifts versus major life events. *Journal of Behavioral Medicine, 4,* 1–39.

Katzung, B. G. (1992). *Basic and clinical Pharmacology* (5th ed.). Norwalk, CT: Lange.

Lacey, J., & Lacey, B. (1962). The law of initial value in the longitudinal study of autonomic constitution. *Annals of the New York Academy of Sciences, 98,* 1257–1290.

Lake, C. R., Ziegler, M., & Kopin, L. (1976). Use of plasma norepinephrine for evaluation of sympathetic neuronal function in man. *Life Sciences, 18,* 1315–1326.

Lazarus, R. S., & Folkman, S. (1984). *Stress, appraisal, and coping.* New York: Springer.

Levi, L. (1975). *Emotions: Their parameters and measurement.* New York: Raven Press.

Malmo, R. B. (1966). Studies of anxiety. In C. Spielberger (Ed.), *Anxiety and behavior* (pp. 157–177). New York: Academic Press.

Malmo, R. B. (1975). *On emotions, needs, and our archaic brain.* New York: Holt, Rinehart & Winston.

Mason, J. W. (1972). Organization of psychoendocrine mechanisms: A review and reconsideration of research. In N. Greenfield & R. Sternbach (Eds.), *Handbook of psychophysiology* (pp. 3–76). New York: Holt, Rinehart & Winston.

McClelland, D. C., Ross, G., & Patel, V. (1985). The effect of an academic examination on salivary norepinephrine and immunoglobulin levels. *Journal of Human Stress, 11,* 52–59.

McNair, D., Lorr, M., & Droppleman, L. (1971). *Profile of mood states manual.* San Diego: Educational and Industrial Testing Service.

McNeil, F. (1996). Psychometric review of Common Grief Response Questionnaire. In B. H. Stamm (Ed.). *Measurement of stress, trauma, and adaptaion.* Lutherville, Maryland; Sidran Press.

Miehlke, A. (1973). *Surgery of the facial nerve.* Philadelphia: Saunders.

Miller, L., & Smith, A. (1982). *The Stress Audit Questionnaire.* Boston: Neuromedical Consultants.

Millon, T. (1981). *Disorders of personality: DSM-III, Axis II.* New York: Wiley.

Millon, T. (1983). *Millon Clinical Multiaxial Inventory manual* (3rd ed.). Minneapolis: National Computer Systems.

Millon, T., Green, C. J., & Meagher, R. B. (1982). *Millon Behavioral Health Inventory manual* (3rd ed.). Minneapolis: National Computer Systems.

Millon, T., Millon, C., Davis, R., & Grossman, S. (2009). *Millon Clinical Multiaxial Inventory–III manual* (4th ed.). Minneapolis, MN: National Computer Systems.

Monroe, S. (1983). Major and minor life events as predictors of psychological distress. *Journal of Behavioral Medicine, 6,* 189–206.

Newman, M. G., Zuellig, A. R., Kachin, K. E., Constantino, M. J., Przeworski, A., Erickson, T., & Cashman-McGrath, L. (2002). Preliminary reliability and validity of the Generalized Anxiety Disorder Questionnaire-IV: A revised self-report diagnostic measure of generalized anxiety disorder. *Behavior Therapy, 33*(2), 215–233.

Nucifora, F., Hall, R., & Everly, G. S., Jr., (2011). Reexamining the role of the traumatic stressor and the trajectory of posttraumatic distress in thewake of disaster. *Disaster Medicine and Public Health Preparednes,s . 5 (supp.2):* S172–175.

Prigerson, H. G., Maciejewski, P. K., Reynolds III, C. F., Bierhals, A. J., Newsom, J. T., Fasiczka, A., Miller, M. (1995). Inventory of complicated grief: A scale to measure maladaptive symptoms of loss. *Psychiatric Research, 59*(1–2), 65–79.

Peek, C. J. (2003). A primer of biofeedback instrumentation. In M. S. Schwartz, F. Andrasik (Eds.), *Biofeedback: A Practitioner's Guide* (pp.43-87). New York: Guilford.

Rosenberg, S., Hayes, J., & Peterson, R. (1987). Revising the Seriousness of Illness Rating Scale. *International Journal of Psychiatry in Medicine, 17*, 85–92.

Rubin, L. R. (1977). *Reanimation of the paralyzed face.* St. Louis, MD: Mosby.

Sarason, I., Johnson, J., & Siegel, J. (1978). Assessing the impact of life changes. *Journal of Consulting and Clinical Psychology, 46*, 932–946.

Schwartz, M. S., & Andrasik, F. (2003). *Biofeedback: A practitioner's guide* (3rd ed.). New York: Guilford.

Schwartz, G., Fair, P., Mandel, M., Salt, P., Mieske, M., & Klerman, G. (1978). Facial electromyography in the assessment of improvement in depression. *Psychosomatic Medicine, 40*, 355–360.

Selye, H. (1976). *Stress in health and disease.* Boston: Butterworth.

Shagass, C., & Malmo, R. (1954). Psychodynamic themes and localized muscular tension during psychotherapy. *Psychosomatic Medicine, 16*, 295–313.

Shalev, A., Peri, T., Canetti, L., & Schreiber, S. (1996). Predictors of PTSD in injured survivors of trauma: A prospective study. *American Journal of Psychiatry, 153*, 219–225.

Smith, M. L., Glass, G. V., & Miller, T. I. (1980). *The benefits of psychotherapy.* Baltimore: Johns Hopkins University Press.

Spielberger, C. D., Gorsuch, R., & Luchene, R. (1970). *The STAI manual.* Palo Alto, CA: Consulting Psychologists Press.

Stamm, B. H. (1996). *Measurement of stress, trauma, and adaptation.* Lutherville, MD: Sidran Press.

Stern, R., Ray, W., & Davis, C. (1980). *Psychophysiological recording.* New York: Oxford University Press.

Stoyva, J. M. (1979). Musculoskeletal and stress-related disorders. In O. Pomerleau & J. Brady (Eds.), *Behavioral medicine* (pp. 155–176). Baltimore: Williams & Wilkins.

Taylor, J. (1953). A scale for manifest anxiety. *Journal of Abnormal and Social Psychology, 45*, 285–290.

UCLA Laboratory for Stress Assessment and Research. (n.d.). Stress and adversity Invetory (STRAIN). Retreived from: http://www.uclastresslab.org/products/strain–stress-and-adversity-inventory

Weil, J. (1974). *A neurophysiological model of emotional and intentional behavior.* Springfield, IL: Charles C. Thomas.

Weiss, D., & Marmar, C. (October, 1993). *The impact of debriefings on emergency services personnel workers: Effects of site and service.* San Antonio, Texas: International Society for Traumatic Stress Studies Annual Meeting.

Wilder, J. (1950). The law of initial values. *Psychosomatic Medicine, 12*, 392–401.

Wolfe, J., & Kimerling, R. (1998). Assessment of PTSD and gender. In J. Wilson & T. M. Keene (Eds.), *Assessing psychological trauma and PTSD.* New York: Plenum.

Wyler, R. A., Masuda, M., & Holmes, T. H. (1968). Seriousness of illness rating scale. *Journal of Psychosomatic Research, 11*, 363–374.

Zuckerman, M. (1960). The development of an affect adjective checklist for the measurement of anxiety. *Journal of Consulting Psychology, 24*, 457–462.

Zuckerman, M., & Lubin, B. (1965). *Manual for the Multiple Affect Adjective Checklist.* San Diego: Educational and Industrial Testing Service.

Chapter 6
Personologic Diathesis and Human Stress

Where malignant disease is concerned it may be more important to understand what kind of patient has the disease rather than what kind of disease the patient has.

Sir William Osler, M.D.

Recall from Chap. 2 that the manner in which an individual chooses to perceive and interpret his or her environment (cognitive interpretation) serves as the single most important determinant of whether the stress response will be elicited in response to a psychosocial stressor. We may then argue that the *consistent* manner in which an individual perceives and interprets the environment, in addition to the aggregation of consistent attitudes, values, and behavior patterns, serves as an operational definition of the construct of "personality." If we accept such a proposition, it becomes reasonable to assume that there may well exist individuals whose consistent personality traits, including cognitive interpretations regarding their environment, may predispose them to excessive elicitation of the stress response and, therefore, increased risk of stress-related disease. Such personality-based predispositions for stress may exist in the form of personologic diatheses, such as cognitive distortions, persistent irrational expectations, "ego" vulnerabilities, and/or consistent stress-producing overt behavior patterns.

If indeed one's personologic idiosyncrasies can predispose to excessive stress arousal, it behooves the clinician to familiarize him or herself with the common manifestations of such personologic predispositions. Investigations into such relationships between personality factors and stress arousal have typically taken one of two perspectives.

1. Historically, investigations into the relation between personality and stress have focused upon highly *specific* personality traits that appear to predispose individuals to highly *specific* diseases, without consideration of the global personality structure within which those traits reside (Alexander, 1950; Dunbar, 1935).

G.S. Everly and J.M. Lating, *A Clinical Guide to the Treatment of the Human Stress Response*, DOI 10.1007/978-1-4614-5538-7_6, © Springer Science+Business Media New York 2013

2. Investigations have pursued the proposition that there exist consistent, personality-based predispositions, that is, "vulnerabilities" unique to and inherent within each and every basic personality pattern (Millon, 1996; Millon, Crossman, Meagher, Millon, & Everly, 1999). Collectively, these characterological susceptibilities serve as a form of Achilles' heel, referred to here as *a personologic diathesis,* serving, under the right set of circumstances, to predispose one to the elicitation of the stress response and a host of subsequent stress-related disorders (Everly, 1987; Frances, 1982; Millon & Everly, 1985). These characterological susceptibilities may exist in the form of "ego" vulnerabilities, consistent cognitive distortions, expectations, and repeated stress-producing behaviors. Such an approach tends not to focus on specific traits and their association with specific diseases, but rather sees each different personality style or pattern as possessing a personologic diathesis consisting of an aggregation of personality-based susceptibilities to stress. Let us pursue these notions further.

Historical Foundations

When one first thinks of the relation between personality and stress, the Type A coronary-prone behavior pattern invariably comes to mind (Friedman & Rosenman, 1974). Yet the search for the stress-prone personality far predates the discovery of the Type A pattern.

The work of Dunbar (1935) represents one of the earliest and most noteworthy efforts at formulating psychosomatic theory based upon personality profiles. Dunbar described various personality profiles that seemed to be predisposed to specific stress-related diseases. For example, from her perspective, the hypertensive patient could be seen as characterologically shy, reserved, rigid, yet possessing the propensity for "Volcanic eruptions of feelings." The migraine patient, on the other hand, could be seen as perfectionistic and overachievement oriented.

As noted earlier in this volume, the conflict theory of French and Alexander (Alexander, 1950) argued that persons prone to repeated characterological conflicts are prone to specific stress-related disorders.

In addition to the work of Dunbar and Alexander, there were other early contributions from the analytically oriented theorists, yet early interest waned, with rather low reliability among the findings of the various theorists. Similarly, even reliable findings contributed only minimal variation to the overall disease process. Thus, research into the relationship between personality and disease significantly diminished for over a decade until interest was rekindled by cardiologists Friedman and Rosenman (1974) in their investigations into the Type A coronary-prone behavior pattern.

Friedman (1969) described the Type A pattern as a characteristic "action—emotion complex" exhibited by individuals engaged in a chronic struggle to "obtain an unlimited number of poorly defined things from their environment in the shortest period of time." Originally, the Type A pattern was believed to constitute chronic time urgency, competitiveness, polyphasic behavior, and poorly planned, often impulsive behavior (Friedman & Rosenman, 1974). The Type A pattern has also been described as consisting of primary traits of time urgency, hostility, ambition, and immoderation. Friedman and Rosenman also described secondary traits of impatience, aggression, competitiveness, and denial.

The original search for the Type A pattern was, indeed, a search for a consistent behavior pattern that predisposed to premature coronary artery disease. When diagnosed via the standardized structured interview technique, the Type A pattern has consistently shown a relation with coronary artery disease (see Powell, 1984; Shepherd & Weiss, 1987; Williams, 1984; Williams et al., 1980). Major investigations that have failed to uncover a relationship between coronary heart disease and the Type A pattern have generally used techniques other than the structured interview to assess the pattern (Everly & Sobelman, 1987; Shepherd & Weiss). The use of diverse measurement technologies may have inadvertently added to the confusion surrounding the nature of the Type A pattern (Everly & Sobelman). Indeed, the pursuit of the Type A pattern has taken on a life of its own, so much so that individuals invariably ask if there is such a thing as a "good" Type A pattern. By definition, the answer to such a question must be "no," if one only remembers that the original quest for the Type A pattern was actually a search for a behavior pattern that predisposes to premature coronary heart disease. Considering this point, how could there be a "good" Type A?

The relation between Type A behavior and coronary heart disease has prompted researchers to conduct various components analyses in search of the pathogenic core of the Type A pattern (Powell, 1984; Williams, 1984; Williams et al., 1980). Such endeavors have uncovered myriad Type A constituents that serve to clarify further the nature of the pattern.

Figure 6.1 represents an integration of findings reported as part of the "second generation" of Type A research designed to better understand the constituents of coronary-prone behavior (Powell, 1984; Williams, 1984, 1986; Williams et al., 1980). It portrays a deeply rooted personologic insecurity as the foundation of the Type A pattern. That characterological insecurity is thought to give rise to an extraordinary need for power and achievement, perhaps as a means of compensating for or contradicting the feelings of insecurity. Power and achievement are related to control, and it has been found that Type A individuals possess not only high achievement motives but also an extraordinary need for control. The need for control and the fear of the loss of control may then account for the observed impatience, time urgency, polyphasic behavior, competitiveness, and related traits that Type A persons exhibit. Studies by Williams and his colleagues have suggested that chronic hostility and cynicism may be an important psychological factor in the increased coronary risk that Type A individuals exhibit. Dembroski and Costa (1988) reviewed the assessment of the Type A pattern and noted that the "global" Type A pattern is not a good predictor of heart disease, but the hostility component may play a critical pathogenic role.

Research has also shown that Type A individuals exhibit extraordinary physiological reactivity when confronted with a psychosocial challenge.

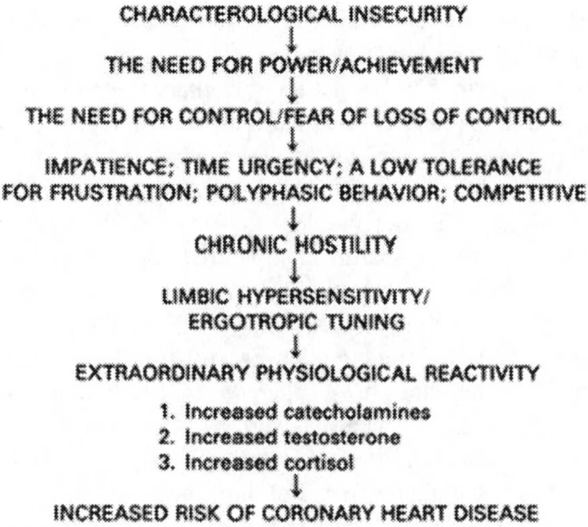

Fig. 6.1 An integrative
model of Type A
characteristics

CHARACTEROLOGICAL INSECURITY
↓
THE NEED FOR POWER/ACHIEVEMENT
↓
THE NEED FOR CONTROL/FEAR OF LOSS OF CONTROL
↓
IMPATIENCE; TIME URGENCY; A LOW TOLERANCE
FOR FRUSTRATION; POLYPHASIC BEHAVIOR; COMPETITIVE
↓
CHRONIC HOSTILITY
↓
LIMBIC HYPERSENSITIVITY/
ERGOTROPIC TUNING
↓
EXTRAORDINARY PHYSIOLOGICAL REACTIVITY

1. Increased catecholamines
2. Increased testosterone
3. Increased cortisol
↓
INCREASED RISK OF CORONARY HEART DISEASE

That reactivity has been shown to be manifest in increased release of catecholamines, testosterone, and cortisol—all well-known atherogenic agents. The physiological reactivity, according to the work of Everly (1985b), may well be based upon some form of limbic system hypersensitivity, or what Gellhorn (1967) has called the "ergotropic tuning phenomenon." Finally, the unusually high levels of circulating catecholamine, cortisol, and testosterone appear to be directly related to the increased risk of coronary artery disease manifested by Type A males. It should be noted that, at rest, the Type A individual manifests no significant differences in catecholamine, testosterone, or cortisol secretion when compared with non-Type A individuals. Only upon psychosocial challenge are the aforementioned differences seen to emerge.

The Type A pattern remains a promising area for continued research into the relationship between personality and disease, especially stress-related disease. It will be recalled that the catecholamines, testosterone, and cortisol are all key stress-responding hormones. The interested reader should refer to Shepherd and Weiss (1987) for an early yet important review.

The next major contribution to the stress and personality phenomenon comes from Suzanne Kobasa, who investigated personality characteristics that seem to act as a buffer between individuals and the pathogenic mechanisms of excessive stress. Her research investigated the domain of "hardiness," that is, characterological factors that appear to mitigate the stress response. Kobasa (1979) and Kobasa & Puccetti (1983) defined hardiness as the aggregation of three factors:

1. Commitment, that is, the tendency to involve oneself in experiences in meaningful ways.
2. Control, that is, the tendency to believe and act as if one has some influence over one's life.
3. Challenge, that is, the belief that change is a positive and normal characteristic of life.

The hardiness research has shown that individuals who demonstrate a commitment to self, family, work, and/or other important values; a sense of control over their lives; and the ability to see life change as an opportunity will experience fewer stress-related diseases/illnesses even though they may find themselves in environments laden with stressor stimuli.

The hardiness construct is indeed a tempting concept to entertain. This formulation has received a serious challenge from Lazarus and Folkman (1984), however, who argue that there is a paucity of systematic studies that examine the relation between antecedent variables and health. Conclusions, they suggest, are typically formulated on the basis of inference with regard to coping mechanisms. They argue that Kobasa's conclusions about hardiness are based on tenuous inferences about coping mechanisms generated through the use of questionable measurement technologies.

It seems clear that factors such as those described in the hardiness research may indeed play an important role in mitigating otherwise pathogenic circumstances. Nevertheless, it may be useful to better operationalize these factors before employing such notions in psychotherapeutic formulations.

No review of historical foundations in personality and stress research would be complete without mentioning the oldest longitudinal research investigation, specifically, the relationship between personality and disease. The Johns Hopkins Precursors Study (see Thomas & McCabe, 1980) seeks to answer the question "Do individuals have distinctive personal characteristics in youth that precede premature disease and death?" The Precursors Study cohort consisted of 1,337 graduates of the Johns Hopkins School of Medicine between the years of 1948 and 1964. Thomas and McCabe investigated, via self-report, consistent "habits of nervous tension" (HNT) and subsequent disease.

> Compared with those of the healthy group, the overall HNT patterns were significantly different for the cancer, coronary occlusion, mental illness and suicide groups. ... It therefore appears that youthful reactions to stress as self-reported in a checklist of habits of nervous tension reflect individual psychobiological differences that are linked with future health or disease. (p. 137)

Thus, in the most liberal interpretation of personality, the Precursors Study continues to reveal links between what may be argued to be characterological traits and the subsequent formation of disease.

Indeed, in a meta-analytic investigation in search of the "disease-prone personality," Friedman and Booth-Kewley (1987) reviewed a research base including *Psychological Abstracts* and *Index Medicus*. Focusing upon psychosomatic disease processes, the authors found 229 studies, of which 101 were ultimately used in the meta-analysis. They conclude: "The results point to the probable existence of a generic 'disease-prone' personality that involves depression, anger/hostility, anxiety, and possibly other aspects of personality" (p. 539).

Let us now turn to a discussion of more recent trends in personality research as it pertains to excessive stress arousal.

The Principle of Personologic Primacy

Should the patient with passive-dependent traits presenting with a stress-induced chronic migraine headache syndrome be treated in the same manner as the patient with histrionic traits and a migraine syndrome of equal severity? Should the patient with avoidant traits and a panic disorder be treated in the same manner as a patient with compulsive traits and a diagnosed panic disorder of equal intensity? A growing body of evidence argues that the answer to both questions is "no" (Millon, Krueger, & Simonsen, 2010; Millon, 2011).

Theoretical (Everly, 1987; Widiger & Frances, 1985; Millon & Davis, 2011), as well as empirical evidence (Kayser, Robinson, Nies, & Howard, 1985; Millon et al., 1999; Strupp, 1980; Taylor & Abrams, 1975) suggests that clinical and subclinical personality patterns may be a uniquely important factor in the diagnosis and treatment of many psychiatric and stress-related disorders. More specifically, the "principle of personologic primacy" as proposed by Everly (1987) denotes that personologic style plays a uniquely important role in the following:

1. The consistent propensity to create psychosocial stressors (via some diathesis).
2. The phenomenological course of psychiatric and stress-related disorders.
3. Diagnostic refinement of major psychiatric syndromes.
4. Psychotherapeutic, as well as psychopharmacological, treatment responsiveness.
5. The long-term prognosis for many psychiatric and stress-related disorders.

The "principle of personologic primacy" further argues that basic personality patterns and their respective hosts of idiosyncratic interpretational predispositions (i.e., personologic diatheses) for stress and other clinical syndromes serve as phenomenological foundations from which major stress-related illnesses and psychiatric syndromes may emerge. Thus, such syndromes are best understood as pathological extensions of potentially malignant personologic undergirdings, for example, consistent cognitive distortions, irrational expectations, "ego" vulnerabilities, unfounded assumptions, and the like (Everly, 1987; Millon & Everly, 1985; Millon et al., 1999; Millon & Davis, 2011). Adverse environmental events, psychoactive drug reactions, and physical and/or psychological trauma may serve as sufficient impetus to cause the personologic substructure to express itself in pathological clinical manifestations such as headaches, panic attacks, and hypertensive and acute tachycardic episodes mediated through the physiological stress response (Chap. 2).

In summary, with regard to stress-related disorders, the "principle of personologic primacy" may be understood as suggesting that (1) a patient's *chronic* propensity to interpret the environment cognitively in such a manner as to engender the stress response with extraordinary frequency is more likely than not to be a function of a personality-based predisposition (diathesis); similarly, (2) a chronic and consistent pattern of elicitation of the stress response is perhaps best viewed more as a manifestation of a dysfunctional characterological predisposition, rather than merely one's exposure to a series of consistently hostile environments. This brings us to the natural corollary of the "principle of personologic primacy": personality-based psychotherapy.

Personologic Psychotherapy and Stress-Related Disorders

If, indeed, we accept personality as playing an important role in the etiology of stress-related disease, then we might logically assume that it must play some role in the treatment of such disease as well. Everly (1987) has introduced the concept of "personologic psychotherapy" as one way of recognizing the role that personality may play in treatment formulation. According to Everly, personologic psychotherapy represents a metatherapeutic approach to the treatment of psychiatric as well as stress-related disorders. More specifically, it is the embodiment of the belief that in most chronic psychiatric and stress-related syndromes, a dysfunctional personologic style supports these syndromes and, therefore, must also become a target for therapeutic intervention, if the chronic nature of the problem is to be addressed. Similarly, the concept of "personologic psychotherapy" embodies the belief that treating only the symptoms of *chronic, recurrent* clinical syndromes may in many cases be analogous to palliatively attending to a clinical veneer while ignoring an important aspect of the etiological malignancy (see also Millon et al., 1999).

The theoretical basis for "personologic psychotherapy" is Millon's biosocial learning theory (Millon, 1988, 1996). It is referred to as a metatherapy because the specific manner in which the personologic dysfunction is treated is left to the discretion of the treating therapist.

With specific attention to stress-related disorders, personologic psychotherapy is broadly interpreted to suggest that in addition to treating the florid symptoms of *chronic* stress-related disorders, it is necessary to direct some aspect of therapeutic effort toward the personologic predispositions (diatheses) that may be serving to sustain the chronic stress-related disorder.

Let us examine one example of how these concepts may be used in treatment planning with a patient who can be said to possess a dependent characterological style while manifesting a chronic and more florid stress-related gastrointestinal (GI) dysfunction. According to the theoretical basis (Millon & Everly, 1985; Millon, 2011), a major sustaining mechanism in a chronically dependent character structure is an extraordinary need for interpersonal affection, affiliation, and support. Such an individual is most vulnerable to chronic stress when this critical need is denied or perhaps only jeopardized. In such a scenario, alleviation of the stress-related GI symptomatology may serve to address only the immediate medical concern. If, indeed, symptom removal has been the only outcome achieved in treatment, then nothing has been done to preclude recurrent GI dysfunction. On the other hand, therapy directed with personologic considerations in mind would certainly consider the potentially self-sustaining mechanisms of extraordinary dependency needs and target the dependent pattern as an additional focus for therapy. Once again, the specific therapeutic technology employed remains at the discretion of the therapist.

The principle of personologic primacy and its therapeutic corollary by no means dictate that formal psychotherapy needs to be conducted in all stress-related disorders. Certainly, there are acute stress-related manifestations that may have little or no etiological basis in personality-related dysfunction. Similarly, "psychotherapeutic" change may well be realized on the basis of therapies not traditionally seen as being "psychotherapeutic" in nature, such as relaxation training and biofeedback therapy (Adler & Morrissey-Adler, 1983; Green & Green, 1983; Murphy & Donovan, 1984). Such therapies commonly yield outcomes such as an improved sense of self-efficacy, a more internal locus of control, improved self-esteem, and what has been called by some a state of "cultivated low arousal" (Adler & Morrissey-Adler; Green & Green; Sarnoff, 1982; Stoyva & Budzynski, 1974).

Millon's Personality Theory and Stress

Preceding sections in this chapter have argued basically two points: (1) that personality type is related to disease, including stress-related disease, and (2) that treatment planning for stress-related diseases should take into consideration the undergirding personality structure if treatment is to be considered complete. It has also been argued that different personalities possess relatively unique characterological "vulnerabilities," or personologic diatheses, which serve as characterological "weak points" for the initiation of pathogenic stress mechanisms should environmental conditions support such development. Yet one factor that has served to limit the progression of the field of research related to personality and stress is the lack of a coherent superordinate theory of personality from which to extend relational investigations. This is in contrast to the traditional search for unique and specific independent personality factors, such as the Type A pattern.

The biosocial learning theory of personality is a theoretically sound but, more important, clinically useful perspective from which to examine the role that personality plays in the initiation and prolongation of the human stress response (Millon, 2011). A comprehensive review of Millon's theory is beyond the scope of this chapter. Interested readers should refer to Millon (2011). A brief description of his basic personality styles will be presented below.

Considering the realm of "normal" personologic styles, Millon (Millon & Everly, 1985) suggests that there exist eight basic and theoretically pure styles. These normal styles are fundamentally adaptive under most circumstances. Yet each one of these styles will be considered to possess, as part of its intrinsic constituency, idiosyncratic "vulnerabilities" or uniqueness that can serve to predispose to excessive stress arousal under the proper set of environmental circumstances.

A brief review of these eight normal styles seems appropriate at this point. We label each of the styles (with one exception) with the traditional diagnostic terms. The reader must keep in mind, however, that although the terms used will be those most commonly associated with personality "disorders," the present discussion refers NOT to personality disorders but to the *"normal"* personologic variants.

The individual with an *aggressive* personality has difficulty trusting others. He or she tends to usurp the rights of others and to be defensively self-centered. Action-oriented and highly independent, the behavioral style of the personality is forceful. The individual often displays intimidating interpersonal conduct and angry affective expressions, yet the self-perception is one of assertiveness. There is a significant need to control and dominate the environment. The basic, sustaining reinforcement pattern is that of negative reinforcement, in which the individual strives to avoid a loss of control, humiliation, and any position or status that is perceived as being inferior.

The individual with a *narcissistic* personality, even in its normal variation, has difficulty postponing gratification. The person is passively independent, and a poised behavioral appearance is usually manifest. Interpersonal conduct is usually seen as being unempathic, and the affective expression may be seen as serene. The self-perception of the narcissist is one of confidence. Narcissistic individuals seem preoccupied with being seen as unique or special. Such persons often resort to creating illusions of extraordinary competence or influence. They usually are so self-absorbed as to be incapable of seeing any point of view other than their own. This lack of empathy often leads to poor interpersonal communications and shallow relationships. The basic reinforcement pattern is that of positive reinforcement, wherein these individuals act to secure for themselves a position of "entitlement."

The *histrionic* personality is driven by a need for approval, affection, affiliation, and support. Histrionic individuals project an animated, sociable, sometimes dramatic, appearance. An exaggerated affective expression is often present. These individuals are often seen as superficial. However, boredom, especially interpersonal boredom, often plagues the person with histrionic traits. With a flair for the drama in life, the histrionic personality moves about searching for approval, yet it seems that this search is never-ending. Thus, these individuals tend to pursue activities that make them the center of attention. The basic sustaining reinforcement pattern is positive, in which support, approval, and affiliation are inherently reinforcing.

The *schizoid* personality style is described as a characterological pattern typified by a passive behavioral appearance and detached, unobtrusive interpersonal conduct, manifesting a rather bland affective expression. The self-perception of the character style is one of placidity. The individual with a schizoid personality style, juxtaposed to the histrionic style, expresses virtually no desire for interpersonal affiliation or support. The classic prototype of the "lone wolf," this individual appears to view interpersonal exchange as a burdensome process. The schizoid seeks isolation as a defense against excess stimulus bombardment and a sense of being overwhelmed. Thus, the reinforcement pattern of the schizoid can be said to be negative.

The *compulsive* personality is a highly respectful personologic style. Driven by the need to behave in a socially acceptable manner, and to avoid making mistakes, individuals with a compulsive personality walk the "straight and narrow." They consistently adhere to foredrawn rules and regulations, ethics and mores. They often appear as rigid and inflexible, tending to suppress emotions and any signs of distress. These people are most comfortable with the concrete things in life. The abstract and ambiguous are to be avoided as sources of distress. Their sustaining pattern of reinforcement is negative; that is, their behavior is driven by the need to avoid making mistakes and being perceived as socially inappropriate.

The *avoidant* personality desires social affiliation and support yet is so afraid of social rejection that social avoidance becomes a way of life. Shy and withdrawing, individuals with an avoidant personality remain extraordinarily sensitive and vigilant to anything that resembles interpersonal rejection. The sustaining pattern of reinforcement appears to be negative, that is, the avoidance of interpersonal rejection and/or humiliation.

The *dependent* personality is driven by the search for support. Unlike the histrionic style, which actively attracts approval and support, the dependent personality acquiesces to gain affection and support. The chronic pattern of submissiveness and passivity often prohibits the natural development of independent skills and autonomous behaviors. The sustaining pattern of reinforcement is dual, that is, both positive and negative reinforcement. The negative reinforcement is revealed as a pattern in which submissiveness "earns" the affection and support of others, thereby, through a negative reinforcement pattern, avoiding the penultimate stressor—rejection, abandonment, and interpersonal isolation.

The *passive–aggressive* personality, in its pure form, is ambivalent. In many ways it represents an adolescent, from a maturational perspective, in an adult's body. The individual with a passive–aggressive personality desires interpersonal independence but lacks the skills required to function in such a manner. This causes the individual to resort to a dependent reinforcement pattern, yet not without considerable dissonance. Such individuals tend to behave aggressively, but lacking the "adult" skills of assertiveness, cannot risk rejection, so they are aggressive in a hidden, cloaked, or "passive" manner. The sustaining reinforcement pattern for these individuals is negative. Their chronic pessimism, negativism, and interpersonal "game playing" seem to provide rewards of some kind, especially when they can see others fail, compromise, or become as negative or cynical about the world as they are. Indeed, perhaps misery does love company. More important, the passive–aggressive manipulation allows the person to avoid a sense of interpersonal impotence and dependence.

These, then, are the theoretically "pure" personologic styles as described by Millon (Millon & Everly, 1985). In reality, it should be noted that most people are combinations of two or three of these styles. Furthermore, to reiterate, each of the aforementioned personality styles can be said to be fundamentally "normal" and *not* to be considered a personality disorder, despite the descriptive labels usually used in conjunction with a personality disorder.

Returning to the issue of the human stress response, the notion of personologic psychotherapy as it pertains to the treatment of stress arousal argues that some degree of therapeutic effort needs to be directed toward the unique qualities and/or sustaining reinforcement patterns of the personality being treated, because it is felt that some idiosyncratic qualities or vulnerabilities may play a significant role in the etiology of chronic stress syndromes. Using Millon's schema, it may be argued that each of the eight basic personality styles possesses its own intrinsic personologic diathesis, that is, factors inherent in the personality that may serve to contribute to extraordinary stress arousal. These factors are listed in Table 6.1. From a clinical perspective, we hope that enumeration of these factors will assist the clinician in (1) understanding how personologic factors may contribute to chronic stress arousal syndromes and (2) targeting psychotherapeutic efforts toward the personologic foundations of excessive stress, that is, the unique vulnerabilities and/or sustaining mechanisms as described in the preceding text or in Table 6.1.

Table 6.1 Personologic diatheses and stress

Personality style	Sustaining reinforcement pattern	Consistent personality factors that contribute to extraordinary arousal
Aggressive	R−	1. Need to exert control of, and to vigilantly monitor, the environment
		2. Being placed in a position of having to rely on, or trust, other individuals
		3. Fear of being taken advantage of and efforts to avoid that
		4. Fear of being humiliated, and efforts to avoid that
		5. Assumption that "only the strong survive"' and the persistent efforts to be "strong"
Narcissistic	R+	1. Inability to postpone gratification
		2. Fear of not being seen as "special"
		3. Need to create illusions of extraordinary competence
		4. Inability to empathize with others, leading to consistently poor communications
		5. Assumption that others will recognize him/her as "special"
Histrionic	R−	1. Interpersonal instability
		2. Fear of a loss of affection
		3. Fear of a loss of support or actual rejection
		4. Frequent changes in life events
		5. Need for interpersonal approval
		6. Belief that he/she must earn, or "perform" for interpersonal affection, approval, and support
Dependent	R−	1. Fear of the loss of interpersonal support
		2. Fear of the loss of affection or of actual rejection
		3. Chronic submissiveness and inability to be assertive when desired
		4. Fear and avoidance of interpersonal confrontation
Passive-aggressive	R−	1. Desire to behave in a manner contrary to previous learning history
		2. Inability to act assertively
		3. Chronic tendency to compare self to others
		4. Chronic negativism
		5. "Successes" of peer group
		6. Actual failure or rejection

(continued)

Table 6.1 (continued)

Personality style	Sustaining reinforcement pattern	Consistent personality factors that contribute to extraordinary arousal
Compulsive	R−	1. Efforts to maintain rigid self-control 2. Change 3. Coping with abstract or ambiguous situations 4. Decision making when options are not clear 5. Unclear directions 6. The "gray areas" of rules and policies 7. Fear of making a mistake 8. Need for, and excessive efforts to, earn approval 9. Fear of social disapproval 10. Belief that emotions should be suppressed 11. Assumption that others share compulsive traits and will act accordingly 12. Waste (e.g., to time, money, effort) 13. Risk taking
Avoidant	R−	1. Interpersonal intrusion 2. Fear of interpersonal rejection 3. Need to remain highly vigilant 4. Lack of interpersonal support 5. Actual rejection 6. Interpersonal hypersensitivity
Schizoid	R−	1. Interpersonal intrusion 2. Lack of interpersonal support 3. Hyperstimulation

Summary

In this chapter, the focus has been upon the role that personality plays in the initiation, prolongation, and ultimate treatment of the human stress response. Let us review the main points:

1. There is a commonly held belief that in the case of *chronic* stress arousal and stress-related diseases, one's personality serves to play a significant role from an etiological, as well as therapeutic, perspective.
2. Historically, investigations have focused upon *specific* personality traits and *specific* disease formation (Alexander, 1950; Dunbar, 1935).
3. More contemporary perspectives have chosen to look within the global personality for characterological vulnerabilities, that is, personologic diathesis, for extraordinary stress arousal and a subsequent host of stress-related diseases (Everly, 1987; Frances, 1982; Millon, 1996).

4. The principle of personologic primacy argues that consistent characterological traits serve to undergird and therefore play a unique role in the patient's propensity to create psychosocial stressors. Such factors play a major role in treatment planning and responsiveness (Everly, 1987; Frances & Hale, 1984) as well.
5. The notion of "personologic psychotherapy" is the natural corollary of the principle of personologic primacy and basically argues that even in chronic stress-related disorders, characterological traits require therapeutic attention and therefore should be considered in treatment planning (Everly, 1987; Millon et al., 1999; Millon, 2011).
6. When attempting to better understand and concretize the role of personologic vulnerabilities as factors that predispose to extraordinary stress arousal, Millon's biosocial learning theory of personality serves as a theoretically cogent and clinically practical framework from which to operate. Table 6.1 describes common personologic factors that serve to contribute to extraordinary stress arousal within each of Millon's basic eight "normal" personality formulations. An understanding of these factors serves to foster a better understanding of *chronic* stress arousal and its subsequent disorders, and to facilitate treatment planning and intervention when one looks beyond the florid symptoms of excessive stress arousal.
7. A final point needs to be reiterated before this chapter is brought to a close. We have indeed attempted to sensitize the reader to the belief that personality traits play an important role in the nature and treatment of the human stress response. That is *not* to say, however, that formal psychotherapy needs to be an integral aspect of all stress treatment/stress management paradigms. Processes such as relaxation training, biofeedback, and even health education practices are clearly capable, in some instances, of altering dysfunctional practices. Yet there are instances where chronic, stress-related diseases are a direct function of personologic disturbances such as dysfunctional self-esteem, persistent cognitive distortions, irrational assumptions, inappropriate expectations of self and others, and so on. In such cases, some concerted psychotherapeutic effort would clearly be indicated. The most effective "mix" of therapeutic technologies (e.g., relaxation training, psychotherapy, hypnosis) remains to be determined by the therapist on a case-by-case basis. It is clearly beyond the scope of this volume to dictate such guidelines.

References

Adler, C., & Morrissey-Adler, S. (1983). Strategies in general psychiatry. In J. Basmajian (Ed.), *Biofeedback* (pp. 239–254). Baltimore, MD: Williams & Wilkins.

Alexander, F. (1950). *Psychosomatic medium*. New York, NY: Norton.

Dembroski, T., & Costa, P. (1988). Assessment of coronary-prone behavior. *Annals of Behavioral Medicine, 10,* 60–63.

Dunbar, H. F. (1935). *Emotions and bodily changes*. New York, NY: Columbia University Press.

Everly, G. S., Jr. (1985b, November). *Biological foundations of psychiatric sequelae in trauma and stress-related "disorders of arousal."* Paper presented to the 8th National Trauma Symposium, Baltimore, MD.

Everly, G. S., Jr. (1987). The principle of personologic primacy. In C. Green (Ed.), *Proceedings of the conference on the Millon Clinical Inventories* (pp. 3–7). Minneapolis, MN: National Computer Systems.

Everly, G. S., Jr., & Sobelman, S. H. (1987). *The assessment of the human stress response: Neurological, biochemical, and psychological foundations.* New York, NY: American Management Systems Press.

Frances, A. (1982). Categorical and dimensional systems of personality diagnosis. *Comprehensive Psychiatry, 23,* 516–527.

Frances, A., & Hale, R. (1984). Determining how a depressed woman's personality affects the choice of treatment. *Hospital and Community Psychiatry, 35,* 883–884.

Friedman, M. (1969). *Pathogenesis of coronary artery disease.* New York, NY: McGraw-Hill.

Friedman, H., & Booth-Kewley, S. (1987). The "disease-prone personality". *American Psychologist, 42,* 539–555.

Friedman, M., & Rosenman, R. (1974). *Type A behavior and your heart.* New York, NY: Knopf.

Gellhorn, E. (1967). *Principles of autonomic-somatic integrations.* Minneapolis, MN: University of Minnesota Press.

Green, E., & Green, A. (1983). General and specific applications of thermal biofeedback. In J. V. Basmajian (Ed.), *Biofeedback* (pp. 211–797). Baltimore, MD: Williams & Wilkins.

Kayser, A., Robinson, D., Nies, A., & Howard, D. (1985). Response to phenelzine among depressed patients with features of hysteroid dysphoria. *American Journal of Psychiatry, 142,* 486–488.

Kobasa, S. (1979). Stressful life events, personality, and health. *Journal of Personality and Social Psychology, 37,* 1–11.

Kobasa, S., & Puccetti, M. (1983). Personality and social resources in stress resistance. *Journal of Personality and Social Psychology, 45,* 839–850.

Lazarus, R. S., & Folkman, S. (1984). *Stress, appraisal, and coping.* New York: Springer.

Millon, T. (1988). Personalogic psychotherapy: Ten commandements for a posteclectic approach to integrative treatment. *Psychotherapy: Theory, Research, Practice, Training, 25*(2), 209–219.

Millon, T. (1996). *Disorders of personality* (2nd ed.). New York: Wiley.

Millon, T. (2011). *Disorders of personality* (3rd ed.). Hoboken, NJ: Wiley.

Millon, T., Crossman, S., Meagher, S., Millon, C., & Everly, G. S., Jr. (1999). *Personality-guided therapy.* New York: Wiley.

Millon, T., & Everly, G. S., Jr. (1985). *Personality and its disorders.* New York: Wiley.

Millon, T., Krueger, R. F., & Simonsen, E. (2010). *Contemporary directions in psychopathology.* NY: Guilford.

Murphy, M., & Donovan, S. (1984). *Contemporary meditation research.* San Francisco: Esalen Institute.

Powell, L. (1984). Type A behavior pattern: An update on conceptual assessment and intervention research. *Behavioral Medicine Update, 6,* 7–10.

Sarnoff, D. (1982). Biofeedback: New uses in counseling. *Personnel and Guidance Journal, 60,* 357–360.

Shepherd, J., & Weiss, S. (Eds.). (1987). Behavioral medicine and cardiovascular disease. *Circulation, 76* (entire Monograph 6).

Stoyva, J. M., & Budzynski, T. H. (1974). Cultivated low-arousal: An anti-stress response? In L. DiCara (Ed.), *Recent advances in limbic and autonomic nervous systems research* (pp. 369–394). New York: Plenum Press.

Strupp, H. H. (1980). Success and failure in time-limited psychotherapy. *Archives of General Psychiatry, 37,* 947–954.

Taylor, M., & Abrams, R. (1975). Acute mania. *Archives of General Psychiatry, 32,* 863–865.

Thomas, C., & McCabe, L. (1980). Precursors of premature disease and death: Habits of nervous tension. *Johns Hopkins Medical Journal, 147*, 137–145.

Widiger, T., & Frances, A. (1985). Axis II personality disorders. *Hospital and Community Psychiatry, 36*, 619–627.

Williams, R. B. (1984). Type A behavior and coronary artery disease. *Behavioral Medicine Update, 6*, 29–33.

Williams, R. B. (1986). Patterns of reactivity and stress. In K. Matthews, R. R. Williams, S. B. Manuck, B. Faulkner, T. Dembroski, T. Detre, & S. M. Weiss (Eds.), *Handbook of stress, reactivity, and cardiovascular disease* (pp. 109–125). New York: Wiley.

Williams, R. B., Haney, T., Lee, K., Kong, Y., Blumenthal, J., & Whalen, R. (1980). Type A behavior, hostility, and artherosclerosis. *Psychosomatic Medicine, 42*, 539–549.

Chapter 7
Resilience: The Final Frontier

The history of stress management has largely been reactive. By that we mean stress management was initially conceived of as a means to manage stress that had become "excessive." More forward thinkers also saw that stress management could be proactive and preventive in nature as the construct evolved. We may be standing at the point in the evolution of the stress management construct where we can see the last iteration, i.e., its "final frontier." From our 57 combined year perspective having watched this field emerge and evolve, we believe the final frontier in the science and practice of stress management is human resilience.

Resilience Defined

Human resilience may be thought of as the ability to positively adapt to and/or rebound from significant adversity and distress. Psychologists have studied resilience for years; however, their primary research foci has been either on studying children who manage to thrive in adversity or on the recovery from traumatic events.

In a review of runaway children who showed remarkable resilience, several factors emerged as protective according to William, Lindsey, Kurtz, and Jarvis (2001). These protective factors include determination and persistence, optimism, orientation to problem solving, ability to find purpose in life, and caring for oneself. According to The Northwest Regional Educational Laboratory, *Fostering Resiliency* [available online: http://www.nwrel.org/pirc/hot9.html], children who develop competence, despite adversity and difficult conditions while growing up, appear to share the following qualities:

1. A sense of self-esteem and self-efficacy
2. An action-oriented approach to obstacles or challenges
3. The ability to see an obstacle as a problem that can be engaged, changed, overcome, or at least endured

G.S. Everly and J.M. Lating, *A Clinical Guide to the Treatment of the Human Stress Response*, DOI 10.1007/978-1-4614-5538-7_7,
© Springer Science+Business Media New York 2013

4. Reasonable persistence, with an ability to know when "enough is enough"
5. Flexible problem solving and stress management tactics

There is now, however, an emerging field of research that focuses on studying resiliency within adults from the perspectives of primary prevention (immunity to distress) as well as secondary prevention (the ability to rebound from debilitation). But given the relative paucity of research on resilience, there has yet to emerge a complete consensus as to the nature of resiliency and how to create it.

(Bonanno (2004), for example, defines resilience as the ability of adults to maintain relatively stable and healthy levels of psychological and physical functioning after having been exposed to potentially disruptive or traumatic events. While the majority of adults will face a traumatic experience at some point in their lives, Bonanno argues that most do not succumb to a traumatic stress disorder. This suggests the existence of a functional resiliency that may not be well understood. Bonanno asserts, "...theorists working in this area have often underestimated or misunderstood resilience, viewing it either as a pathological state or as something seen only in rare and exceptionally healthy individuals" (p. 20). Bonanno suggests that factors such as hardiness, self-enhancement, repressive coping (emotional dissociation), and positive emotions may undergird effective resilience.

Haglund, Cooper, Southwick, and Charney (2007) provide one of the most succinct analyses of the various components of resilience. They identify six primary factors that may protect against and aid in recovery from extreme or traumatic stress: (1) actively facing fears and trying to solve problems; (2) regular physical exercise; (3) optimism; (4) following a moral compass; (5) promoting social support, nurturing friendships, and seeking role models; and (6) being open minded and flexible in the way one thinks about problems, or avoiding rigid and dogmatic thinking.

Lastly, Reivich and Shatte (2002) define resilience as the ability to "persevere and adapt when things go awry" (p. 1). They argue that resilience resides in the domain of cognitive appraisal, a theme we have discussed in this volume and indeed much of our model is predicated upon. Theory and controlled empirical investigations alike appear to converge on the conclusion that the response to any stressful event will be greatly influenced by the appraisal of the situation, the ability to attach a constructive meaning to the experience, the ability to foresee an effective means of coping with the challenges of a given situation, and the ability to ultimately incorporate the experience into some overarching belief system or schema (Everly, 1980; Everly & Lating, 2004; Reivich & Shatte; Smith, Davey, & Everly, 2007). A series of research studies was conducted to empirically examine the viability of the putative deterministic role of appraisal in health and work-related outcomes (Smith, Davey, & Everly, 1995, Smith, Davy, et al. 2006, 2007; Smith & Everly, 1990; Smith, Everly, & Johns, 1993). In a number of investigations, acute cognitive or affective indicators were predictive of physical health outcomes as well as work-related outcomes such as job satisfaction, turnover intention, and burnout. Replicated results indicate that adverse life events are not as important in the ultimate determination of physical health, psychological health, job satisfaction, job performance, and the desire to change jobs as are the cognitive or affective indicia associated with those events (Everly, Davy, Smith, Lating, & Nucifora, 2011; Everly, Smith, & Lating, 2009).

The Johns Hopkins Model of Resiliency

One integrative model contributing heuristic value to the construct of resilience is the Johns Hopkins Tripartite Model of Resistance, Resilience, and Recovery (henceforth, the Hopkins Model), which embraces the distinction between protective factors and rebound capability (Kaminsky, McCabe, Langlieb, & Everly, 2007; Nucifora, Langlieb, Siegal, Everly, & Kaminsky, 2007; Nucifora, Hall, & Everly, 2011). The Hopkins model describes *resistance* as the "ability of an individual, a group, an organization, or even an entire population to withstand manifestations of clinical distress, impairment, or dysfunction associated with critical incidents, terrorism, and even mass disasters." One could think of resistance as a form of "psychological immunity to distress and dysfunction" (Nucifora et al., 2007, p. 534). *Resilience*, in this model, refers to "the ability of an individual, a group, an organization, or even an entire population, to *rapidly and effectively rebound* from psychological and/or behavioral perturbations associated with critical incidents, terrorism, and even mass disasters" (Kaminsky et al.). Finally, *recovery* refers to observed improvement following the application of treatment and rehabilitative procedures. The Hopkins Model views the notion of self-efficacy and self-confidence as essential elements in resistance and resilience. These elements are supported in prior research as being central features of resilience (Connor & Davidson, 2003; Kobasa, 1979; Nucifora et al., 2007; Rutter, 1985), and derivatively in more recent research (Everly et al., 2011; Everly, Smith, & Lating, 2009; Everly & Links, in press).

Seven Characteristics of Highly Resilient People

In an effort to integrate previous theory and research in human resilience, Everly (2009; Everly, Strouse, & Everly, 2010) offers a distillation of findings in an effort to better inform the enhancement of human resilience. We believe that the defining elements of human resilience reside in seven core characteristics, all of which can be learned: (1) innovative, nondogmatic thinking, (2) decisiveness, (3) tenacity, (4) interpersonal connectedness, (5) honestly and integrity, (6) self-control, and (7) optimism and a positive perspective on life. Let's take a closer look at each.

Innovation and creative thinking are often essential element in resilience. The ability to see old problems from a new perspective is the key to overcome hindrances that stifle others. Sometimes referred to as "out of the box" thinking, innovative thinking is characterized by highly flexible, nondogmatic cognitive processes. Such cognitive processing can result in a new level of decision-making efficacy. The key platform upon which innovative thinking rests is the belief that a solution can always be found.

Once a decision has been reached, it is essential to act decisively. Many people wait for the "moment of absolute certainty." Sadly the moment of absolute certainty seldom comes, or when it does, it's often too late. The hesitancy that typifies nonresilient decision making is often the fear of making a mistake, or failing. A cognitive reframing that is sometimes used to help people get over such a block is the reminder, "Anything worth having is worth failing for." The corollary to decisive action, however, is the necessity to take responsibility for one's actions. Taking responsibility is difficult especially if the action led to an undesirable outcome.

Sometimes, making a decision and acting on it in a timely manner is still not enough to warrant being considered resilient. Tenacity is essential. Great American success stories are replete with the theme of tenacity. In many cases it was not the genius that predicted success, it was the tenacity. Take the case of the electric light bulb. The first electric light was invented in 1800 by Humphry Davy, an English scientist. He successfully electrified a carbon filament with a battery. Unfortunately, the filament burned out too quickly to have practical value. In 1879, Thomas Edison discovered that a carbon cotton filament in an oxygen-free glass bulb that glowed for up to 40 h. This new bulb required relatively low levels of electricity and could be produced for a large market. With further time, Edison created a bulb that could glow for over 1,200 h. And what was the difference between Davy on one hand and Edison on the other? Edison persevered in his testing until he found the right combination of filament and bulb. But, according to Edison himself, it required over 6,000 failed experiments to arrive at the right combination.

As Abraham Lincoln learned numerous failures often precede remarkable victories. In 1833, Lincoln failed in business, but was elected to the Illinois state legislature in 1834. In 1835, he lost his "sweetheart." In 1836 he suffered a "nervous breakdown." In 1838 he was re-elected to the Illinois legislature. In 1843, Lincoln was defeated for a congressional nomination, but was elected in 1846. In 1848, he lost renomination. In 1854, Lincoln was defeated in his run for the US Senate and then defeated for nomination for vice president in 1856. In 1858, Lincoln was again defeated for US Senate. In 1860, Abraham Lincoln was elected 16th President of the USA. Finally, On July 4th 1863, in the little town of Gettysburg, Pennsylvania, President Abraham Lincoln delivered in about two and one half minutes one of the greatest presentations of American oratory, his Gettysburg Address, wherein his words resound with tenacity and optimism.

Interpersonal connectedness and support may be the single most powerful predictor of human resilience. In real estate, the mantra is location, location, location. In the military, the mantra is "unit cohesion, unit cohesion, unit cohesion." In the social and business worlds, sometimes it really is *whom* you know, *whom* you know, *whom* you know that counts, and how strong the bond of affinity. The benefits of interpersonal support have been known for over a century. Charles Darwin, writing in 1871, noted, that a tribe whose members were always ready to aid one another and to sacrifice themselves for the common good would be victorious over most other tribes.

One of the founding fathers of the field of psychosomatic medicine was a Johns Hopkins trained physician by the name of Stewart Wolf. While Dr. Wolf made many important contributions, one of his greatest was his study of Roseta, Pennsylvania and is summarized in his book, *"The Power of Clan: The Influences of Human Relationships on Heart Disease."* The book told the story of the socially cohesive community of Roseta and Dr. Wolf's amazing 25-year investigation of the health of its inhabitants. That which made Roseta a medical marvel was that its inhabitants possessed significant risk factors for heart disease such as smoking, high cholesterol diets, and a sedentary lifestyle. Despite these risk factors occurring at a prevalence equal to surrounding towns, the inhabitants appeared to possess an immunity to heart disease compared to their neighbors. The death rate from heart disease was less than half that of surrounding towns! Dr. Wolf discovered that the protective factor was not in the water, nor the air, but was in the people themselves. Research revealed that social cohesiveness, traditional family values, a family-oriented social structure (where three and even four generations could reside in the same household), and emotional support imparted immunity from heart disease. The people of Roseta shared a strong Italian heritage. They practiced the same religion. They shared a strong sense of community identity and civic pride. Unfortunately, with time, the young adults embraced suburban living and with the rise of suburban living, the residents of Roseta slowly abandoned the mutually supportive family oriented social structure and as they did the prevalence of heart disease ultimately rose so as to be equivalent to that of surrounding towns. The immunity that a shared identity, mutual values, and social cohesion had afforded was lost.

Having just read of the importance of interpersonal support, one must wonder what characteristics are likely to engender the support of others? We believe among the most compelling is integrity. Integrity is the quality of doing that which is right. It is considering not only what is good for you but also what is good for others as well. Integrity isn't just a situation by situation process of decision making, it is a consistent way of living. When we see it in others, we usually admire it. Integrity engenders trust. It makes us feel safe. Mahatma Gandhi said that there are seven things that will destroy society: wealth without work; pleasure without conscience; knowledge without character; religion without sacrifice; politics without principle; science without humanity; business without ethics.

Self-discipline and self-control is another factor we believe engenders resilience. Perhaps the single most dangerous action one can take is the impulsive action. Road rage, airline rage, certain types of gambling, and even certain types of domestic violence may be related to the inability to practice self-control. On the other hand, we know certain health promoting behaviors detailed in this volume, such as relaxation training, physical exercise, and practicing good nutrition require a certain self-discipline that many simply find too challenging to practice consistently. Sadly these health promoting practices seem to engender resilience (and resistance) as we have discussed previously.

The seventh and final core characteristic of personal resilience we believe is optimism and positive thinking. Optimism is the tendency to take the most positive or hopeful view of matters. It is the tendency to expect the best outcome, and it is the belief that good prevails over evil. Optimistic people are more perseverant and resilient than are pessimists. Optimistic people tend to be more task oriented and committed to success than are pessimistic people. Optimistic people appear to tolerate adversity to a greater extent than do pessimists. The optimist always has a reason to look forward to another day. Recent research (Everly & Links, in press) suggests there may be two types of optimism: passive and active. Passive optimism consists of "hoping" things will turn out well in the future. Active optimism is "acting" in a manner to increase the likelihood that things will indeed turn out well in the future. Active optimism has been described as a "mandate" to create a positive future.

In his groundbreaking book *Learned Optimism*, Dr. Martin Seligman (Seligman, 1998) argues that optimists get depressed less often, they are higher achievers, and they are physically healthier than pessimistic people. In his another book, *The Optimistic Child*, Dr. Seligman (Seligman, Reivich, Jaycox, & Gillham, 1995) makes the case that depression has become a virtual epidemic that has gradually increased over the years to the point that in one research investigation the incidence of a depressive disorder was found to be 9% in a sample of 3,000 adolescent children in southeastern USA. Prior to 1960, depression was relatively rare, reported mostly by middle-aged women. Now depression appears in both males and females as early as middle school and its prevalence increases as one ages. Seligman (Seligman et al.) notes, "Our society has changed from an achieving society to a feel-good society. Up until the 1960s, achievement was the most important goal to instill in our children. This goal was overtaken by the twin goals of happiness and self-esteem" (p. 40). Now you might read this and say, "What's wrong with happiness and self-esteem?" The answer is nothing, as long as they are built upon a foundation of something more substantial than the mere desire to possess them. Seligman argues that we cannot directly teach lasting self-esteem, rather he says, "self-esteem is caused by…successes and failures in the world" (p. 35).

Self-Efficacy

Seligman has shown that people can be taught optimistic behaviors. The world's leading expert on self-efficacy is Dr Albert Bandura. Bandura's work is summarized in his magnum opus on self-efficacy and human agency authored in 1997 entitled *Self-efficacy: The exercise of control*. Bandura defines the perception of self-efficacy as the belief in one's own ability to exercise control in a meaningful and positive way.

Albert Bandura (1977, 1982a, b, 1997), renowned for his social cognitive theory of human behavior, focuses on a cognitive locus of appraisal to help account for maladaptive stimulus–response interactions. A major construct in his more than 20 years of work is the concept of self-efficacy, which he defines as "beliefs in one's capabilities to organize and execute the courses of action required to produce given attainments" (1997, p. 3). Thus, efficacy beliefs or appraisals of competence and control influence behaviors, thoughts, feelings, and emotions. Individuals possessing a high sense of self-efficacy are often task oriented and utilize multifaceted, integrative problem-solving skills to enhance successful outcomes when dealing with psychosocial stressors. Conversely, people with limited self-efficacy may perceive psychosocial stressors as unmanageable and are more likely to dwell on perceived deficiencies, which generates increased stress and diminishes potential problem-solving energy, lowers aspirations, and weakens commitments.

Bandura (1997) posits that people's beliefs concerning their efficacy are determined by four principal influences:

1. Enactive mastery experiences or performance accomplishments are considered the most powerful source of self-efficacy, because mastery is based on actual success.
2. Vicarious experiences (observational learning, modeling, imitation) increases confidence as people observe behaviors of others, noting contingencies of behavior, and then use this information to form expectancies of their own behavior. An observer's perception of characteristic similarity between him- or herself and the model is an important factor in vicarious experiences.
3. Verbal or social persuasion utilizes expressions of faith in one's competence. The impact of verbal persuasion is less profound than the previous two sources; however, when applied in combination with vicarious and enactive techniques, the influence of self-efficacy is more effective.
4. Finally, physiological and affective states influence self-efficacy, in that comfortable physiological sensations and positive affect are likely to enhance one's confidence in a given situation.

Thus, self-efficacy is the belief in one's ability to organize and execute the courses of action required to achieve necessary and desired goals. This perception of control, or influence, Bandura points out, is an essential aspect of life itself; "People guide their lives by their beliefs of personal efficacy" (p. 3). He goes on to note:

> People's beliefs in their efficacy have diverse effects. Such beliefs influence the courses of action people choose to pursue, how much effort they put forth in given endeavors, how long they will persevere in the face of obstacles and failures... (Bandura, 1997, p. 3).

Personal and group resiliency, for the most part, appears to rest largely upon this notion of self-efficacy.

Hardiness

Before leaving the discussion of individual resilience, we should mention the construct of "hardiness." Suzanne Kobasa, investigated personality characteristics that seem to act as a buffer between individuals and the pathogenic mechanisms of excessive stress. Her research investigated the domain of "hardiness," that is, characterological factors that appear to mitigate the stress response. Originally, Kobasa (1979; Kobasa & Puccetti, 1983) defined hardiness as the aggregation of three factors:

1. Commitment, that is, the tendency to involve oneself in experiences in meaningful ways.
2. Control, that is, the tendency to believe and act as if one has some influence over one's life.
3. Challenge, that is, the belief that change is a positive and normal characteristic of life.

The hardiness research has shown that individuals who demonstrate a commitment to self, family, work, and/or other important values; a sense of control over their lives; and the ability to see life change as an opportunity will experience fewer stress-related diseases/illnesses even though they may find themselves in environments laden with stressor stimuli.

Resilient Leadership and the Culture of Resilience

The previous section addressed what we believe to be the core the elements of personal resilience. But human resilience is not resigned to be an individual practice. Resilience can extend to groups, organizations, and communities. Historically, the family system has been an excellent platform upon which to study and promote resilience. It can serve as a proxy for the study of communities and organizations of all kinds. McCubbin and McCubbin (1988) argued that there are three things resilient families do that less resilient families fail to do:

1. They believe in the family unit. They believe in the importance of family cohesion. They believe in their ability to support and protect one another, and they are optimistic about their ability to achieve family goals.
2. They celebrate key family events, such as birthdays and anniversaries.
3. They create and uphold rituals and routines.

Finally, the critical factors that appear to assist families to rebound from adversity include a sense of family identity and cohesion, good family communications, adherence to family routines and traditions, optimism, and self-efficacy of the family unit and the ability for the family to advocate for itself (McCubbin, McCubbin, Thompson, Han, & Allen, 1997).

The key to the successful and resilient families, organizations, and communities appears to be the creation of a "culture of resilience." Simply stated, the culture of resilience is an environment wherein resistance and resilience are, not only fostered but also are the core fabric of the culture itself. The question then arises as how to create a culture of resilience.

Everly, Strouse, and Everly (2010) postulate that the best way to create the culture of resilience is through resilient leadership. Resilient leadership practices serve as the catalyst that inspires others to exhibit resistance and resilience and to exceed their own expectations. It helps create a culture of resilience wherein adversity is seen as opportunity and support is omnipresent. Based upon the observations of Malcom Gladwell (2000) and consistent with his "Law of the Few," resilient leaders can create the "tipping point" that changes an entire culture. Using a military model, the tipping point for changing the culture would be having roughly 20% of the population of a group practicing resilient leadership, although this might vary according to the organization. But for those 20% to have a maximum impact they must be unique. They should meet three criteria (1) have credibility, (2) be information conduits (usually frontline supervisors), and (3) be willing to promote the success of others. Consistent with our previous discussions, Everly et al. (2010) argue that four characteristics are essential to communicate resilient leadership and to foster the development of a culture of resilience: (1) optimism, (2) decisiveness, (3) integrity, and (4) open communications.

Positive Psychology

Finally, it is important that we frame our discussion of human resilience within another construct. The foregoing discussions of "optimism" and human resilience may be viewed within the broader perspective of "positive psychology." The science of positive psychology is a recent designation predicated on fundamental issues such as happiness, well-being, excellence, and optimal human functioning, among others (Seligman & Csikszentmihalyi, 2000). In essence, the focus of positive psychology is on what makes life worth living for individuals, families, and communities. What Seligman and Csikszentmihalyi note, however, is that since World War II, the emphasis of psychology as a science has been on assessing and treating mental illness. At the start of a new millennium, they suggest that we have reached a time in our history when we should formalize our research efforts to understand systematically what makes individuals and communities flourish. It will be interesting to observe the empirical and theoretical impact of positive psychology over the next several years, both within and outside of the social sciences. We recognize and appreciate that positive psychology should not be construed as a subtype of cognitive therapy (Seligman, personal communication, June 2000); rather, positive psychology is a far broader construct that may indeed be fostered via the use of cognitively based techniques as well as other processes mentioned within the current chapter.

Summary

In this chapter we have introduced and reviewed core concepts related to human resilience. Here we review the main concepts:

1. The history of stress management has largely been reactive. By that we mean stress management was initially conceived of as a means to manage stress that had become "excessive." We now argue that the final frontier in this endeavor is the quest to be more proactive. The term resilience benefits from nonpathological orientation and connotation.
2. The Johns Hopkins' Model of Resistance, Resilience, Recovery serves to lend heuristic value in the creation of a continuum of care, something that was heretofore lacking.
3. We believe that the defining elements of human resilience reside in seven core characteristics, all of which can be learned: (1) innovative, nondogmatic thinking, (2) decisiveness, (3) tenacity, (4) interpersonal connectedness, (5) honesty and integrity, (6) self-control, and (7) optimism and a positive perspective on life.

4. The key to the successful and resilient families, organizations, and communities appears to be the creation of a "culture of resilience." Simply stated, the culture of resilience is an environment wherein resistance and resilience are, not only fostered but also are the core fabric of the culture itself. The question then arises as how to create a culture of resilience.
5. Everly et al. (2010) postulate that the best way to create the culture of resilience is through resilient leadership. Resilient leadership practices serve as the catalyst that inspires others to exhibit resistance and resilience and to exceed their own expectations. It helps create a culture of resilience wherein adversity is seen as opportunity and support is omnipresent. They argue that four characteristics are essential to communicate resilient leadership and to foster the development of a culture of resilience: (1) optimism, (2) decisiveness, (3) integrity, and (4) open communications.
6. Albert Bandura points out that "self-efficacy is an essential aspect of life itself; "People guide their lives by their beliefs of personal efficacy" (p. 3). He goes on to note:
   "People' s beliefs in their efficacy have diverse effects. Such beliefs influence the courses of action people choose to pursue, how much effort they put forth in given endeavors, how long they will persevere in the face of obstacles and failures…" (Bandura, 1997, p. 3). Bandura has described four sources that affect the perception of self-efficacy and are particularly relevant in terms of the building of stress resilience. They are as follows:
   (a) Self-efficacy by doing things successfully.
   (b) Self-efficacy by watching others be successful.
   (c) Self-efficacy through coaching, encouragement, support.
   (d) Self-efficacy through self-regulation. These serve as an important foundation for human resilience.
7. Suzanne Kobasa' early research on hardiness revealed that individuals who demonstrate a commitment to self, family, work, and/or other important values; a sense of control over their lives; and the ability to see life change as an opportunity will experience fewer stress-related diseases/illnesses even though they may find themselves in environments laden with stressor stimuli.
8. Finally, the entire notion of human resilience may best be understood within the overarching construct of positive psychology.

References

Bandura, A. (1977). Self-efficacy: Toward a unifying theory of behavioral change. *Psychological Review, 84*, 191–215.
Bandura, A. (1982a). Self-efficacy mechanism in human agency. *The American Psychologist, 37*, 122–147.
Bandura, A. (1982b). The self and mechanisms of agency. In J. Suls (Ed.), *Psychological perspectives on the self* (pp. 3–39). Hillsdale, NJ: Erlbaum.

Bandura, A. (1997). *Self-efficacy: The exercise of control*. New York, NY: Freeman.

Bonanno, G. A. (2004). Loss, trauma, and human resilience: Have we underestimated the human capacity to thrive after extremely aversive events? *The American Psychologist, 59*(1), 20–28.

Connor, K. M., & Davidson, J. R. T. (2003). Development of a new resilience scale: The Connor-Davidson Resilience Scale (DC-RISC). *Depression and Anxiety, 18*(2), 76–82.

Everly, G. S., Jr. (1980). *The nature and treatment of the human stress response*. New York, NY: Plenum.

Everly, G. S., Jr. (2009). *The resilient child*. New York, NY: DiaMedica.

Everly, G. S., Jr., Davy, J. A., Smith, K. J., Lating, J. M., & Nucifora, F. C., Jr. (2011). A defining aspect of human resilience in the workplace: A structural modeling approach. *Disaster Medicine and Public Health Preparedness, 5*(2), 98–105.

Everly, G. S., Jr., & Lating, J. M. (2004). *Personality guided therapy of posttraumatic stress disorder*. Washington, DC: American Psychological Association.

Everly, G. S., Jr. & Links, A. (in press). Resiliency: A qualitative analysis of law enforcement and Elite military personnel. In D. Paton, J. Violanti (Eds.), *Working in high risk environments: Developing sustained resiliency*. Springfield, IL: CC Thomas.

Everly, G. S., Jr., Smith, K. J., & Lating, J. M. (2009). A rationale for cognitively-based resilience and psychological first aid (PFA) training: A structural modeling analysis. *International Journal of Emergency Mental Health, 11*(4), 249–262.

Everly, G. S., Jr., Strouse, D. A., & Everly, G. S., III. (2010). *The secrets of resilient leadership*. New York, NY: DiaMedica.

Gladwell, M. (2000). *Tipping point*. New York, NY: Little Brown.

Haglund, M., Cooper, N., Southwick, S., & Charney, D. (2007). 6 keys to resilience for PTSD and everyday life. *Current Psychiatry, 6*, 23–30.

Kaminsky, M. J., McCabe, O. L., Langlieb, A., & Everly, G. S., Jr. (2007). An evidence-informed model of human resistance, resilience, & recovery: The Johns Hopkins' outcomes-driven paradigm for disaster mental health services. *Brief Therapy and Crisis Intervention, 7*, 1–11.

Kobasa, S. (1979). Stressful life events, personality, and health. *Journal of Personality and Social Psychology, 37*, 1–11.

Kobasa, S., & Puccetti, M. (1983). Personality and social resources in stress resistance. *Journal of Personality and Social Psychology, 45*, 839–850.

McCubbin, H. I., & McCubbin, M. A. (1988). Typologies of resilient families: Emerging roles of social class and ethnicity. *Family Relations, 37*, 247–254.

McCubbin, H. I., McCubbin, M., Thompson, A. I., Han, S., & Allen, C. T. (1997). *Families under stress: What makes them resilient*. Paper presented to the American Association of Family and Consumer Sciences. Washington, D. C. June 22, 1997

Nucifora, F., Hall, R., & Everly, G. S., Jr., (2011). Reexamining the role of the traumatic stressor and the trajectory of posttraumatic distress in thewake of disaster. *Disaster Medicine and Public Health Preparednes,s . 5 (supp.2):* S172-175.

Nucifora, F., Jr., Langlieb, A. M., Siegal, E., Everly, G. S., Jr., & Kaminsky, M. (2007). Building resistance, resilience, and recovery in the wake of school and workplace violence. *Disaster Medicine and Public Health Preparedness, 1(supp.1)*, 533–537.

Reivich, K., & Shatte, A. (2002). *The resilience factor: 7 essential skills for overcoming life's inevitable obstacles*. New York, NY: Broadway Books.

Rutter, M. (1985). Resilience in the face of adversity. *British Journal of Psychiatry, 147*, 598–611.

Seligman, M. (1998). *Learned optimism*. New York, NY: Pocket Books.

Seligman, M. E. P., & Csikszentmihalyi, M. (2000). Positive psychology: An introduction. *American Psychologist, 55*(1), 5–14.

Seligman, M. E. P., Reivich, K., Jaycox, L., & Gillham, J. (1995). *The optimistic child*. New York: Houghton-Mifflin.

Smith, K. J., Davy, J. A., & Everly, G. S., Jr. (1995). An examination of the antecedents of job dissatisfaction and turnover intentions among CPAs in public accounting. *Accounting Enquiries, 5*(1), 99–142.

Smith, K. J., Davy, J. A., & Everly, G. S., Jr. (2006). Stress arousal and burnout: A construct distinctiveness evaluation. *Proceedings of the 2006 Annual Meeting of the American Accounting Association*. Washington, DC.

Smith, K. J., Davy, J. A., & Everly, G. S., Jr. (2007). An assessment of the contribution of stress arousal to the beyond the role stress model. *Advances in Accounting Behavioral Research, 10,* 127–158.

Smith, K. J., & Everly, G. S., Jr. (1990). An intra- and inter occupational analysis of stress among accounting academicians. *Behavioral Research in Accounting, 2*(154), 173.

Smith, K. J., Everly, G. S., & Johns, T. (1993). The role of stress arousal in the dynamics of the stressor-to-illness process among accountants. *Contemporary Accounting Research, 9,* 432–449.

William, N. R., Lindsey, E. W., Kurtz, P. D., & Jarvis, S. (2001). From trauma to resiliency: Lessons from runaway and homeless youth. *Journal of Youth Studies, 4,* 233–253.

Part II
The Treatment of the Human Stress Response

Part II is the second of three major sections in this book. It is dedicated to the presentation of not only reviews of therapeutic technologies but also does so in adherence to the overarching systems model of treatment that was introduced in Chap. 2.

Chapter 8 begins our description of therapeutic options by providing a brief overview of the role of psychotherapy in the mitigation and treatment of human stress. The reader should note that Chap. 8 is not a "how to" guide for conducting a psychotherapeutic intervention, rather that is reserved for original treatment manuals. Our goal is to simply sensitize the reader to the role that psychotherapy, from a cognitive perspective, may play in the overall treatment plan.

Chapter 9 entitled "A Neurophysiological Rationale for the Use of the Relaxation Response" is a unique foray into the scientific foundations of relaxation-based interventions, some of which have been employed for centuries.

Chapters 10–12 provide step-by-step guidelines for the use of meditation, respiration, and muscle relaxation.

Chapters 13 and 14 continue the discussion of specific therapeutic interventions such as hypnosis and biofeedback, respectively.

Chapter 15 "Physical Exercise and the Human Stress Response" reviews physical exercise as both preventive and therapeutic. As Walter Cannon noted, stress may be thought of as the "fight or flight" response, i.e., a mechanism that better prepares the individual for physical activity and exertion.

Chapter 16 reviews advances in the pharmacologic treatment of human stress.

Chapter 8
Psychotherapy: A Cognitive Perspective

I'm an old man and have known a great many troubles,
but most of them never happened.

Mark Twain

Having provided the reader with what we feel is a comprehensive review of the phenomenology of the human stress response, this chapter begins our focus upon therapeutic intervention.

Like beauty, a stressor resides in the eye of the beholder. It should be clear by now that the patient's cognitive interpretation of the environment leads to the formation of a psychosocial stressor from an otherwise neutral stimulus. This concept has resulted in more eloquent phrasing such as "There are no things good or bad, but thinking makes them so" (Shakespeare); "It is not what happens to you that matters, but how you take it" (Hans Selye); "Men are disturbed not by things, but by the views which they take of them" (Epictetus); "No one can make you feel inferior without your consent" (Eleanor Roosevelt).

If one accepts the concept that the primary determinant of any given psychosocial stressor is the cognitive interpretation or appraisal of that stimulus (as argued in Chap. 2), then it seems reasonable to assume that a useful therapy in treating stress-related disorders might be a psychotherapeutic effort directed toward the cognitive-interpretational domain. Although clearly not the only psychotherapeutic technique or approach of value in treating excessive stress, psychotherapy with cognitive restructuring or reinterpretation as a goal seems applicable, particularly in the treatment of pathogenic stress-response syndromes.

As noted in the preface to this volume, and in the introduction to Part II, the unique purpose of this text is to provide the reader with the physiological foundations and phenomenological processes of the human stress response, and then to offer a neurophysiological rationale along with practical protocols for employing specific relaxation techniques. Therefore, while we acknowledge the potential benefits in providing exhaustive protocols for each of the following cognitive-based psychotherapy strategies, the goal of this chapter is not to provide a "how-to"

G.S. Everly and J.M. Lating, *A Clinical Guide to the Treatment*
of the Human Stress Response, DOI 10.1007/978-1-4614-5538-7_8,
© Springer Science+Business Media New York 2013

manual of cognitively-based therapies. Excellent practitioner-oriented guides are available elsewhere (see Beck & Beck, 2011; Beck & Emery, 1985; Dobson, 2010; Fairburn, 2008; Meichenbaum, 1985; Meichenbaum & Jaremko, 1983). Rather, it is our hope that this chapter will sensitize the reader to the critical role that cognition plays in the initiation and prolongation of human stress and to the important role of cognitively-based therapies in the treatment of stress-related problems.

In an effort to help sensitize the reader to the role of cognition in mitigating the impact of the stress, and before reviewing the various cognitive models, we would like to present what we believe to be one of the seminal and most fascinating research studies depicting this phenomenon. Previous research has demonstrated that breathing carbon dioxide (CO_2)-enriched air (e.g., 5.5% CO_2-enriched) can provoke panic attacks in a majority of patients with panic disorder. While most evidence has focused on the biochemical effects of 5.5% CO_2, Sanderson, Rapee, and Barlow (1989), noting that "fear of losing control" was reported as the most intense symptom during a panic attack, examined the influence of instilling an illusion of cognitive control in 20 patients exposed to 5.5% CO_2-enriched air for 15 min.

Prior to being exposed to the enriched air, all participants were told that a box located directly in front of them *might* light up during the exposure. They were also informed that when this box was lit, they would be able to decrease the amount of CO_2, if desired, by turning a dial attached to the chairs in which they were sitting. All were encouraged, however, to lower the CO_2 only if they felt that it was absolutely necessary. In actuality, the dial had no effect on the deliverance of CO_2. For half of the participants, the light box was randomly illuminated periodically throughout their CO_2 exposure, whereas for the other participants, the light never came on. Participants who believed they could not control the quantity of CO_2 (no-light participants) reported a greater number of symptoms and intensity of panic compared to the participants who believed they could control the CO_2. In fact, 80% of the participants in the "no illusion of control" group reported that they experienced a panic attack compared to only 20% in the "illusion of control" group.

Cognitive Primacy

The cognitive primacy postulation is the perspective accepted within this volume. This viewpoint became apparent in Chap. 2, where we noted that the individual's interpretation of the environment is the primary determinant in the elicitation of the stress response in reaction to a psychosocial stressor. A similar yet more extensive view is summarized by Roseman (1984), who states, "A cognitive approach to the causation of emotion assumes that it is the interpretation of events rather than events per se that determine which emotion will be felt" (p. 14).

Although when discussing the stress and emotions of flight crews dealing with the threat of war, Grinker and Spiegel (1945) were two of the first researchers to refer to the notion of appraisal, Magda Arnold (1960) was the most explicit of the early theorists in support of cognitive primacy. She concluded that emotions are caused by the "appraisal" of the stimuli that one encounters. Given the perception of some environmental stimulus, subsequent emotions are a function, not of the stimulus per se but of the cognitive interpretation (appraisal) of that stimulus. Thus, Arnold was the first person to systematically state that there is a cognitive-mediational approach to the study of emotions, with appraisal as the core construct.

Lazarus first used the term *appraisal* in 1964, and by 1966 it became the essence of his theory of psychological stress (Lazarus, 1966). He and his colleagues extended Arnold's work to recognize the role of initial appraisal of a given environmental stimulus but added the notion of reappraisal, which entails the cognitive interpretation of one's perceived ability to handle, cope with, or benefit from exposure to the stimulus. This work became known as the transactional model, and as described by Coyne and Holroyd (1982):

> The Lazarus group applies the concept of appraisal to the person's continually reevaluated judgments about demands and constraints in transactions with the environment and options and resources for meeting them. A key assumption of the model is that these evaluations determine the person's stress reaction, the emotions experienced, and adaptational outcomes. (p. 108)

Thus, the Lazarus group emphasized first a primary appraisal ("Is this situation a threat, challenge, or aversion?") and then a secondary one ("Can I cope or benefit from it?") in the origin of human adult emotions.

The basic position of the primacy of cognition in the cognitive–affective relation is held by numerous theorists and researchers (Arnold, 1960, 1984; Chang, 1998; Dewe, 1992; Hemenover & Dienstbier, 1996; Lazarus, 1966, 1999; Levine, 1996; Peeters, Buunk, & Schaufeli, 1995; Terry, Tonge, & Callan, 1995). To reiterate, the cognitive primacy perspective argues "that cognitive activity is a 'necessary' as well as sufficient condition of emotion" (Lazarus, 1982, p. 1019). More specifically, cognitive activity here refers to "cognitive appraisal," the role of which is to mediate the relations between people and their environments. In a monograph on stress and emotion, Lazarus (1999) succinctly notes that "emotions are the product of reason in that they flow from how we appraise what is happening in our lives. In effect, the way we evaluate an event determines how we react emotionally. This is what it means to speak of cognitive mediation" (p. 87). Commenting on the cognitive perspectives, Dobson and Shaw (1995) note that "they share an assumption that it is the perception of events, rather than events themselves, that mediates the response to different circumstances and ultimately determines the quality of adaptation of individuals" (p. 159). More recently, Hofmann, Asmundson, and Beck (2011) note that "negative emotions and harmful behaviors are products of dysfunctional thoughts and cognitive distortions" (p. 2)

Although the preponderance of stress researchers supports the notion of cognitive primacy, not all writers have agreed. During the 1980s, Zajonc and Lazarus had vigorous literary disagreements regarding the merits of cognitive primacy. Zajonc (1984) argued that an affective reaction could occur independently or without cognitive participation under certain circumstances (e.g., phylogenetic and ontogenetic primacy, separation of neuroanatomical structures for affect and cognition, the periodic lack of correlation between appraisal and affect, the formation of new affective reactions established without apparent appraisal, and the consideration that affective states can be induced by noncognitive procedures), but Lazarus was able to provide effective rebuttals for each contention. In the 1990s, Parkinson and Manstead (1992) presented a critique of appraisal theory; however, Lazarus's (1999) response to their criticism suggests that their points of disagreement are actually quite narrow and that they generally accept most of his theory on stress and emotion. He acknowledges that a definitive empirical separation of appraisal and emotion is arduous due to the obvious methodological limitations; however, he contends that more empirical support is offered for cognitive primacy than for any other theories. Lazarus further contends that the theory of cognitive primacy should not be discarded unless one is prepared to offer a more encompassing and effective alternative explanation. Most researchers continue to agree that a more effective alternative explanation to cognitive primacy is yet to come.

Cognitive-Based Psychotherapy

According to Bandura (1997, 1982a, b), the primary factor in the determination of a stressful event is the individual's *perceived* inefficiency in coping with or controlling a potentially aversive event. We now review several models of cognitively based psychotherapeutic interventions that may be employed to alter the patient's perception (cognitive interpretation) of an environmental transaction that might be seen as potentially aversive.

Ellis's Model

Modern cognitive therapy is considered to have emerged in 1955, when Albert Ellis developed rational-emotive therapy (RET; Arnkoff & Glass, 1992). Ellis (1971, 1973, 1984, 1991) has proposed that individuals often acquire irrational or illogical cognitive interpretations or beliefs about themselves or their environment. The extent to which these beliefs are irrational and important corresponds to the amount of emotional distress experienced by the individual. Ellis believes that the emotional disturbance experienced by the individual can be summarized using the following "A-B-C" model:

$$A \rightarrow B \rightarrow C$$
Activating experience   Belief   Emotional consequence

In Condition A, some environmental transaction involving the individual occurs (e.g., he or she is late for an appointment). In Condition B, the person generates

Table 8.1 Disputing irrational beliefs

1. What irrational belief needs to be disputed?
2. Can this belief be rationally supported?
3. What evidence exists for the falseness of this belief?
4. Does an evidence exist for the truth of this belief?
5. What worse things could *actually* happen to me if my initial experience (activating experience) does not end favorably?
6. What good things can I make happen even if my initial experience does not end favorably?

some "irrational" belief about him- or herself based on the original experience (e.g., "I'm stupid, worthless, incompetent for being late"). Condition C represents the emotional consequence (e.g., guilt, depression, shame, or anxiety) that results, not from the experience itself (A) but directly from the irrational belief (B). Ellis then employs his model of RET, which consists of adding a "D" to the A-B-C paradigm, representing a conscious effort to "dispute" the irrational cognitive belief that resulted in the emotional distress. The RET therapist may use techniques such as debating, role playing, social skills training, and bibliotherapy to challenge the individual's beliefs, often in a confrontational, forceful fashion. Therefore, regardless of the techniques used, the overall psychotherapeutic goal is to alter the individual's interpretation. Ellis has delineated a series of questions to assist in the disputation of irrational beliefs (see Table 8.1).

Beck's Cognitive Therapy Model

The cognitive therapy process of Aaron T. Beck is considered the second major cognitive restructuring therapy (Arnkoff & Glass, 1992). Similar to RET, cognitive therapy assists the client in identifying maladaptive thinking and persuades him or her to develop a more adaptive view. However, whereas RET is more philosophically driven (Ellis, 1995), Beck's cognitive therapy is more empirically based and focuses on whether thoughts and beliefs are realistic compared to whether they are rational (Meichenbaum, 1995). As Beck (1995) notes,

> Based on my clinical observations and some systematic clinical studies and experiments, I theorized that there was a thinking disorder at the core of the psychiatric syndromes such as depression and anxiety. This disorder was reflected in a systematic bias in the way the patients interpreted particular experiences. (vii)

Beck differentiates between three types of cognitions that may be involved in disrupted thinking: automatic thoughts, schemas, and cognitive distortions. Automatic thoughts are considered a "surface level" cognition that is brought to awareness quickly and readily, and leads directly to the individual's emotional and behavioral responses. Cognitive schemas are thought of as internal models of aspects of the self and the environment, and are used to process information. They often lead individuals with emotional problems to develop perceptions of threat, loss, or danger. Cognitive distortions serve in essence as a link between dysfunctional schemas and automatic thoughts. For example, when new information is processed cognitively, the material may be biased or skewed in order to make it consistent with a current schema.

Then, to challenge the patient's maladaptive thinking, Beck encourages the use of a Socratic dialogue, which relies on the ability of the treating therapist to ask questions in a probing manner that allows the patient to answer in a way to persuade *him-* or *herself* to think differently. Beck and Emery (1985) describe in elaborate detail how cognitive restructuring principles can be used in the treatment of anxiety and stress-related disorders: "Anxious patients in the simplest terms believe, 'Something bad is going to happen that I won't be able to handle.' The cognitive therapist uses three basic strategies or questions to help the patient restructure this thinking" (p. 200):

1. What is the evidence supporting the conclusion currently held by the patient?
2. What is another way of looking at the same situation but reaching some other conclusion?
3. What will happen if, indeed, the currently held conclusion/opinion is correct?

While examining each of these three strategic questions, it is important to keep in mind that individual differences may affect a patient's responses. It is also worth acknowledging that the therapist may need to employ all three strategies throughout therapy.

1. *What is the evidence?* One goal of this strategy is to analyze the patient's cognitive patterns and search for "faulty logic." Therapists may help patients to correct faulty logic and ideas through questioning techniques that may allow them better to clarify the meaning(s) and definitions of the problem. According to Beck (1993), individuals experiencing stress reactions tend to personalize events not relevant to them (egocentrism) and interpret situations in global and absolute terms. Therefore, the following are typical questions used to improve the patient's ability to process information and test reality:

- What is the evidence supporting this conclusion?
- What is the evidence against this conclusion?
- Are you oversimplifying causal relationships?
- Are you confusing habits or commonly held opinions with fact?
- Are your interpretations too far removed from your actual experiences?
- Are you thinking in "all-or-nothing" terms (i.e., black–white, either–or, on–off, or all-or-none types of decisions and outcome)?
- Are your conclusions in any way extreme or exaggerated?
- Are you taking selected examples out of context and basing you conclusion on such information?
- Is the source of information reliable?
- Is your thinking in terms of certainties rather than probabilities?
- Are you confusing low-probability with high-probability events?
- Are you basing your conclusions on feelings or values rather than facts?
- Are you focusing on irrelevant factors in forming your conclusions?

- Through the use of such questions, patterns of faulty reasoning, such as projections, exaggerations, and negative attributions, may be discovered and corrected.

2. *What is another way of looking at it?* The goal of this strategy is to help the patient generate alternative interpretations in lieu of the interpretation currently held. Strategies such as increasing both objectivity and perspective, and shifting or diverting cognitive set (Beck, 1993) may lead to reattribution, diminishing the significance of the environmental transaction, or even restructuring the transaction to find something positive in the event.

3. *So what if it happens?* The goal of this strategy is to help the patient "decatastrophize" the environmental transaction as well as to develop coping strategies and problem-solving skills. It will be recalled from the multidimensional treatment model that "environmental engineering" (Girdano, Everly, & Dusek, 1997) and "problem solving" are merely terms that describe the therapeutic processes of this third strategic phase of therapy as described by Beck and Emery (1985). These authors suggest that "therapist and patient collaboratively develop a variety of strategies that the person can use" (p. 208). Ultimately, the goal of therapy is to allow the patient to develop autonomous skills in each of the three strategic areas mentioned previously. The notions of "environmental engineering" and "problem solving" will be more formally integrated in the next model—Meichenbaum's stress inoculation training mode.

Meichenbaum's Stress Inoculation Training

Using the principles contained in his classic text, *Cognitive-Behavior Modification*, Meichenbaum (1977) developed a specialized, cognitively based therapy for the treatment of excessive stress in a therapeutic formulation called "stress inoculation training" (SIT).

Meichenbaum (1993), reflecting on 20 years of SIT, notes:

> In short, SIT helps clients acquire sufficient knowledge, self-understanding, and coping skills to facilitate better ways of handling expected stressful encounters. SIT combines elements of Socratic and didactic teaching, client self-monitoring, cognitive restructuring, problem solving, self-instructional and relaxation training, behavioral and imagined rehearsal, and environmental change. With regard to the notion of environmental change, SIT recognizes that stress is transactional in nature. (p. 381)

The SIT paradigm consists of an overlapping, three-phase intervention (Meichenbaum, 2007). The first phase, the initial conceptualization phase, includes the development of a collaborative relationship between the client and trainer through the use of Socratic exchanges. The overall objectives of this phase include data collection and education to help clients reconceptualize their stressful experiences in a more hopeful and empowered manner.

In the second phase of SIT, coping and problem-solving skills are taught and rehearsed. Table 8.2 provides examples of self-statements that may be used as coping techniques. Skills acquisition in this phase encompasses more than self-statements.

Table 8.2 Examples of coping self-statements rehearsed in stress inoculation training

Preparing for a stressor
- What is it you have to do?
- You can develop a plan to deal with it
- Just think about what you can do about it. That's better than getting anxious
- No negative self-statements: Just think rationally
- Don't worry: Worry won't help anything
- Maybe what you think is anxiety is eagerness to confront the stressor

Confronting and handling a stressor
- Just "psych" yourself up—you can meet this challenge
- You can convince yourself to do it. You can reason your fear away
- One step at a time: You can handle the situation
- Don't think about fear; just think about what you have to do. Stay relevant
- This anxiety is what the doctor said you would feel. It's reminder to use your coping exercises
- This tenseness can be an ally; a cue to cope
- Relax; you're in control. Take a slow deep breath
- Ah, good

Coping with the feeling of being overwhelmed
- When fear comes, just pause
- Keep the focus on the present; what is it you have to do?
- Label your fear from 0 to 10 and watch it change
- You should expect your fear to rise
- Don't try to eliminate fear totally; just keep it manageable

Reinforcing self-statements
- It worked; you did it
- Wait until you tell your therapist (or group) about this
- It wasn't as bad as you expected
- You made more out of your fear than it was worth
- Your damn ideas—that's the problem. When you control them, you control your fear
- It's getting better each time you use the procedures
- You can be pleased with progress you're making
- You did it!

Source: D. Meichenbaum (1977). *Cognitive Behavior Modification*. Copyright by Plenum Press. Reprinted by permission.

Assertion training, anger control, study skills, parenting, and relaxation may be incorporated.

The third phase of SIT, application and follow-through, allows patients to apply the skills acquired in the preceding two phases across situations with increasing levels of actual stress. Therefore, techniques such as modeling, role playing, and in vivo exposure are used, as well as features of relapse prevention. The follow-up component allows for future extension of SIT uses.

These three phases of SIT are enumerated in greater detail in Table 8.3. (A valuable guide for practitioners on the use of SIT is also available; see Meichenbaum, 1985, 2007.)

Table 8.3 Flowchart of stress inoculation training

Phase One: Conceptualization

(a) Data collection—integration

- Identify determinants of problem via interview, image-based reconstruction, self-monitoring, psychological and environmental assessments, and behavioral observance
- Allow the client to tell his or her own story and help the description to be broken down into behaviorally specific terms
- Formulate treatment plan. Have the client establish short-term, intermediate, and long-term behaviorally specific goals
- Introduce integrative conceptual model

(b) Assessment skills training

- Distinguish between performance failure and skill deficit
- Train clients to analyze problems independently (e.g., conduct situational and developmental analyses and to seek disconfirmatory data)
- Formulate a reconceptualization of the client's stress while encouraging the client and bringing to light his or her strength's and bolstering feelings of resourcefulness

Phase Two: Skills Acquisition and Rehearsal

(a) Skills training

- Training instrumental coping skills (e.g., communication assertion, anxiety management, problem solving, relaxation training, parenting, study skills)
- Train emotionally focused palliative coping skills (e.g., perspective-taking, attention diversion, use of social supports, adaptive affect expression, relaxation)
- Aim to develop an extensive repertoire of coping responses to facilitate flexible responding

(b) Skills rehearsal

- Promote smooth integration and execution of coping responses via imagery and role play
- Use coping modeling including collaborative discussion, practice and feedback
- Use self-instructional training to develop internal mediators to self-regulate coping responses

Phase Three: Application and Follow-Through

(a) Induce application of skills

- Prepare for application using coping imagery, using early stress cues as signals for coping
- Role-play-anticipated stressful situations and encourage adoption of "role play" attitude in real world
- Exposure to in-session-graded stressors
- Use of graded exposure and other response induction aids to foster in vivo responding and building self-efficacy
- Use relapse prevention procedures (e.g., identifying high-risk situations, anticipate possible stressful reactions, and practice coping responses)

(b) Maintenance and generalization

- Slowly phase out treatment and arrange follow-up sessions and review
- Involve others in client's life (e.g., parents, spouse, doctors) and encourage the use of peer and self-help groups
- Encourage the client to coach someone with a similar problem
- Build a sense of coping self-efficacy in relation to situations clients sees as high risk, as well as developing coping strategies to deal with recovery from failures and setbacks

General guidelines for training

- Attend to referral and intake process

(continued)

Table 8.3 (continued)

- Establish realistic expectations regarding course and outcome of therapy
- Foster optimism and confidence by structuring incremental success experiences
- Respond to stalled progress with problem solving versus labeling client resistant

Sources: Adapted from "Stress Inoculation Training: Toward a Paradigm for Training Coping Skills" by D. Meichenbaum and R. Cameron in *Stress Reduction and Prevention* (p. 121) edited by D. Meichenbaum and M. E. Jaremko. Copyright 1983 by Plenum Press, and D. Meichenbaum (2007) Stress inoculation training. A preventative and treatment approach. In P. M. Lehrer, R. L. Woolfolk, & W. E. Sime (Eds). *Principles and practice of stress management* (3rd ed., pp. 506–507). New York: Guilford

Meichenbaum's SIT training is of special interest in this volume because it manifests the belief that stress management is most effective when it is flexible and multidimensional. Similarly, SIT allows us to integrate the concept of "environmental engineering" as delineated in the treatment model described in the introduction to Part II. The term *environmental engineering*, it will be recalled, is borrowed from the work of Girdano, Dusek, and Everly (2001) as it was first described in 1979, and refers to any conscious attempts at manipulating environmental factors to reduce one's exposure to stressor events. Both proactive, environmental change and reactive problem solving must be included under this heading. The reader will observe that there are different points within the model wherein problem solving, or any other form of environmental engineering, is obviously applicable.

As implied earlier, one of the real strengths of SIT is its inherent flexibility, structured as it is around a cognitive foundation. SIT has been demonstrated to be of value in the control of anger, test anxiety, phobias, general stress, pain, surgical anxiety, essential hypertension, and PTSD (see Meichenbaum, 1985, 1993 and D'Arienzo, 2010).

Acceptance and Commitment Therapy

In the past decade, there has been a flourishing of a "third wave" of psychotherapeutic models that focus on the relevance of distressing thoughts and emotions, and emphasize concepts such as mindfulness, acceptance, cognitive defusion, and spirituality in treatment (Hayes, 2004). Acceptance and Commitment Therapy (ACT; Hayes, Strosahl, & Wilson, 1999) is one of the more prominent of these therapies. Although we appreciate that ACT is more closely aligned with the basic tenets of traditional cognitive-behavioral therapy (CBT) (Forman & Herbert, 2009), the emergence of ACT, particularly its cognitive foundation warrants a brief review in this volume.

As noted by Hayes (2004), "Theoretically speaking, ACT is rigorously behavioral, but yet is based on a comprehensive empirical analysis of human cognition" (p. 640). More recently, Hayes and his colleagues describe that "ACT is an overarching model of key intervention and change processes, linked to a research program on the nature of language and cognition, to a pragmatic philosophy of science, and to a model of how to speed scientific development…a contextual behavioral science

(CBS) approach" (Hayes, Levin, Plumb-Vilardaga, Villatte, & Pistorello, 2011, in press). ACT is based primarily on Relational Frame Theory (RFT; Hayes et al., 2011), which adheres to the basic tenet that human language and cognition are based on how events are mutually combined and related to each other based on arbitrary cues not just on their formal properties, and grounded in functional contextualism that in essence "conceptualizes psychological events as a set of ongoing interactions between whole organisms and historically and situationally defined contexts" (Hayes, 2004 p.646). In other words, ACT considers that actions are whole events and that their meaning is established only with consideration of the established contextual function, relational frames, and meaning of an event both historically and situationally, and not just solely on its occurrence (Hayes et al., 2011). This is thought to be one of the differences between ACT and traditional cognitive therapy, which is considered by ACT therapists to be more mechanistic (i.e., a bivariate causal chain or link between cognitions and behaviors that does not require an explanation of the cognitions' origins) (Herbert & Forman, 2011). In contrast, ACT therapists, while accepting the possible causal role of cognitions, assert that it is relevant to explore and examine external factors, including environmental and others that are manipulable, that serve as the origin of cognitions (Herbert & Forman, 2011). More specifically, "thoughts may be related to particular emotional and overt behavioral events, but only in historical and situational contexts that give rise both to these thoughts and to their relation to subsequent emotions and actions" (in press).

According to Hayes and colleagues (2006, 2011), there are six core processes or psychological skills associated with ACT interventions, including, (1) *acceptance* (actively embracing experiences in the moment without attempting to alter content or frequency); (2) *cognitive defusion* (changing one's interaction or relation to cognitions by considering or creating other contexts that diminish their literal interpretive quality or unhelpfulness; taking thoughts literally without considering the process of thinking itself) (3) *being present or in contact with the present moment* (continual nonjudgmental and direct occurrences to allow actions to be consistent with held values), (4) *self as context* (being aware of one's experiences without attachment to them, thus fostering acceptance); (5) *values* (clarifying goals and objectives in order to allow actions to produce these goals and the barriers that keep one from them); and (6) *committed action* (being focused on moving toward aspired goals, working through barriers, and having an action plan). According to the ACT perspective, distress or psychopathology is the result of taking cognitions literally and being focused on problem solving despite its questionable benefit. In general, this is referred to as "psychological inflexibility" and the primary goal of ACT intervention is to become more fully aware of the here and now and applying the core processes through various exercises to increase flexibility (Hayes et al., 2011).

A 2009 meta-analysis of 18 randomized control studies of ACT with a total sample size of 917 participants (Powers, Zum V rde Sive V rding, & Emmelkamp, 2009) revealed overall that ACT was superior to control conditions (waiting list, treatment as usual, psychological placebo) with an effect size of 0.42. The results revealed that participants receiving ACT were more improved than 66% of participants in the control condition, but ACT was not more effective than control conditions for distress problems. Moreover, the data revealed that ACT was not more effective than the established treatments of CBT or CT. Also relevant to this volume, a randomized comparative intervention study of ACT, SIT and waitlist control in a sample of 107 employees of local working individuals with above average levels of distress revealed that ACT and SIT were equally effective in reducing distress over a 3-month time frame (Flaxman & Bond, 2010).

Summary

This chapter has reviewed the first of the specific therapeutic interventions we present in this edition for the treatment of pathogenic human stress.

In this chapter, we have focused on the role that psychotherapy can play in treating excessive stress. Reflecting the biases of the epiphenomenological model of human stress constructed in Chap. 2, we have chosen to provide a brief overview of cognitive-based psychotherapeutic interventions. The main points in this chapter are:

1. Referring back to Fig. 2.6, this chapter acknowledges the primary role that cognition plays in the initiation and propagation of a psychosocially induced stress response.
2. The genesis and features of "cognitive primacy" (the notion that affect is subsequent to cognition), as well as updates and critiques of the theory, are reviewed.
3. The rational-emotive therapy of Ellis (1971, 1973, 1984, 1991) is introduced as the first of modern, cognitive-based psychotherapeutic interventions to challenge and alter dysfunctional cognitions. Its core assumption is that individuals who suffer excessive stress may have a proclivity, albeit pathogenic, to accept irrational or otherwise inappropriate beliefs about environmental transactions. This propensity can be corrected by teaching the patient to "dispute" his or her irrational beliefs as they give rise to excessive stress arousal.
4. Beck's cognitive therapy is considered the second major cognitive restructuring therapy. It is viewed as a broader spectrum cognitive intervention that not only focuses on inappropriate cognitive patterns but also assists the patient in developing other coping and problem-solving activities. Three basic therapeutic strategies are employed to assist in cognitive restructuring: (1) analyzing the nature of any evidence that affected the individual's cognitive interpretation, (2) generating alternative interpretations via cognitive reattribution and searching for positive aspects inherent in the environmental transaction ("the silver lining"), and (3) developing environmental engineering, adaptive coping strategies, and useful problem-solving techniques.
5. The broadest spectrum cognitive-based stress management intervention extends well beyond psychotherapy and is referred to as "stress inoculation training." In the paradigm developed by Meichenbaum (1977, 1985, 1993, 2007), the intervention consists of three basic stages: (1) data collection and education, (2) skills acquisition, and (3) application and follow-through to a real-world setting. The multiple components of this approach are delineated in Table 8.3.

6. Cognitive-based interventions have demonstrated their utility in the treatment of a wide array of problems, including anger, pain, phobias, anxiety, general stress arousal, headaches, and PTSD (see Meichenbaum, 1985, Table 8.1).
7. Acceptance and Commitment Therapy focuses on the relevance of distressing thoughts and emotions, and emphasizes how acceptance, cognitive diffusion, being present, using one's self as a context (i.e., being aware of experiences without attaching to them), clarifying goals and objectives (i.e., values) and being committed to an action plan are associated with successful intervention (Hayes et al., 2006, 2011).

References

Arnkoff, D. B., & Glass, C. R. (1992). Cognitive therapy and psychotherapy integration. In D. Freedheim (Ed.), *History of psychotherapy: A century of change* (pp. 657–694). Washington, DC: American Psychological Association.

Arnold, M. B. (1960). *Emotion and personality* (Vol. 2). New York, NY: Columbia University Press.

Arnold, M. (1984). *Memory and the brain*. Hillsdale, NJ: Erlbaum.

Bandura, A. (1982a). Self-efficacy mechanism in human agency. *The American Psychologist, 37*, 122–147.

Bandura, A. (1982b). The self and mechanisms of agency. In J. Suls (Ed.), *Psychological perspectives on the self* (pp. 3–39). Hillsdale, NJ: Erlbaum.

Bandura, A. (1997). *Self-efficacy: The exercise of control*. New York, NY: Freeman.

Beck, A. T. (1993). Cognitive approaches to stress. In P. M. Lehrer & R. L. Woolfolk (Eds.), *Principles and practices of stress management* (2nd ed., pp. 333–372). New York, NY: Guilford.

Beck, A. T. (1995). Foreword. In J. S. Beck (Ed.), *Cognitive therapy: Basics and beyond* (p. vii). New York, NY: Guilford.

Beck, J. S., & Beck, A. T. (2011). *Cognitive behavior therapy: Basics and beyond* (2nd ed.). New York, NY: Guilford.

Beck, A., & Emery, G. (1985). *Anxiety disorders and phobias: A cognitive perspective*. New York, NY: Basic Books.

Chang, E. C. (1998). Dispositional optimism and primary and secondary appraisal of a stressor: Controlling for confounding influences and relations to coping and psychological and physical adjustment. *Journal of Personality and Social Psychology, 74*, 1109–1120.

Coyne, J. C., & Holroyd, K. (1982). Stress, coping, and illness. In T. Millon, C. Green, & R. Meagher (Eds.), *Handbook of clinical health psychology* (pp. 103–128). New York, NY: Plenum Press.

D'Arienzo, J. A. (2010). Inoculation training for trauma and stress-related disorders. In S. S. Fehr (Ed.), *101 interventions in group therapy* (pp. 431–435). New York, NY: Routledge/Taylor & Francis Group.

Dewe, P. J. (1992). The appraisal process: Exploring the role of meaning, importance, control, and coping in work stress. *Anxiety, Stress, and Coping, 5*, 95–109.

Dobson, K. S. (2010). *Handbook of cognitive-behavioral therapies* (3rd ed.). New York, NY: Guilford.

Dobson, K. S., & Shaw, B. F. (1995). Cognitive therapies in practice. In B. Bongar & L. E. Bentler (Eds.), *Comprehensive textbook of psychotherapies: Theory and practice* (pp. 159–172). New York, NY: Oxford University Press.

Ellis, A. (1971). Emotional disturbance and its treatment in a nutshell. *Canadian Counselor, 5*, 168–171.

Ellis, A. (1973). *Humanistic psychology: The rational-emotive approach*. New York, NY: Julian.

Ellis, A. (1984). The use of hypnosis with rational-emotive therapy. *Journal of Integrative and Eclectic Psychotherapy, 2*, 15–22.

Ellis, A. (1991). The revised ABC's of rational-emotive therapy (RET). *Journal of Rational-Emotive and Cognitive-Behavior Therapy, 9*, 139–177.

Ellis, A. (1995). Reflections on rational-emotive therapy (RET). *Journal of Rational-Emotive and Cognitive-Behavior Therapy, 9*, 139–177.

Fairburn, C. G. (2008). *Cognitive behavior therapy and eating disorders*. New York, NY: Guilford.

Flaxman, P. E., & Bond, F. W. (2010). A randomized worksite comparison of acceptance and commitment therapy and stress inoculation training. *Behavior Research and Therapy, 48*, 816–820.

Forman, E. M., & Herbert, J. D. (2009). New directions in cognitive behavior therapy: Acceptance-based therapies. In W. O'Donohue & J. E. Fisher (Eds.), *General principles and empirically supported techniques of cognitive behavior therapy* (pp. 102–114). Hoboken, NJ: Wiley.

Girdano, D. A., Everly, G. S., Jr., & Dusek, D. E. (1997). *Controlling stress and tension* (5th ed.). Boston, MA: Allyn & Bacon.

Girdano, D., Dusek, D., & Everly, G. (2009). Controlling stress and tension. San Francisco, CA: Pearson Benjamin Cummings.

Grinker, R. R., & Spiegel, J. P. (1945). War neuroses in flying personnel overseas and after return to the U.S.A. *American Journal of Psychiatry, 101*, 619–624.

Hayes, S. C. (2004). Acceptance and Commitment Therapy, Relational Frame Theory, and the third wave of behavioral and cognitive therapies. *Behavior Therapy, 35*, 639–665.

Hayes, S. C., Levin, M. E., Plumb-Vilardaga, J., Villatte, J. L., & Pistorello, J. (2011). Acceptance and Commitment Therapy and Contextual Behavioral Science: Examining the progress of a distinctive model of behavioral and cognitive therapy. *Behavior Therapy,* Available online: http://www.sciencedirect.com/science/article/pii/S0005789411000669

Hayes, S. C., Luoma, J. B., Bond, F. W., Masuda, A., & Lillis, J. (2006). Acceptance and Commitment Therapy: Model, processes and outcomes. *Behavior Research and Therapy, 44*, 1–25.

Hayes, S. C., Strosahl, K. D., & Wilson, K. G. (1999). *Acceptance and commitment therapy: An experiential approach to behavior change*. New York, NY: Guilford Press.

Hemenover, S. H., & Dienstbier, R. A. (1996). The effects of an appraisal manipulation: Affect, intrusive cognitions, and performance for two cognitive tasks. *Motivation and Emotion, 20*, 319–340.

Herbert, J. D., & Forman, E. M. (2011). Caution: the differences between CT and ACT may be larger (and smaller) than they appear. *Behavior Therapy,* Available online: http://www.science-direct.com/science/article/pii/S0005789411000712

Hofmann, S. G., Asmundson, G. J. G., & Beck, A. T. (2011). The science of cognitive therapy. *Behavior Therapy,* 1–14. Retreived from: http://www.sciencedirect.com/science/article/pii/S0005789411000591

Lazarus, R. S. (1966). *Psychological stress and the coping process*. New York: McGraw-Hill.

Lazarus, R. S. (1982). Thoughts on the relations between emotions and cognition. *American Psychologist, 37*, 1019–1024.

Lazarus, R. S. (1999). *Stress and emotion: A new synthesis*. New York: Springer.

Levine, L. J. (1996). The anatomy of disappointment: A natural test of appraisal models of sadness, anger, and hope. *Cognition and Emotion, 10*, 337–359.

Meichenbaum, D. (1977). *Cognitive-behavior modification*. New York: Plenum Press.

Meichenbaum, D. (1985). *Stress innoculation training*. New York: Plenum Press.

Meichenbaum, D. (1993). Stress inoculation training: A 20-year update. In P. M. Lehrer & R. L. Woolfolk (Eds.), *Principles and practice of stress management* (2nd ed., pp. 373–406). New York: Guilford.

Meichenbaum, D. (1995). Changing conceptions of cognitive behavior modification: Retrospect and prospect. In M. Mahoney (Ed.), *Cognitive and constructive psychotherapies: Theory, research, and practice* (pp. 20–26). New York: Springer.

Meichenbaum, D. (2007). Stress inoculation training. A preventative and treatment approach. In P. M. Lehrer, R. L. Woolfolk, & W. E. Sime (Eds.) *Principles and practice of stress mamangement* (3rd ed., pp. 497–516. New York: Guilford

Meichenbaum, D., & Jaremko, M. (1983). *Stress reduction and prevention*. New York: Plenum Press.

Parkinson, B., & Manstead, A. S. R. (1992). Appraisal as a cause of emotion. In M.Clark (Ed.), *Emotion* (pp. 122–149). Newbury Park, CA: Sage.

Peeters, M. C. W., Buunk, B. P., & Schaufeli, W. B. (1995). The role of attributions in the cognitive appraisal of work-related stressful events: An event-recording approach. *Work and Stress, 9*, 463–474.

Powers, M. B., Zum V rde Sive V rding, M. D., & Emmelkamp, P. M. G. (2009). Acceptance and Commitment Therapy: A meta-analytic review. *Psychotherapy and Psychosomatics, 78*, 73–80.

Roseman, L. (1984). Cognitive determinants of emotion. In P. Shaver (Ed.), *Review of personality and social psychology* (pp. 11–36). Beverly Hills, CA: Sage.

Sanderson, W. C., Rapee, R. M., & Barlow, D. H. (1989). The influence of an illusion of control on panic attacks induced via inhalation of 5.5% carbon dioxide-enriched air. *Archives of General Psychiatry, 46*, 157–162.

Terry, D. J., Tonge, L., & Callan, V. J. (1995). Employee adjustment to stress: The role of coping resources, situational factors, and coping resources. *Anxiety, Stress, and Coping, 8*, 1–24.

Zajonc, R. B. (1984). On the primacy of affect. *American Psychologist, 39*(2), 117–123.

Chapter 9
A Neurophysiological Rationale for the Use of the Relaxation Response: Neurological Desensitization

Since the original applications of behavioral technologies to the treatment of disease, it has been observed that the elicitation of what Benson (1975) has called the "relaxation response" has proved useful in the treatment of a wide variety of psychiatric and stress-related somatic diseases (Benson, 1974; Caudill, Schnable, Zuttermeister, Benson, & Friedman, 1991; Chen et al., 2009; Domar, Seidel, & Benson, 1990; Dunford & Thompson, 2010; Forbes, et al., 2008; Hellman, 1990; Kutz, Borysenko, & Benson, 1985; Lavey & Taylor, 1985; Mackereth, Booth, Hillier, & Caress, 2009; Manzoni, Pagnini, Castelnuovo, & Molinari, 2008; Moturi & Avis, 2010; Rausch, Gramilin, & Auerbach, 2006; Shapiro & Giber, 1978). The relaxation response is perhaps best understood as a psychophysiological state of hypoarousal engendered by a multitude of diverse technologies (e.g., meditation, neuromuscular relaxation, hypnosis). Research into the relaxation response as a therapeutic mechanism and its clinical proliferation have been hampered, however, by a lack of conceptual clarity regarding its therapeutic foundations and/ or its mechanisms of action. This chapter will explore the physiological and psychological foundations of the relaxation response to set the stage for discussions in subsequent chapters of specific therapeutic technologies (e.g., meditation, neuromuscular relaxation) used to elicit the relaxation response for the treatment of stress-related diseases.

The specific aims of this chapter are: (1) to explore the psychophysiological foundations of the relaxation response as a possible rationale for the use of the relaxation response as a primary therapy as well as an adjunctive therapy in the treatment of pathogenic stress arousal (while remaining aware of the fact that in some cases specific end-organ symptoms may initially require medical stabilization or amelioration); (2) to gain insight into the counterintuitive and antireductionistic observation that a single therapeutic mechanism (i.e., the relaxation response) can be of value in treating a wide and disparate variety of psychiatric and stress-related somatic disorders; and (3) to consider the relaxation response as a natural treatment for anxiety and excessive stress arousal—a treatment intrinsically antithetical to the very nature of pathogenic stress arousal.

G.S. Everly and J.M. Lating, *A Clinical Guide to the Treatment of the Human Stress Response*, DOI 10.1007/978-1-4614-5538-7_9,
© Springer Science+Business Media New York 2013

In order to formulate such a view of the relaxation response as a therapeutic mechanism, it first becomes necessary to reformulate the common perspective on psychiatric and stress-related somatic disorders.

Disorders of Arousal

Traditionally, science has classified diseases on the basis of their cause or their end-organ symptoms or signs. The American Psychiatric Association's *Diagnostic and Statistical Manual of Mental Disorders* (DSM-IV-TR; American Psychiatric Association, 2000) is replete with examples of both. Regarding classification by "cause," for example, adjustment disorders are "caused" by the inability to adjust to new situations; viral disorders are caused by viruses; and bacteriological disorders are caused by bacteria. Regarding classification by symptoms, on the other hand, mood disorders are characterized by affective symptom complexes, and anxiety disorders are characterized by anxious symptomatology. The posttraumatic stress disorder is classified by both its cause (trauma) *and* its symptoms (stress). Seldom in our nosological quests, however, do we bother to consider other, less obvious, taxonomic criteria, even though these "latent taxa" might be far more utilitarian. Such a taxonomic consideration is derived from the work of Meehl (1973).

Based on an integration of the work of Selye (1976), Gellhorn (1967), Gray (1982), and Post (Post & Ballenger, 1981), it has been proposed that various anxiety and stress-related diseases be viewed in light of a new taxonomic perspective (Everly, 1985b; Everly & Benson, 1989). Evidence indicates that numerous psychiatric and somatic stress-related diseases possess a latent yet common denominator that serves nosologically as a latent taxonomic criterion—"latent taxon" for short. It has been proposed that this latent taxon is pathognomonic arousal. Thus, such disorders may be referred to collectively as "disorders of arousal." Despite a wide variety of etiological stimuli, and an even wider variety of symptom complexes, these disorders are best seen as but variations on a theme of a pathognomonic hypersensitivity for, or an overall characteristic of, arousal.

More specifically, the "disorders of arousal" concept is based on a corpus of evidence indicating that a major homogenizing phenomenological constituent of these disorders is a limbic-system-based neurological hypersensitivity; that is, a lowered threshold for excitation and/or a pathognomonic status of excess arousal within the limbic circuitry or its neurological, neuroendocrine, and/or endocrine efferent limbs. This neurological hypersensitivity is then capable of giving rise to a host of psychiatric and stress-related somatic disorders as noted in Chaps. 3 and 4 (see Fig. 9.1). These disorders are referred to collectively as "disorders of arousal."

Fig. 9.1 Limbic
hypersensitivity
phenomenon: The latent
taxon in stress-related
"disorders of arousal"

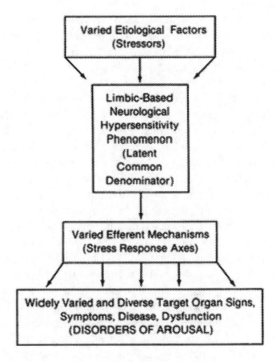

Psychiatric Disorders of Arousal

Over the years, clinical psychiatry anecdotes have well documented the notion that anxiety disorders and stress-related syndromes seem to be characterized by what appears to be an increased vulnerability to frustrating, challenging, or sympathomimetic stimuli. This phenomenon is best thought of as a hypersensitivity for stimulation; a sort of neurological sensitization combined with a lowered activation threshold for emotional arousal. Such reports of sensitization or hyperreactivity are consistent with the well-documented activity and function of the limbic system and its major neurological, neuroendocrine, and endocrine efferents (Cannon, 1929; Gray, 1982; MacLean, 1949; Nauta & Domesick, 1982).

In a seminal paper, Papez (1937) boldly discussed the rhinencephalon as the anatomical basis for emotional arousal. He considered the mammillary bodies, fornix, hippocampus, cingulate cortex, and anterior thalamic nuclei as key elements in a then-proposed mechanism of emotion. In a description of Papez's model, Papez notes:

> Neural activity representing the emotional processes originating in the cortex would be passed along into the hippocampus, the fornix, the mammillary bodies, and the anterior nuclei of the thalamus and would finally be projected onto the receptive region of the "emotional cortex" (i.e., the cingulate cortex). From the cingulate cortex, activity representing emotional processes could pass into other regions of the cerebral cortex and add emotional coloring to psychic processes occurring elsewhere. (p. 55)

The "Papez Circuit," as it came to be called, was modified as a contributor to human emotional arousal by MacLean (1949), who developed the notion of a "limbic system" (the term *limbic* is derived from limbus, which means border and refers to the fact that this system serves to undergird the cerebral neocortices). MacLean (1949) hypothesized that in addition to the basic circuitry of Papez, the amygdala, septum, and associated areas were best understood as a "system" of integrated anatomical structures that were implicated not only in emotional expression but also in the aggregation of all sensory stimulation with affect, and that ultimately provide for emotional expression, or "discharge." Such discharge would have profound potential to affect not only mental health but also physical health. According to MacLean, "This region of the brain appears to be so strategically situated as to be able to correlate every form of internal and external perception. And ... has many strong connections with the hypothalamus for discharging its impressions." (p. 351). It should be noted that the hypothalamus and hippocampus are still thought to be the prime sites of integration for visceral efferent arousal discharge (LeDoux, 1992; Reiman et al., 1986; Van Hoesen, 1982; for more recent research see, Streeter, Gerbarg, Saper, Ciraulo, & Brown, 2012; Feder, Charney, & Collins, 2011).

Finally, the work of Nauta (Nauta, 1979; Nauta & Domesick, 1982) further refined and clarified our understanding of the vital role that the limbic system plays in emotional arousal, the integration of internal and external stimulation, and the process of hypothalamically mediated "psychosomatic" processes. His work supports the conclusion that sensory input is integrated and processed via limbic structures such as the amygdala, the hippocampus, and cingulate gyrus and that such limbic structures have the potential for upward and downward efferent projections. Such projections are likely to exert influence over neocortical as well as hypothalamic, neuroendocrine, and endocrine processes.

It is important to note at this juncture that the limbic system receives efferent impulses from, as well as sending afferent impulses to, brain-stem structures—more specifically the reticular activating system and the locus coeruleus. The reticular activating system (RAS) may be thought of as a system of projections with responsibility for nonspecific arousal of the entire cerebrum. The locus coeruleus (LC) represents an aggregation of 20,000–30,000 cells responsible for 50–70% of the norepinephrine in the human brain (Redmond, 1979). Its activity is highly associated with worry, threat, and flight behavior. The reciprocal connections that the LC has with prefrontal and limbic structures suggest cognitive, affective, and LC activities are intimately interwoven (Gellhorn, 1967; Redmond) and collectively may play key etiologic roles in psychiatric and somatic disorders (Doane, 1986; Gellhorn & Loofbourrow, 1963; Gloor, 1986; Post, 1986; Post & Ballenger, 1981).

The American Psychiatric Association's own DSM-III, DSM-III-R, DSM-IV, and DSM-IV-TR have included references to criteria such as hyper-alertness, hypersensitivity, and autonomic nervous system hyperactivity in the diagnosis of anxiety-related disorders. Considerable evidence that these symptoms arise from the limbic circuitry comes from benzodiazepine and other behavioral pharmacological research (Carr & Sheehan, 1984; Gray, 1982; Pinna, Costa, Guidotti, 2009)

Table 9.1 Psychiatric disorders related to arousal

1. Anxiety disorders (posttraumatic stress disorder, panic disorders, and diffuse generalized anxiety disorders)
2. Adjustment disorders (with anxious mood and with mixed emotional features)
3. Various primary and secondary affective disorders (especially fast-cycling bipolar disorders and secondary reactive depression)
4. Addictive disorders (cocaine, amphetamine, nicotine)
5. Temporal lobe disorders
6. Acute atypical psychotic decompensation
7. Alcohol withdrawal ($X > 6$ years alcoholism)

as well as neurotransmitter research (Mefferd, 1979; Nordquist & Oreland, 2010). Even major reviews of the etiology, diagnosis, and treatment of anxiety disorders implicate subcortically initiated arousal and reactivity as core features of anxiety disorders (Aggleton, 1992; Barlow & Beck, 1984; Carr & Sheehan, 1984; Friedman, Charney, & Deutch, 1995; Gorman, Dillon, Fyer, Liebowitz, & Klein, 1985; Shader, 1984; Shin & Liberson, 2011).

Anxiety disorders are not the only psychiatric disorders wherein arousal plays a significant role. Post and his co-workers (Post, 1985; Post & Ballenger, 1981; Post, Uhde, Putnam, Ballenger, & Berrettini, 1982; more recently, Simon, Kaufman, Musch, Kischkel, & Kathmann, 2010) have cogently argued that limbic hypersensitivity ("sensitization") underlies various primary and secondary affective disorders. They conclude that "sensitization models provide a conceptual approach to previously inexplicable clinical phenomena in the longitudinal course of affective illness" (p. 191). Neurological sensitization is also believed to underlie various functional psychoses, personality disorders, posttraumatic reactions, addictive disorders, and withdrawal syndromes (Aggleton, 1992; Monroe, 1970; 1982; Post, 1985; Post & Ballenger, 1981; Post, Weiss, & Smith, 1995; van der Kolk, Greenberg, Boyd, & Krystal, 1985; more recently Savitz & Drevets, 2009). Similarly, Gellhorn and Loofburrow (1963) implicated propensities for excessive limbic excitation in a host of emotional disorders (see Table 9.1).

The sensitization phenomenon may be based upon one or more of six mechanisms (Cain, 1992; Everly, 1993; Gloor, 1992):

1. Augmentation of excitatory neurotransmitters.
2. Declination of inhibitory neurotransmitters.
3. Augmentation of micromorphological structures (especially amygdaloidal and hippocampal).
4. Changes in the biochemical bases of neuronal activation (e.g., augmentation of phosphoproteins and/or changes on the transduction mechanism *c-fos* so as to change the genetic message within the neuron's nucleus).
5. Increased neuromuscular arousal.
6. Repetitive cognitive excitation.

Somatic Disorders of Arousal

The psychiatric domain is not the only arena within which pathogenic arousal may manifest itself. Many stress-related "medical" syndromes contain a core arousal constituent. A review by Lown et al. (1976) concluded that ventricular fibrillation in the absence of coronary heart disease may be related to increased sympathetic tone or activity. Similarly, evidence indicates that increased sympathetic tone and sympathetic hyperreactivity may be key etiological factors in the development of psychophysiological essential hypertension (Eliot, 1979; Gellhorn, 1964a; Grassi & Esler, 1999; Henry & Stephens, 1977; Steptoe, 1981; Suter, 1986). Other cardiovascular diseases implicated as having pathogenic arousal as a key etiological factor include nonischemic myofibrillar degeneration (Corley, 1985; Eliot), coronary artery disease (Corley; Eliot; Henry & Stephens, 1977; see Manuck & Krantz, 1984, for a more conservative interpretation; more recently, Moulapoulos, 2009), sudden death (Corley; Eliot; Steptoe, 1981), and migraine headaches (Mehlsteibl, Schankin, Herin, Sostak, & Straube, 2011) and Raynaud's disease (Suter, 1986; Cooke & Marshall, 2005). Gellhorn (1967), Weil (1974), and Malmo (1975) have implicated excessive sympathetic tone as a major etiological factor in a host of muscle contraction syndromes and dysfunctions including muscle contraction headaches and fibromyalgia (Sarzi-Puttini, Atzeni, & Cazzola, 2010). Finally, there is some evidence that peptic ulcers (Wolf, 1985), irritable bowel syndrome (Latimer, 1985), and other gastrointestinal disorders may be related to an excessive propensity for arousal (Dotevall, 1985; Henke, 1992; see Table 9.2).

In summary, pathognomonic hypersensitivity within the limbic circuitry as a common denominator within a host of otherwise widely disparate disorders seems to warrant the proposed taxonomic reconsideration, that is, the disorders of arousal taxonomy. It may well be that research will ultimately show that disorders of arousal actually include all stress-related psychosomatic disorders (see Friedman & Schnurr, 1995; Heninger, 1995; Williams, 1995; Chrousos, 2009).

Table 9.2 Somatic disorders related to arousal

1. Hypertension
2. Stress-related ventricular fibrillation
3. Nonischemic myofibrillar degeneration
4. Stress-related coronary artery disease
5. Migraine headaches
6. Raynaud's disease
7. Muscle contradiction headaches
8. Non-head-related muscle contraction dysfunctions
9. Peptic ulcer
10. Irritable bowel syndrome

The Neurological Foundations of Limbic Hypersensitivity and the Disorders of Arousal

Ergotropic Tuning

Within this chapter, it has been argued that a limbic-system-based neurological hypersensitivity to stimulation and a propensity for sustained arousal undergirds a host of psychiatric and stress-related somatic disorders, herein called "disorders of arousal." The work of Gellhorn not only documented the existence of complex autonomic nervous system–neocortical–limbic–somatic integration (Gellhorn, 1957; 1967) but also later served as one of the most coherent and cogent explanations of the pathognomonic arousal described in this chapter. Over four decades ago, Gellhorn described a hypothalamically based "ergotropic tuning" process as the neurophysiological basis for affective lability, ANS hyperfunction, anxiety, stress arousal, and related emotional disorders (Gellhorn, 1965; 1967; Gellhorn & Loofburrow, 1963). Gellhorn has stated:

> It is a matter of everyday experience that a person's reaction to a given situation depends very much upon his own mental, physical, and emotional state. One might be said to be "set" to respond in a given manner. In the same fashion the autonomic response to a given stimulus may at one time be predominantly sympathetic and may at another time be predominantly parasympathetic. ... The sensitization of autonomic centers has been designated "tuning" and we speak of sympathetic tuning and parasympathetic tuning... and refers merely to the "sensitization" or "facilitation" of particular centers of the brain. (Gellhorn & Loofburrow, 1963, pp. 90–91)

Gellhorn chose the term *ergotropic tuning* to describe a preferential pattern of SNS responsiveness. Such a neurological status could then serve as the basis for a host of psychiatric and stress-related somatic disorders.

From an etiological perspective, Gellhorn (1965) states: "In the waking state the ergotropic division of the autonomic is dominant and responds primarily to environmental stimuli. If these stimuli are very strong or follow each other at short intervals, the tone and reactivity of the sympathetic system increases" (pp. 494–495). Thus, either extremely intense, acute (traumatic) sympathetic stimulation or chronically repeated, intermittent lower level sympathetic stimulation, both of which can be environmental in origin, can lead to SNS hyperfunction. Such sympathetic activity, according to Gellhorn, creates a condition of sympathetic neurological hypersensitivity, called ergotropic tuning, which serves as the neurological predisposition, or even etiological factor, associated with the psychophysiological sequelae observed in anxiety, stress, and related disorders of arousal.

Several mechanisms may sustain the ergotropically tuned status. Gellhorn (1964a, b) has provided cogent documentation that discharge from limbic centers sends neural impulses in two simultaneous directions: (1) to neocortical targets and (2) to the skeletal musculature via pyramidal and extrapyramidal projections (see also Gellhorn & Loofburrow, 1963). The neocortical centers then send impulses back to the limbic areas and to the locus coeruleus by way of noradrenergic and other pathways, thus sustaining limbic activity. Simultaneously, neuromuscular proprioceptive impulses (indicative of neuromuscular status) from afferent muscle spindle projections ascend primarily via the dorsal root and reticular activating system, ultimately projecting not only to cerebellar targets but also to limbic and neocortical targets. Such proprioceptive bombardment further excites target areas and sets into motion a complex mechanism of positive neurological feedback, sustaining and potentially intensifying ergotropic tone (Gellhorn, 1964a, b; 1965; 1967).

Thus, we see that Gellhorn has proposed a model and empirically demonstrated that intimate neocortical–hypothalamic–somatic relationships exist that use the limbic system as a central "hub" for efferent projections to the neocortex and somatic musculature as well as an afferent target for neocortical, proprioceptive, interoceptive, and brain-stem impulses. This configuration creates a functional, potentially self-sustaining mechanism of affective and ergotropic arousal. It certainly seems reasonable that such a mechanism could play a major role in chronic anxiety and stress-related disorders of arousal.

Neurological Reverberation and Charging

Weil (1974) has developed a model somewhat similar to that of Gellhorn. In fact, Weil makes brief reference to the work of Gellhorn in his construction of a neurophysiological model of emotional behavior.

Weil notes, in agreement with Gellhorn, that the activation thresholds of the ANS (particularly hypothalamic nuclei), as well as limbic centers, can be altered. Instead of the concepts of sympathetic and parasympathetic systems, Weil uses a parallel but broader construction, that of arousal and tranquilizing systems, respectively. He calls the facilitation of activation within these systems, "charging." With regard to the concept of neurological hypersensitivity, Weil notes that two major processes can be effective in "charging the arousal system" in the human organism: (1) high-intensity stimulation and/or (2) increased rate of repeated stimulation. The processes that appear to underlie the charging of the arousal system as well as the mechanisms that could serve to sustain such a neurological status seem to be (1) the neuromuscular proprioceptive system, as described earlier, and (2) intrinsic neuronal reverberation. Regarding the latter, Weil (1974) notes:

> The reciprocal association of the hypothalamus with the midbrain and the thalamic reticular formation makes possible the establishment of intrinsic reverberating circuits. Such hypothalamic reticular circuits are in a position to be set into motion by extrinsic impulses reaching the reticular formation. They provide a neuroanatomical basis for the maintenance of a reverberating supply of impulses to reticular nonspecific activation even during a momentary reduction or deficiency of extrinsic input. (p. 37)

Thus, we see that Weil's notion of charging is similar to Gellhorn's notion of tuning. Weil's formulation seems somewhat broader in the neurological mechanisms it encompasses, yet narrower in its implications for emotional and behavioral disorders. Points of agreement can be found, however, in the recognition of the fact that neurological hypersensitivity (i.e., a lowered threshold for activating limbic, autonomic, and hypothalamic effector systems) can be achieved through environmental stimulation and proprioceptive stimulation when presented in either an acute and intense (trauma-like) manner or in a lower level yet chronically repeated exposure pattern. Once achieved, such a status of lowered activation threshold could serve as a self-sustaining neurological basis for emotional and psychophysiological dysfunction.

Neuromuscular Set-Point Theory

In reviewing Gellhorn's and Weil's notions of tuning and charging theory, respectively, and the neurological mechanisms that support them, one is impressed with the central role that the striated musculature plays in sensitizing and maintaining hypersensitivity (ergotropic status). The work of Malmo seems appropriate to introduce at this juncture, for it deals directly with the role of striated muscles in psychophysiological and anxiety disorders. In a brief but cogent treatise, Malmo (1975) summarizes his classic studies on the prolonged activation of the striated musculature of anxiety patients following stressor presentation, compared with nonanxiety patients exposed to the same stressor. The work of Gellhorn clearly demonstrated that the striated muscles were target organs for limbic arousal. Malmo and his colleagues found that select groups of individuals who possessed arousal disorders, such as anxiety, seemed to demonstrate somewhat higher baseline levels of muscle tension when compared with nonpatients. More important, however, upon the presentation of a stressor stimulus, the muscle tension of the patient population reached higher levels of peak amplitude and subsequently took significantly longer to return to baseline levels once the stressor was removed. This phenomenon was interpreted by Malmo as being indicative of a defect in homeostatic mechanisms following arousal in such patients.

Malmo offered two possible mechanisms that might explain the observed homeostatic dysfunction: one neural, the other biochemical. He cites the research of Jasper (1949), who discovered that direct stimulation of the motor cortex created not only the expected electromyographic activity in the target muscle but also an "after discharge" in that muscle. The after discharge may be thought of as a residual depolarization of the neurons in the absence of direct exogenous stimulation. However, when Jasper simultaneously stimulated the thalamic–reticular system, the after discharge was eliminated. These data suggest that the thalamic–reticular system may play a role in dampening, or inhibiting, excess neuromuscular activation. Malmo then extended Jasper's work to his own and used it as a model to explain the homeostatic dysfunction observed in his own studies. Malmo saw Jasper's discovery as the homeostatic mechanism that was most likely dysfunctional in anxiety patients (i.e., a mechanism protracting neuromuscular excitation in stressful situations). More specifically, he argues that this neural inhibitory system represents a "set point" similar to that of a thermostat. This neural set point may be designed to dampen excessive muscular activity, thus preventing excessive strain. He notes that in cases where muscles are extremely tense and corresponding proprioceptive activity is sufficiently strong (i.e., exceeding the tolerances of the set point), the inhibitory neurons would be activated, thus reducing lingering peripheral muscular after-charge activity. He further notes:

> Such a system as this would work well in providing for extra muscular exertion to meet emergencies; and by the return of the set point to normal afterwards, the motor system would have a built-in protection against excessive strain. If, however, extremely demanding life situations are prolonged ... it seems the setpoint "sticks" at the higher (above normal) level even when the individual is removed to a quiet environment. This then would be a neural mechanism that could account for the "persistence" of anxiety and the accompanying increase in muscular activity. (Malmo, 1975, pp. 152–153)

Malmo places the most emphasis on this neural mechanism in explaining the homeostatic dysfunction seen in anxiety patients, yet he does briefly mention a biochemical–neurological process that has played a central role in the formulation of current thinking on arousal disorders. Malmo notes that muscle tension leads to increased levels of lactic acid (a by-product of anaerobic metabolism). Furthermore, he notes research by Pitts and McClure (1967) clearly demonstrating that lactate infusions had panicogenic properties for panic anxiety patients but had none for nonanxiety patients. It has been postulated that panic patients metabolize lactate normally, thus suggesting a neural receptor hypersensitivity existing somewhere in their CNS as the etiological site for this dysfunction. The lactate infusion data are similar to those obtained by inhalation of 5% CO_2, thus demonstrating panicogenic properties for this agent as well. The specific mechanism by which these agents induce panic attacks is unclear at this time. Interested readers should refer to Carr and Sheehan (1984), Gorman, Dillon, Fyer, Liebowitz, and Klein (1985), and Liebowitz et al. (1984). The major point of clinical interest, however, is that Gellhorn and Weil, as well as Malmo, have shown mechanisms by which anxiety and stress may lead to chronically contracted muscles and that these muscles (while under chronic anaerobic contraction) may produce a by-product (lactic acid) that may have anxiogenic properties of a biochemical nature in addition to the anxiogenic properties of excessive proprioceptive bombardment of the brain stem, limbic system, and neocortex. Thus, there appears to be remarkable agreement from researchers in diverse fields as to the probability that neurological hypersensitivity underlies anxiety and stress-related disorders of a chronic nature.

Models of Neuronal Plasticity

In an attempt to understand the phenomenon of neurological hypersensitivity at the most basic structural levels, this section briefly reviews popular models of neuronal plasticity. It should be noted that the phenomenon of neural plasticity appears to be evolving from the role of explanatory construct to useful clinical phenomenon, largely as our understanding of this once vague notion has similarly evolved. In this section we briefly follow that evolution.

The concept of *kindling* represents one of the most popular models of plasticity and neurological hypersensitivity in clinical literature. *Kindling* is a term originally conceived of to identify the process by which repeated stimulation of limbic structures leads to a lowered convulsive threshold (limbic ictus) and to a propensity for spontaneous activation of such structures, with resultant affective lability, ANS hyperfunction, and behavioral disturbances (Goddard, McIntyre, & Leech, 1969; Joy, 1985; Post, 1985; Post, Uhde, Putnam, Ballenger, & Berrettini, 1982). Kindling-like processes have been implicated in a host of behavioral and psychopathological conditions (Cain, 1992; Gloor, 1992; Mann, 1992; Monroe, 1970; Post & Ballenger, 1981; Reynolds, 1992; McFarlane, 2010).

Shader (1984) has stated, "With regard to anxiety disorders, one might speculate that kindling processes … could increase attack-like firing from a source such as the locus coeruleus" (p. 14). Redmond and Huang (1979) support such a conclusion by suggesting that panic disorders are predicated on a lowered firing threshold at the locus coeruleus. Such discharge could then arouse limbic and cortical structures on the basis of ventral and dorsal adrenergic efferent projections arising from the locus coeruleus. Monroe (1982) has provided evidence that certain episodic behavioral disorders may be based on a kindling-like limbic ictus. He notes, "As it is known that environmental events can induce synchronized electrical activity within the limbic system, this also provides an explanation of why environmental stress might sensitize patients to acute exacerbations of an ictal illness" (p. 713). Monroe (1970; 1982) implicates explosive behavioral tirades, impulsively destructive behavior, extreme affective lability, and episodic psychotic behavior in such a neurological dysfunction. According to van der Kolk, Greenberg, Boyd, and Krystal (1985), "Long-term augmentation of LC (locus coeruleus) pathways following trauma underlies the repetitive intrusive recollections and nightmares that plague patients with PTSD (posttraumatic stress disorder)" (p. 318).

Post et al. (1982) have taken the kindling model and extrapolated from it, stating, "Kindling and related sensitization models may also be useful conceptual approaches to understanding the development of psychopathology in the absence of seizure discharges" (p. 719). They report data that demonstrate the ability of adrenergic and dopaminergic agonists to sensitize animals and humans to behavioral hyperactivity and especially affective disorders. They refer to this phenomenon as "behavioral sensitization" rather than kindling because no ictal status is obtained as an end point. Rather, the achieved end point represents a lowered depolarization threshold and an increased propensity for spontaneous activation of limbic and related circuitry (Post, Weiss, & Smith, 1995).

According to Racine, Tuff and Zaide (1976), "Except for neural development and learning, the kindling phenomenon may be the most robust example of neural plasticity in the mammalian nervous system" (p. 19). Indeed, models of learning and memory may serve as tools for understanding the biology of kindling-like phenomena. Goddard and Douglas (1976) conducted a series of investigations designed to see if the "engram" model of memory had applicability in the understanding of the kindling phenomenon. They concluded:

> Thus it would appear that kindling is caused, in part, by a lasting potentiation of excitatory synapses. More work is needed to decide whether the changes are pre-synaptic or in the post-synaptic membrane, whether they are accompanied by alteration in synaptic morphology... Our answer to the question: does the engram of kindling model the engram of normal long term memory? is yes. (pp. 14–15)

Lynch and his colleagues at the University of California have sought to clarify this mechanism and have identified postsynaptic processes as the likely target area. Their research in long-term neuronal potentiation revealed a functional augmentation in the dendritic spines of stimulated neuronal pathways. More specifically, such changes included a 33% increase in synaptic contacts, as well as a decrease in the length and width variation of the dendritic spines (Deadwyler, Gribkoff, Cotman & Lynch, 1976; Lee, Schottler, Oliver & Lynch, 1980). Rosenzweig and Leiman (1982) have suggested that the number of dendritic spines as well as the postsynaptic membrane area may be increased in such neural plasticity. Delanoy, Tucci and Gold (1983) pharmacologically stimulated the dentate granule cells in rats and found a kindling-like neurological hypersensitivity to result. Similar agonists have been shown to enhance state-dependent learning.

Joy's superb review of the nature and effects of kindling (1985) summarizes the potential alterations in biological substrata that may be involved in the kindling phenomenon. He notes that "kindling produces important changes in neuronal function and connectivity" (p. 46) and continues:

> One would expect that these changes would have morphological or neurochemical correlates. Increased connectivity could result from a morphological rearrangement of neuronal circuits, perhaps from collateral sprouting and new synapse formation. Alternatively, it could result from a modification of existing synapses, perhaps by the growth of presynaptic terminals or by an increase in the postsynaptic receptive surface or number of receptors, (p. 49)

Whatever the biological alteration underlying the neuronal plasticity associated with limbic system neurological hypersensitivity, the phenomenon: (1) appears to be inducible on the basis of repeated, intermittent stimulation (Delanoy et al., 1983), with the optimal interval between stimulations to induce kindling being about 24 h (Monroe, 1982); (2) appears to last for hours, days, and even months (Deadwyler et al., 1976; Fifková & van Harreveld, 1977; Goddard & Douglas, 1976; Monroe, 1982); (3) appears to show at least some tendency to decay over a period of days of months in the absence of continued stimulation if the initial stimulation was insufficient to cause permanent alteration (Fifková & van Harreveld, 1977; Joy, 1985); and (4) appears to be inducible on the basis of environmental, psychosocial, pharmacological, and/or electrical stimulation (Black et al., 1987; Doane, 1986; Monroe, 1970; Post, 1986; Post, Weiss & Smith, 1995; Sorg & Kalivas, 1995).

In summary, the preceding sections have argued for the existence of a group of disorders that share a latent yet common denominator of limbic-based neurological hypersensitivity and arousal. The neurology of this "common thread" has been

Fig. 9.2 Limbic
hypersensitivity phenomenon
(LHP)

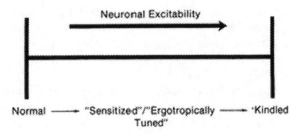

discussed in some detail. Figure 9.2 graphically depicts the hypersensitivity phenomenon.

The etiological and/or sustaining mechanisms of the limbic-system-based neurological hypersensitivity that serves to undergird the disorders of arousal may be summarized into six basic categories:

1. Increased excitatory neurotransmitter activity within the limbic circuitry (Black et al., 1987; Post, 1985; Post & Ballenger, 1981; Post, Rubinow, & Ballenger, 1986; Post, Weiss & Smith, 1995; Sorg & Kalivas, 1995).
2. Declination of inhibitory neurotransmitters and/or receptors (Cain, 1992; see Everly, 1993).
3. Augmentation of micromorphological structures (especially amygdaloidal and hippocampal) (Cain, 1992; Post, Weiss & Smith, 1995; see Everly, 1993).
4. Changes in the biochemical bases of neuronal activation (e.g., augmentation of phosphoproteins and/or changes on the transduction mechanism *c-fos* so as to change the genetic message within the neuron's nucleus) (Cain, 1992; Sorg & Kalivas, 1995).
5. Increased arousal of neuromuscular efferents, with resultant increased proprioceptive bombardment of the limbic system (especially amygdaloid and hippocampal nuclei) (Gellhorn, 1964a, b; 1968; Malmo, 1975; Weil, 1974).
6. Repetitive cognitive excitation (Gellhorn, 1964a, b; Gellhorn, 1968; Gellhorn & Loofburrow, 1963; Post, Rubinow & Ballenger, 1986).

The important point to keep in mind here is that these mechanisms appear to be inducible and responsive to environmental, psychosocial, pharmacological, and/or electrical stimulation (Castren & Rantamaki, 2010; McEwen, 2011). If, indeed, a group of psychiatric and somatic diseases exist that differ in their end-organ symptoms yet share a common pathogenic thread of neurological hypersensitivity and arousal, a therapy for the etiological and sustaining mechanisms of such disorders of arousal seems almost too obvious. If we look beyond the multitude of varied symptoms and signs that characterize these numerous disorders to the common yet latent taxonomic criterion of limbic-based neural hypersensitivity, it becomes obvious that, at least in theory, antiarousal therapies are "ideal" for achieving a neurological desensitization and amelioration of the core mechanism of pathogenesis in all of these disorders. Any such therapy, therefore, should prove of value in treating not only the *symptoms* of these varied disorders (assuming the symptoms have not become self-perpetuating) but also the *causal mechanisms* of neurological hypersensitivity and psychophysiological arousal also. Ironically, Gellhorn and Loofburrow (1963) noted nearly 40 years ago, "If it were possible to alter the autonomic reactivity at the hypothalamic level important therapeutic results might be obtained" (p. 90).

McEwen (2011) masterfully summarizes the notion that learning and other environmental exposures affect neural structures. He notes that excessive stress results in reduced neurogenesis and even dendritic shrinkage, especially in the hippocampal regions. Interventions that reduce stress arousal, especially cortisol saturation might prove neuroprotective. Physical exercise, mental exercise, and even selective serotonergic reuptake inhibitors may exert neuroprotective and even neurogenic effects. It is an easy extrapolation to hypothesize that relaxation techniques might have a similar effect.

The Relaxation Response

The preceding sections have argued that there exists a host of psychiatric and stress-related somatic disorders that, although diverse in their end-organ symptomatology, share a latent common thread of limbicogenic hypersensitivity (i.e., a propensity for hyperreactivity and/ or sustained psychophysiological activation). These disorders have been referred to as "disorders of arousal." The available data suggest that these disorders may possess the following key etiological or sustaining constituents: (1) increased excitatory neurotransmitter activity, (2) increased neuromuscular arousal, and (3) repetitive cognitive excitation. It would seem reasonable that in order for a therapeutic intervention to work effectively to ameliorate these disorders, it should work in such a way as to neurologically desensitize and reduce overall activity within the limbic circuitry. This can be achieved by (1) reducing excitatory neurotransmitter responsivity, (2) reducing neuromuscular arousal, and (3) reducing cognitive excitation. Just such an antiarousal therapy has been uniquely captured in Benson's concept of the "relaxation response," a natural antiarousal psychophysiological phenomenon intrinsically antithetical to the mechanisms that undergird the "disorders of arousal" (Benson, 1975; Benson, Beary & Carol, 1974; Hellman, Budd, Borysenko, McClelland, & Benson, 1990).

Current evidence fails to indicate reliably that there is a best way of eliciting the relaxation response; furthermore, there is no reliable evidence that only one or two specific diseases may show superior therapeutic improvement from its application (Lehrer, Woolfolk & Sime, 2007). Indeed, many technologies are available to elicit the relaxation response, such as mantra meditation, progressive relaxation, presuggestion hypnosis, and prayer (Benson, 1983; 1985), and a wide variety of diverse diseases seem amenable to its therapeutic effect (Benson, 1985; Hellman et al., 1990; Lavey & Taylor, 1985; Lehrer, 1995; Lehrer et al., 2007; Murphy & Donovan, 1988; Shapiro & Giber, 1978).

The Physiology of the Relaxation Response

The physiology of the relaxation response is fundamentally a physiology of hypoarousal, and much of its therapeutic effect derives from this quality. According to Gellhorn, relaxation is a result of a "loss in ergotropic tone of the hypothalamus, [and] a diminution of hypothalamic-cortical discharges" (Gellhorn & Kiely, 1972, p. 404). In agreement with Gellhorn, Taylor (1978) has suggested that relaxation involves a decrease in the arousability of the central nervous system. According to Benson (1983), "The relaxation response results in physiological changes which are thought to characterize an integrated hypothalamic function. These physiological changes are consistent with generalized decreased sympathetic nervous system activity" (p. 282). A more current reinterpretation might be that the relaxation response represents a neurological "desensitization" of the limbic system and/or its sympathetic efferents.

Specific empirical investigations have traditionally shown the elicitation of the relaxation response to result in decreases in O_2 consumption and CO_2 elimination, with no change in the respiratory quotient. Other similar changes include a reduction in heart and respiratory rates with a similar reduction in arterial blood lactate (Benson, 1983; 1985). All of these alterations are consistent with a decrease in central and peripheral adrenergic excitation (Benson, 1985; Delmonte, 1984). Yet the actual mechanisms appear more complex. Research has failed to show reductions consistently in circulating adrenergic catecholamines (Michaels, Haber, & McCann, 1976). In fact, it has been observed that plasma norepinephrine may actually increase as a result of the elicitation of the relaxation response (Hoffman et al., 1982; Lang, Dehof, Meurer, & Kaufmann, 1979). Yet more recent investigations into this seeming paradox reveal that although there may be more norepinephrine available, a diminished adrenergic responsivity actually occurs at the end organ itself (Hoffman et al.; Lehmann et al., 1986). In effect, the relaxation response has shown evidence of exerting effects consistent with those of an adrenergic end-organ blocking agent (Benson, 1983; 1985; Lehmann et al. 1986).

Behavioral psychophysiological studies support the notion that the relaxation response is capable of dampening a form of adrenergic responsivity. In one study, Allen (1981) used a 2,700-Hz tone at 90 dB for a duration of 0.7 s to trigger what was assumed to be posterior hypothalamically mediated arousal in 653 subjects. He found that after training in the relaxation response for a period of approximately 10 weeks, participants demonstrated a dampened psychophysiological responsivity to the auditory stressor. The results of Allen's study are basically in concert with those of Goleman and Schwartz (1976), who compared the stress reactivity of 30 experienced meditators with that of 30 control subjects. Results indicated that recovery from a 12-min video stressor was more rapid among the experienced meditators when compared with the control participants. A study by English and Baker (1983) used a cold pressor to induce arousal and then measured blood pressure recovery time among 36 participants. All participants participated in a 4-week progressive relaxation program and then were submitted to a repetition of the cold pressor.

Results indicated that relaxation training did not reduce cardiovascular response during the stressor but did facilitate a more rapid recovery within the domain of measured blood pressure.

Similar results regarding facilitated psychophysiological recovery as described in this section have been found by Praeger-Decker and Decker (1980) and by Michaels, Parra, McCann and Vander (1979). Although not totally concordant, these studies in the aggregate still suggest that the elicitation of the relaxation response serves to reduce forms of excessive arousal (Benson & Friedman, 1985; Delmonte, 1984). Complete agreement among observers remains entangled, however, in methodological and phenomenological complexities. The interested reader is referred to Suler (1985), Delmonte, Shapiro (1985), and Benson and Friedman (1985) for a useful debate of this topic.

Having addressed the notion of arousal responsivity and the relaxation response, we now consider the issue of neuromuscular arousal. Gellhorn (1964b) notes that "states of abnormal emotional tension are alleviated in various 'relaxation' therapies through reducing proprioceptive impulses which impinge on the posterior hypothalamus and maintain the cerebral cortex in an abnormal state of excitation" (p. 457). Gellhorn (1958a; b; 1964a, b) and Weil (1974) have clearly documented the existing interconnections between the neuromuscular system and the limbic circuitry. Similarly, they have argued that reductions of neuromuscular tone achieved by the elicitation of the relaxation response would be of value in reducing abnormal states of limbic sensitivity and excitation. The primary mechanism of mediation used to achieve such a neurological desensitization, Gellhorn and Weil argue, is the reduction of proprioceptive stimulation to the limbic system.

Finally, Averill (1973), Benson (1983; 1985), Gellhorn (1958b; 1967; Gellhorn & Kiely, 1972), and Lazarus and Folkman (1984) all agree that cognitive distortion, rumination, and overall cognitive excitation can give rise to states of ergotropic and generalized psychophysiological arousal. Similarly, evidence shows that a reduction in cognitive arousal via the relaxation response contributes to a reduction in ergotropic tone and a neurological desensitization effect as well as a reduction in dysphoric psychological states (Benson, 1985; Klajner, Hartman & Sobell, 1984; Kutz, Borysenko, & Benson, 1985; Lavey & Taylor, 1985; Shapiro & Giber, 1978).

The "psychotherapeutic effect" of the relaxation response has been hypothesized to be derived from a sense of "mental calmness" (Rachman, 1968), a sense of "control" (Klajner, Hartman & Sobell, 1984; Stoyva & Anderson, 1982), and a reduction of cognitive–affective rumination (Gellhorn, 1964b; Gellhorn & Loofburrow, 1963). In reviewing the evidence for the psychotherapeutic value of the relaxation response, one is struck by the recurrent theme of an increase in "self-efficacy" derived from consistent practice of the relaxation response, as well as the sense of control engendered by the physiological auto-regulatory skills developed (Bandura, 1977; Romano, 1982; Sarnoff, 1982; Shapiro & Giber, 1978).

This point is especially well made by Green and Green (1977), Hamberger and Lohr (1984), and Stoyva and Anderson (1982). Bandura (1982b), however, has done the most to develop this theme. He notes that the most powerful tool for combating perceptions of low self-efficacy and helplessness appears to be experience. Furthermore, he has shown that perceptions of self-efficacy can actually influence SNS activity, as well as subsequent performance. He concludes, "Treatments that eliminate emotional arousal ... heighten perceived efficacy with corresponding improvements in performance" (Bandura, 1982b, p. 28). The relaxation response appears to be just such a treatment.

Selecting a Relaxation Technique

As noted earlier in this chapter, many different techniques/strategies can engender the relaxation response. Such therapeutic technologies include meditation, neuro-muscular relaxation, controlled breathing, imagery, and hypnosis. As Lehrer, Woolfolk and Sime (2007) point out, research has shown there to be no single, best relaxation technology; nor has any one stress-related disorder proved to be the most responsive to therapeutic amelioration by any specific relaxation technique. Not all relaxation techniques, however, are equally efficacious. The answer to this seeming paradox resides in the concept of individual differences.

"Inadequate recognition of individual differences is a methodological deficiency that has seriously slowed psychological research" (Tart, 1975, p. 140). Indeed, few outcomes in the behavioral sciences are a result of "main effects"; rather, "interaction effects" usually explain far more clinical variation.

So how does the clinician know what relaxation technology to employ? What treatment will be the most useful? Rather than ascribe main effects to therapies, perhaps the individual patient should be given primary consideration, as discussed in Chap. 6. If, then, the relaxation response can be engendered via numerous techniques, with none showing generic superiority, then the clinician should select the relaxation technique that best meets the interacting needs of patient, therapist, setting, and disorder (Paul, 1967). Unfortunately, there are no algorithmic models to guide the clinician to this end. Nevertheless, a review of Chap. 6, or texts such as that of Millon and Everly (1985) or Millon (2011), will serve to give the clinician insight into personologic differences. For example, compulsive persons may respond well to structured, directive therapy interventions (e.g., biofeedback), whereas avoidant–defensive persons may respond better to less structured technologies.

In the final analysis, it may be that the most powerful stress management/behavioral medicine programs are multicomponent programs with aspects that functionally address (1) neurological hypersensitivity via neural desensitization practices, (2) neuromuscular hypertension, and (3) pathogenic cognitive reiteration. Such a program was established by Herbert Benson (1979; 1996; Kutz et al., 1985) and evolved into a multidimensional "mind–body" behavioral medicine program through the input of Ian Kutz, Joan Borysenko, Margaret Caudill, Alice Domar, and others, and has been found to be effective in the treatment of a wide variety of "disorders of arousal" (Caudill, 1994; Caudill et al., 1991; Domar et al., 1990; 1992; Hellman, 1990; Hellman et al., 1990; more recently, Dusek & Benson, 2009). Benson's formulations and clinical applications clearly represent "watershed" ideas that have evolved into the "gold standard" of clinical stress management programs.

Clinical Precautions and Undesirable Side Effects

It was assumed that the clinical use of the relaxation response was a totally harmless therapeutic intervention, but data have argued to the contrary.

Luthe (1969) was perhaps the first to point out that the relaxation response should be used with caution. A pioneer in self-regulatory therapies, Luthe has compiled an impressive list of precautions for such therapies. They include psychotic states, dissociative reactions, paranoid ideation, dysfunctional thyroid conditions, and "disagreeable cardiac and vasomotor reactions."

Stroebel (1979), another pioneer in self-regulatory therapies (especially biofeedback), has argued that fragile ego structures serve as precautions for self-regulatory interventions. Heide and Borkovec (1983) observed in 30.8% of their progressive neuromuscular relaxation patients, and in 53.8% of their meditation patients, clinical evidence of anxiety reactions during preliminary training. Edinger (1982), on the other hand, reported that undesirable side effects arose from relaxation training in 3–4% of the clinical cases surveyed.

These disparate reports led Everly, Spollen, Hackman, and Kobran (1987) to conduct a survey analysis of clinical practitioners who use relaxation training as a major component of their practice. Data were obtained from a national survey of 133 clinicians reporting on over 71,000 patients and over 700,000 patient hours. The results indicated that anxiety reactions occurred about 1.0% of the time; muscle tension headaches resulted about 0.8% of the time; a freeing of repressed ideation resulted about 0.7% of the time; and undesirable depersonalization resulted about 0.7% of the time from the elicitation of the relaxation response or some other form of self-regulatory therapy.

Based on the research of Luthe (1969), Stroebel (1979), Emmons (1978), and Everly et al. (1987), there are five major areas of concern in the elicitation of the relaxation response.

Loss of Reality Contact

The loss of reality contact during the elicitation of the relaxation response includes dissociative states, hallucinations, delusions, and perhaps paresthesias. Care should be taken when treating patients who suffer from affective or thought-disturbance psychoses or who use nonpsychotic fantasy excessively. In such conditions, the use of deep relaxation may exacerbate the problem.

Drug Reactions

Clinical evidence has clearly indicated that the induction of the relaxation response may actually intensify the effects of any medication or other chemical substance that the patient may be taking. Of special concern would be patients taking insulin, sedatives/hypnotics, or cardiovascular medications. All such patients should be carefully monitored medically (although in many cases, chronic relaxation may ultimately result in long-term reductions in required use of medications).

Panic States

Panic state reactions are characterized by high levels of anxiety concerning the loss of control, insecurity, and, in some cases, seduction. Diffuse, free-floating worry, and apprehension have also been observed. With such patients it is generally more desirable to provide a more concrete relaxation paradigm (such as neuromuscular techniques or biofeedback) rather than the abstract relaxation paradigms (such as meditation). Similarly, it is important to assure the patient that he or she is really always in control—even in the states of "passive attention," which will be discussed in the following chapter on meditation.

Premature Freeing of Repressed Ideation

It is not uncommon for deeply repressed thoughts and emotions to be released into the patient's consciousness in response to a deeply relaxed state. Although in some psychotherapeutic paradigms such reactions are considered desirable, such reactions could be perceived as destructive by the patient if unexpected and/or too intense to be dealt with constructively at that point in the therapeutic process. Before implementation of relaxation techniques, the clinician may wish to inform the patient of the possibility that such ideation may arise. Similarly, the clinician must be prepared to render support should such thoughts emerge (see Adler & Morrissey-Adler, 1983; Glueck & Stroebel, 1978).

Excessive Trophotropic States

In some instances, relaxation techniques that intended to be therapeutic may induce an excessively lowered state of psychophysiological functioning. If this occurs, several phenomena may result:

1. *Temporary Hypotensive State.* This acute state of lowered blood pressure may cause dizziness, headaches, or momentary fainting, particularly if the patient rushes to stand up following the relaxation session. The clinician should know

the patient's history of resting blood pressure before employing relaxation techniques. Caution should be used if the patient's resting blood pressure is lower than 90 mmHg systolic and 50 mmHg diastolic. Dizziness and fainting can often be aborted if the patient is instructed to open his or her eyes and to stretch and look around the room at the first signs of uncomfortable lightheadedness. Similarly, the patient should be told to wait 1–3 min before standing up following the relaxation session.

2. *Temporary Hypoglycemic State.* This condition of low blood sugar may follow the inducement of the trophotropic state and most likely last until the patient eats. Deep relaxation, like exercise, appears to have an insulin-like action, and may induce such an action if the patient has a tendency for such conditions, or has not eaten properly that day. The acute hypoglycemic state just described may result in symptoms similar to the hypotensive condition.

3. *Fatigue.* Although relaxation techniques are known to create a refreshed feeling of vigor in many patients, a very few have reported feeling tired after relaxation practice. This is a highly unusual result and may be linked to an over-striving to relax on the part of the patient. The clinician should inform the patient that the best outcome in any attempt at relaxation is achieved when the patient *allows* relaxation to occur, rather than making it happen.

Summary

Earlier in this chapter, we suggested that the disorders of arousal described earlier might be treated effectively if limbic hypersensitivity and related factors could be reduced. Operationally, this meant achieving a reduction in (1) adrenergic cate-cholamine activity and responsiveness, (2) neuromuscular arousal, and (3) pathogenic cognitive processes, such as rumination and perceptions of powerlessness and a lack of control. We have reviewed the concept of the relaxation response as described by Benson and found it to be capable of achieving all three of the aforementioned therapeutic goals necessary for the successful treatment of the stress-related psychiatric and somatic disorders of arousal. Thus, it would appear that a cogent rationale for the use of techniques that engender the relaxation response in the treatment of the human stress response has emerged. To briefly review, this chapter has suggested the following:

1. Neuronal hypersensitivity for excitation residing within the limbic system may be a latent common denominator serving to undergird a host of stress-related psychiatric and somatic disorders.
2. These disorders, in the aggregate, have been referred to as "disorders of arousal" by Everly and Benson (Everly, 1985b; Everly & Benson, 1989).
3. The relaxation response, as described by Benson, represents a broad-spectrum psychophysiological phenomenon antithetical to the stress-related disorders of arousal.

4. As such, the relaxation response may be a valuable tool in the treatment of all of the disorders of arousal, despite their wide varieties of etiological mechanisms and their diverse target organ symptom complexes.
5. There is no best relaxation technology. Clinicians should consider the interaction of the needs of the patient, therapist, setting, and disorder in the selection of the technology for the elicitation of the relaxation response.
6. Contrary to popular opinion, the elicitation of the relaxation response is not without its precautions and undesirable side effects. Precautions include patients with psychotic disorders, major affective disorders, patients on pharmacotherapy, and those with dysfunctional thyroid conditions, fragile ego structure, and delusion conditions. Undesirable side effects appear to occur between 3 and 4% of the time (Edinger, 1982; Everly et al. (1987)) and include depersonalization, excessive trophotropic states, anxiety reactions, freeing of repressed ideation, and headaches.

In summary, this chapter has reviewed in detail the neurophysiology of the limbic system and the relaxation response. The notion of the disorders of arousal has also been introduced. In effect, we see the emergence of a rationale for using the relaxation response in the treatment of a multitude of diseases spanning a wide spectrum of traditional diagnostic boundaries—something counterintuitive to traditional, linear, Pasteurian conceptualization.

Thus, we hope that this chapter has given new credibility and importance to therapeutic technologies such as meditation, controlled respiration, and, especially, progressive neuromuscular relaxation exercises (given the important role of proprioception in the prolongation of stress-related disorders). With these points in mind, let us now move to a discussion of techniques that engender the relaxation response and see how they can be used in the treatment of all stress-related disorders of arousal described in this chapter and in Chap. 4.

References

Adler, C., & Morrissey-Adler, S. (1983). Strategies in general psychiatry. In J. Basmajian (Ed.), *Biofeedback* (pp. 239–254). Baltimore, MD: Williams & Wilkins.

Aggleton, J. P. (Ed.). (1992). *The amygdala*. New York, NY: Wiley-Liss.

Allen, R. (1981). Controlling stress and tension. *The Journal of School Health, 17*, 360–364.

American Psychiatric Association. (2000). *Diagnostic and statistical manual of mental disorders* (4th ed. Text revision). Washington, DC: Author

Averill, J. (1973). Personal control over aversive stimuli and its relationship to stress. *Psychological Bulletin, 80*, 286–307.

Bandura, A. (1977). Self-efficacy: Toward a unifying theory of behavioral change. *Psychological Review, 84*, 191–215.

Bandura, A. (1982b). The self and mechanisms of agency. In J. Suls (Ed.), *Psychological perspectives on the self* (pp. 3–39). Hillsdale, NJ: Erlbaum.

Barlow, D., & Beck, J. (1984). The psychosocial treatment of anxiety disorders. In J. B. Williams & R. Spitzer (Eds.), *Psychotherapy research* (pp. 29–69). New York, NY: Guilford.

Benson, H. (1975). *The relaxation response*. New York, NY: Morrow.

Benson, H. (1979). *The mind body effect*. New York, NY: Simon and Schuster.
Benson, H. (1983). The relaxation response: Its subjective and objective historical precedents and physiology. *Trends in Neuroscience, 6*, 281–284.
Benson, H. (1985). *Beyond the relaxation response: How to harness the healing power of your personal beliefs*. New York, NY: Berkley Books.
Benson, H. (1996). *Timeless healing: The power and biology of belief*. New York, NY: Scribner.
Benson, H., Beary, J., & Carol, M. (1974). The relaxation response. *Psychiatry, 37*, 37–46.
Benson, H., & Friedman, R. (1985). A rebuttal to the conclusions of David S Holme's article: Meditation and somatic arousal reduction. *American Psychologist, 40*, 725–728.
Black, I., Adler, J., Dreyfus, C., Friedman, W., Laganuna, E., & Roach, A. (1987). Biochemistry of information storage in the nervous system. *Science, 236*, 1263–1268.
Cain, D. P. (1992). Kindling and the amygdala. In J. P. Aggleton (Ed.), *The amygdala* (pp. 539–560). New York, NY: Wiley-Liss.
Cannon, W. B. (1929). *Bodily changes in pain, fear, hunger, and rage*. New York, NY: Appleton.
Carr, D., & Sheehan, D. (1984). Panic anxiety: A new biological model. *The Journal of Clinical Psychiatry, 45*, 323–330.
Castren, E., & Rantamaki, T. (2010). The role of BDNF and its receptors in depression and antidepressant drug action: Reactivation of developmental plasticity. *Developmental Neurobiology, 70*, 289–297.
Caudill, M. (1994). *Managing pain before it manages you*. New York, NY: Guilford.
Caudill, M., Schnable, R., Zuttermeister, P., Benson, H., & Friedman, R. (1991). Decreased clinic utilization by chronic pain patients. *The Clinical Journal of Pain, 7*, 305–310.
Chen, W. C., Chu, H., Lu, R. B., Chou, Y. H., Chen, C. H., & Chang, Y. C., et al. (2009). Efficacy of progressive muscle relaxation training in reducing anxiety in patients with acute schizophrenia. *Journal of Clinical Nursing, 18*(15), 2187–2196.
Chrousos, G. P. (2009). Stress and disorders of the stress system. *Nature Reviews Endocrinology, 5*, 374–381.
Cooke, J. P., & Marshall, J. M. (2005). Mechanisms of Raynaud's disease. *Vascular Medicine, 10*, 293–307.
Corley, K. (1985). Psychopathology of stress. In S. Burchfield (Ed.), *Stress* (pp. 185–206). New York, NY: Hemisphere.
Deadwyler, S., Gribkoff, V., Cotman, D., & Lynch, G. (1976). Long-lasting chances in the spontaneous activity of hippocampal neurons following stimulation of the entorhinal cortex. *Brain Research Bulletin, 169*, 1–7.
Delanoy, R., Tucci, D., & Gold, P. (1983). Amphetamine effects on LTP in dendate granule cells. *Pharmacology, Biochemistry, and Behavior, 18*, 137–139.
Delmonte, M. (1984). Physiological concomitants of meditation practice. *International Journal of Psychosomatics, 31*, 23–36.
Doane, B. (1986). Clinical psychiatry and the physiodynamics of the limbic system. In B. Doane & K. Livingston (Eds.), *The limbic system* (pp. 285–315). New York, NY: Raven Press.
Domar, A., Seidel, M., & Benson, H. (1990). The mind body program for infertility. *Infertility and Sterility, 53*, 246–249.
Domar, A., Zuttermeister, P., Seibel, M., & Benson, H. (1992). Psychological improvement in infertile women after behavioral treatment. *Infertility and Sterility, 55*, 144–147.
Dotevall, G. (1985). *Stress and the common gastrointestinal disorders*. New York, NY: Praeger.
Dunford, E., & Thompson, M. (2010). Relaxation and mindfulness in pain: A review. *British Journal of Pain, 4*(1), 18–22.
Dusek, J. A., & Benson, H. (2009). Mind-body medicine: A model of the comparative clinical impact of the acute stress and relaxation responses. *Minnesota Medicine, 92*(5), 47–50.
Edinger, J. (1982). Incidence and significance of relaxation treatment side effects. *Behavior Therapist, 5*, 137–138.
Eliot, R. (1979). *Stress and the major cardiovascular diseases*. Mt. Kisco, NY: Futura.

Emmons, M. (1978). *The inner source: A guide to meditative therapy*. San Luis Obispo, CA: Impact.

English, E., & Baker, T. (1983). Relaxation training and cardiovascular response to experimental stressors. *Health Psychology, 2*, 239–259.

Everly, G. S., Jr. (1985b, November). *Biological foundations of psychiatric sequelae in trauma and stress-related "disorders of arousal."* Paper presented to the 8th National Trauma Symposium, Baltimore, MD.

Everly, G. S., Jr. (1993). Psychotraumatology: A two-factor formulation of posttraumatic stress disorder. *Integrative Physiology and Behavioral Science, 28*, 270–278.

Everly, G. S., Jr., & Benson, H. (1989). Disorders of arousal and the relaxation response. *International Journal of Psychosomatics, 36*, 15–21.

Everly, G. S., Jr., Spollen, M., Hackman, A., & Kobran, E. (1987). Undesirable side-effects and self-regulatory therapies. In *Proceedings of the Eighteenth Annual Meeting of the Biofeedback Society of America* (pp. 166–167).

Feder, A., Charney, D., & Collins, K. (2011). Neurobiology of resilience. In S. M. Southwick, D. Charnery, & M. J. Friedman (Eds.), *Resilience and mental health: Challenges across the lifespan* (pp. 1–29). Cambridge, UK: Cambridge University Press.

Fifková, E., & van Harreveld, A. (1977). Long-lasting morphological changes in dendritic spines of dentate granular cells following stimulation of the entorhinal area. *Journal of Neurocytology, 6*(2), 211–230.

Forbes, B., Akturk, C., Cummer-Nacco, C., Gaither, P., Gotz, J., Harper, A., & Hartsell, K. (2008). Using intergrative yoga therapeutics in the treatment of comorbid anxiety and depression. *International Journal of Yoga Therapy, 18*(1), 87–95.

Friedman, M. J., Charney, D., & Deutch, A. (Eds.). (1995). *Neurobiological, and clinical consequences of stress*. Philadelphia, PA: Lippincott-Raven.

Friedman, M. J., & Schnurr, P. P. (1995). The relationship between trauma, postraumatic stress disorder, and physical health. In M. J. Friedman, D. Charney, & A. Deutch (Eds.), *Neurobiological, and clinical consequences of stress* (pp. 507–526). Philadelphia, PA: Lippincott-Raven.

Gellhorn, E. (1957). *Autonomic imbalance and the hypothalamus*. Minneapolis, MN: University of Minnesota Press.

Gellhorn, E. (1958a). The physiological basis of neuromuscular relaxation. *Archives of Internal Medicine, 102*, 392–399.

Gellhorn, E. (1958b). The influence of curare on hypothalamic excitability and the electroencephalogram. *Electroencephalography and Clinical Neurophysiology, 10*, 697–703.

Gellhorn, E. (1964a). Motion and emotion. *Psychological Review, 71*, 457–472.

Gellhorn, E. (1964b). Sympathetic reactivity in hypertension. *Acta Neurovegetative, 26*, 35–44.

Gellhorn, E. (1965). The neurophysiological basis of anxiety. *Perspectives in Biology and Medicine, 8*, 488–515.

Gellhorn, E. (1967). *Principles of autonomic-somatic integrations*. Minneapolis, MN: University of Minnesota Press.

Gellhorn, E. (1968). Central nervous system tuning and its implications for neuropsychiatry. *Journal of Nervous and Mental Disease, 147*, 148–162.

Gellhorn, E., & Kiely, W. (1972). Mystical states of consciousness. *Journal of Nervous and Mental Disease, 154*, 399–405.

Gellhorn, E., & Loofburrow, G. (1963). *Emotions and emotional disorders*. New York, NY: Harper & Row.

Gloor, P. (1986). Role of the human limbic system in perception, memory, and affect. In B. Doane & K. Livingston (Eds.), *The limbic system* (pp. 159–169). New York, NY: Raven Press.

Gloor, P. (1992). Role of the amygdala in temporal lobe epiepsy. In J. P. Aggleton (Ed.), *The amygdala* (pp. 561–574). New York, NY: Wiley-Liss.

Glueck, G., & Stroebel, C. (1975). Biofeedback and meditation in the treatment of psychiatric illness. *Comprehensive Psychiatry, 16*, 309.

Goddard, G., & Douglas, R. (1976). Does the engram of kindling model the engram of normal long-term memory? In J. Wads (Ed.), *Kindling* (pp. 1–18). New York, NY: Raven Press.

Goddard, G., McIntyre, D., & Leech, C. (1969). A permanent change in brain function resulting from daily electrical stimulation. *Experimental Neurology, 25,* 295–330.

Goleman, D., & Schwartz, G. (1976). Meditation as an intervention in stress reactivity. *Journal of Consulting and Clinical Psychology, 15,* 110–111.

Gorman, J., Dillon, D., Fyer, A., Liebowitz, M., & Klein, D. (1985). The lactate infusion model. *Psychopharmacology Bulletin, 21,* 428–433.

Grassi, G., & Esler, M. (1999). How to assess sympathetic activity in humans. *Journal of Hypertension, 17,* 719–734.

Gray, J. (1982). *The neuropsychology of anxiety.* New York, NY: Oxford University Press.

Green, E., & Green, A. (1977). *Beyond biofeedback.* San Francisco, CA: Delta.

Hamberger, L., & Lohr, I. (1984). *Stress and stress management.* New York, NY: Springer.

Heide, F., & Borkovec, T. (1983). Relaxation induced anxiety. *Journal of Consulting and Clinical Psychology, 51,* 171–182.

Hellman, C. (1990). Overview of behavioral medicine. Practical Reviews in Psychiatry, Audiocassette volume 14.

Hellman, C. J., Budd, M., Borysenko, J., McClelland, D. C., & Benson, H. (1990). A study of the effectiveness of two group behavioral medicine interventions for patients with psychosomatic complaints. *Behavioral Medicine, 16,* 165–173.

Heninger, G. R. (1995). Neuroimmunology of stress. In M. J. Friedman, D. Charney, & A. Deutch (Eds.), *Neurobiological, and clinical consequences of stress* (pp. 381–402). Philadelphia: Lippincott-Raven.

Henke, P. G. (1992). Stomach pathology and the amygdala. In J. P. Aggleton (Ed.), *The amygdala* (pp. 323–338). New York, NY: Wiley-Liss.

Henry, J. P., & Stephens, P. (1977). *Stress, health, and the social environment.* New York, NY: Springer-Verlag.

Hoffman, J., Benson, H., Arns, P., Stainbrook, G., Landsberg, L., Young, J., & Gill, A. (1982). Reduced sympathetic relaxation response. *Science, 215,* 190–192.

Jasper, H. (1949). Diffuse projection systems. *Electroencephalography and Clinical Neuropsychology, 1,* 405–420.

Joy, R. (1985). The effects of neurotoxicants on kindling and kindled seizures. *Fundamental and Applied Toxicology, 5,* 41–65.

Klajner, F., Hartman, L., & Sobell, M. (1984). Treatment of substance abuse by relaxation training. *Addictive Behaviors, 9,* 41–55.

Kutz, I., Borysenko, J., & Benson, H. (1985). Meditation and psychotherapy. *American Journal of Psychiatry, 142,* 1–8.

Lang, R., Dehof, K., Meurer, K., & Kaufmann, W. (1979). Sympathetic activity and transcendental meditation. *Journal of Neural Transmission, 44,* 117–135.

Latimer, P. (1985). Irritable bowel syndrome. In W. Dorfman & L. Cristofar (Eds.), *Psychosomatic illness review* (pp. 61–75). New York: Macmillan.

Lavey, R., & Taylor, C. (1985). The nature of relaxation therapy. In S. Burchfield (Ed.), *Stress* (pp. 329–358). New York: Hemisphere.

Lazarus, R. S., & Folkman, S. (1984). *Stress, appraisal, and coping.* New York: Springer.

LeDoux, J. E. (1992). Emotion and the amygdala. In J. P. Aggleton (Ed.), *The amygdala* (pp. 339–352). New York: Wiley-Liss.

Lee, K., Schottler, F., Oliver, M., & Lynch, G. (1980). Brief bursts of high-frequency stimulation produce two types of structural change in rat hippocampus. *Journal of Neurophysiology, 44,* 247–258.

Lehmann, J., Goodale, I., & Benson, H. (1986). Reduced pupillarysensitivity to topicalphenyleph-rine associated with the relaxation response. *Journal of Human Stress, 12,* 101–104.

Lehrer, P. M. (1995). Recent research findings on stress management techniques. *Directions in Clinical Psychology, 5,* whole issue 9.

Lehrer, P. M., Woolfolk, R. L., & Sime, W. E. (2007). *Principles and Practice of Stress Management* (3rd ed.). New York, NY: The Guildford Press.

Liebowitz, M., Quitkin, F. M., Stewart, J. W., McGrath, P. J., Harrison, W., Rabkin, J. G., Tricamo, E., Markowitz, J. S., & Klein, D. F. (1984). Psychopharmacologic validation of atypical depression. *Journal of Clinical Psychiatry, 45*(7), 22–25.

Lown, B., Temte, J. V., Reich, P., Gaughan, C., Regestein, Q., & Hai, H. (1976). Basis for recurring ventricular fibrillation in the absence of coronary heart disease and its management. *New England Journal of Medicine, 294*, 623–629.

Luthe, W. (Ed.). (1969). *Autogenic therapy* (Vol. I–VI). New York: Grune & Stratton.

Mackereth, P. A., Booth, K., Hillier, V. F., & Caress, A. (2009). Reflexology and progressive muscle relaxation training for people with multiple sclerosis: a crossover trial. *Complementary Therapies in Clinical Practice, 15*(1), 14–21.

MacLean, P. D. (1949). Psychosomatic disease and the "visceral brain. *Psychosomatic Medicine, 11*, 338–353.

Malmo, R. B. (1975). *On emotions, needs, and our archaic brain*. New York: Holt, Rinehart & Winston.

Mann, D. M. A. (1992). The neuropathology of the amygdala in ageing and in dementia. In J. P. Aggleton (Ed.), *The amygdala* (pp. 561–574). New York: Wiley-Liss.

Manuck, S., & Krantz, D. (1984). Psychophysiologic reactivity in coronary artery disease. *Behavioral Medicine Update, 6*, 11–15.

Manzoni, G. M., Pagnini, F., Castelnuovo, G., & Molinari, E. (2008). Relaxation training for anxiety: A ten-years systematic review with meta-analysis. *BMC Psychiatry, 8*, 41.

McEwen, B. (2011, April 1). Protection and damage by mediators of stress and adaptation: Central role of the brain. Invited paper presented to the Academy of the Harvard Medical School. Boston: MA.

McFarlane, A. C. (2010). The long-term costs of traumatic stress: intertwined physical and psychological consquences. *World Psychiatry, 9*(1), 3–10.

Meehl, P. (1973). *Psychodiagnosis*. NewYork: Norton.

Mefferd, R. (1979). The developing biological concept of anxiety. In W. Fann, I. Karacan, A. D. Porkorny, & R. L. Williams (Eds.), *Phenomenology and treatment of anxiety* (pp. 111–124). New York: Spectrum.

Mehlsteibl, D., Schankin, C., Herin, P., Sostak, P., & Straube, A. (2011). Anxiety disorders in headache patients in a specialised clinic: prevalence and symptoms in comparison to patients in a general neurological clinic. *Journal of Headache and Pain, 12*(3), 323–329.

Michaels, R., Haber, M., & McCann, D. (1976). Evaluation of transcendental meditation as a method of reducing stress. *Science, 192*, 1242–1244.

Michaels, R., Parra, J., McCann, D., & Vander, A. (1979). Renin, cortisol, and aldosterone during Transcendental Meditation. *Psychosomatic Medicine, 41*, 49–54.

Millon, T. (2011). *Disorders of Personality*. Hoboken, NJ: Wiley.

Millon, T., & Everly, G. S., Jr. (1985). *Personality and its disorders*. New York: Wiley.

Monroe, R. (1970). *Episodic behavioral disorders*. Cambridge, MA: Harvard University Press.

Monroe, R. (1982). Limbic ictus and atypical psychosis. *Journal of Nervous and Mental Disease, 170*, 711–716.

Moturi, S., & Avis, K. (2010). Assessment and treatment of common pediatric sleep disorders. *Psychiatry, 7*(6), 24–37.

Moulapoulos, S. D. (2009). Do we need a routine mental stress test for ischemic heart disease and arrhythmias? *Hellenic Journal of Cardiology, 50*, 167–169.

Murphy, M., & Donovan, S. (1988). *The physical and psychological effects of meditation* (2nd ed.). San Rafael, CA: Esalen Institute Study of Exceptional Functioning.

Nauta, W. (1979). Expanding borders of the limbic system concept. In T. Rasmussen & R. Marino (Eds.), *Functional neurosurgery* (pp. 7–23). New York: Raven Press.

Nauta, W., & Domesick, V. (1982). Neural associations of the limbic system. In A. Beckman (Ed.), *Neural substrates of behavior* (pp. 3–29). New York: Spectrum.

Nordquist, N., & Oreland, L. (2010). Serotonin, genetic variability, behavior, and psychiatric disorders. *Upsala Jounral of Medical Sciences, 115*(1), 2–10.

Papez, J. (1937). A proposed mechanism of emotion. *Archives of Neurology and Psychiatry, 38*, 725–743.

Paul, G. (1967). Strategy of outcome research in psychotherapy. *Journal of Consulting and Clinical Psychology, 31*, 109–118.

Pinna, G., Costa, E., & Guidotti, A. (2009). SSRIs act as selective brain steroidogenic stimulants (SBSSs) at low doses that are inactice on 5-HT reuptake. *Current Opinions in Pharmacology, 9*(1), 24–30.

Pitts, F., & McClure, J. (1967). Lactate metabolism in anxiety neurosis. *New England Journal of Medicine, 277*, 1329–1336.

Post, R. (1985). Stress sensitization, kindling, and conditioning. *Behavioral and Brain Sciences, 8*, 372–373.

Post, R. (1986). Does limbic system dysfunction play a role in affective illness? In B. Doane & K. Livingston (Eds.), *The limbic system* (pp. 229–249). New York: Raven Press.

Post, R., & Ballenger, J. (1981). Kindling models for the progressive development of psychopathology. In H. van Pragg (Ed.), *Handbook of biological psychiatry* (pp. 609–651). New York: Marcel Dekker.

Post, R., Rubinow, D., & Ballenger, J. (1986). Conditioning and sensitisation in the longitudinal course of affective illness. *British Journal of Psychiatry, 149*, 191–201.

Post, R., Uhde, T., Putnam, F., Ballenger, J., & Berrettini, W. (1982). Kindling and carbamazepine in affective illness. *Journal of Nervous and Mental Disease, 170*, 717–731.

Post, R. M., Weiss, S., & Smith, M. (1995). Sensitization and kindling. In M. J. Friedmean, D. Charney, & A. Deutch (Eds.), *Neurobiological, and clinical consequences of stress* (pp. 203–224). Philadelphia: Lippincott-Raven.

Praeger-Decker, I., & Decker, W. (1980). Efficacy of muscle relaxation in combating stress. *Health Education, 11*, 39–42.

Rachman, S. (1968). The effect of muscular relaxation or desensitization therapy. *Behavior Therapy and Research, 6*, 159–166.

Racine, R., Tuff, L., & Zaide, J. (1976). Kindling unit discharge patterns and neural plasticity. In J. Wada & R. Ross (Eds.), *Kindling* (pp. 19–39). New York: Raven Press.

Rausch, S. M., Gramilin, S. E., & Auerbach, S. M. (2006). Effects of a single session of large-group meditation and progressive muscle relaxation training on stress reduction, reactivity, and recovery. *International Journal of Stress Management, 13*(3), 273–290.

Redmond, D. E. (1979). New and old evidence for the involvement of a brain norepinephrine system in anxiety. In W. Fann, I. Karacan, A. Pikomey, & R. Williams (Eds.), *Phenomenology and treatment of anxiety* (pp. 153–204). New York: Spectrum.

Redmond, D. E., & Huang, Y. (1979). New evidence for a locus ceruleus–norepinephrine connection with anxiety. *Life Sciences, 25*, 2149–2162.

Reiman, E., Raichle, M. E., Robins, E., Butler, F. K., Herscovitch, P., Fox, P., & Perlmutter, J. (1986). The application of positron emission tomography to the study of panic disorder. *American Journal of Psychiatry, 143*, 469–477.

Reynolds, G. P. (1992). The amygdala and the neurochemistry of schizophrenia. In J. P. Aggleton (Ed.), *The amygdala* (pp. 561–574). New York: Wiley-Liss.

Romano, J. (1982). Biofeedback training and therapeutic gains. *Personnel and Guidance Journal, 60*, 473–475.

Rosenzweig, M., & Leiman, A. (1982). *Physiological psychology*. Lexington, MA: Heath.

Sarnoff, D. (1982). Biofeedback: New uses in counseling. *Personnel and Guidance Journal, 60*, 357–360.

Sarzi-Puttini, P., Atzeni, F., & Cazzola, M. (2010). Neuroendocrine therapy of fibromyalgia syndrome: an update. *Annals of the New York Academy of Science, 1193*(1), 91–97.

Savitz, J., & Drevets, W. C. (2009). Bipolar and major depressive disorder: neuroimaging the developmental-degenerative divide. *Neuroscience and Biobehavioral Reviews, 33*(5), 669–771.

Selye, H. (1976). *Stress in health and disease*. Boston: Butterworth.

Shader, R. (1984). Epidemiologic and family studies. *Psychosomatics, 25(Suppl.),* 10–15.

Shapiro, D. H. (1985). Clinical use of meditation as a self-regulation strategy. *American Psychologist, 40*, 719–722.

Shapiro, D. H., & Giber, D. (1978). Meditation and psychotherapeutic effects. *Archives of General Psychiatry, 35*, 294–302.

Shin, L. M., & Liberzon, I. (2011). The neurocircuitry of fear, stress, and anxiety disorders. *Focus, 9*(3), 311–334.

Simon, D., Kaufman, C., Musch, K., Kischkel, E., & Kathmann, N. (2010). Fronto-striato-limbic hyperactivation in obsessive-compulsive disorder during individually tailored symptom provocation. *Psychophysiology, 47*, 728–738.

Sorg, B. A., & Kalivas, P. (1995). Stress and neuronal sensitization. In M. J. Friedman, D. Charney, & A. Deutch (Eds.), *Neurobiological, and clinical consequences of stress* (pp. 83–102). Philadelphia: Lippincott-Raven.

Steptoe, A. (1981). *Psychological factors in cardiovascular disorders*. New York: Academic Press.

Stoyva, J. M., & Anderson, C. (1982). A coping-rest model of relaxation and stress management. In L. Goldberger & S. Breznitz (Eds.), *Handbook of Stress* (pp. 745–763). New York: Free Press.

Streeter, C. C., Gerbarg, P. L., Saper, R. B., Ciraulo, D. A., & Brown, R. P. (2012). Effects of yoga on the automonic nervous system, gamma-aminobutyric acid, and allostatsis in epilepsy, depression, and post-traumatic stress disorder. *Medical Hypotheses, 78*(5), 571–579.

Stroebel, C. F. (1979, November). *Non-specific effects and psychodynamic issues in self-regulatory techniques*. Paper presented at the Johns Hopkins Conference in Clinical Biofeedback, Baltimore, MD.

Suler, J. R. (1985). Meditation and somatic arousal reduction: A comment on Holme's review. *American Psychologist, 40*, 717.

Suter, S. (1986). *Health psychophysiology*. Hillsdale, NJ: Erlbaum.

Tart, C. (1975). *States of consciousness*. New York: Dutton.

Taylor, C. B. (1978). Relaxation training and related techniques. In W. S. Agras (Ed.), *Behavioral modification* (pp. 30–52). Boston: Little, Brown.

van der Kolk, B. A., Greenberg, M., Boyd, H., & Krystal, J. (1985). Inescapable shock, neurotransmitters, and addition to trauma. *Biological Psychiatry, 20*, 314–325.

Van Hoesen, G. W. (1982). The para-hippocampal gyrus. *Trends in Neuroscience, 5*, 345–350.

Weil, J. (1974). *A neurophysiological model of emotional and intentional behavior*. Springfield, IL: Charles C. Thomas.

Williams, R. B. (1995). Somatic consequences of stress. In M. J. Friedman, D. Charney, & A. Deutch (Eds.), *Neurobiological, and clinical consequences of stress* (pp. 381–402). Philadelphia: Lippincott-Raven.

Wolf, S. (1985). Peptic ulcer. In W. Dorfman & L. Cristofar (Eds.), *Psychosomatic illness review* (pp. 52–60). New York: Macmillan.

Chapter 10
Meditation

Chapter 9 provided a rationale for the use of the relaxation response in the treatment of stress-related disorders. We now explore several techniques used to create the relaxation response. The purpose of this chapter is to provide a clinically relevant introduction to meditation.

In our culture, *meditation* refers to the act of thinking, planning, pondering, or reflecting. Our Western definitions are, however, not representative of the essence of the Eastern notion of meditation, in whose tradition, meditation is a process by which one attains "enlightenment." It is a growth-producing experience along intellectual, philosophical, and existential dimensions. Given the focus of our text, we use the term *meditation* to mean, quite simply, the autogenic practice of a genre of techniques that have the potential for inducing the relaxation response in the participant through the use of a repetitive focal device. Inherent in the success of using these procedures is achieving a mental state characterized by a non-ego-centered and nonintrusive mode of thought processing. According to Sethi (1989), meditation provides an "attempt to achieve a blissful state where stress has lost all its negative psychophysiological impacts" (p. 10).

History of Meditation

It is difficult to trace the history of meditation without considering it within the context of religion (Braboszcz, Hahusseau, & Delorme, 2010). The origins of religion date back to prehistoric times, and data suggest that it was common practice for older civilizations to use repetitive, rhythmic chants and sacrificial offerings (e.g., gold, food, animals, or sometimes humans) in attempts to appease the gods (Joseph, 1998). Therefore, a legacy of strong religious beliefs is used to instill a calming, relaxing effect on the mind, often at the expense of imposing fear on the worshipers.

G.S. Everly and J.M. Lating, *A Clinical Guide to the Treatment of the Human Stress Response*, DOI 10.1007/978-1-4614-5538-7_10, © Springer Science+Business Media New York 2013

Some of the earliest written records on meditation come from the Hindu traditions of Vedantism around 1500 B.C.E. These records consist of scriptures called Vedas, which discuss the meditative traditions of ancient India. Around 500 to 600 B.C.E., other forms of meditation developed, such as the Taoist in China and the Buddhist in India. From 1000 C.E. to 1100 C.E., the Zen form of meditation, called "zazen," gained popularity in Japan.

In Christianity, the use of repetitive prayers to effect a calming response spread by word of mouth. One of these earliest prayers, recorded in the fourteenth century on Mount Athos in Greece (Benson & Stuart, 1993), required participants to concentrate on their breathing and to repeat to themselves on each exhalation, "Lord Jesus Christ, have mercy on me." Like other meditative practices, participants were instructed to discard intrusive thoughts passively and return to the repetitive prayer (Benson & Stuart, 1993). Until the eighteenth century in the Western Hemisphere, medicine was the domain of the church, and monks treated the majority of physical and emotional symptoms. Thus, chanting and repetitious prayers may be considered the beginnings of formal meditative practices specifically designed to mitigate stress and anxiety (Joseph, 1998).

Meditation was introduced to the western world in 1920 by Indian spiritualist Paramahansa Yogananda (Hussain & Bhushan, 2010). However, in the 1960s, a form of "westernized" style in the Hindu tradition called "transcendental meditation" (TM) was started in the USA by Maharishi Mahesh Yogi. TM gained immense popularity in America during a time of political and social unrest and activism. Part of TM's appeal was its secular emphasis, its elimination of unnecessary elements of traditional yoga practices, and its relative simplicity of initiation. Meditation has flourished in the USA in the past several decades, and its practice is recognized as one of the top ten most commonly used forms of complementary and alternative medicine (CAM) therapy as noted by the National Center for Complementary and Alternative Medicine (NCCAM) (Barnes, Powell-Griner, McFann, & Nahin, 2002; Barnes, Bloom, & Nahin, 2008). In fact, a national survey 9.4% of respondents indicated that they had meditated in the past year (NCCAM, 2010). It is worth noting that although the preponderance of the literature on meditation attests to its relaxing effects, some literature suggests that meditation may have widely differing effects on consciousness and the body, including the potential, under some circumstances, for physiological arousal (Cortright, 1997).

Types of Meditation

As mentioned earlier, and for the purpose of our text, we refer to the practice of meditation as a group of techniques or procedures that have the potential of inducing the relaxation response. There are many meditation techniques that are practiced; however, they are usually grouped into two basic approaches—concentrative meditations and mindfulness/insight meditations (Hart, 2007; Hussain & Bhushan, 2010). Concentration meditation techniques involve focusing on specific mental or sensory activity (Cahn & Polich, 2006), an example being TM, whereas mindfulness meditation, according to Jon Kabat-Zinn (founder of the Center for Mindfulness at the University of Massachusetts Medical School), is defined as "moment-to-moment-awareness" in paying attention to senses, thoughts, and physical sensations (Kabat-Zinn, 1990). Walsh and Shapiro (2006) acknowledge that training and maintenance of attention, either in a narrowing of focus in concentrative meditation, or broadening of perceptivity in mindfulness meditation, is a common characteristic of both forms. Regardless of the general type, one element seemingly consistent with all forms of meditative practice is a stimulus, or thing, on which the meditator focuses his or her awareness. Olendzki (2009) describes meditation "as focusing the mind to a single point, unifying it, and placing it upon a particular object" (p. 38), and according to Naranjo and Ornstein (1971), this stimulus is something to "dwell upon," in effect, a focal device.

Therefore, for our purpose, meditative techniques may be categorized by the nature of their focal devices. Using this criterion, there are four general forms of meditative techniques:

1. *Mental Repetition.* This form of focal device involves dwelling on some mental event. The classic example of a mentally repetitive focal device is the "mantra," a word, phrase, or mystical sound that is repeated over and over, usually silently to oneself. We include chanting in this category as well. TM uses a mantra format, with the mantra chosen from a list of Sanskrit words. Benson (1975) and Benson and Stuart, 1993) employs neutral words such as *one, peace,* or *love* to evoke the relaxation response. One Tibetan Buddhist mantra in verse form is "Om mani padme hum." In Sikh meditation, the word *Vahiguru,* which literally means "wonderful light," is repeated for 10–20 min daily, and Hare Krishna practitioners repeat the 16-word mantra, "Hare Krishna Hare Krishna, Krishna Krishna Hare Hare, Hare Rama Hare Rama, Rama Rama Hare Hare," 1,728 times a day, keeping count with their prayer beads.

2. *Physical Repetition.* This form of focal device involves focusing one's awareness on some physical act. An ancient Yogic (Hindu) style of repetitive meditation focuses on the physically repetitive act of breathing. There are many different approaches to Yoga (which means "union"), and one of them, Hatha Yoga, uses various forms of breath control and breath counting (called *pranayama).* Hatha Yoga focuses on physical education, and the aspect most recognized by the public involves the practice of postures (called *asanas*). The Moslem Sufis are known for their practice of continuous, circular dancing or whirling. The name "whirling dervishes" was given to the ancient practitioners of this style. Finally, the popularity of jogging in the USA has given rise to the study of the effects of such activity. One effect reported by some joggers, either on the open road or on a treadmill, is a meditative-like experience, which could be caused by repetitive breathing or the repetitive sounds of feet pounding on the ground or treadmill.

3. *Problem Contemplation.* This focal device involves attempting to solve a problem with paradoxical components. The Zen *koan* is the classic example. In this case, a seemingly paradoxical problem or riddle is presented for contemplation.

"What is the sound of one hand clapping?" is a commonly used *koan.* Koans are intended to foster meditators to remove themselves from a thought-based state of consciousness and access pure awareness of the present moment.

4. *Visual Concentration.* This focal device involves visually focusing on an image— a picture, a candle flame, a leaf, a relaxing scene, or anything else. The *mandala,* a geometric design that features a square within a circle, representing the union of humanity within the universe, is often used in Eastern cultures for visual concentration.

Mechanisms of Action

Even after more than 40 years of scientific study (Braboszcz et al., 2010), the exact mechanisms underlying meditation remain unclear. However, as noted, the focal device or stimulus to "dwell upon," considered the common and essential link between various forms of meditation, appears to be a potential source of applied exploration (Benson, 1975; Benson & Stuart, 1993; Glueck & Stroebel, 1975, 1978; Naranjo & Ornstein, 1971; Ornstein, 1972).

Not long after its introduction to Western culture, researchers proposed that the focal device appears to prepare the neocortex for a shift from the normally domi-nant, analytic, ego-centered mode of thought processing (associated with left brain activity) to the intuitive, non-ego-centered mode of thought processing (associated with the brain's right neocortical hemisphere) (see Davidson, 1976; Naranjo & Ornstein, 1971; Ornstein, 1972). When the focal device is successfully employed, the brain's order of processing appears to be altered. "When the rational (analytic) mind is silenced, the intuitive mode produces extraordinary awareness" (Capra, 1975, p. 26). This awareness, or heightened attention, is the goal of all meditative techniques.

In the last edition of this text, we focused on the proposed shift from the "left" hemisphere to the "right" hemisphere of the brain that was thought to occur as a result of mediation. Cahn and Polich (2006) in reviewing lateralized EEG measures suggested that "meditation practice may alter the fundamental electrical balance between the cerebral hemispheres to modulate individual differences in affective experience" (p. 188), but noted that additional studies are needed to support this tenet. However, in the last decade, there have been tremendous advances in assess-ing the underlying anatomical correlates of medication using sophisticated imagery techniques. Hözel et al. (2011a, 2011b) provide a comprehensive review of this topic, so the interested reader is referred to this work. What follows is a brief summary and expansion in some areas of the major findings noted by Hözel, her colleagues, and others.

In the past 20 years, research has suggested that in individuals who have a pro-clivity to react positively and let go rapidly of negative emotions, their baseline electrical activity of the brain exhibits more left-sided anterior activation compared to those who harbor more negative emotions (Davidson, 2004). A recent study on

26 participants being taught meditation and practicing over a 5-week training period for an average of just more than 6 h showed a significantly greater leftward shift in frontal EEG asymmetry when compared to a waitlist control group, a pattern suggestive of more positive emotions and occurring without the need for years of meditative practice (Moyer et al., 2011). Data have shown that during the onset of meditation, there is increased activation in the putamen (the area of the brain involved in part in coordinating automatic behaviors) and motor cortex, while there is less overall activity in the right hemisphere (mainly in the medial part of the right occipital and parietal lobes and precuneus) (Baeretsen et al., 2010). In this same study, sustained meditation was shown to activate the head of the left caudate nucleus, while deactivations occurred mostly in the white matter of the right hemisphere (primarily in the posterior part of the occipito-pariteto-temporal area, as well as in the frontal lobes).

Neuroimaging studies focusing on attention have also shown that when compared with matched controls (age, gender, education) experienced meditators showed greater activation in the rostral part of the anterior cingulated cortex (ACC), which is thought to enable and sustain executive attention (Hölzel et al., 2007). Structural MRI studies indicate that experienced meditators have greater cortical thickness in the dorsal ACC compared with controls (Grant, Courtemanche, Duerden, Duncan, & Rainville, 2010) and increased white matter integrity in the ACC (Tang et al., 2010). Electroencephalographic data are consistent with frontal midline theta brain wave activity (see Chap. 14) during meditation (Aftanas & Golocheikine, 2002), which is associated with ACC activity and has implications for the use of meditation to treat disorders such as ADHD (Passarotti, Sweeney & Pavuluri, 2010) and bipolar disorder (Fountoulakis, Giannakopoulos, Kovari & Bouras, 2008). When compared to controls, meditators had greater cortical thickness and more gray matter concentration in the right anterior insula, which is associated with increased body awareness (Hölzel et al., 2007; Lazar et al., 2005).

Other studies have implicated meditation in the improvement of emotional regulation, such that meditation decreases negative mood (Jha, Stanley, Kiyonaga, Wong, & Gelfand, 2010) and enhances positive mood (Jain et al., 2007). From a neurophysiological perspective, increased activation of regions in the prefrontal cortex and decreased activation of the amygdala have been shown to successfully regulate affective responses (Harenski & Hamann, 2006), and neuroimaging studies have shown where mindfulness meditation has shown increased prefrontal activation and improved prefrontal control over the amygdala (Creswell, Way, Eisenberger, & Lieberman, 2007). Other data suggest that emotional control and regulation may depend on the amount of training and expertise of the meditator (Brefczynski-Lewis, Lutz, Schaefer, Levinson, & Davidson, 2007).

A study comparing 16 pre- and 14 posttreatment patients diagnosed with primary generalized social anxiety disorder (SAD) who underwent 8 weeks of mindfulness-based stress reduction (MBSR) showed improvements in anxiety and depression symptoms and reduced amygdala activity (Goldin & Gross, 2010). Hözel et al. (2011a, 2011b) demonstrated in a sample of 26 participants with high reported scores on the Perceived Stress Scale (PSS) who underwent 8 weeks of MBSR that reduced scores on PSS were correlated positively with decreases in gray matter density in the right amygdala. Additionally, a high-resolution MRI study of 44 participants (22 active meditation practitioners and 22 controls) showed that meditators, who averaged 24.2 years of practice, had larger gray matter volumes in the right orbito-frontal cortex and the right hippocampus, both of these being implicated in emotional regulation (Luders, Toga, Lepore, & Gaser, 2009). Hözel et al. (2011a, 2011b) in a longitudinal study of 16 participants with no meditation experience recently demonstrated increased gray matter concentrations in the left hippocampus after only 8 weeks of MBSR when compared to 17 control participants. In this same study participants also evinced increased gray matter concentration in the posterior cingulated cortex and the temporo-parietal junction, suggesting along with the increased concentration of gray matter in the hippocampus, an ability that is consistent with meditative teachings to alter one's internal perspective (Buckner & Carroll, 2007).

Other EEG data, despite being far from conclusive, have implicated increases in theta wave activity (often associated with a daydreaming-like state) and alpha wave activity (associated with relaxation) and decreases in overall frequency (Andersen, 2000; Cahn & Polich, 2006; Chiesa & Serretti, 2010). Some studies suggest that higher theta and alpha activity may be related to years of practice, the meditative technique used (as compared to concentrative meditation techniques, mindfulness meditation produced greater theta activity), and slower baseline EEG frequency in long-term meditators (Aftanas & Golocheikine, 2002; Andersen, 2000; Dunn, Hartigan, & Mikulas, 1999).

Austin (1998), in an earlier summary of EEG data, acknowledges that episodes of "microawakening" and "microsleep" (going directly from sleeping to waking back to sleep again, without the usual stepwise progression of surface EEG findings) are common during meditation. He further suggests that this implies that the brain may pass suddenly through its brain wave activity, and that "during meditation, some unstable fragments of physiological mechanisms seem to be briefly 'loosened' and are then available to recombine in new, unexpected ways" (p. 93).

Part of this recombining may lead to the state of "extraordinary awareness" alluded to earlier. This state has been called many things. In the East, it is called *nirvana* or *satori*. A liberal translation of these words means "enlightenment." Similar translations for this state include "truth consciousness" or "being-cognition." In the early Western World, those few individuals who understood it used the term *supraconsciousness* or the "cosmic consciousness." Benson (1975) and Benson and Stuart (1993) has called this state the "relaxation response," as described in the preceding chapter.

Although modern research investigations continue to attempt to qualify the neurophysiology of this supraconscious state, results continue to remain inconclusive. Part of the difficulty in gathering more conclusive results is participant selection. Most participants in meditation studies are considered beginners by traditional standards. As noted previously, data suggest that possible neurophysiological explanations include simultaneous EEG amplitude increases and decreases in various parts of the brain, particularly in alpha and theta waves, and primarily occur in individuals with many years of meditative experience (Aftanas & Golocheikine, 2002; Andresen, 2000; Jevning, Wallace, & Beidebach, 1992; Walsh, 1996).

It is important to emphasize that meditation and the achievement of the supra-conscious state are not always the same! It should be made abundantly clear to the patient that meditation is the process, or series of techniques, that the meditator employs to achieve the goal of attaining the relaxation response and its associated supraconsciousness.

Therapeutic Hallmarks

As just mentioned, the "extraordinary awareness" of the relaxation response, or supra-consciousness state, is the desired goal of the devoted practitioners of all meditative styles. However, it is important for the clinician *and* the patient alike to understand that achievement of this state is never assured, and that this state may not be achieved every time, even by very experienced meditators. Given this, the question must then arise, "Is the time spent in the meditative session wasted if the meditator is unable to achieve the supraconscious state?" The answer to this question is a resounding No! Positive therapeutic growth can be achieved without reaching the supraconscious state. The rationale for this statement lies in the fact there exist several "therapeutic hallmarks" inherent in the process of meditation as one approaches the supraconscious state. While Shapiro (1978), in his seminal work, discusses five steps in the meditative process: (1) difficulty in breathing, (2) wandering mind, (3) relaxation, (4) detached observation, and (5) higher state of consciousness, and Austin (2006) describes five stages in the meditative process to mitigate distractibility, we have chosen to describe and expand upon the hallmarks we see in the meditative process.

The first and most fundamental of these hallmarks resides in practice itself. Even the ancient Hindu and Zen scriptures on meditation acknowledge that the attempt to achieve the supraconscious state is far more important than actually reaching it. By simply taking time to meditate, the patient is making a conscious effort to improve his or her health and reduce the effects of excessive stress. Similarly, by emphasiz-ing to the patient the importance of simply meditating, rather than achieving the supraconscious state, the clinician removes much of the competitive, or success-versus-failure, component in this process. Meditation is an art; however, as noted by Austin (2006), "one problem is that it takes such a long time to become art*less*" (p. 14). As summarized nicely by Kabat-Zinn (1993), "Practice simply means invit-ing yourself to embody calmness, mindfulness, and equanimity right here, right now, in this moment, as best you can" (p. 267). Moreover, as noted by Hözel et al. (2011a, 2011b), mindfulness practice requires that the meditator expose him or her-self to whatever is present in his or her field of awareness, accept it, and refrain from engaging in internal reactivity, including cognitive avoidance, toward it. In many ways this mindfulness approach parallels the behavioral therapy technique of expo-sure therapy (Öst, 1997).

The second hallmark is a noticeable increase in somatic relaxation: a decline in oxygen consumption by about 20–32% (Sarang & Telles, 2006; Telles, Reddy, & Nagendra, 2000) and a lowering of respiratory rate of more than 50%

(Arambula, Pepper, Kawakami & Gibney, 2001), reduced sensitivity to CO_2 (Kesterson & Clinch, 1989), acute decline of adrenocortical activity (Bevan, 1980), decreases in galvanic skin response (GSR) activity, sympathetic nervous system reactivity, electromyographic (EMG) reactivity and cortisol levels (Mohan, Sharma, & Bijlani, 2011), and decreases in heart rate and blood pressure (Murphy & Donovan, 1988; Ospina et al., 2007; Shapiro & Walsh, 1984). The combination of these and other physiological factors leads to an autogenically induced state of somatic relaxation. This awakened state of hypometabolic functioning referred to in the literature is therapeutic in that (1) the body is placed into a mode equal or superior to sleep with regard to the restorative functions performed (Jevning et al., 1992; Orme-Johnson & Farrow, 1978) and (2) ergotropic stimulation of afferent proprioceptive impulses is reduced, and trophotropic responses are enhanced (Davidson, 1976; Gellhorn & Kiely, 1972).

The third hallmark is that of detached observation (Astin, 1997; and see Shapiro, 1978). In the Indian scriptures, this is described as a state in which the meditators remain "a spectator resting in him-or herself" as he observes his environment. In this state egoless, passive state of observation, the meditator simply "coexists" with the environment rather than confronting or attempting to master it. It is a nonanalytic, intuitive state. One similar experience that many individuals have had is that of "highway hypnosis," a state often experienced by individuals driving on monotonous expressways. At one point they may notice that they are at Exit 6; in what seems a mere moment later, they may notice they are at Exit 16 yet have no immediate recollection of the 10 intervening exits. Many refer to this as a "daydreaming state." It is important to note that the driver of the car is fully capable of driving; this is not a sleep state. Had an emergency arisen, the driver would have been able to react appropriately. Therefore, the clinician should explain that this state is not one of lethargy or total passivity, which happens to be a concern for many patients.

The final step in the meditative experience is the "supraconscious state" or *nirvana*. This appears to be a summation of all the previous states except that it is more intense. Davidson (1976) and Sethi (1989) and Austin (2006) have characterized its nature:

1. A positive mood (tranquility, peace of mind)
2. A dissolving of worry and anxiety
3. An experience of unity, or oneness, with the environment; what the ancients called the joining of microcosm (human) with macrocosm (universe)
4. A sense of ineffability (being inexpressible or transcendent)
5. A feeling of active peace
6. An alteration in time–space relationships
7. An enhanced sense of reality and meanings
8. A development of new creative energy
9. Paradoxicality, that is, acceptance of things that seem paradoxical in ordinary consciousness
10. A state of "no-mind" in which the natural flow of mental states and actions are void of all egocentric intrusions

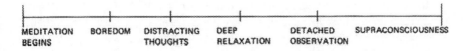

Fig. 10.1 A meditative continuum

Given that most clinicians receive myriad questions concerning the active nature of meditation, we have placed some common experiences on a continuum (see Fig. 10.1). This continuum of meditative experiences is not completely progressive from one discrete state to the next. A meditator may progress from any one state to another and then back again. Also, varying degrees of depth may be experienced within each state. Note, specifically, that boredom and distracting thoughts often precede more positive effects. The clinician should explain to the patient that this is a natural occurrence, and that he or she should be tolerant when this happens and simply return his or her concentration to the focal device.

As mentioned earlier, the meditator should be discouraged from evaluating the meditative sessions in a success–failure paradigm. Simple, descriptive reports to the clinician are useful to monitor the course of the activity for a period of 2–3 weeks. A daily log might be kept by the patient, as long as it is descriptive and not evaluative.

Research on the Clinical Applications and Effects of Meditation

Well-controlled research studies on the clinical effectiveness of meditation are available [see Austin (1998) for an earlier review, and Chiesa and Serretti (2010), Fortney and Taylor (2010), and Rubia (2009) for more recent reviews]. These studies recognize a potentially wide range of stress-related therapeutic applications for meditation. One general area of benefit entails strategies for refocusing or retraining attention. As noted by Sethi (1989) in his influential text,

> The importance of strategic meditation (SM), in enabling cognitive shift, becomes a crucial tool in allocation of attention as a resource for stress management. This proposition is based on the conceptualization that consciousness is a cybernetic system that can be managed through attention via strategic choice (meditation). (p. 86)

Other, specific meditative and mindfulness techniques have been found useful for the following:

1. In the treatment of generalized autonomic arousal and excessive ergotrophic tone or emotional distress (Astin, 1997; Benson, 1985; Burns, Lee, & Brown, 2011; Shapiro, Schwartz, & Bonner, 1998; Young & Baime, 2010)
2. In the treatment of anxiety disorders (Goldin, Ramel, & Gross, 2009; Kabat-Zinn et al., 1992; Lehrer & Woolfolk, 1984; Miller, Fletcher, & Kabat-Zinn, 1995;

Rahul & Joseph, 2009; Ramel, Goldin, Carmona, & McQuaid, 2004) and anxiety related to schizophrenia (Brown, Davis, LaRoco, & Strasburger, 2010); "enhancement," and "well-being" (Benson, 1985; Carmody & Baer, 2008; Coppola & Spector, 2009; Davidson, Kabat-Zinn, Schumacher, Rosenkranz, Muller, & Santorellli, 2003; Kutz, Borysenko, & Benson, 1985; Smith, Compton, & West, 1995)

3. In the treatment of psoriasis (Gaston, Crombez & Dupuis, 1989; Kabat-Zinn et al., 1998)

4. In the treatment of migraines (Wachholtz & Pargament, 2008).

5. For treatment of binge eating (Kristeller & Hallett, 1999)

6. As an adjunct in the treatment of cancer patients (Ando et al., 2009; Brennan & Stevens, 1998; Carlson, Speca, Patel, & Goodey, 2004; Gawler, 1998; Matousek & Dobkin, 2010; Smith, Richardson, Hoffman & Pilkington, 2005; Tácon, 2003) and their partners (Birnie, Garland & Carlson, 2010)

7. To reduce the impact of patients with fibromyalgia (Kaplan, Goldenberg & Galvin-Nadeau, 1993; Lush et al., 2009)

8. In the regulation of chronic pain (Kabat-Zinn, Lipworth & Burney, 1985; Plews-Ogan, Owens, Goodman, Wolfe & Schorling, 2005; Rosenzweig et al., 2010) and as an adjunct to palliative care in a hospice setting (Bruce & Davies, 2005)

9. As an intervention for patients with myocardial infarction (MI) or coronary artery disease (CAD) (Buselli & Stuart, 1999; Tácon , McComb, Caldera, & Randolph, 2003; Zamarra, Schneider, Besseghini, Robinson, & Salerno, 1996; Zeidan, Johnson, Gordon, & Goolkasian, 2010)

10. As an adjunct in the treatment of essential hypertension (Barnes, Schneider, Alexander, & Staggers, 1997; Benson, Beary, & Carol, 1974; Sothers & Anchor, 1989)

11. As an adjunct in the treatment of drug and alcohol abuse (Brooks, 1994; Gelderloos, Walton, Orme-Johnson, & Alexander, 1991; Zgierska et al., 2008)

12. In the treatment of rheumatoid arthritis (Pradhan et al., 2007; Zautra et al., 2008)

13. As an adjunct in the treatment of HIV-1 (Cresswell, Myers, Cole & Irwin, 2009)

14. As an adjunct to the treatment of type 2 diabetes (Rosenzweig et al., 2007)

15. In the treatment of symptoms of anxiety and PTSD associated with disaster relief (Waelde et al., 2008) or in survivors of child abuse (Kimbrough, Magyari, Langenberg, Chesney & Berman, 2010).

16. As a complementary treatment for tinnitus (Mazzoli, 2011).

17. As an adjunct in the treatment of ADHD (Black, Milam & Sussman, 2009; Zylowska et al., 2008)

Having provided a rationale for the clinical use of meditation, we now examine its implementation.

How to Implement Meditation

The following discussion is provided as a guide to the clinical use of meditation.

Preparation

In addition to the general precautions for relaxation mentioned in an earlier chapter, the following preparations are important for the implementation of meditation:

1. Determine whether the patient has any specific contraindications for the use of meditation. For example, affective or thought disorders may possibly be exacerbated by meditation. Similarly, the clinician should use care with patients who demonstrate a tendency to employ nonpsychotic fantasy, as in the schizoid personality. There are also possible instances of muscle or gastrointestinal spasms. It should also be noted that some compulsive or action-oriented individuals appear to have greater difficulty in learning to meditate effectively than do less compulsive individuals. Boredom and distracting thoughts appear to compete with meditation.
2. Inquire into the patient's previous knowledge or experience in meditation. Pay particular attention to any mention of cultic or religious aspects. These are the most common misconceptions that patients find troublesome. Some may feel that by meditating, they will be performing a sacrilegious act.
3. Provide the patient with a basic explanation of meditation.
4. Describe to the patient the proper environment for the practice of meditation (see next section).

Components

In his original book, *The Relaxation Response,* and in later reviews and updates of his work, Benson (1975, 1996, 2000; Benson & Stuart, 1993) describes the following basic components in successful meditation:

1. A quiet environment
2. A mental device
3. A passive attitude
4. A comfortable position

In elaborating and expanding Benson's paradigm to some extent, the first condition we recommend is a *quiet environment,* absent of external stimuli that would compete with the meditative process. Many patients state that it is impossible to find such a place. If this is so, then some creativity may be needed. The patient may wish to use music or environmental recordings to "mask" distractions. For example, the steady hum of a fan or an air conditioner may effectively drown out noise. If this is not possible, the patient may choose to cover his or her eyes and/or use earplugs to reduce external stimulation.

The second condition (for physically passive meditation) is a *comfortable position.* Muscle tension can be disruptive to the meditative process. When first learning, the patient should have most of his or her weight supported. The notable exceptions would be the head and neck. By keeping the spine straight, and the head and neck unsupported, there will be sufficient muscle tension to keep the patient from falling asleep. If the patient does continually falls asleep during meditation, then he or she should use a posture that requires greater muscle tension.

The third condition, a *focal device*, is the link between all forms of meditation, even the physically active forms, as discussed earlier. The focal device appears to act by allowing the brain to alter it normal mode of processing.

The fourth condition, a *passive attitude*, has been called "passive volition" or "passive attention" by some. Benson (1975) states that this "passive attitude is perhaps the most important element" (p. 113). With this attitude, the patient "allows" the meditative act to occur rather than striving to control the meditative process. As Benson and Stuart (1993) have noted, "Don't worry about how well you're doing. When other thoughts come to mind, simply say to yourself, 'Oh, well,' and gently return to the repetition [focal device]" (p. 240).

If the patient is unable to adopt this attitude, he or she will ask questions:

"Am I doing this correctly?"—usually indicative of concern regarding performance.

"How long does this take?"—usually indicative of concern for time.

"What is a *good* level of proficiency?"—usually indicative of concern for performance outcome rather than process.

"Should I try to remember everything I feel?"—usually indicative of overanalysis.

The more the patient dwells on such thoughts, the less successful he or she will be. Distracting thoughts are completely normal during the meditative process and are to be expected. However, adoption of a passive attitude allows the patient to recognize distracting thoughts and simply return concentration to the focal device.

The fifth and final condition that we would recognize is a *receptive psychophysiological environment.* By this we mean a set of internal psychophysiological conditions that will allow the patient to meditate. It has been noted, for example, that psychophysiologically aroused patients have a very low success rate when they attempt to meditate. Therefore, it may be necessary to teach the patients to put themselves in a more "receptive condition" for meditating (this applies to biofeedback, hypnosis, and guided imagery as well). To achieve this receptive condition, the patient may wish to use a few neuromuscular relaxation techniques before the meditation, in order to reduce excessive muscle tension. We have recommended in some circumstances that the patient take a hot bath before meditating. In fact, some patients have reported high levels of success when they meditate while sitting in a hot tub. We have found this infrequently mentioned concept of psychophysiological receptivity to be a critical variable in many clinical experiences. Therefore, the meditative continuum is expanded (Fig. 10.1) to include this variable (see Fig. 10.2).

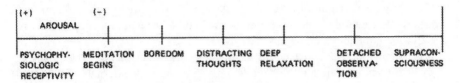

Fig. 10.2 Arousal and the meditative continuum

Example Protocol

This section provides an example of a protocol for a physically passive, mantra-like form of meditation. Use it as a guideline and make necessary revisions in the margins in order to tailor the protocol to your specific needs.

Background Information. The purpose is to familiarize you with the use of meditation as a way of reducing the stress in your life. These instructions consist of background information and specific directions for the use of four techniques from which you may choose in order to meditate. Follow all the instructions closely. Later you may wish to modify a part of the technique to fit a personal preference or situation, but in the initial learning phase, you should do all the exercises exactly as instructed. Once you have chosen one of the meditative techniques, employ that technique as instructed for 15 to 20 min of uninterrupted meditation once or twice a day.

Some people, not familiar with the nature and origins of meditation, confuse its pure form with its possible uses. There are important differences. The techniques of meditation presented here are derived from ancient Eastern philosophies that have then been blended with modern relaxation and stress-reduction techniques. Although some of the techniques were used in the practice of specific religions, to say that meditation is a religious practice is like saying wine is a religious instrument simply because in many religions wine is used in the ceremonies. Meditation is a technique of quieting the mind, which, of course, is a necessary prerequisite for reducing anxiety and tension.

As taught here, a quiet mind is an end in itself. What you do with this valuable skill is, of course, up to you.

The fundamentals of meditation are often misunderstood, as meditation itself is difficult to define. It is not a physiological state. Nor is it any specific psychological feeling or a religion. Rather, as used here, meditation is a technique so basic that it has transcended time, cultures, races, religions, and ideologies. The physiological, psychological, and philosophical goals of meditation cannot be achieved without training, and mastery of technique cannot be achieved except through continued practice.

Although there are many types of meditation, the most popular meditative techniques in Western society are derived from specific practices of ancient Yoga and Zen. Each type of meditation represents a variation of purpose and technique. Those presented here are thought to be the best suited for stress reduction. The technique is the easiest to learn and the one most devoid of cultic, religious, and spiritual overtones. It is complete and can be all the meditation one will ever need; or, it may serve as an introduction to more specific types.

There are several essential steps you should follow when learning to meditate.

A first essential step is to find a quiet environment, both external and internal. A quiet room away from others who are not meditating is essential, especially while learning. Take the phone off the hook, or at least go into a room without one. Generally, do whatever can be done to reduce external noise. If you cannot completely eliminate the noise, which is often the case in busy households or in college dorms, and so forth, use ear plugs. Play a record or tape of some soft instrumental sounds, or use any of the numerous environmental sound recordings that are commercially available. Even the steady hum of a fan or an air conditioner can effectively block out, or mask, external noise. You may also wish to turn down, or completely off, any lights in the room. Now that you have quieted your external environment, the next essential step is to work on quieting your internal environment. One way is to reduce muscle tension, which represents one of the biggest obstacles to successful meditation. Spend some time relaxing your muscles. One way is to reduce muscle tension is to sit comfortably, you may not feel like a real meditator unless you are sitting in the Eastern, cross-legged lotus position, but that takes a great deal of flexibility and training. For now, sit comfortably on the floor, or, better yet, sit in a straight-backed, comfortable chair, feet on the floor, legs not crossed, hands resting on the thighs, with fingers slightly opened, not interlocked. You should sit still, but remember, meditation is not a trance. If you are uncomfortable or feel too much pressure on any one spot, move. If you have an itch, scratch. Do not assume a tight inflexible position or attitude. Relax. It is best not to lie down or support your head, or you will tend to fall asleep. Keep the head, neck, and spine in a straight vertical line. A small but significant amount of muscle tension is needed to maintain this posture, and this effort helps prevent sleep from occurring, while at the same time creating an optimal position for learning to meditate.

There are many types of meditation. Some focus on inner forces, inner power, or self-identity. Others focus on external things, such as words, lights, or sounds. Meditation is simply a natural process. And though techniques may differ, the core experience is essentially the same. The basic meditative experience involves concentrating passively on some stimulus, whether it be a word, an image, your breath, or nothing at all. The stimulus acts as a vehicle to keep distracting thoughts out of your mind. And yet, the harder you concentrate on the stimulus, the harder it is to meditate. Although this sounds confusing, it is true, simply because meditation is a "passive" activity. You must allow the stimulus, whatever it is, to interact passively with you. You must learn to concentrate passively on your stimulus. The skill of passive concentration takes time to develop—so don't be discouraged if it seems difficult for the first few weeks. Just continue to practice.

Actual Instruction. You are now ready to begin the actual instruction. To begin with, close your eyes. Notice the quietness. Much of our sensory input comes in through our eyes. Just by closing your eyes, you can do much to quiet the mind.

The Use of Breath Concentration. What we are going to do now is clear our minds. Not of all thoughts, but of ongoing thoughts that use the imagination to increase stress arousal. Focus on your breathing. Shift your awareness from the hectic external world to the quiet and relaxing internal world.

As you breathe in, think in. Let the air out. Think out. In and out. Concentrate on your breathing. Think in. Think out. Breath in through your nose and let the air out through the mouth very effortlessly. Just open your mouth and let the air flow out. Do not force it. Become involved with the breathing process. Concentrate on your breathing. In and out. Now, each time you breathe in, I want you to feel how cold the air is, and each time you breathe out, feel how warm and moist the air is. Do that now. (*Pause 30 s.*)

The Use of One. Now we would like to replace the concentration on breathing with the use of a mantra. A mantra is a vehicle that is often a word or phrase to help keep your mind from wandering back to daydreams. An example of a mantra, suggested by Herbert Benson in his book *The Relaxation Response,* is simply the word *one* (o-n-e). This is a soft, noncultic word that has little meaning as a number. Every time you breathe out, say the word *one* to yourself. Say *one. One.* Say it softly. *One.* Say the word *one* without moving your lips. Say it yet more softly, until it becomes just a mental thought. (*Pause 75 s here.*)

The Use of Om. The word *one* is an example of a mantra: a vehicle to help clear your mind. By concentrating on a word without emotion or significance, your mind's order of processing begins to change. The mind begins to wander, with a quieter, more subtle state of consciousness. Many people like to use words from the ancient Sanskrit language, feeling that they represent soft sounds with spiritual significances that can also be used as a focus for contemplation. The universal mantra is the word *om;* spelled o-m, it also means one. Each time you breathe out say the word *om. Om. Om.* Breathe softly and normally, but now do not concentrate on your breathing. Repeat the mantra in your mind. Just think of saying it. Do not actually move your lips. Just think of it. Do not concentrate on your breathing. Let the mantra repeat itself in your mind. Do not force it. Just let it flow. Gradually the mantra will fade. The mind will be quiet. Occasionally, the quiet will be broken by sporadic thoughts. Let them come. Experience them, then let them leave your mind as quickly as they entered, by simply going stronger to your mantra. Let us now use *om* as a mantra. Say the word *om, om.* (*Pause here 75 s.*) Remember, the mantra is a vehicle to help clear the mind when you cannot do so without it. Also remember, keep your movements to a minimum, but if you are uncomfortable, move. If you are worried about time, look at a clock. Discomfort or anxiety will prevent full attainment of the relaxed state.

The Use of Counting. A final mantra that you may select if you find your mind wandering too much requires a little more concentration than the three previous meditation techniques.

As you breathe out, begin to count backward from 10 to 1. Say a single number to yourself each time you exhale. As you say the number, try to picture that number in your "mind's eye." When you reach 1, go back to 10 and start over. Let us do that now. (*Pause here 3 min.*)

Reawaken. Now I want to bring attention back to yourself and the world around you. I will count from 1 to 10. With each number you will feel your mind become more and more awake and your body more and more refreshed. When I reach 10, open your eyes, and you will feel the best you've felt all day—you will feel alert, refreshed, full of energy, and eager to resume your activities. Let us begin: 1–2 you are beginning to feel more alert, 3–4–5 you are more and more awake, 6–7 now begin to stretch your hands and feet, 8 now begin to stretch your arms and legs, 9–10 open your eyes *now!* You feel alert, awake; your mind is clear and your body refreshed.

Having read the preceding example, please note the following points:

1. In the example, the patient was given four different mantras from which to choose. Such "freedom of choice" may increase clinical effectiveness. It is important to ask the patient which mantra was best for him or her, and why. Such questions foster introspection and self-understanding.
2. The meditation example contains a *reawaken* step, as does the neuromuscular relaxation example in Chap. 12.
3. The clinician should indicate, at some point, when the patient should meditate. We have found once or twice a day to be sufficient, 15–20 min in duration for each session. As with neuromuscular relaxation, before lunch or before dinner is generally the best time to meditate, although practice in the morning may provide a relaxing start for the entire day.

Summary

In this chapter we discussed the first of several techniques that can be used to engender the relaxation response, specifically, the technique of meditation. Let us review several of the focal points:

1. The history of meditation is rich, vast, and provides the rationale for its clinical applications.
2. The two basic approaches to meditation are concentrative and mindfulness/insight.
3. The practice of meditation is one way to engender a relaxation response. We will review other techniques in later chapters (e.g., neuromuscular relaxation, controlled respiration).
4. Enhanced neuroimaging techniques in the last decade have added to the growing knowledge of anatomical structures associated with meditation.
5. The "supraconscious state," as described in this chapter, may be considered one of the end points or therapeutic hallmarks along a meditative continuum within the relaxation response.
6. Research has now clearly shown that the relaxation response, as engendered by the practice of meditation via a focal device, can be useful in the treatment of a wide variety of stress-related disorders.

7. Within this chapter, a typical protocol for teaching meditation has been provided. The clinician should tailor it to the personal needs of each patient when practical.
8. Finally, it is advisable to always practice meditation, or any other relaxation technique, in an office setting before assigning it as homework. This gives you the opportunity to (1) observe whether the technique is done properly, and (2) talk with the patient about his or her experiences.

References

Aftanas, L. I., & Golocheikine, S. A. (2002). Non-linear dynamic complexity of the human EEG during meditation. *Neuroscience Letters, 330*, 143–146.

Andersen, J. (2000). Meditation meets behavioural medicine: The story of experimental research on meditation. *Journal of Consciousness Studies, 7*, 17–73.

Ando, M., Morita, T. Akechi, T., Ito, S. Tanaka, M., Ifuku, Y., & Nakayama, T. (2009). The efficacy of mindfulness-based meditation therapy on anxiety, depression, and spirituality in Japanese patients with cancer. *Journal of Palliative Medicine, 12*(12), 1091–1094.

Arambula, P., Pepper, E., Kawakami, M., & Gibney, K. H. (2001). The physiological correltate of Kundalini Yoga meditation: A study of a Yoga master. *Applied Psychophysiology and Biofeedback, 26*, 142–153.

Astin, J. A. (1997). Stress reduction through mindfulness meditation: Effects on psychological symptomatology, sense of control, and spiritual experiences. *Psychotherapy and Psychosomalics, 66*(2), 97–106.

Austin, J. H. (1998). *Zen and the brain: Toward an understanding of meditation and consciousness.* Cambridge, MA: MIT Press.

Austin, J. H. (2006). *Zen-brain reflections.* Cambridge, MA: MIT Press.

Baeretsen, K. B., Stödkilde-Jörgensen, H., Sommerlund, B. Hartmann, T., Damsgaard-Madsen, J., Fosnæs, M., & Green, A. C. (2010). An investigation of brain processes supporting meditation. *Cognitive Processing, 11*, 57–84.

Barnes, P. M., Bloom, B., & Nahin, R. L. (2008). Complementary and alternative medicine use among adults: United States, 2007. *National Health Statistics Report, 12*, 1–24.

Barnes, P., Powell-Griner, E., McFann, K., & Nahin, R. (2002). *CDC advance data report #343: Complementary and alternative medicine use among adults: United States, 2002.* Washington, DC: U.S. Government.

Barnes, V., Schneider, R., Alexander, C., & Staggers, F. (1997). Stress, stress reduction, and hypertension in African Americans: An update and review. *Journal of the National Medical Association, 7*, 464–476.

Benson, H. (1975). *The relaxation response.* New York, NY: Morrow.

Benson, H. (1985). *Beyond the relaxation response: How to harness the healing power of your personal beliefs.* New York, NY: Berkley Books.

Benson, H. (1996). *Timeless healing: The power and biology of belief.* New York, NY: Scribner.

Benson, H. (with Klipper, M. Z.) (2000). *The relaxation response.* New York, NY: HarperCollins

Benson, H., Beary, J., & Carol, M. (1974). The relaxation response. *Psychiatry, 37*, 37–46.

Benson, H., & Stuart, E. (1993). *The wellness book.* New York, NY: Fireside.

Bevan, A. J. W. (1980). Endocrine changes in transcendental meditation. *Clinical and Experimental Pharmacology and Physiology, 7*(1), 75–76.

Birnie, K., Garland, S. N., & Carlson, L. E. (2010). Psychological benefits for cancer patients and their partners participating in mindfulness-based stress reduction (MBSR). *Psycho-Oncology, 19*(9), 1004–1009.

Black, D. S., Milam, J., & Sussman, S. (2009). Sitting-meditation interventions among youth: A review of treatment efficacy. *Pediatrics, 124*(3), e532–e541.

Braboszcz, C., Hahusseau, S., & Delorme, A. (2010). Meditation and neuroscience: From basic research to clinical practice. In R. Carlstedt (Ed.), *Integrative clinical psychology, psychiatry and behavioral medicine: Perspectives, practices and research* (pp. 1910–1929). New York, NY: Springer.

Brefczynski-Lewis, J. A., Lutz, A., Schaefer, H. S., Levinson, D. B., & Davidson, R. J. (2007). Neural correlates of attentional expertise in long-term meditation practitioners. *Proceedings of the National Academy of Sciences of the United States of America, 104*, 11483–11488.

Brennan, D., & Stevens, J. (1998). A grounded theory approach towards understanding the self perceived effects of meditation on people being treated for cancer. *The Australian Journal of Holistic Nursing, 5*(2), 20–26.

Brooks, J. (1994). The application of Maharishi Ayur-Veda to mental health and substance abuse treatment. *Alcoholism Treatment Quarterly, 11*(3–4), 395–411.

Brown, L. F., Davis, L. W., LaRocco, V. A., & Strasburger, A. (2010). Participant perspectives on mindfulness meditation training for anxiety in schizophrenia. *American Journal of Psychiatric Rehabilitation, 13*(3), 224–242.

Bruce, A., & Davies, B. (2005). Mindfulness in hospice care: Practicing meditation-in-action. *Qualitative Health Research, 15*, 1329–1344.

Buckner, R. L., & Carroll, D. C. (2007). Self-projection and the brain. *Trends in Cognitive Sciences, 11*, 49–57.

Burns, J. L., Lee, R. M., & Brown, L. J. (2011). The effect of meditation on self-reported measures of stress, anxiety, depression, and perfectionism in a college population. *Journal of College Student Psychotherapy, 25*(2), 132–144.

Buselli, E. F., & Stuart, E. M. (1999). Influence of psychosocial factors and biopsychosocial interventions on outcomes after myocardial infarction. *Journal of Cardiovascular Nursing, 13*(3), 60–72.

Cahn, B. R., & Polich, J. (2006). Meditation states and traits: EEG, ERP, and neuroimaging studies. *Psychological Bulletin, 132*, 180–211.

Capra, F. (1975). *The tao of physics*. Boulder, CO: Shambala.

Carlson, L. E., Speca, M., Patel, K. D., & Goodey, E. (2004). Mindfulness-based stress reduction in relation to quality of life, mood, symptoms of stress and levels of cortisol, dehydroepiandrosterone sulfate (DHEAS), and melatonin in breast and prostate cancer outpatients. *Psychoneuroendocrinology, 29*, 448–474.

Carmody, J., & Baer, R. A. (2008). Relationships between mindfulness practice and levels of mindfulness, medical and psychological symptoms and well-being in a mindfulness-based stress reduction program. *Journal of Behavioral Medicine, 31*, 22–33.

Chiesa, A., & Serretti, A. (2010). A systematic review of neurobiological and clinical features of mindfulness meditations. *Psychological Medicine, 40*, 1239–1252.

Coppola, F., & Spector, D. (2009). Natural stress relief meditation as a tool for reducing anxiety and increasing self-actualization. *Social Behavior and Personality, 37*(3), 307–312.

Cortright, B. (1997). *Psychotherapy and spirit: Theory and practice in transpersonal psychotherapy*. Albany, NY: State University of New York Press.

Cresswell, J. D., Myers, H. F., Cole, S. W., & Irwin, M. R. (2009). Mindfulness meditation training effects on CD4+ T lymphocytes in HIV-1 infected adults: A small randomized controlled trial. *Brain, Behavior, and Immunity, 23*(2), 184–188.

Creswell, J. D., Way, B. M., Eisenberger, N. I., & Lieberman, M. D. (2007). Neural correlates of disositional mindfulness during affect labeling. *Psychosomatic Medicine, 69*, 560–565.

Davidson, J. (1976). The physiology of meditation and mystical states of consciousness. *Perspectives in Biology and Medicine, 19*, 345–379.

Davidson, R. J. (2004). Well-being and affective style: neural substrates and biobehavioral correlates. *Philosophical Transactions of the Royal Society, 359*(1449), 1395–1411.

Davidson, R. J., Kabat-Zinn, J., Schumacher, J., Rosenkranz, M., Muller, D., Santorelli, S., Sheridan, J. F. (2003). Alterations in brain and immune function produced by mindfulness meditation. *Psychosomatic Medicine, 65*, 564–570.

Dunn, B. R., Hartigan, J. A., & Mikulas, W. L. (1999). Concentration and mindfulness meditations: Unique forms of consciousness? *Applied Psychophysiology and Biofeedback, 24*, 147–165.

Fortney, L., & Taylor, M. (2010). Meditation in medical practice: A review of the evidence and practice. *Primary Care: Clinics in Office Practice, 37*, 81–90.

Fountoulakis, K. N., Giannakopoulos, P., Kovari, E., & Bouras, C. (2008). Assessing the role of cingulate cortex in bipolar disorder: Neuropathological, structural and functional imaging data. *Brain Research Reviews, 59*, 9–21.

Gaston, L., Crombez, J. C., & Dupuis, G. (1989). An imagery and meditation technique in the treatment of psoriasis: A case study using an A-B-A design. *Journal of Mental Imagery, 13*(1), 31–38.

Gawler, I. (1998). The creative power of imagery: Specific techniques for people affected by cancer. *Australian Journal of Clinical Hypnotherapy and Hypnosis, 19*(1), 17–30.

Gelderloos, P., Walton, K. G., Orme-Johnson, D. W., & Alexander, C. N. (1991). Effectiveness of the transcendental meditation program in preventing a substance misuse: A review. *International Journal of the Addictions, 26*(3), 293–325.

Gellhorn, E., & Kiely, W. (1972). Mystical states of consciousness. *Journal of Nervous and Mental Disease, 154*, 399–405.

Glueck, G., & Stroebel, C. (1975). Biofeedback and meditation in the treatment of psychiatric illness. *Comprehensive Psychiatry, 16*, 309.

Glueck, B., & Stroebel, C. (1978). Psychophysiological correlates of relaxation. In A. Sugerman & R. Tarter (Eds.), *Expanding dimensions of consciousness* (pp. 99–129). New York, NY: Springer.

Goldin, P. R., & Gross, J. J. (2010). Effects of mindfulness-based stress reduction (MBSR) on emotion regulation in social anxiety disorder. *Emotion, 10*, 83–91.

Goldin, P. R., Ramel, W., & Gross, J. J. (2009). Mindfulness meditation training and self-referential processing in Social Anxiety Disorder: Behavioral and neural effects. *Journal of Cognitive Psychotherapy: An International Quarterly, 23*(3), 242–257.

Grant, J. A., Courtemanche, J., Duerden, E. G., Duncan, G. H., & Rainville, P. (2010). Cortical thickness and pain sensitivity in Zen meditators. *Emotion, 10*, 43–53.

Harenski, C. L., & Hamann, S. (2006). Neural correlates of regulation negative emotions related to moral violations. *NeuroImage, 30*, 313–324.

Hart, J. (2007). Clinical applications for meditation: A review and recommendations. *Alternative & Complementary Therapies, 13*(1), 24–29.

Hölzel, B. K., Carmody, J., Vangel, M., Congleton, C., Yerramsetti, S. M., Gard, T., & Lazar, S. W. (2011a). Mindfulness practice leads to increases in regional brain gray matter density. *Psychiatry Research, 191*, 36–43.

Hölzel, B. K., Lazar, S. W., Gard, T., Schuman-Olivier, Z., Bago, D. R., & Ott, U. (2011b). How does mindfulness meditation work? Proposing mechanisms of action from a conceptual and neural perspective. *Perspectives on Psychological Science, 6*, 537–559.

Hölzel, B. K., Ott, U., Hempel, H., Hackl, A., Wolf, K., Stark, R., & Vaitl, D. (2007). Differential engagement of anterior cingulated and adjacent medial frontal cortex in adept meditators and nonmeditators. *Neuroscience Letters, 421*, 16–21.

Hussain, D., & Bhushan, B. (2010). Psychology of meditation and health: Present status and future directions. *International Journal of Psychology and Psychological Therapy, 10*(3), 439–451.

Jain, S., Shapiro, S. L., Swanick, S., Roesch, S. C., Mills, P. J., Bell, I., & Schwartz, G. E. (2007). A randomized controlled trial of mindfulness meditation versus relaxation training: Effects on distress, positive states of mind, rumination, and distraction. *Annals of Behavioral Medicine, 33*, 11–21.

Jevning, R., Wallace, R. K., & Beidebach, M. (1992). The physiology of meditation: A review. A wakeful hypometabolic integrated response. *Neuroscience and Biobehavioral Reviews, 16*, 415–424.

Jha, A. P., Stanley, E. A., Kiyonaga, A., Wong, L., & Gelfand, L. (2010). Examining the protective effects of mindfulness training on working memory capacity and affective experience. *Emotion, 10*, 54–64.

Joseph, M. (1998). The effect of strong religious beliefs on coping with stress. *Stress Medicine, 14*, 219–224.

Kabat-Zinn, J. (1990). *Fill catastrophe living: Using the wisdom of your body and mind to face stress, pain, and illness*. New York, NY: Random House.

Kabat-Zinn, J. (1993). Mindfulness meditation: Health benefits of an ancient Buddhist practice. In D. Coleman &J. Gurin (Eds.), *Mind–body medicine: How to use your mind for better health* (pp. 259–275). Yonkers, NY: Consumer Reports Books.

Kabat-Zinn, J., Lipworth, L., & Burney, R. (1985). The clinical use of mindfulness meditation for the self-regulation of chronic pain. *Journal of Behavioral Medicine, 8*(2), 163–190.

Kabat-Zinn, J., Massion, A. O., Kristeller, J., Peterson, L. G., Fletcher, K. E., Pbert, L., Santorelli, S. F. (1992). Effectiveness of a meditation based stress reduction program in the treatment of anxiety disorders. *American Journal of Psychiatry, 149*, 936–943.

Kabat-Zinn.J., Wheeler, E., Light, T., Skillings, A., Scharf, M.J., Cropley, T. G., Bernhard, J. D. (1998). Influence of a mindfulness meditation-based stress reduction intervention on rates of skin clearing in patients with moderate to severe psoriasis undergoing phototherapy (UVB) and photochemotherapy (PUVA). *Psychosomatic Medicine, 60*(5), 625–632.

Kaplan, K. H., Goldenberg, D. L., & Galvin-Nadeau, M. (1993). The impact of a meditation-based stress reduction program on fibromyalgia. *General Hospital Psychiatry, 15*(5), 284–289.

Kesterson, J., & Clinch, N. F. (1989). Metabolic rate, respiratory exchange ratio and apneas during meditation. *American Journal of Physiology, 256*(3, Pt. 2), R632-R638.

Kimbrough, E., Magyari, T., Langenberg, P., Chesney, M., & Berman, B. (2010). Mindfulness intervention for child abuse survivors. *Journal of Clinical Psychology, 66*(1), 17–33.

Kristeller, J., & Hallett, B. C. (1999). An exploratory study of a meditation-based intervention for binge eating disorder. *Journal of Health Psychology, 4*(3), 357–363.

Kutz, I., Borysenko, J., & Benson, H. (1985). Meditation and psychotherapy. *American Journal of Psychiatry, 142*, 1–8.

Lazar, S. W., Kerr, C. E., Wasserman, R. H., Gray, J. R., Greve, D. N., Treatdway, M. T., & Fischl, B. (2005). Meditation experience is associated with increased cortical thickness. *NeuroReport, 16*, 1893–1897.

Lehrer, P. M., & Woolfolk, R. (1984). Are stress reduction techniques interchangable, or do they specific effects? In R. Woolfolk & P. Lehrer (Eds.), *Principles and practice of stress management* (pp. 404–477). New York: Guilford.

Luders, E., Toga, A. W., Lepore, N., & Gaser, C. (2009). The underlying anatomical correlates of long-term meditation: Larger hippocampal and frontal volumes of gray matter. *NeuroImage, 45*, 672–678.

Lush, E., Salmon, P., Floyd, A., Studts, J. L., Weissbecker, I., & Sephton, S. E. (2009). Mindfulness meditation for symptom reduction in fibromyalgia: Psychophysiological correlates. *Journal of Clinical Psychology in Medical Settings, 16*(2), 200–207.

Matousek, R. H., & Dobkin, P. L. (2010). Weathering storms: A cohort study of how participation in a mindfulness-based stress reduction program benefits women after breast cancer treatment. *Current Oncology, 17*(4), 62–70.

Mazzoli, M. (2011). Complementary tinnitus therapies. In A. R. Møller, B. Langguth, D. De Ridder, & T. Kleinjung (Eds.) *Textbook of tinnitus* (pp. 733–747). New York: Springer

Miller, J. J., Fletcher, K., & Kabat-Zinn, J. (1995). Three-year follow-up and clinical implications of a mindfulness meditation-based stress reduction intervention in the treatment of anxiety disorders. *General Hospital Psychiatry, 17*(3), 192–200.

Mohan, A., Sharma, R., & Bijlani, R. L. (2011). Effect of meditation on stress-induced changes in cognitive functions. *Journal of Alternative and Complementary Medicine, 17*(3), 207–212.

Moyer, C. A., Donnelly, M. P. W., Anderson, J. C., Valek, K. C., Huckaby, S. J., Wiederholt, D. A., … Rice, B. L. (2011). Frontal electroencephalographic asymmetry associated with positive emotion is produced by very brief meditation training. *Psychological Science, 22*(10), 1277–1279

Murphy, M., & Donovan, S. (1988). *The physical and psychological effects of meditation* (2nd ed.). San Rafael, CA: Esalen Institute Study of Exceptional Functioning.

Naranjo, C., & Ornstein, R. (1971). *On the psychology of meditation*. New York: Viking.

NCCAM (2010). *Meditation: An introduction*. Retrieved from: http://nccam.nih.gov/health/meditation/overview.htm

Olendzki, A. (2009). Mindfulness and meditation. In F. Didonna (Ed.), *Clinical handbook of mindfulness* (pp. 37–44). New York: Springer.

Orme-Johnson, D., & Farrow, J. (1978). *Scientific research on the transcendental meditation program [Collected paper]*. New York: Maharishi International University Press.

Ornstein, R. E. (1972). *The psychology of consciousness*. Oxford, England: Penguin.

Ospina, M. B., Bond, K, Karkhaneh, M., Tjosvold, L., Vandermeer, B., Liang, Y., ... Klassen, T. P. Meditation practices for health: state of the research.*Evidence Report/Technology Assessment (Full Report) 2007*. 1–263

Öst, L. G. (1997). Rapid treatment of specific phobias. In G. C. L. Davey (Ed.), *Phobias: A handbook of theory, research, and treatment* (pp. 227–247). Chichester, UK: John Wiley.

Passarotti, A. M., Sweeney, J. A., & Pavuluri, M. N. (2010). Emotion processing influences working memory circuits in pediatric bipolar disorder and attention-deficit/hyperactivity disorder. *Journal of the American Academy of Child & Adolescent Psychiatry, 49*, 1064–1080.

Plews-Ogan, M., Owens, J. E., Goodman, M., Wolfe, P., & Schorling, J. (2005). A pilot study evaluating mindfulness-based stress reduction and massage for the management of chronic pain. *Journal of General Internal Medicine, 20*(12), 1136–1138.

Pradhan, E. K., Baumgarten, M., Langenberg, P., Handwerger, B. Gilpin, A. K., Magyari, T., ... Berman, B. M. (2007) Effect of mindfulness-based stress reduction in rheumatoid arthritis patients. *Arthritis Care & Research, 57,* 1134–1142

Rahul, A. G., & Joseph, M. I. (2009). Influence of meditation on anxiety. *Indian Journal of Community Psychology, 5*(2), 228–234.

Ramel, W., Goldin, P. R., Carmona, P. E., & McQuaid, J. R. (2004). The effects of mindfulness meditation on cognitive process and affect in patients with past deparession. *Cognitive Therapy and Research, 28*, 433–455.

Rosenzweig, S., Greeson, J. M., Reibel, D. K., Green, J. S., Jasser, S. A., & Beasley, D. (2010). Mindfulness-based stress reduction for chronic pain conditions: Variation in treatment outcomes and role of home meditation practice. *Journal of Psychosomatic Research, 68*, 29–36.

Rosenzweig, S., Reibel, D. K., Greeson, J. M., Edman, J. S., Jasser, S. A., McMearty, K. D., & Goldstein, B. J. (2007). Mindfulness-based stress reduction is associated with improved glycemic control in type 2 diabetes mellitus: A pilot study. *Alternative Therapies, 13*(5), 36–38.

Rubia, K. (2009). The neurobiology of meditation and its clinical effectiveness in psychiatric disorders. *Biological Psychology, 82*, 1–11.

Sarang, P. S., & Telles, S. (2006). Oxygen consumption and respiration during and after two yoga relaxation techniques. *Applied Psychophysiology and Biofeedback, 31*(2), 143–153.

Sethi, A. S. (1989). *Meditation as an intervention in stress reactivity*. New York: American Management Services Press.

Shapiro, D. H. (1978). *Precision nirvana*. Englewood Cliffs, NJ: Prentice-Hall.

Shapiro, S. L., Schwartz, G. E., & Bonner, G. (1998). Effects of mindfulness-based stress reduction on medical and premedical students. *Journal of Behavioral Medicine, 21*(6), 581–599.

Shapiro, D. H., & Walsh, R. N. (Eds.). (1984). *Meditation: Classic and contemporary perspectives*. New York: Aldine.

Smith, W. P., Compton, W. C., & West, W. B. (1995). Meditation as an adjunct to a happiness enhancement program. *Journal of Clinical Psychology, 51*(2), 269–273.

Smith, J. E., Richardson, J., Hoffman, C., & Pilkington, K. (2005). Mindfulness-based stress reduction as supportive therapy in cancer care: Systematic review. *Journal of Advanced Nursing, 52*, 315–327.

Sothers, K., & Anchor, K. (1989). Prevention and treatment of essential hypertension with meditation-related methods. *Medical Psychotherapy: An International Journal, 2*, 137–156.

Tácon, A. M. (2003). Meditation as a complementary therapy in cancer. *Family Community Health, 26*(1), 64–73.

Tácon, A. M., McComb, J., Caldera, Y., & Randolph, P. (2003). Mindfulness meditation, anxiety reduction, and heart disease. *A pilot study. Family Community Health, 26*, 25–33.

Tang, Y. Y., Lu, Q., Geng, X., Stein, E. A., Yang, Y., & Posner, M. I. (2010). Short-term meditation induces white matter changes in the anterior cingulate. *Proceedings of the National Academy of Sciences of the United States of America, 107*, 15649–15652.

Telles, S., Reddy, S. K., & Nagendra, H. R. (2000). Oxygen Consumption and respiration following two yoga relaxation techniques. *Applied Psychophysiology and Biofeedback, 25*(4), 221–227.

Wachholtz, A. B., & Pargament, K. I. (2008). Migraines and meditation: Does spirituality matter? *Journal of Behavioral Medicine, 31*(4), 351–366.

Waelde, L. C., Uddo, M., Marquett, R., Ropelato, M., Freightman, S., Pardo, A., & Salazar, J. (2008). A pilot study of meditation for mental health workers following Hurricane Katrina. *Journal of Traumatic Stress, 21*(5), 497–500.

Walsh, R. (1996). Meditation research: The state of the art. In B. Scotton, A. Chinen, & J. Battista (Eds.), *Textbook of transpersonal psychiatry and psychology* (pp. 167–175). New York: Basic Books.

Walsh, R., & Shapiro, S. L. (2006). The meeting of meditative disciplines and Western psychology. *American Psychologist, 61*, 227–239.

Young, L. A., & Baime, M. J. (2010). Mindfulness-based stress reduction: Effect on emotional distress in older adults. *Complementary Health Practice Review, 15*(2), 59–64.

Zamarra, J. W., Schneider, R. H., Besseghini, I., Robinson, D. K., & Salerno, J. W. (1996). Usefulness of the transcendental meditation program in the treatment of patients with coronary artery disease. *American Journal of Cardiology, 77*(10), 867–870.

Zautra, A. J., Davis, M. C., Reich, J. W., Nicassario, P., Tennen, H., Finan, P., … Irwin, M. R. (2008). Comparison of cognitive behavioral and mindfulness meditation interventions on adaptation to rheumatoid arthritis for patients with and without history of recurrent depression. *Journal of Consulting and Clinical Psychology, 76*(3), 408–421

Zeidan, F., Johnson, S. K., Gordon, N. S., & Goolkasian, P. (2010). Effects of brief and sham mindfulness meditation on mood and cardiovascular variables. *The Journal of Alternative and Complementary Medicine, 16*(8), 867–873.

Zgierska, A., Rabago, D., Zuelsdorff, M., Coe, C., Miller, M., & Fleming, M. (2008). Mindfulness meditation for alcohol relapse prevention: A feasibility pilot study. *Journal of Addiction Medicine, 2*(3), 165–173.

Zylowska, L., Ackerman, D. L., Yang, M. H., Futrell, J. L., Horton, N. L., Hale, T. S., … Smalley, S. L. (2008). Mindfulness meditation training in adults and adolescents with ADHD: A feasibility study. *Journal of Attention Disorders, 11*(6), 737–746

Chapter 11
Voluntary Control of Respiration Patterns

Controlled respiration is one of the oldest and certainly the single, most efficient acute intervention for the mitigation and treatment of excessive stress. Any clinician treating patients who manifest excessive stress syndromes should consider controlled respiration as a potentially suitable intervention for virtually all patients. The purpose of this chapter is to discuss the uses of voluntary control of *respiration patterns* in the treatment of excessive stress. As used in this text, this term refers to the process by which the patient exerts voluntary control over his or her breathing pattern—in effect, breath control. There are hundreds of diverse patterns of controlled respiration; we examine several that we feel have particular introductory utility for the clinician concerned with the treatment of the stress response. The exercises presented in this chapter are by no means inclusive. We have simply chosen several patterns that are simple to learn and effective. Again, the goal of voluntary, controlled respiration in the treatment of excessive stress is to have the patient voluntarily alter his or her rhythmic pattern of breathing to create a more relaxed state.

History

As mentioned earlier, voluntary control of respiration patterns (breath control) is perhaps the oldest stress-reduction technique known. It has been used for thousands of years to reduce anxiety and to promote a generalized state of relaxation. The history of voluntary breath control dates back centuries before Christ. References to voluntary breath control for obtaining a relaxation state can be found in the Hindu tradition of Hatha Yoga. In fact, "the word *hatha* itself comes from the Sanskrit root *ha,* meaning sun, and *tha,* meaning moon, and refers to the incoming and outgoing breaths in breathing" (Sethi 1989, p. 69). Thus, Hatha Yoga (the yoga of postures) is built on various patterns of breathing known as *pranayama.* The term *prana* literally means "life force," and *ayama* means "to prolong." Therefore, *pranayama,* which consists of three phases: "puraka" (inhalation), "kumbhaka" (retention), and

G.S. Everly and J.M. Lating, *A Clinical Guide to the Treatment of the Human Stress Response*, DOI 10.1007/978-1-4614-5538-7_11,
© Springer Science+Business Media New York 2013

"rechaka" (exhalation) (Jerath, Edry, Barnes, & Jerath, 2006) loosely translates into prolonged breath control or breath restraint (Fried, 1993; Telles & Naveen, 2008), and more than 3,000 years ago, yogis proclaimed that "life is in the breath."

While in ancient India breath control was developing in the Hindu tradition, the Chinese were practicing it as well. The development of the movement arts of T'ai Chi and Kung Fu both included controlled breathing as an essential component. These "martial arts" continue to enjoy enhanced popularity in the USA.

Perhaps the most widely used form of breath control today is the procedure for "natural" childbirth, in which various types of controlled breathing are used to reduce pain for the mother during delivery and to facilitate the descent of the child through the birth canal (Spiby, Slade, Escott, Henderson, & Fraser, 2003).

In this chapter, we focus on the voluntary, controlled breathing patterns that seem most useful as general aids to relaxation, without any specific goal other than common stress reduction.

Basic Patterns of Breathing

In this section, we briefly describe the fundamentals involved in the breathing process by examining the four phases of the respiratory cycle and describing three basic types of breathing.

According to Hewitt (1977), and elaborated upon by Fried (1993), Austin (1998), and more recently Drummond (2010), four distinct phases of the breathing cycle are relevant in learning voluntary control of respiration patterns (the clinician may find this cursory phasic division useful in teaching any form of deep-breathing technique):

1. *Inhalation or inspiration.* Incidentally, it is no coincidence that the word *inspiration* is used to recognize the connective link between breathing and vital energy (i.e., we all have at times felt "inspired" by a creative idea or an influential other). Inhalation occurs as air is taken into the nose or mouth, descends via the trachea, the bronchi, and bronchioles, and finally inflates the alveoli, which are the air sacs constituting the major portions of the lobes of the lungs. As the lungs expand, their stretch receptors tighten, which in turn sends inhibitory signals from the vagus nerve to the brain stem, signaling inhalation to stop.
2. *The pause that follows inhalation.* During this pause, the lungs remain inflated.
3. *Exhalation or expiration.* Again, note the connection between breathing and life force in the term *expiration*. For example, when someone passes away, we say that they have expired, or that they have breathed their last breath: in essence, that their life energy is now gone. Exhalation occurs as the lungs are deflated, emptying the waste gases from the alveoli.
4. *The pause that follows the exhalation phase.* During this phase, the lungs are at rest in a deflated state.

Rama, Ballentine, and Hymes (1998) describe three basic types of breathing that differ primarily according to the nature of the inhalation initiating the breathing cycle: clavicular, thoracic, and diaphragmatic.

The clavicular breath, the shortest and shallowest of the three, can be observed as a slight vertical elevation of the clavicles, combined with a slight expansion of the thoracic cage upon inhalation.

The thoracic breath represents (in varying degrees) a deeper breath—deeper in the sense that a greater amount of air is inhaled, more alveoli are inflated, and the lobes of the lungs are expanded to a greater degree. It is initiated by activation of the intercostal muscles, which expand the thoracic cage up and outward. The thoracic breath can be observed as a greater expansion of the thoracic cage, followed by an elevation of the clavicles on inhalation. Thoracic breathing is the most common breathing pattern.

Finally, the diaphragmatic breath represents the deepest of all the breaths, with the most air inhaled and the greatest number of alveoli inflated. In addition, for the first time, the lowest levels of the lungs are inflated. The lower third of the lungs contains the greater part of the blood when the individual stands vertically; therefore, the diaphragmatic breath oxygenates a greater quantity of blood per breathing cycle than the other types of breathing. During the diaphragmatic breath, the diaphragm (a thin, dome-shaped sheet of muscle that separates the chest cavity and the abdomen) flattens downward during inhalation. This causes the abdominal muscles to relax and rise, and push the organs in the abdominal cavity forward, which creates a partial vacuum and allows air to descend into the lungs. Thus, the movement of the diaphragm becomes the major cause of the deep inhalation. The full diaphragmatic breath may be observed as the abdominal cavity expands outward, followed by expansion of the thoracic cage, and, finally, elevation of the clavicles.

Variations of the diaphragmatic breath are considered by many to be the simplest and most effective form of controlled respiration in the reduction of excessive stress. Therefore, we limit our discussion to the role of diaphragmatic patterns in reducing excessive stress. It would, however, be helpful to the clinician to learn to identify all the three basic patterns of breathing.

Mechanisms of Action

Although the specific mechanisms involved in stress reduction via breath control may differ from technique to technique, a general therapeutic factor is thought to be the ability of the diaphragmatic breath to induce a temporary trophotropic state. Jerath and colleagues (2006) note that the tone of the sympathetic and parasympathetic nervous systems is greatly affected by the process of respiration. Harvey (1978) recognizes that "diaphragmatic breathing stimulates both the solar plexus and the right vagus nerve in a manner that enervates the parasympathetic nervous system, thus facilitating full relaxation" (p. 14).

Expiration is also thought to affect the relaxation response. In fact, the mere act of breathing out may increase parasympathetic tone (Ballentine, 1976) and serve to slightly decrease neural firing in the amygdala and hippocampus (Austin, 2006; Frysinger & Harper, 1989). Moreover, prolonged expiration, along with quieter breathing, may further reduce neural firing in the amygdala that could lead to physiological calming (Zhang, Harper, & Ni, 1986). It is notable that during most types of diaphragmatic breathing, expiration is protracted. Interestingly, the normal person spends less time breathing in (about 43%) than breathing out; however, monks practicing the meditative art of zazen have been known to increase the exhalation phase of their respiratory cycle to around 75% (Austin, 1998). In patients practicing guided imagery, Austin (2006) notes that when successful they have been able to slow their respiration to 3–5 breaths per minute. He also notes that breathing techniques that prolong exhalation may increase the inhibitory tone of the vagus nerve and reduce respiratory drive in the brain stem. Additionally, deep, slow diaphragmatic breathing is considered to initiate inhibitory signals in lung tissue that overall may lead "to changes in the autonomic nervous system and a resultant condition characterized by reduced metabolism and parasympathetic dominance" (Telles & Naveen, 2008, p. 72).

Independent of the predominately physiological mechanisms, voluntary breath control may prove therapeutic from a cognitive perspective as well. The rationale for this statement comes from the supposition that concentration on respiration patterns may serve to enhance a perception of internal control, along with ways to compete with obsessive thought patterns, and maybe even compulsive behaviors. More recently, studies have assessed how the respiratory system may be involved in the activation of the fear network, composed of the prefrontal cortex, the amygdala, the hippocampus, and the subsequent brainstem projections, in patients suffering with panic disorder (de Carvalho, Rozenthal, & Nardi, 2010; Nardi, Freire, & Zin, 2009). In addition, it has been hypothesized how slow breathing exercises that increase parasympathetic tone might be effective in reducing seizure frequency in those with refractory epilepsy (Yuen & Sander, 2010).

Clinical Research

One of the seminal studies related to the efficacy of breathing training is on 105 male patients awaiting imminent electric shocks to the hand. Those who were instructed to regulate their breathing to only eight breaths per minute evidenced lower subjective arousal, and less change in skin resistance and finger pulse volume than control participants who were not taught respiratory control (McCaul, Sollmon, & Holmes, 1979).

1. Use of deep breathing meditation was effective in mitigating the effects of stress and test anxiety in a sample of 64 post-baccalaureate premedical students (Paul, Elam, & Verhulst, 2007).
2. Controlled breathing has been used effectively as part of the treatment of children and adults with asthma (Chiang, Ma, Huang, Tseng, & Hsueh, 2009; Meuret, Ritz, Wilhelm, & Roth, 2007), and slow, regular diaphragmatic breathing has been shown to reduce the potential of hyperventilation in asthma patients and improve quality of life (Thomas et al., 2003).

3. The benefits of controlled breathing have been observed in 76 post-MI patients (van Dixhoorn, 1998), in patients experiencing non-cardiac chest pain (Van Peski-Oosterbaan, Spinhoven, van Rood, Van der Does, & Bruschke, 1997), and in children experiencing chest pain (Lipsitz, Gur, Albano, & Sherman, 2011).
4. Cognitive-behavioral interventions for panic disorder, which reliably entail breathing retraining, have been associated with decreased frequency and intensity of attacks (Meuret, Wilhelm & Roth, 2004). In a recent meta-analysis of 42 studies assessing the treatment of panic disorder, with and without agoraphobia, Sánchez-Meca, Rosa-Alcázar, Marín-Martínez, & Gómez-Conesa (2010) reported that the combination of exposure, relaxation training, and breathing retraining provides the best evidence for treating panic disorder.
5. Breathing retraining has also been implemented in cognitive-behavioral program used to treat PTSD (Mueser, Rosenberg, & Rosenberg, 2009).

How to Implement

Voluntary breath control appears to be the most flexible of the interventions for the reduction of excessive stress. It can be used under a wide variety of environmental and behavioral conditions.

Despite its versatility, voluntary breath control should be used with precautions. When breathing is used as a meditative device, the precautions discussed in the chapter on meditation are relevant. The primary precaution, relatively unique to voluntary breath control, is regarding hyperventilation. Simply defined, hyperventilation is a condition in which the patient's rate and depth of breathing is too much for the body's needs at a particular time. Hyperventilation can quickly create the condition of hypocapnia, a decreased production and availability of CO_2. Hypocapnia results in decreased blood flow to the extremities and to the brain (Fried, 1993). The symptoms of hyperventilation, which include dizziness, panic, fatigue, feelings of suffocation, chest pain, stomach cramps, racing heart, trembling, loss of consciousness, tenseness, hot flashes, and nausea, overlap considerably with the symptoms of stress and anxiety. Many of these symptoms could appear after several minutes of prolonged hyperventilation. According to Grossman and DeSwart (1984), dizziness, tiredness, and feelings of suffocation and panic are the most commonly reported hyperventilation symptoms.

Fried (1993) offers the following insights, recommendations, and additional precautions in the use of diaphragmatic breathing:

1. Some individuals with a high stress profile may unknowingly hold their diaphragm in a partially contracted position; therefore, diaphragmatic breathing may initially produce cramps.
2. If pain or discomfort is experienced due to muscle or tissue injury, then the diaphragmatic breathing exercise should be stopped.
3. In cases where metabolic acidosis may occur, such as severe hypoglycemia, kidney disease, heart disease, or diabetes, approval from a physician should be acquired before beginning diaphragmatic breathing.

4. Since diaphragmatic breathing may significantly lower blood pressure, individuals with normally low blood pressure or syncope should use the technique cautiously.

Since the publication of the last edition of this text, there has been increased treatment interest in the use of voluntary hyperventilation that involves having a patient breath "fast and deep" and to focus on "exhaling hard" from 18 to 60 breaths/ min for 1–3 min (Meuret, Ritz, Wilhelm, & Roth, 2005). Most clinical applications of voluntary hyperventilation are associated with breathing training that is designed to induce and then mitigate acute decreases in arterial pCO_2 by breathing more diaphragmatically (Craske, Barlow, & Meadows, 2000). Even though not all data support the use of voluntary hyperventilation tests to diagnose or assess hyperventilation syndrome (Hornsveld, Garssen, Fiedeldij Dop, van Spiegel, & de Haes, 1996), voluntary hyperventilation is an integral part of the cognitive-behavioral technique of interoceptive exposure (IE) used in the treatment of panic disorder. IE involves having patients repeatedly induce, experience, and attend to their feared sensations, such as dizziness, feelings of suffocation, heart palpitations, and shortness of breath, and to then challenge their catastrophic thinking, to understand the physiological mechanisms involved in the response, and to learn to accept their anxiety so that the physiological arousal sensations do not result in panic and avoidance (Lee et al., 2006; Otto, Powers, & Fischmann, 2005; Stewart & Watt, 2008).

Predicated on a breathing method developed over the past 25 years in Europe, van Dixhoorn (2007, 2008) has offered an integrative systems and process model of breathing, known as whole-body breathing that incorporates elements of direct respiratory retraining, as well as indirect approaches of respiratory modification for breath training and relaxation. According to the systems approach, respiration has two functions: regulation of mental and physical tension, and provision of information regarding internal tension. Van Dixhoorn's (2008) approach offers patients a range of treatment modalities and techniques (e.g., breathing, self-talk, postural changes, mental images), as well as broad treatment goals (e.g., lower arousal, attentional shift; renewal of energy or balance, increased body awareness, organization of functional movement that follows the skeletal structure; cognitive restructuring, and functional breathing). In addition, whole-body breathing relies on information gathered and observed from a first-person as well as a third-person (or external observer) perspective. The whole-body approach and its suggestions should be considered when reviewing the exercises below.

Listed below are three diaphragmatic breathing exercises reported to be useful in promoting a more relaxed state. In teaching any form of diaphragmatic breathing, the clinician must monitor the activities of the patient to assure proper techniques. Hewitt (1977) offers the following guidelines, which we believe are still appropriate for all forms of diaphragmatic breathing:

> You fill the lungs to a point of fullness without strain or discomfort (p. 90). If after retention [of the inhalation] the air bursts out noisely, the suspension has been overprolonged; the air should be released in a steady smooth stream… Similarly, following the empty pause, the air should unhurriedly and quietly begin its ascent of the nostrils [as the new inhalation begins]. (p. 73)

We consider these general guidelines useful to avoid patients' over breathing, as well as other inappropriate breathing practices. These guidelines should be followed when instructing a patient in each of the following three breathing exercises.

Breathing Exercise 1

This breathing technique may be thought of as a "complete breath." In fact, variations of this breath appear with similar names in the Yogic literature. The technique is extremely simple to complete. In order to assist the clinician in teaching the exercise to patients, we present the four phases of breath described by Hewitt (1977).

Inhalation. The inhalation should begin through the nose if possible. The nose is preferred to the mouth because of its ability to filter and warm the incoming air. On inhalation, the abdomen should begin to move outward, followed by expansion of the chest. The length of the inhalation should be 2 to 3 s (or to some point less than that in which the lungs and chest expand without discomfort).

Pause after inhalation. There should be no pause. Inhalation should transfer smoothly into the beginning of exhalation.

Exhalation. Here, the air is expired (through the mouth or the nose, whichever is more comfortable). The length of this exhalation should be 2–3 s.

Pause after exhalation. This pause should last only 1 s, then inhalation should begin again in a smooth manner. We have found that this exercise can be repeated by many patients for several minutes without the initiation of hyperventilation. However, patients should usually be instructed to stop when lightheadedness occurs.

Breathing Exercise 2

This breathing exercise may be thought of as a form of "counting breath," of which variations appear in the Yogic literature. The term *counting* is applied to this exercise because the patient is asked literally to count to him- or herself the number of seconds each of the four phases of the exercise will last. In order to assist the clinician in teaching this exercise, we present the four phases of breathing described by Hewitt (1977).

Inhalation. The inhalation should begin through the nose if possible. The abdomen should begin to move outward, followed by expansion of the chest. The length of the inhalation should be 2 s (or to some point less than that in which the lungs and chest expand without discomfort). The length of the inhalation should be counted silently, as 1,000; 2,000; etc.

Pause after inhalation. There should be a pause here, following the 2-s inhalation. The counted pause here should be 1 s in duration.

Pause after Exhalation. This counted pause should last 1 s. The next inhalation should follow smoothly. We have found that this exercise can be repeated by many patients for several minutes without the occurrence of hyperventilation. However, patients should usually be instructed to stop when light-headedness occurs.

Breathing Exercise 3

This technique, developed by G. S. Everly, is designed to rapidly induce (within 30–60 s) a state of relaxation. Research has shown it to be effective in reducing muscle tension and subjective reports of anxiety, as well as having some potential for reducing heart rate (see Everly, 1979b, c; Vanderhoof, 1980). The following description is presented as if instructing a patient:

> During the course of an average day, many of us find ourselves in anxiety-producing situations. Our heart rates increase, our stomachs may become upset, and our thoughts may race uncontrollably through our minds. It is during such episodes that we require fast-acting relief from our stressful reactions. The brief exercise described below has been found effective in reducing most of the stress reaction that we suffer from during acute exposures to stressors—it is, in effect, a quick way to "calm down" in the face of a stressful situation.

The basic mechanism for stress reduction in this exercise involves deep breathing. The procedure is as follows:

Step 1. Assume a comfortable position. Rest your left hand (palm down) on top of your abdomen, over your navel. Now place your right hand so that it rests comfortably on your left. Your eyes can remain open. However, it is usually easier to complete Step 2 with your eyes closed (see Fig. 11.1).

Step 2. Imagine a hollow bottle, or pouch, lying internally beneath the point at which your hands are resting. Begin to inhale. As you inhale imagine that the air is entering through your nose and descending to fill that internal pouch. Your hands will rise as you fill the pouch with air. As you continue to inhale, imagine the pouch being filled to the top. Your rib cage and upper chest will continue the wavelike rise that began at your navel. The total length of your inhalation should be two seconds for the first week or two, then possibly lengthening to two and a half or three seconds as you progress in skill development (see Fig. 11.2).

Step 3. Hold your breath. Keep the air inside the pouch. Repeat to yourself the phrase, "My body is calm." This step should last no more than 2 s.

Step 4. Slowly begin to exhale—to empty the pouch. As you do, repeat to yourself the phrase, "My body is quiet." As you exhale, you will feel your raised abdomen and chest recede. This step should last as long as the two preceding steps, or may last one second longer, after a week or two of practice. (*Note.* Step 1 need only be used during the first week or so, as you learn to breathe deeply. Once you master that skill, you may omit that step.) Repeat this four-step exercise three to five times in succession. Should you begin to feel light-headed, stop at that point. If light-headedness recurs

Fig. 11.1 Step 1

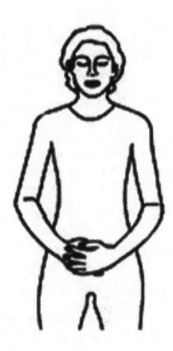

Fig. 11.2 Step 2

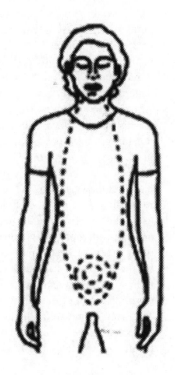

with continued practice, simply shorten the length of the inhalation and/or decrease the number of times you repeat the exercise in succession.

Practice this exercise 10–20 times a day. Make it a ritual in the morning, afternoon, and evening, as well as during stressful situations. Because this form of relaxation is a skill, it is important to practice at least 10–20 times a day. At first you may not notice any on-the-spot relaxation. However, after a week or two of regular practice, you will increase your capabilities to relax temporarily. Remember, you must *practice regularly* if you are to master this skill. Regular, consistent practice of these daily exercises will ultimately lead to the development of a more calm and relaxed attitude—a sort of anti-stress attitude—and when you do have stressful moments, they will be far less severe.

Summary

This chapter has presented a discussion of voluntary, controlled patterns of respiration for use in reducing excessive stress. As mentioned earlier, the goal of voluntary respiration in the treatment of excessive stress is to have the patient voluntarily alter his or her rhythmic pattern of breathing to create a more relaxed state.

1. Dating back to centuries before Christ, there is a rich and lengthy history of using breath control as a means to enhance relaxation.
2. There are three basic types of breathing patterns—clavicular, thoracic, and diaphragmatic. The first two are associated with (and may stimulate) a sympathetic response. The latter is associated with (and may stimulate) a parasympathetic response (see Ballentine, 1976). It has been found useful for the clinician to learn to recognize these patterns in patients and to teach them how to recognize these patterns in themselves.
3. Although the literature (especially that of Yoga) presents myriad diverse respiratory techniques for relaxation, we have focused in this chapter on diaphragmatic breathing. This emphasis is based on the conclusion that variations of diaphragmatic breathing are the simplest to teach and among the most effective for achieving a relaxed psychophysiological state. For these reasons, the clinician may find the variations of the diaphragmatic pattern most useful.
4. In the final analysis, the clinician needs to assess the suitability of using voluntary, controlled respiration with each patient on a case-by-case basis. The clinician may attempt to teach the three different exercises presented in this chapter in order to assess which may be of most utility. These variations of diaphragmatic breathing are not provided as a prescription, but as a sample of breath control techniques that have been beneficial in reducing excessive stress. Many other useful variations exist (see Fried, 1993; Hewitt, 1977; van Dixhoorn, 2007).
5. The primary precaution in the use of breath control in stress reduction regards the hyperventilation reaction. This is usually not a problem when the patient uses breathing exercises (such as those described in this chapter) for short time

durations and ceases if light-headedness ensues. The Yogic literature reports that no more than 15 min of any hour should be spent in *pranayama* practice. Again, this topic should be addressed with patients individually.

6. In conclusion, Patel (1993) states that "if breath influences both the body and the mind, not only physical, mental, and emotional states are reflected in the pattern of breath, but through breathing we can also influence our physical, psychological, and spiritual well-being" (p. 119). This analysis certainly seems accurate. Additionally, teaching breath control may serve to enhance an overall perception of enhanced personal control.

References

Austin, J. H. (1998). *Zen and the brain: Toward an understanding of meditation and consciousness.* Cambridge, MA: MIT Press.

Austin, J. H. (2006). *Zen-brain reflections.* Cambridge, MA: MIT Press.

Ballentine, R. (1976). *Science of breath.* Glenview, IL: Himalayan International Institute.

Chiang, L. C., Ma, W. F., Huang, J. L., Tseng, L. F., & Hsueh, K. C. (2009). Effect of relaxation-breathing training on anxiety and asthma signs/symptoms of children with moderate-to-severe asthma: A randomized controlled trial. *International Journal of Nursing Studies, 46,* 1061–1070.

Craske, M. G., Barlow, D. H., & Meadows, E. A. (2000). *Mastery of your anxiety and panic: Therapist guide for anxiety, panic and agoraphobia (MAP-3).* San Antonio, TX: Graywind/ Psychological Corporation.

de Carvalho, M. R., Rozenthal, M., & Nardi, A. E. (2010). The fear circuitry in panic disorder and its modulation by cognitive-behaviour therapy interventions. *World Journal of Biological Psychiatry, 11*(2), 188–198.

Drummond, G. (2010). Like breathing out and breathing in...*The Journal of Physiology, 588*(18), 3345.

Everly, G. S., Jr. (1979b). Technique for the immediate reduction of psychophysiological reactivity. *Health Education, 10,* 44.

Everly, G. S., Jr. (1979c). A psychophysiological technique for the rapid onset of a trophotropic state. *IRCS Journal of Medical Science, 7,* 423.

Fried, R. (1993). The role of respiration in stress and stress control: Toward a theory of stress as a hypoxic phenomenon. In P. M. Lehrer & R. L. Woolfolk (Eds.), *Principles and practice of stress management* (2nd ed., pp. 301–331). New York, NY: Guilford.

Frysinger, R., & Harper, R. (1989). Cardiac and respiratory correlations with unit discharge in human amygdala and hippocampus. *Electroencephalography and Clinical Neurophysiology, 72,* 463–470.

Grossman, P., & DeSwart, J. C. G. (1984). Diagnosis of hyperventilation syndrome on the basis of reported complaints. *Journal of Psychosomatic Research, 28,* 97–104.

Harvey, J. (1978). Diaphragmatic breathing: A practical technique for breath control. *Behavior Therapist, 1,* 13–14.

Hewitt, J. (1977). *The complete yoga book.* New York, NY: Schocken.

Hornsveld, H. K., Garssen, B., Fiedeldij Dop, M. J. C., van Spiegel, P., & de Haes, J. C. J. M. (1996). Double-blind placebo-controlled study of the hyperventilation provocation test and the validity of the hyperventilation syndrome. *The Lancet, 348,* 152–158.

Jerath, R., Edry, J. W., Barnes, V. A., & Jerath, V. (2006). Physiology of long pranayamic breathing: Neural respiratory elements may provide a mechanism that explains how slow deep breathing shifts the autonomic nervous system. *Medical Hypotheses, 67,* 566–571.

Lee, K., Noda, Y., Nakano, Y., Ogawa, S., Kinoshita, Y., Funayama, T., & Furukawa, T. A. (2006). Interoceptive hypsensitivity and interceptive exposure in patients with panic disorder: Specificity and effectiveness. *BMC Psychiatry, 6*, 32.

Lipsitz, J. D., Gur, M., Albano, A. M., & Sherman, B. (2011). A psychological intervention for pediatric chest pain: Development and open trial. *Journal of Developmental and Behavioral Pediatrics, 32*(2), 153–157.

McCaul, K., Solomon, S., & Holmes, D. (1979). The effects of paced respiration and expectations on physiological responses to threat. *Journal of Personality and Social Psychology, 37*, 564–571.

Meuret, A. E., Ritz, T., Wilhelm, F. H., & Roth, W. T. (2005). Voluntary hyperventilation in the treatment of panic disorder – functions of hyperventilation, their implications for breathing training, and recommendations for standardization. *Clinical Psychology Review, 25*, 285–306.

Meuret, A. E., Ritz, T., Wilhelm, F. H., & Roth, W. T. (2007). Targeting pCO2 in Asthma: Pilot evaluation of a capnometry-assisted breathing training. *Applied Psychophysiological Biofeedback, 32*, 99.

Meuret, A. E., Wilhelm, F. H., & Roth, W. T. (2004). Respiratory feedback for treating panic disorder. *Journal of Clinical Psychology/In Session, 60*, 197–207.

Mueser, K. T., Rosenberg, S. D., & Rosenberg, H. J. (2009). *Treatment of posttraumatic stress disorder in special populations: A cognitive restructuring program.* Washington, DC: American Psychological Association.

Nardi, A. E., Freire, R. C., & Zin, W. A. (2009). Panic disorder and control of breathing. *Respiratory Physiology & Neurobiology, 167*(1), 133–143.

Otto, M. W., Powers, M. B., & Fischmann, D. (2005). Emotional exposure in the treatment of substance use disorders: Conceptual model, evidence, and future direction. *Clinical Psychology Review, 25*, 824–839.

Patel, C. (1993). Yoga-based therapy. In P. M. Lehrer & R. L. Woolfolk (Eds.), *Principles and practice of stress management* (2nd ed., pp. 89–137). New York: Guilford.

Paul, G., Elam, B., & Verhulst, S. J. (2007). A longitudinal study of students' perceptions of using deep breathing meditation to reduce testing stresses. *Teaching and Learning in Medicine, 19*(3), 287–292.

Rama, S., Balltentine, R., & Hymes, A. (1998). *Science of breath: A practical guide.* Honesdale, PA: Himalayian Institute Press.

Sánchez-Meca, J., Rosa-Alcázar, A. I., Marín-Martínez, F., & Gómez-Conesa, A. (2010). Psychological treatment of panic disorder with or without agoraphobia: A meta-analysis. *Clinical Psychology Review, 30*(1), 37–50.

Sethi, A. S. (1989). *Meditation as an intervention in stress reactivity.* New York: American Management Services Press.

Spiby, H., Slade, P., Escott, D., Henderson, B., & Fraser, R. B. (2003). Selected coping strategies in labor: An investigation of women's experiences. *Birth: Issues in Perinatal Care, 30*(3), 189–194.

Stewart, S. H., & Watt, M. C. (2008). Introduction to the special issue on interoceptive exposure in the treatment of anxiety and related disorders: Novel applications and mechanisms of action. *Journal of Cognitive Psychotherapy: An International Quarterly, 22*(4), 291–302.

Telles, S., & Naveen, K. V. (2008). Voluntary breath in yoga: Its relevance and physiological effects. *Biofeedback, 36*(2), 70–73.

Thomas, M., McKinley, R. K., Freeman, E., Foy, C., Prodger, P., & Price, D. (2003). Breathing retraining for dysfunctional breathing in asthma: A randomized controlled trial. *Thorax, 58*, 110–115.

van Dixhoorn, J. (1998). Cardiorespiratory effects of breathing and relaxation instruction in myocardial infarction patients. *Biological Psychology, 49*(1–2), 123–135.

van Dixhoorn, J. (2007). Whole-body breathing: A systems perspective on respiratory retraining. In P. M. Lehrer, R. L. Woolfolk, & W. E. Sime (Eds.), *Principles and practice of stress management* (3rd ed., pp. 291–332). New York: Guiford.

van Dixhoorn, J. (2008). Whole-body breathing. *Biofeedback, 36*, 54–58.

Van Peski-Oosterbaan, A. S., Spinhoven, P., van Rood, Y., Van der Does, W. A. J., & Bruschke, A. J. V. (1997). Cognitive behavioural therapy for unexplained noncardiac chest pain: A pilot study. *Behavioural and Cognitive Psychotherapy, 25*(4), 339–350.

Vanderhoof, L. (1980). *The effects of a simple relaxation technique on stress during pelvic examinations.* Unpublished master's thesis, University of Maryland School of Nursing, Baltimore.

Yuen, A. W. C., & Sander, J. W. (2010). Can slow breathing exercises improve seizure control in people with refractory epilepsy? A hypothesis. *Epilepsy & Behavior, 18*(4), 331–334.

Zhang, J., Harper, R., & Ni, H. (1986). Cryogenic blockade of the central nucleus of the amygdala attenuates aversively conditioned blood pressure and respiratory responses. *Brain Research, 386*, 136–145.

Chapter 12
Neuromuscular Relaxation

Chapter 9 presented a neurophysiological rationale for the use of relaxation response in the treatment of stress-related disorders. In developing that rationale, we reviewed the research efforts of Gellhorn (1958a, b, 1964b, 1967), Weil (1974), and Malmo (1975). A reader of these respective literatures is likely to be impressed by the convergence these independent authors reached regarding the critically central role that the neuromuscular system plays in the determination of emotional and stress-related manifestations. Yet it was Gellhorn (1958a, b, 1964b) who, through a series of well-designed experiments, demonstrated that the nuclear origin of the SNS, the posterior hypothalamus, is dramatically affected by neuromuscular proprioceptive feedback from the skeletal musculature. Such findings led him (1964b) to conclude "that states of abnormal emotional tension are alleviated in various "relaxation" therapies which impinge on the posterior hypothalamus" (p. 457). This chapter explores the clinical corollary of this notion.

The purpose of this chapter is to provide a clinically useful introduction to a genre of interventions termed *neuromuscular relaxation* (NMR). As used here, this term refers to a process by which an individual can perform a series of exercises to reduce the neural activity (*neuro*) and contractile tension in striate skeletal muscles (*muscular*). This process usually consists of isotonic and/or isometric muscular contractions performed by the patient with initial instruction from the clinician. The proper practice of NMR ultimately leads to the elicitation of the relaxation response.

History

The NMR procedure presented in this chapter comes from four primary sources: (1) the "progressive relaxation" procedures developed byJacobson (1970), (2) the research of Bernstein and Borkovec (1973), (3) research protocols developed by this text's senior author, and (4) the clinical work of Bhalla (1980) applying neuromuscular interventions to the field of physical medicine and stress.

G.S. Everly and J.M. Lating, *A Clinical Guide to the Treatment of the Human Stress Response*, DOI 10.1007/978-1-4614-5538-7_12,
© Springer Science+Business Media New York 2013

Edmund Jacobson is often considered the originator of relaxation techniques. His distinguished career took him from undergraduate studies at Northwestern to Harvard, where he worked with William James, among others, and received his PhD in 1910, to a fellowship with Edward Titchner at Cornell, and finally to Rush Medical School (part of the University of Chicago). After receiving his MD, Jacobson did psychophysiological research until his death in 1983 (see Gessel, 1989, for a biographic article of Jacobson). According to Gessel, Jacobson's "contributions, taken in their totality, create the basis for a comprehensive discipline of neuromuscular psychophysiology" (p. 5).

Early research by Jacobson and his colleague Carlson on the knee-jerk reflex led to the observation that in participants who appeared most deeply relaxed, the knee-jerk reflex was absent or noticeably diminished (Gessel, 1989). This type of work led Jacobson (1938) to conclude that striated muscle tension plays a major role in anxiety states. By teaching individuals to reduce striated muscle tension, Jacobson reported success in reducing subjective reports of anxiety. Later work in the area of mind–body functioning led Jacobson to hypothesize that all thought occurs with collateral skeletal muscle activity of varying, and often extremely low, response amplitudes. As Jacobson stated, "It might be naive to say that we think with our muscles, but it would be inaccurate to say that we think without them" (cited in McGuigan & Lehrer, 2007, p. 58).

Gellhorn (1958b, 1964b), who was particularly impressed with Jacobson's research, offered a neurophysiological rationale for the use of progressive relaxation in the treatment of stress-related disorders. After the 1940s, Charles Atlas developed a program of muscular "dynamic tension" for general health, but the model developed by Jacobson gained greater popularity among practicing clinicians.

Jacobson called his system "progressive relaxation." It consists of a series of exercises in which the patient tenses (contracts) and then relaxes selected muscles and muscle groups so as to achieve the desired state of deep relaxation. Jacobson considered his procedure "progressive" for the following reasons:

1. The patient learns progressively to relax the neuromuscular activity (tension) in the selected muscle. This process may require several minutes to achieve maximal NMR in any selected muscle.
2. The patient tenses and then relaxes selected muscles in the body in such a manner as to progress through the principal muscle groups, until the entire body, or selected body area, is relaxed.
3. With continued daily practice, the patient tends progressively to develop a "habit of repose" (1978, p. 161)—a less stressful, less excitable attitude.

Progressive relaxation gained considerable popularity when Wolpe (1958) used the same basic relaxation system in his phobia treatment called "systematic desensitization." This treatment paradigm, which is a classic behavioral therapeutic intervention, consists of relaxing the patient before and during exposure to a hierarchy of anxiety-evoking stimuli. Wolpe has successfully employed the tenet that an individual cannot concurrently be relaxed and anxious; that is, relaxation acts to inhibit a stress response. A comprehensive, excellent review of Jacobson's work is that of McGuigan and Lehrer (2007).

Mechanisms of Action

Jacobson (1978) argues that the main therapeutic actions of the NMR system reside in having the patient *learn* the difference between tension and relaxation. This learning is based on having the patient enhance his or her awareness of proprioceptive neuromuscular impulses that originate at the peripheral muscular levels and increase with striated muscle tension. These afferent proprioceptive impulses are major determiners of chronic diffuse anxiety and overall stressful sympathetic arousal, according to Jacobson. This conclusion is supported by the research of Gellhorn, who demonstrated the critical role played by afferent proprioceptive impulses from the muscle spindles in the determination of generalized ergotropic tone (Gellhorn, 1958a,b, 1964b, 1967). The neuromuscular mechanisms of action were discussed in detail in Chap. 9. Please refer back to the work of Gellhorn, Malmo, and Weil discussed in that chapter.

Once the patient learns adequate neuromuscular awareness, he or she may then effectively learn to reduce excessive muscle tension by consciously and progressively "letting go," or reducing the degree of contraction in the selected muscles. It has been argued that it is difficult for "unpracticed" individuals to achieve a similar degree of conscious relaxation, because they are not educated in the sensations of tension versus conscious deep relaxation—as a result, measurable "residual tension" remains during conscious efforts to relax.

Empirical support for the impact of progressive muscle relaxation on the endocrine and immune systems comes from a study of undergraduates who either received or did not receive Abbreviated Progressive Relaxation Training and then had salivary cortisol and salivary immunoglobulin A (sIgA) measured (Pawlow & Jones, 2005). Compared to the 14 control participants, the 41 participants who received the one-hour relaxation intervention had lower post-intervention salivary cortisol levels and higher levels of post-intervention sIgA concentration and secretion rates. A study of 30 volunteers by Lowe, Bland, Greenman, Kirkpatrick, and Lowe (2001) demonstrated a similar increase in IgA, accompanied by decreased heart rate and cortisol following four weekly sessions of progressive relaxation training for 15 participants, compared to the 15 neutral control participants (who received a shipping weather forecast).

Other studies on progressive relaxation have suggested that there are two principal therapeutic components at work. Although it is generally accepted that the traditional Jacobsonian concept of *learned awareness* of the differences between the tension of contraction and relaxation experienced on the release of contraction is an important therapeutic component, there may be more. It has been suggested that the actual procedure of *contracting* a muscle before attempting to relax it may add impetus to the total amount of relaxation achieved in that muscle, over and above the process of learned awareness (Borkovec, Grayson, & Cooper, 1978).

Research on Clinical Applications and Effects

A review of research and clinical literature on the genre of techniques considered part of NMR (including Jacobson's procedures) reveals myriad stress-related therapeutic applications. Specifically, neuromuscular or progressive relaxation has been suggested to be effective for the following:

1. Non-insulin-dependent diabetes mellitus (Henry, Wilson, Bruce, Chisholm, & Rawling, 1997).
2. Peptic ulcers (Thankachan & Mishra, 1996).
3. Bronchial asthma (Nickel et al., 2005).
4. Chronic tension headache (Sadoughi, Nouri, Kajbaf, Akkashe, & Molavi, 2009)
5. Pain (Chen & Francis, 2010; Pavlek, 2008).
6. Tinnitus (Jakes, Hallam, Rachman, & Hinchcliffe, 1986).
7. Psychobiological well-being during pregnancy (Urech et al., 2010).
8. Anxiety reduction in patients with acute schizophrenia (Chen et al., 2009) and in debilitating test anxiety among medical students (Powell, 2004).
9. Assistance in the treatment of cancer chemotherapy (Carey & Burish, 1987; de Carvalho, Matins, dos Santos, 2007; Demiralp, Oflaz, & Komurcu, 2010).
10. Symptom severity associated with PTSD (Zucker, Samuelson, Muench, Greenberg, & Gervitz, 2009).
11. Assistance in the treatment of HIV infection and AIDS (Kocsis, 1996).
12. Buffering the negative impact of watching the news (Szabo & Hopkinson, 2007).
13. Children and adolescents overcoming stress (Klien, 2008).

Manzoni, Pagnini, Castelnuovo, & Molinari (2008) reported the results of a 10-year meta-analytic review of 27 studies that assessed relaxation training (including Jacobson's progressive relaxation) for anxiety. Their results showed a medium–large effect size (Cohen's d of 0.57 for within analysis and 0.51 for the between group analysis), and the authors concluded that there is consistent and significant efficacy in using relaxation training in mitigating anxiety.

Given these research findings, it seems that NMR strategies may be an effective component in a variety of treatment programs designed to mitigate the impact of both chronic stress and stress that exacerbates a disease process. We now present a structure for clinical implementation.

How to Implement a Physically Active Form of Neuromuscular Relaxation: Preparation

To review, NMR represents a series of exercises during which the participant tenses (contracts) and then releases (relaxes) selected muscles in a predetermined and orderly manner. Some preliminary activities that the clinician should perform before implementing the procedure are as follows:

1. In addition to the general precautions for relaxation mentioned in an earlier chapter, determine whether the patient has any muscular or neuromuscular contraindications: for example, nerve problems, weak or damaged muscles, or skeletal problems that would be enhanced through the neuromuscular exercises. When in doubt, avoid that specific muscle group until a qualified opinion can be obtained.
2. Ask about the patient's previous knowledge or experience of NMR techniques. Because the clinician must consider whether such knowledge or experience will facilitate or be detrimental to the current treatment situation, it is usually helpful to discuss in relative detail any previous exposure that the patient may have had with NMR techniques.
3. Provide the patient with background and rationale for use of NMR techniques.
4. Discuss with the patient the proper environment for the practice of NMR techniques: (a) quiet, comfortable surroundings; darkened, if possible, in order to enhance concentration on bodily sensations; (b) loose clothing; remove contact lenses, glasses, and shoes if desired; (c) body supported as much as possible (with the exception of neck and head, if the patient falls asleep inadvertently).
5. Educate the patient about the difference between the desired muscle "tension" and undesirable muscle "strain." Tension is indicated by a tightened, somewhat uncomfortable, sensation in the muscles being tensed. Strain is indicated by any pain in the muscle, joints, and tendons, as well as any uncontrolled trembling in the muscles. Strain is actually excessive muscle tension.
6. Instruct the patient in proper breathing: Do not hold the breath while tensing muscles. Instead, breathe normally, or inhale on tensing and exhale on relaxing the muscles.
7. Before beginning the actual protocol with the patient, informally demonstrate all the exercises you will be employing. Take this opportunity to answer any questions that the patient may have.
8. Finally, explain to the patient exactly "how" you will provide the instructions. For example, "In the case of each muscle group that we focus upon, I will always carefully describe the relaxation exercise to you first, before you actually do the exercise. Therefore, don't begin the exercise until I say, 'Ready? Begin.'"

The order of these steps may vary. In order to facilitate awareness of some of this preliminary information, the clinician may present a handout to patients.

How to Implement Neuromuscular Relaxation: Procedure

Whenever possible, begin the total protocol with the lowest areas of the body to be relaxed and end with the face, because once a muscle has been tensed and then relaxed, we attempt to ensure that it is not inadvertently retensed. The quasi-voluntary muscles of the face are the most susceptible to retensing; therefore, we relax them last to eliminate the opportunity.

The Sequential Steps to Follow for Each Muscle Being Relaxed

Once the clinician is ready to initiate the actual protocol, he or she should be sure to follow a fundamental sequence of steps for *each* muscle group.

Step 1. Describe to the patient the specific muscle(s) to be tensed and how it/they will be contracted. "We are now going to tense the muscles in the calf. To begin, I'd like you to leave your toes flat on the floor and raise both of your heels as high as you can."

Step 2. Have the patient initiate the response with some predetermined cue: "Ready? Begin."

Step 3. Have the patient hold the contraction for 3 to 5 s. During this time, you may wish to encourage the patient to exert an even greater effort: "Raise your toes higher, higher, even higher."

Step 4. Signal the patient to relax the concentration: "And now relax."

Step 5. Facilitate the patient's awareness of the muscles just relaxed by having him or her search for feelings of relaxation: "Now sense how the backs of your legs feel. Are they warm, tingling? Do they feel heavy? Search for the feelings."

Step 6. The clinician may wish to encourage further relaxation: "Now let the muscles relax even more. They are heavier and heavier and heavier."

Step 7. Pause at least 5–10 s after each exercise to allow the patient to experience relaxation. Pause 15–20 s after each major muscle group.

Step 8. When possible, go directly to the opposing set of muscles. In this case, it would involve leaving the heels flat on the floor and raising the toes as high as possible.

Example Protocol

The following brief protocol includes previously discussed components. See whether you can identify the major preliminary activities (only a few can be included in this example) and the sequenced steps (some sample muscle groups have only six or seven of the steps to avoid monotony).

As you read the example, make notes in the margins provided as to what changes you might make in order to make the protocol more effective for your needs in teaching a general NMR protocol.

Background Information. As early as 1908, researchers at Harvard University discovered that stress and anxiety are related to muscle tension. Muscle tension is created by a shortening or contraction of muscle fibers. The relationship between stress and anxiety, on one hand, and muscle tension, on the other, is such that if you are able to reduce muscle tension, stress and anxiety will be reduced as well.

Progressive NMR is a tool that you can use to reduce muscle tension and, therefore, stress and anxiety. It is a progressive system by which you can systematically tense and then relax major muscle groups in your body, in an orderly manner, so as to achieve a state of total relaxation. This total relaxation is made possible by two important processes.

First, by tensing a muscle and then relaxing it, you will actually receive a sort of running start, in order to achieve a greater degree of muscular relaxation than would normally be obtainable.

Second, by tensing a muscle and then relaxing it, you are able to compare and contrast muscular tension and muscular relaxation. Therefore, we see that the basic premises underlying your muscular relaxation are as follows:

1. Stress and anxiety are related to muscular tension.
2. When you reduce muscular tension, a significant reduction in stress and anxiety will be achieved as well.
3. NMR provides you with the unique opportunity to compare and contrast tension with relaxation.
4. NMR has been proven to be a powerful tool that can be used to achieve relaxation and peace of mind. However, relaxation is an active skill and, like any skill, it must be practiced. The mistake that most individuals make is to rush through this relaxation procedure. NMR works, but it takes practice and patience to succeed. But, after all, aren't your health and well-being worth at least 15 min a day?

Preliminary Instructions. Before beginning the progressive NMR procedure, let us review some basic considerations. First, find a quiet place without interruptions or glaring lights. You should find a comfortable chair to relax, though you will also find progressive relaxation useful when performed lying in bed in order to help you fall asleep at night. Loosen tight articles of clothing. Glasses, jewelry, and contact lenses should be removed.

Second, the progressive NMR system requires you to tense each set of muscles for two periods, lasting about 5 s each. However, it is possible to tense each set of muscles up to several times if you continue to feel residual tension. Muscular tension is not equal to muscular strain. They are not the same. You will know that you have strained a muscle if you feel pain in the muscle or any of the joints around it, or if it begins to shiver or tremble uncontrollably. In either case, these should be signs to you to employ a lesser degree of tension, or simply avoid that exercise. The entire NMR procedure lasts about 20–30 min, should you wish to relax your entire body. The time may be less if you choose to relax only a few muscles groups.

Last, do not hold your breath during contractions. Breathe normally, or inhale as you tense and exhale as you release the tension.

Actual Instructions. You are now ready to relax progressively the major muscle groups in your body, in order to achieve a state of total relaxation. I would like you to settle back and get very, very comfortable. You may loosen or remove any tight articles of clothing, such as shoes or coats, ties, or glasses. You should also remove contact lenses. Try to get very, very comfortable. I would like you to close your eyes. Just sit back and close your eyes. Begin by directing your attention to your breathing. The breath is the body's metronome. So let us become aware of the metronome. As you inhale, become aware of how the air comes in through your nostrils and down into your lungs, and how your stomach and chest expand, and how they recede as you exhale. Concentrate on your breathing. (*Provide 30 s pause here.*)

In the case of each muscle group that we focus on, I shall always carefully describe the relaxation exercise to you first, before you are actually to do the exercise. Therefore, do not begin the exercise described until I say, "Ready? Begin."

Chest. Let us begin with the chest. At my request, and not before, I would like you to take a very, very deep breath. Breathe in all the air around you. Let us do that now. Ready? Begin. Take a very deep breath. A very deep breath; hold it… and relax. Just exhale all the air from your lungs and resume your normal breathing. Did you notice tension in your chest as you inhaled? Did you notice relaxation as you exhaled? If you had to, could you describe the difference between tension and relaxation? Let us keep that in mind as we repeat this exercise. Ready? Begin. Inhale very deeply, very deeply. Hold it, and relax. Just exhale and resume your normal breathing. Could you feel the tension that time? Could you feel the relaxation? Try to concentrate on that difference in all the muscle groups that we shall be attending to. (*Always pause 5–10 s between exercises.*)

Lower legs. Let us go now to the lower legs and the muscles in the calf. Before we begin, place both your feet flat on the floor. Now, to engage in this exercise, I should like you simply to leave your toes flat on the floor, and raise both your heels at the same time as high as they will go. Ready? Begin. Raise your heels. Raise them both very high (see Fig. 12.1). Hold it, and relax. Just let them fall gently back to the floor. You should have felt some contraction in the back of your calves. Let us repeat this exercise. Ready? Begin. Raise the heels high. Hold it, and relax. As you relax, you may feel some tingling, some warmth, perhaps some heaviness as the muscle becomes loose and relaxed. To work the opposite set of muscles, leave both your heels flat on the floor, point both sets of your toes very high. Point them as high as you can toward the ceiling. This is the same motion that you would make if you lifted your foot off the accelerator pedal in your car (see Fig. 12.2). Except that, we shall do both feet at the same time. Let us do that now. Ready? Begin. Raise the toes very high. Hold it, and relax. Now let us repeat this exercise. Ready? Begin. Raise the toes high. Hold it, and relax. You should feel some tingling or heaviness in your

Fig. 12.1 Raising heels

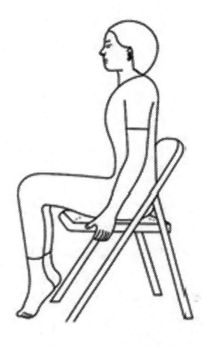

Fig. 12.2 Raising toes

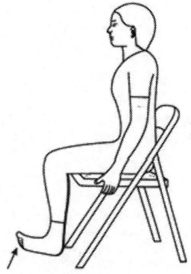

lower legs. That feeling is there. You must simply search for it. So take a moment and try to feel that tingling, warmth, or perhaps that heaviness that tells you that your muscles are now relaxed. Let those muscles become looser and heavier, and even heavier. (*Pause for 20 s.*)

Thighs and stomach. The next set of muscles that we shall concentrate on is those of the thigh. This exercise is a simple one. At my request, I should like you simply to

Fig. 12.3 Extending legs

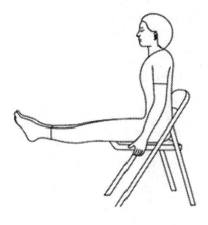

Fig. 12.4 Digging heels

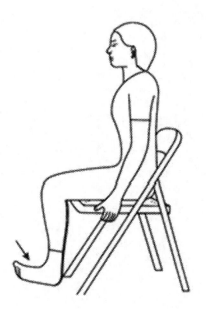

extend both your legs out in front of you as straight as you can (see Fig. 12.3). (*If this is uncomfortable for the patient, let him or her exercise one leg at a time.*) Remember to leave your calves loose. Do not tense them. Let us do that now. Ready? Begin. Straighten both your legs out in front of you. Very straight. Hold it, and relax. Just let the feet fall gently to the floor. Did you feel tension in the top of your thighs? Let us repeat this exercise. Ready? Begin. Straighten both your legs out. Hold it, and relax. To work the opposite set of muscles, I should like you to imagine that you are at the beach and are digging your heels down into the sand (see Fig. 12.4). Ready? Begin. Dig your feet down into the floor. Harder. And relax. Now let us repeat this exercise. Ready? Begin. Dig your heels down into the floor and relax. Now the top of your legs should feel relaxed. Let them become more and more relaxed—more and more relaxed. Concentrate on that feeling now. (*Pause here 20 s.*)

Fig. 12.5 Clenching fists

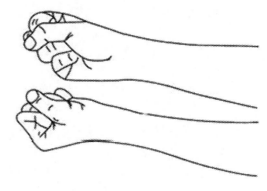

Fig. 12.6 Spreading fingers

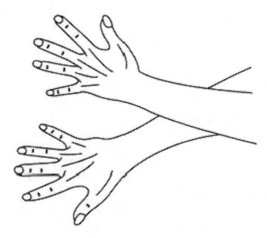

Hands and arms. Let us move now to the hands. The first thing that I should like you to do, with both your hands at the same time, is make very tight fists (See Fig. 12.5). Tighten your fists and arms together. Ready? Begin. Clench your fists very tightly. Tighter. Hold it, and relax. This exercise is excellent if you type or do a lot of writing during the day. Now let us repeat. Ready? Begin. Clench both your fists very tightly. Hold it, and relax. To work the opposing muscles, simply spread your fingers as wide as you can (see Fig. 12.6). Ready? Begin. Spread your fingers very wide. Wider. Hold it, and relax. Now let us repeat this exercise. Ready? Begin. Spread the fingers wide. Wider. Widest of all. Hold it, and relax. Concentrate on the warmth or tingling in your hands and forearms. (*Pause here 20 s.*)

Shoulders. Now let us work on the shoulders. We tend to store a lot of our tension and stress in our shoulders. This exercise simply consists of shrugging your shoulders vertically up toward your ears. Imagine trying to touch your ear lobes with the tops of your shoulders (see Fig. 12.7). Let us do that now. Ready? Begin. Shrug your shoulders up high. Higher than that. Hold it, and relax. Now let us repeat. Ready? Begin.

Fig. 12.7 Raising shoulders

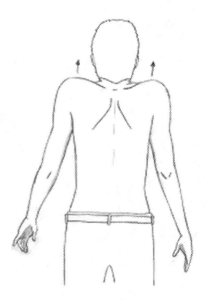

Fig. 12.8 Smiling widely

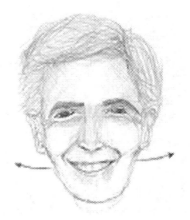

Shrug the shoulders. Higher. Hold it, and relax. Let us repeat this exercise one more time. Ready? Begin. Shrug the shoulders as high as you can. Hold it, and relax. Very good. Now just concentrate on the heaviness in your shoulders. Let your shoulders go, let them completely relax—heavier and heavier. (*Pause here 20 s.*)

Face. Let us move now into the facial region. We shall start with the mouth. The first thing I should like you to do is smile as widely as you possibly can (see Fig. 12.8). An ear-to-ear grin. Ready? Begin. Hold it, and relax. Now let us repeat this exercise. Ready? Begin. Grin very wide. Wider. Hold it, and relax. The opposite set of muscles will be activated when you pucker or purse your lips together, as if

Fig. 12.9 Puckering lips

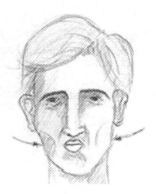

Fig. 12.10 Squinting eyes

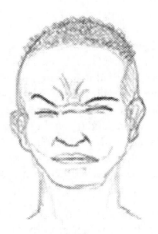

you were trying to give someone a kiss (see Fig. 12.9). Ready? Begin. Pucker the lips together. Purse them together very tightly. Hold it, and relax. Now let us repeat that exercise. Ready? Begin. Purse the lips together. Hold it, and relax. Let your mouth relax. Let the muscles go — let them relax, more and more; even more.

Now let us move up to the eyes. (Be sure to remove contact lenses.) I should like you to keep your eyes closed, but to clench them even tighter. Imagine that you are trying to keep shampoo suds out of your eyes (see Fig. 12.10). Ready? Begin. Clench the eyes tightly, and relax.

Let us repeat this exercise. Ready? Begin. Clench the eyes, tighter. Hold it, and relax.

The last exercise consists simply of raising your eyebrows as high as you can. Now, remember to keep your eyes closed, but raise your eyebrows as high as you can (see Fig. 12.11). Ready? Begin. Raise the eyebrows high. Hold it, and relax. Now let us repeat this exercise. Ready? Begin. Raise the eyebrows higher. Highest of all. Hold it, and relax. Let us pause for a few moments to allow you to feel the relaxation in your face. (*Pause 15 s.*)

Fig. 12.11 Raising eyebrows

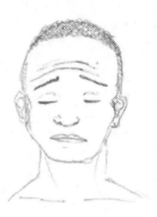

Closure. You have now relaxed most of the major muscles in your body. To make sure that they are all relaxed, I shall go back and name the muscles that we have just activated and just relaxed. And, as I name them, let them go even further into relaxation. You will feel a sense of relaxation descend over your entire body in a warm wave. You will feel the muscular relaxation now in your forehead, and as it goes down into your eyes, down into your cheeks, you can feel the heaviness of relaxation descend into your jaws, into your neck, down through your shoulders, to the chest and arms, to the stomach, into your hands. Relaxation is descending into your legs, into the thighs, and calves, and down to the feet. Your body now feels very heavy. Very relaxed. This is a good feeling. So take a moment and enjoy this feeling of relaxation. (*Pause here 2 min.*)

Reawaken. Now I want you to bring your attention back to yourself and the world around you. I shall count from 1 to 10. With each count, you will feel your mind become more and more awake, and your body more and more refreshed and responsive. When I reach 10, open your eyes, and you will feel the *best* you've felt all day—you will feel alert, refreshed, full of energy, and eager to resume your activities. Let us begin: 1–2 you are beginning to feel more alert, 3–4–5 you are more and more awake, 6–7 now begin to stretch your hands and feet, 8 now begin to stretch your arms and legs, 9–10 open your eyes *now!* You feel alert, awake, your mind is clear and your body refreshed.

Summary

This chapter has presented an introduction to a series of techniques known as *neuromuscular relaxation,* which has been employed in the mitigation of the human stress response. The chapter highlighted the work of Edmund Jacobson, considered by many to be the originator of relaxation training.

The mechanisms of therapeutic action include learning the difference between the feelings of tension and relaxation, which is predicated on enhanced awareness

Table 12.1 Summary checklist of NMR components

Preparation for implementation
1. Identify contraindications and precautions
2. Inquire as to previous knowledge/experience in techniques
3. Provide the patient with background/rationale for use of technique
4. Describe proper environment for practice of technique
5. Instruct the patient regarding the difference between muscle "tension" and muscle "strain"
6. Instruct the patient in proper breathing
7. Informally demonstrate all specific muscular contractions to be used
8. Describe "how" you will provide instruction and cues

Implementation of sequential steps for each muscle being relaxed
1. Describe the specific muscle and "how" it will be contracted
2. Signal the patient to begin contraction
3. Hold contraction and encourage greater contraction
4. Signal the patient to release tension, i.e., relax
5. Facilitate patient awareness of muscles just relaxed through verbal and intonational cues
6. Encourage further relaxation
7. Pause and allow the patient to become aware of sensations
8. Proceed with opposing muscle group, if applicable

of proprioceptive neuromuscular impulses. It has also been suggested that the actual process of contracting a muscle before attempting to relax it may increase the relaxation response beyond learned awareness.

We then reviewed the preparation and actual procedures involved in implementing a series of exercises that are part of a brief NMR protocol. It is not a prescription for use with patients so much as an example of how such a protocol may be created. Usually, greater specificity is included for muscle groups, and even individual muscles, depending on the requirements of the patient. It is worth noting that Jacobson emphasizes the utility of relaxing the facial muscles, particularly the throat, mouth, and eyes, to obtain maximal relaxation. Therefore, far more specialization directed toward those muscle groups may be considered in developing a protocol:

1. The clinician may encourage the patient to develop his or her own personalized protocol. He or she may further encourage or provide the patient with a home practice audiotape.
2. Jacobson's text, *You Must Relax* (1978), Davis, Eshelman, and McKay's *Relaxation and Stress Reduction Workbook* (1988) and Bernstein, Borkovec, and Hazlett-Stevens' (2000) *New Directions in Progressive Relaxation Training: A Guidebook for Helping Professionals* are excellent resources for additional, far more specific exercises. However, in the final analysis, it is the clinician's discretion to assess the suitability of any form of NMR on an individual basis.
3. Table 12.1 may be used as a checklist of important procedural information that should be addressed when teaching NMR to patients. As each step is completed, simply check it off. This same table may be used to evaluate a clinical student's mastery of these procedures. As in the first edition, it is designed to be reprinted from this text and used clinically or in educational settings.

4. Finally, Appendix B contains a different version of NMR, consisting of a physically passive form that uses focused sensory awareness and directed concentration for the reduction of striated muscle tension. The clinician may consider this as a potential clinical alternative to the form of NMR just described.

Acknowledgements We would like to thank David Essien and Andrea N. Everly for their artistic contributions to this chapter.

References

Bernstein, D. A., Borkovec, T. D., & Hazlett-Stevens, H. (2000). *New directions in progressive relaxation training: A guidebook for helping professionals.* Westport, Connecticut: Praeger.

Berstein, D., & Borkovec, T. (1973). *Progressive relaxation training.* Champaign, IL: Research Press.

Bhalla, V. (1980). Neuroendocrine, cardiovascular, and musculoskeletal analyses of a holistic approach to stress reduction. Unpublished doctoral dissertation, University of Maryland, College Park.

Borkovec, T., Grayson, J., & Cooper, K. (1978). Treatment of general tension: Subjective and physiological effects of progressive relaxation. *Journal of Consulting and Clinical Psychology, 46*, 518–526.

Carey, M. P., & Burish, T. G. (1987). Providing relaxation training to cancer chemotherapy patients: A comparison of three delivery techniques. *Journal of Consulting and Clinical Psychology, 55*, 732–737.

Chen, W. C., Chu, H., Lu, R. B., Chou, Y. H., Chen, C. H., Chang, Y. C., & Chou, K. R. (2009). Efficacy of progressive muscle relaxation training in reducing anxiety in patients with acute schizophrenia. *Journal of Clinical Nursing, 18*(15), 2187–2196.

Chen, Y. L. (Elaine), & Francis, A. J. P. (2010). Relaxation and imagery for chronic, nonmalignant pain: Effects on pain symptoms, quality of life, and mental health. *Pain Nursing Management, 11*(3), 159–168.

Davis, M., Eshelman, E. R., & McKay, M. (1988). *Relaxation and stress reduction workbook* (3rd ed.). Oakland, CA: New Harbinger.

de Carvalho, E. C., Martins, F. T. M., & dos Santos, C. B. (2007). A pilot study of a relaxation technique for management of nausea and vomiting in patients receiving cancer chemotherapy. *Cancer Nursing, 30*(2), 163–167.

Demiralp, M., Oflaz, F., & Komurcu, S. (2010). Effects of relaxation training on sleep quality and fatigue in patients with breast cancer undergoing adjuvant chemotherapy. *Journal of Clinical Nursing, 19*, 1073–1083.

Gellhorn, E. (1958a). The physiological basis of neuromuscular relaxation. *Archives of Internal Medicine, 102*, 392–399.

Gellhorn, E. (1958b). The influence of curare on hypothalamic excitability and the electroencephalogram. *Electroencephalography and Clinical Neurophysiology, 10*, 697–703.

Gellhorn, E. (1964b). Sympathetic reactivity in hypertension. *Acta Neurovegetative, 26*, 35–44.

Gellhorn, E. (1967). *Principles of autonomic-somatic integrations.* Minneapolis, MN: University of Minnesota Press.

Gessel, A. H. (1989). Edmund Jacobson, M. D., Ph.D.: The founder of scientific relaxation. *International Journal of Psychosomatics, 36*(1–4), 5–14.

Henry, J. L., Wilson, P. H., Bruce, D. G., Chisholm, D. J., & Rawling, P. J. (1997). Cognitive-behavioural stress management for patients with non-insulin dependent diabetes mellitus. *Psychology, Health and Medicine, 2*(2), 109–118.

Jacobson, E. (1938). *Progressive relaxation.* Chicago: University of Chicago Press.

Jacobson, E. (1970). *Modern treatment of tense patients.* Springfield, IL: Charles C. Thomas.

Jacobson, E. (1978). *You must relax.* New York, NY: McGraw-Hill.

Jakes, S. C., Hallam, R. S., Rachman, S., & Hinchcliffe, R. (1986). The effects of reassurance, relaxation training and distraction on chronic tinnitus sufferers. *Behavioural Research and Therapy, 24,* 497–507.

Klein, R. J. (2008). Ready…, set…, relax!: Relaxation strategies with children and adolescents. In C. A. Malchiodi (Ed.), *Creative interventions with traumatized children* (pp. 302–320). New York: Guilford.

Kocsis, A. (1996). Relaxation. In J. Green & A. McCreaner (Eds.), *Counselling in HIV infection and AIDS* (2nd ed., pp. 270–278). Cambridge, MA: Blackwell Scientific.

Lowe, G., Bland, R., Greenman, J., Kirkpatrick, N., & Lowe, G. (2001). Progressive muscle relaxation and secretory immunoglobulin A. *Psychological Reports, 88,* 912–914.

Malmo, R. B. (1975). *On emotions, needs, and our archaic brain.* New York: Holt, Rinehart & Winston.

Manzoni, G. M., Pagnini, F., Castelnuovo, G., & Molinari, E. (2008). Relaxation training for anxiety: A ten-years systematic review with meta-analysis. *BMC Psychiatry, 8,* 41.

McGuigan, F. J., & Lehrer, P. M. (2007). Progressive relaxation: Origins, principles, and clinical applications. In P. M. Lehrer, R. L. Woolfolk, & W. E. Sime (Eds.), *Principles and practices of stress management* (3rd ed., pp. 57–87). New York: Guilford.

Nickel, C., Kettler, C., Muehlbacher, M., Lahmann, C., Tritt, K., Fartacek, R., … Nickel, M. K. (2005). Effect of progressive muscle relaxation in adolescent female bronchial asthma patients: A randomized, double-blind, controlled study. *Journal of Psychosomatic Research 59*(6), 393–398

Pavlek, M. (2008). Paining out: An integrative pain therapy model. *Clinical Social Work Journal, 36*(4), 385–393.

Pawlow, L. A., & Jones, G. E. (2005). The impact of Abbreviated Progressive Muscle Relaxation on salivary cortisol and salivary immunoglobulin A (sIgA). *Applied Psychophysiology and Biofeedback, 30*(4), 375–387.

Powell, D. H. (2004). Behavioral treatment of debilitating test anxiety among medical students. *Journal of Clinical Psychology, 60*(8), 853–865.

Sadoughi, M., Nouri, A., Kajbaf, M. B., Akkashe, G., & Molavi, H. (2009). Can progressive relaxation training reduce chronic tension headache? *Journal of Iranian Psychologists, 5*(18), 149–158.

Szabo, A., & Hopkinson, K. L. (2007). Negative psychological effects of watching the news in the television: Relaxation or another intervention may be needed to buffer them! *International Journal of Behavioral Medicine, 14,* 57–62.

Thankachan, M. V., & Mishra, H. (1996). Behavioural management with peptic ulcer cases. *Indian Journal of Clinical Psychology, 23*(2), 135–141.

Urech, C., Fink, N. S., Hoesli, I., Wilhelm, F. H., Bitzer, J., & Alder, J. (2010). Effects of relaxation on psychobiological wellbeing during pregnancy: A randomized controlled trial. *Psychoneuroendocrinology, 35*(9), 1348–1355.

Weil, J. (1974). *A neurophysiological model of emotional and intentional behavior.* Springfield, IL: Charles C. Thomas.

Wolpe, J. (1958). *Psychotherapy by reciprocal inhibition.* Stanford, CA: Stanford University Press.

Zucker, T. L., Samuelson, K. W., Muench, F., Greenberg, M. A., & Gevirtz, R. N. (2009). The effects of respiratory sinus arrhythmia biofeedback on heart rate variability and Posttraumatic Stress Disorder symptoms: A pilot study. *Applied Psychophysiology and Biofeedback, 34,* 135–143.

Chapter 13
Hypnosis in the Management of Stress Reactions

Melvin A. Gravitz
Clinical Professor of Psychiatry and Behavioral Sciences,
George Washington University Medical Center, Washington, DC 20036, USA

Roger A. Page
Professor of Psychology, Ohio State University at Lima, Lima, OH 45804, USA

The modality known in modern times as hypnosis has been a useful and recognized remedial method for more than 200 years. Originally conceptualized by Franz Anton Mesmer (1734–1815) as a physical fluid (animal magnetism) that could be transferred from one person to another, that theory has since been discredited; but even today, the fundamental principles and mechanisms underlying hypnosis have not yet been definitively established. Even so, there are useful applications of hypnosis in numerous areas, including stress management.

Historical Perspectives

Originating as a medical dissertation submitted to the University of Vienna in the late 1700s, Mesmer's techniques soon became controversial, even though they were undeniably effective with many of his patients. That was understandable, because the medical establishment was threatened by his thesis that there was only one sickness (so-called magnetic illness) and only one treatment (*animal magnetism,* or *mesmerism,* as it was soon termed). Consequently, he was compelled to relocate to Paris, where, once again, his practice flourished and his techniques proved to be ameliorative for many. Controversy again dogged his steps, however, and his opponents prevailed on the king to initiate an investigation. Two commissions comprising prominent figures in science and medicine conducted a series of generally well-designed studies, although, curiously, they never interviewed Mesmer himself. Their finding, published in 1784, was that no fluid existed. They also concluded that the effectiveness of mesmerism was due to collusion and to deception of naive patients and, above all, to the force of imagination. Since the imagination at that time had no scientific status, Mesmer was labeled a charlatan, and he soon left France in disgrace. To his credit, one of the investigators, Laurent de Jussieu, an eminent botanist, dissented from the majority view and proposed that the imagination could have a therapeutic benefit. Mesmer's method survived him, however, and in France, elsewhere in Europe, and in the newly established USA, a number of followers modified his work and managed to keep mesmerism going for a number of years. During the first decade of the 1800s, several French investigators began using the nomenclature of *hypnotisme,* because they believed that it was a state of sleep, and Hypnos was the name of the ancient Greek god of sleep (Gravitz, 1997). By 1820, however, the modality was dormant.

In the mid-1800s, practitioners in England and elsewhere revived hypnotism (later to be termed *hypnosis*), principally as a form of pain management, but that use also faded as the more acceptable ether and chloroform were developed as surgical anesthetics. News of animal magnetism had earlier been brought to the USA in 1784 by Marquis de Lafayette, a dedicated disciple of Mesmer. Influential opponents, notably Benjamin Franklin, who had chaired one of the French investigative commissions while serving as the first American diplomatic representative to Paris, intervened, with the result that hypnosis did not flourish in the USA until decades later.

In the late 1800s, influenced by the earlier work of the British, notably James Braid, hypnotism was revived in France, and important French scientific figures became involved in practice and research. Within the same time frame, an Austrian physician studying hypnosis in Paris helped launch the new psychotherapy called *psychoanalysis:* this was Sigmund Freud, whose contributions to hypnosis, however, were minimal. By the turn of the century, mainly because of the rise of psychoanalysis, the modality had once again faded in significance, although a number of prominent workers in the field continued their efforts. Among others, these included Pierre Janet and Alfred Binet in France, Morton Prince and Boris Sidis in the USA, Ivan Pavlov in Russia, Albert Moll in Germany, and Charles Baudouin in Switzerland.

There was a brief revival of hypnosis during World War I, when it was employed by both sides as surgical anesthesia and front-line psychotherapy for the so-called shell shock and soldier's heart. These latter reactions to the effects of overwhelming stress became known in later times as combat fatigue and, in more recent years, post-traumatic stress disorder. During the 1920s, Clark L. Hull and Milton H. Erickson helped revive research and clinical interest in the method through their teaching and research. During World War II, clinical hypnosis became an important means of treating stress in the military services, where psychological problems comprised a large percentage of overall causalities. The current wave of professional and scientific interest in hypnosis had its origins in the demonstrated value of the modality during those years. The fact that hypnosis has always returned to the stage of history can be attributed to its undoubted effectiveness in assisting with the management of a wide variety of disorders, including those resulting from inordinate stress.

Hypnosis, Stress, and Mind–Body Interaction

Stress can be either physical or psychological, or, as is usually the case, both. Stress of whatever kind can impact negatively on bodily chemistry and function, as Hans Selye (e.g., 1976) demonstrated many years ago, and there is truly no demarcation between the mind and body—however, one may define those constructs. There are two ways of viewing the implication of these truisms. One is the recognition that psychological forces can result in physical problems. The other is that psychological forces can positively impact the healing process. The demonstrated effectiveness of psychological means, including hypnosis, in treating psychosomatic disorders is a prime example of what is involved here. These considerations have evolved into the current interest in the so-called mind–body interaction, which in turn has generated important, and at times admittedly speculative, thinking about the underlying mechanisms involved. Rossi (1986), in particular, may be cited as a reference for further reading. Throughout these hypotheses, hypnosis has played significant historical and modern roles.

Theories of Hypnosis

A number of theories, at times conflicting, have been proposed (Gravitz, 1991) to explain the process of hypnosis. These have been broadly grouped into state versus non-state positions, and each view has presented scientific findings in support of its stance. A related approach has been the advocacy of either neurophysiological or socio-cognitive perspectives, again, with evidence submitted for both positions. Recently, Gruzelier (2000) has proposed an overarching integration of these various viewpoints: His theory is that hypnosis is an altered state of brain function involving interrelations of, and between, certain brain regions initiated through the intervention of the hypnotist and the situation in which the process is undertaken. He has also emphasized the central role of cognitive and neuropsychological dissociation. Thus, Gruzelier has integrated social and interpersonal contexts, as well as psychological and neurobiological findings, into a comprehensive and coherent system that merits further study.

Despite the absence so far of a generally accepted understanding of the hypnotic process, the modality has proven effective in managing a broad array of problem areas, including stress management. The basis for such applications has been the observation that hypnosis can in many instances facilitate the enhancement of human behaviors and then apply them more effectively on behalf of the individual subject or client, as the case may be. The mechanisms for these applications have included the long-known, hypnotically induced phenomena of enhanced suggestibility, hypermnesia, distortion of the time sense, regression and revivification, response to posthypnotic instructions, dissociation, ideomotor communication, tolerance for distortion of reality, modified physiological processes, and suspension of critical thinking. These phenomena are a function of the individuals' unique talents as hypnotic participants and the source of individual differences.

Hypnosis and Stress

Hypnosis is not a therapy, but a technique to be used as an adjunct to therapy. For example, hypnosis has been used with Ellis's (1962) rational-emotive therapy (RET) by Stanton (1989) to reduce stress in high-school teachers. Ellis (1984) had previously suggested the use of hypnosis with RET to reduce the number of sessions necessary to achieve positive results. Hypnosis has also been used with an extension of RET developed by Tosi (1974) called rational stage directed hypnotherapy (RSDH) to treat pathological non-assertiveness (Gwynne, Tosi, & Howard, 1978) and anxiety neurosis (Tosi, Howard, & Gwynne, 1982). RSDH combines cognitive restructuring, imagery, and hypnosis. A variation of RSDH was also used by Der and Lewington (1990) in the treatment of panic attacks to reduce panic symptoms in stressful situations.

The use of hypnosis with cognitive-behavioral therapies such as Wolpe's (1958) systematic desensitization is far from new: Wolpe and Lazarus (1966) reported using it with a number of their patients. Since then, a few examples of hypnosis used in conjunction with systematic desensitization include both Frankel (1976) and Seif (1982) in treating phobic behavior, Taylor (1985) in treating an obsession, Moore (1965) in treating bronchial asthma, and Barabasz and Spiegel (1989) in treating obesity. The literature is replete with such examples of hypnosis used with various therapies over several decades, including the more traditional insight-oriented therapies (e.g., Brenman & Gill, 1947; Crasilneck & Hall, 1975).

Support for the use of hypnosis as an adjunct to therapy has been mounting. An earlier argument by Holroyd (1987) that hypnosis serves to potentiate psychotherapy has been confirmed by Kirsch and his associates. In an initial meta-analysis of 18 studies, Kirsch, Montgomery, and Sapirstein (1995) found a substantial effect size (mean effect size=0.87 standard deviations) when hypnosis was used as an adjunct to cognitive-behavioral psychotherapy (in the treatment of various presenting problems, including obesity) compared to the same therapy without hypnosis. This effect size is in the order of magnitude found by Smith, Glass, and Miller (1980) for psychotherapy compared to no treatment! Furthermore, long-term follow-ups of the obesity studies (ranging from 2 months to 2 years) indicated that participants who had received hypnosis continued to lose weight after the treatment had ended. These findings were confirmed by a second meta-analysis conducted by Kirsch (1996) that included additional data obtained from two of the original studies, corrected for computational inaccuracies, excluded results from a questionable study, and employed conservative calculation methods. The mean effect size for hypnosis compared to therapy without hypnosis for obesity studies was 0.66 standard deviations for the initial assessment and 0.98 standard deviations for the final assessment, leading Kirsch to conclude, "The addition of hypnosis appears to have a significant and substantial effect on the outcome of cognitive-behavioral treatment for weight reduction and this effect increases over time" (p. 519).

Given the well-established usefulness of hypnosis as a technique, a brief description of a "prototypical" hypnotic induction and suggestions as used in the treatment of stress is appropriate. The typical induction begins with the patient sitting comfortably while focusing on some target. Suggestions for progressive muscle relaxation are given, usually accompanied by counting as a deepening technique, while the patient is instructed to visualize a pleasant scene (e.g., lying on a beach on a warm, sunny day). A word of caution is in order here. Suggestions are most effective when tailored to fit the individual. For example, visualizing a beach may work perfectly well for a given patient, whereas being asked to visualize lying in front of a cozy fire on a cold winter day may produce an adverse reaction if the patient is pyrophobic. This sort of reaction can be easily avoided by administering a checklist of fears, likes and dislikes, and so on, prior to the induction.

Following the induction, the stress-specific suggestions will vary depending upon the patient and the particular treatment regimen employed. For example, one may have a patient recall a pleasant memory while associating this with a cue (e.g., a simple motor act), then instruct the patient to self-present the cue (or perform the motor act) when faced with a stressful situation. Or, one may use a desensitization strategy in which the relaxation achieved through hypnosis is first paired with low stress-producing situations and eventually with high stress-producing situations. For examples of specific suggestions that have a variety of applications not only in psychology but also in medicine and dentistry, the reader is directed to the *Handbook of Hypnotic Suggestions and Metaphors* (1990) edited by Hammond, or *A Syllabus on Hypnosis and a Handbook of Therapeutic Suggestions* (1973) published by the American Society of Clinical Hypnosis Education and Research Foundation.

As we return to the primary focus of this chapter, the use of hypnosis with stress, our review of this body of work indicates that it can somewhat arbitrarily be divided into two broad types, with an admittedly gray area, without a sharp, clear-cut distinction between them. The first type would be studies that have involved reducing stress associated with a variety of *specific* situations (or external stressors). The second would be those studies dealing with stress in general and/or learning techniques to cope with it (stress management). We begin with the former.

In noting that both physical and psychological stressors have the *perception of threat* as a final common pathway for stress response, Bowers and Kelly (1979) created a list of four "generic stressors" that the relevant literature deems threatening and hence stressful: (a) a perceived lack or loss of control (together with related factors such as event uncertainty and unpredictability), (b) the anticipation and occurrence of physical or psychological pain, (c) the loss of close emotional and social supports, and (d) effortful "trying" to avoid aversive stimuli or conditions. (p. 491)

In the following examples, hypnosis was employed and often compared to other techniques in treating individuals exposed to various stressors, ranging from surgeries to college exams.

Enqvist, von Konow, and Bystedt (1995) utilized preoperative hypnosis to reduce stress during maxillofacial surgery, including suggestions to reduce bleeding and edema, and to improve recovery. Compared to control patients, hypnosis patients displayed reduced swelling, fever, and post-operative consumption of anxiolytics.

In a similar vein, Faymonville et al. (1997) conducted a randomized study comparing the effectiveness of hypnosis to stress-reducing strategies (including emotional support, deep breathing/relaxation, and positive emotion induction) in decreasing discomfort during plastic surgery under local anesthesia and intravenous sedation (midazolam and alfentanil) upon request. Patient anxiety, pain, and perceived control before, during, and after surgery, along with postsurgical nausea and vomiting, were recorded. Results showed that the hypnosis patients (during and following surgery) had significantly less anxiety, pain, nausea, and vomiting than controls. They also reported experiencing more intraoperative control. The authors noted that the reduction in anxiety and pain were achieved in spite of the fact that the hypnosis group required significantly less midazolam and alfentanil during surgery! Furthermore, no direct suggestions for analgesia were given.

Another example of hypnosis used to control anxiety in a surgical setting is when oral surgical procedures are necessary in hemophiliacs. These procedures can be extremely stressful to the patient for obvious reasons. Lucas (1975) makes a case for the use of hypnosis, since anxiety can trigger (or complicate an ongoing) hemorrhagic episode, and this tendency (during and following surgery) is decreased considerably if the patient is relaxed and tranquil. An additional benefit is a reduction in pain and capillary bleeding through suggestion.

In a unique intervention for a psychosomatic condition, Gravitz (1995) successfully used a hypnosis-based paradigm to relieve functional infertility in several patients. Verbal suggestions coupled with mental imagery to relax fallopian tube musculature were provided to two patients. Since hypnosis is known to relax muscle tension, it was theorized that the consequent dilation of the tubular lumen would enable an ovum to travel successfully down the fallopian tube and achieve uterine implantation. In both cases, pregnancy resulted within several months.

Two final examples deal with what is commonly called test anxiety, admittedly a less dramatic stressor than surgery, but certainly far from mundane for those experiencing the stress. Boutin and Tosi (1983) employed the previously mentioned technique RSDH in the modification of irrational ideation and test anxiety in female nursing students. Participants were randomly assigned to one of four treatment conditions: RSDH, hypnosis-only treatment, placebo condition, or no-treatment control. Primary treatment was 1 h/week for 6 weeks. Dependent measures included the State-Trait Anxiety Inventory (STAI; Spielberger, 1983) and the Test Anxiety Scale (Sarason, 1957), among others. Results showed a significant advantage for the RSDH and hypnosis-only groups at both post-test and at 2-month follow-up, with RSDH being more effective than hypnosis-only at both test times.

The last example involving test anxiety is a study by Palan and Chandwani (1989) that compared hypnotic suggestions, waking suggestions, and passive relaxation in medical school students. In addition to the suggestions for reduced test anxiety, suggestions were also calculated to enhance self-image and improve study habits (e.g., suggestions that concentration and memory of material would improve). Although results showed that all treatment conditions produced a significant increase in motivation to study, only the hypnosis group reported significant increases in variables such as self-confidence, general health, sleep, and so forth.

The final type of study to be examined deals with reducing stress in general and/ or stress management, i.e., techniques to cope with stress. This type of treatment falls into what Bowers and Kelly (1979), in describing attempts to treat psychosomatic disorders psychologically, called an "intermediate level of specificity... that focuses on the reduction of stress by altering the threatening character of the environment" (p. 494). One way this is typically accomplished is that "patients' resources to deal with threats are increased through some combination of enhancing their ability to relax, to cope with a threat, and to defend themselves more adequately against its stress-producing characteristics". (p. 494)

A list of some stress management techniques *other than hypnosis* includes the following: progressive muscle relaxation (Jacobson, 1970), diaphragmatic breathing (Fried, 1987), meditation (including TM), listening to music, frontalis electromyographic feedback (EMG-FB; Budzynski, Stoyva, & Adler, 1976), distraction (and focused) imagery, and emotional support. Several studies have examined the effectiveness of these techniques compared to controls (usually sitting quietly with eyes closed), hypnosis, or other stress management techniques. For example, Avants, Margolin, and Salovey (1990) compared a brief (20 min) treatment of four different techniques (progressive muscle relaxation, distraction, focused imagery, and listening to music) to sitting quietly and found that only distraction imagery and listening to music reduced anxiety to a greater extent than sitting quietly.

Raskin, Bali, and Peeke (1980) compared the effectiveness of EMG-FB, TM, and progressive relaxation in reducing general anxiety. Although 40% of their participants showed marked anxiety relief, they found no differences between the treatments with respect to efficacy.

In an effort to reduce stress in high-school teachers, Stanton (1989) compared hypnosis combined with Ellis's RET to controls who spent an equal amount of time discussing stress management, with emphasis on cognitive restructuring to promote more rational thinking. Although both groups showed reductions on measures of irrational thinking and stress following treatment, the experimental group showed significantly more improvement than controls. Furthermore, they showed continued improvement at a 1-year follow-up, whereas control group scores were comparable to those immediately following treatment.

Elton (1993) compared the efficacy of hypnosis and hypnosis combined with EMG-FB in the treatment of stress-related conditions, including emotional problems such as frustration, anxiety, and low self-esteem, as well as conditions such as migraines and tension headaches. Although no control group was included, participants' scores on several variables (e.g., state and trait anxiety, self-esteem, and body stress) were compared to their baseline scores following treatment at 12 weeks and again at 24 weeks. Both groups showed significant improvement over baseline on all variables. At week 12, the hypnosis/EMG-FB group showed a significantly greater reduction on trait anxiety (as measured by Spielberger's STAI) than the hypnosis-only group; at week 24, the former group showed a significantly greater reduction in trait and state anxiety, and a greater increase in self-esteem. No significant differences were found between groups on other variables at either 12 or 24 weeks.

In a similar combinatory vein, Sapp (1992) employed relaxation therapy combined with hypnosis in treating anxiety and stress in adults with neurogenic impairment. Several measures of anxiety and stress were significantly reduced both post-test and at 4-week follow-up.

The next three studies explored the use of *self-hypnosis* for stress management, a skill that, once learned, can be practiced outside of the therapist's office, accounting in part for its growing popularity. Soskis, Orne, Orne, and Dinges (1989) taught executives either self-hypnosis or meditation as part of "an organization stress-management program aimed at promoting health through the use of effective coping strategies" (p. 286). Depending upon their group assignment, participants were encouraged to practice self-hypnosis (or meditation) twice daily, 5 days per week for 2 weeks, and then as needed. Telephone follow-ups occurred 1 month and 6 months after the training session. The rate of use dropped equally for both groups over the 6-month follow-up interval (from 90% to 42% for all participants). In addition, the frequently described uses of self-hypnosis or meditation were similar for both groups (e.g., to relax, to aid in sleep onset, to reduce effects of external stressors, etc.), as were problems encountered (e.g., scheduling difficulties, obtaining the necessary privacy, etc.).

Whitehouse et al. (1996) trained first-year medical school students in the use of self-hypnosis as a means of coping with stress and potentially reducing the impact of stress on immune function. Although the self-hypnosis group did not differ from controls with respect to immune function at four measurement times, they did report lower anxiety and stress ratings at exam time, and less variability in the ratings of sleep quality throughout the measurement period.

Finally, Benson et al. (1978) compared self-hypnosis to meditation/relaxation in the treatment of anxious patients in an 8-week follow-up assessment. Both treatments showed moderate (and comparable) success in reducing anxiety at follow-up, with 37.5% of the self-hypnosis group and 31.3% of the meditation/relaxation group showing improvement.

This study, one of only a few thus far reviewed that assessed a key variable that can potentially moderate treatment outcome—hypnotic ability or hypnotizability—is worthy of further attention. To illustrate, Bowers and Kelly (1979) noted that when participants in the Benson et al. (1978) study were divided into low, moderate, and high hypnotic ability based on a pretest assessment, 47.6% (10 out of 21) of the moderate-to-high hypnotizable participants showed significant reductions in anxiety, while only 9.1% (1 out of 11) of low hypnotizable participants showed a comparable reduction. Bowers and Kelly concluded,

> Clearly, differences in hypnotic ability were far more important to treatment outcome than the ritualistic differences of the two therapeutic regimens being compared.... In sum, self-hypnosis and relaxation were equally effective in reducing psychological and physiological manifestations of anxiety in moderate to high hypnotizables, and equally ineffective for low susceptibles. (p. 499)

To reiterate, despite the importance of hypnotizability, few studies have formally assessed it. Although the aforementioned Elton (1993) study did assess hypnotizability, there was no analysis of how it may have affected treatment outcome. Although the Barber Suggestibility Scale (Barber 1969) was used in the Sapp (1992) study, it was administered without a prior hypnotic induction and was therefore a measure of *waking* suggestibility, which correlates only moderately with hypnotic susceptibility. In addition, only a single item was administered in hypnosis. Thus, it is not surprising that hypnotic susceptibility was not related to treatment gains. Finally, Whitehouse et al. (1996) obtained a pretest measure of hypnotizability and found that it was not related to treatment outcome, but their measure of self-hypnosis correlated only a modest 0.42 with a standard susceptibility scale, suggesting that "self-hypnosis and heterohypnosis involve distinctive processes that may render standard heterohypnosis scales... poor predictors of self-hypnosis skill when used on their own". (p. 251)

A series of studies by Pekala and his associates (Pekala & Forbes 1988, 1990; Pekala, Forbes, & Contrisciani, 1988) is relevant to the importance of hypnotizability as a moderating variable. These studies, based on 300 nursing students who experienced progressive relaxation, deep abdominal breathing, and hypnosis, respectively, all following a baseline condition of sitting quietly with eyes closed, revealed not only that techniques such as progressive relaxation and hypnosis are *not* experienced as phenomenologically equivalent but also that the experience is moderated by an individual's hypnotic susceptibility. Specifically, high susceptible participants reported not only more hypnoidal effects than low susceptible across all conditions but also essentially equivalent hypnoidal effects for both progressive relaxation and hypnosis. (This suggests the possibility that high susceptible participants may be experiencing hypnosis, or something akin to it, when engaged in techniques such as progressive relaxation.) The low susceptible participants, however, experienced more hypnoidal effects during progressive relaxation than hypnosis, suggesting that for lows, progressive relaxation may be functioning as an indirect hypnotic technique (i.e., a technique not defined as hypnosis to the subjects, but possibly being hypnotic in nature; Barber, 1977).

Summary

In this chapter, we have discussed the potentially valuable role of hypnosis in the treatment of excessive stress. The information presented can be summarized as follows:

1. Hypnosis has been used for more than 200 years in the treatment of human ailments. It was first introduced by Franz Anton Mesmer; however, his controversial conceptualization of animal magnetism was discredited.
2. Hypnotism was later revived in France and Austria; however, with the rise and popularity of psychoanalysis, hypnosis faded in significance by the end of the twentieth century.
3. Interest in hypnosis was revived following the clinical applications that occurred during World Wars I and II primarily for stress-related disorders. The current interest in hypnosis is credited in part to the successes that occurred during those years.
4. There are a number of theories to explain the hypnotic process. Gruzelier (2000) has recently proposed a viewpoint that comprehensively integrates the social, interpersonal, psychological, and neurobiological contexts.
5. There are also several proposed mechanisms of action responsible for the hypnotic effect, including but not limited to enhanced suggestibility, hypermnesia, distortion of time, regression, and response to posthypnotic instructions.

6. It is important to emphasize that hypnosis is not therapy but a technique used as an adjunct to therapy. Hypnosis has been used with cognitive-behavioral therapies, insight-oriented therapies, rational-emotive therapy (RET), and rational stage directed hypnotherapy (RSDH), which is an extension of RET.

7. The use of hypnosis relative to stress can generally be divided into studies that address two broad categories. The first is the use of hypnosis to reduce stress associated with specific stressors that may fall with the generic categories of (a) loss of control, (b) anticipation of physical or psychological pain, (c) loss of emotional and social support, and (d) attempts to avoid aversive stimuli. Studies examining specific stressors such as surgeries, and college exams are examples of this first category. The second category includes studies examining how hypnosis compares to other stress management techniques such as biofeedback, progressive muscle relaxation, deep breathing, and meditation.

8. In summary, more research is needed that assesses relevant variables such as hypnotizability and expectancies, especially when comparing hypnosis to other stress management techniques. To date, the data suggest that hypnosis is at least as effective, if not more so, than other techniques for reducing stress and helping the individual learn to cope with stress. In addition, the efficacy of hypnosis seems to be enhanced when combined with other techniques such as biofeedback (see Chap. 14).

References

American Society of Clinical Hypnosis. (1973). *A syllabus on hypnosis and a handbook of therapeutic suggestions*. Des Plaines, IL: American Society of Clinical Hypnosis Education and Research Foundation.

Avants, S. K., Margolin, A., & Salovey, P. (1990). Stress management techniques: Anxiety reduction, appeal, and individual differences. *Imagination, Cognition and Personality, 10*, 3–23.

Barabasz, M., & Spiegel, D. (1989). Hypnotizability and weight loss in obese subjects. *The International Journal of Eating Disorders, 8*, 335–341.

Barber, T. X. (1969). *Hypnosis: A scientific approach*. New York, NY: Van Nostrand Reinhold.

Barber, T. X. (1977). Rapid induction analgesia: A clinical report. *The American Journal of Clinical Hypnosis, 19*, 138–147.

Benson, H., Frankel, F. H., Apfel, R., Daniels, M. D., Schniewind, H. E., Nemiah, J. C., Sifneos, P. E., Crassweller, K. D., Greenwood, M., Kotch, J. B., Arns, P. A., & Rosner, B. (1978). Treatment of anxiety: A comparison of the usefulness of self-hypnosis and a meditational relaxation technique: An overview. *Psychotherapy and Psychosomatics, 30*, 229–242.

Boutin, G. E., & Tosi, D. J. (1983). Modification of irrational ideas and test anxiety through rational stage directed hypnotherapy (RSDH). *Journal of Clinical Psychology, 39*, 382–391.

Bowers, K. S., & Kelly, P. (1979). Stress, disease, psychotherapy, and hypnosis. *Journal of Abnormal Psychology, 88*, 490–505.

Brenman, M., & Gill, M. M. (1947). *Hypnotherapy*. New York, NY: Wiley.

Budzynski, T. H., Stoyva, J. M., & Adler, C. S. (1976, September). *The use of feedback-induced muscle relaxation in tension headache: A controlled study*. Paper presented at the Annual Meeting of the American Psychological Association, Miami Beach, FL.

Crasilneck, H. B., & Hall, J. A. (1975). *Clinical hypnosis: Principles and applications*. New York, NY: Grune & Stratton.

Der, D., & Lewington, P. (1990). Rational self-directed hypnotherapy: A treatment for panic attacks. *American Journal of Clinical Hypnosis, 32*, 160–167.

Ellis, A. (1962). *Reason and emotion in psychotherapy*. Secaucus, NJ: Lyle Stuart.

Ellis, A. (1984). The use of hypnosis with rational-emotive therapy. *Journal of Integrative and Eclectic Psychotherapy, 2*, 15–22.

Elton, D. (1993). Combined use of hypnosis and EMG biofeedback in the treatment of stress-induced conditions. *Stress Medicine, 9*, 25–35.

Enqvist, B., Von Konow, L., & Bystedt, H. (1995). Stress reduction, preoperative hypnosis and perioperative suggestion in maxillofacial surgery: Somatic responses and recovery. *Stress Medicine, 11*, 229–233.

Faymonville, M. E., Mambourg, P. H., Joris, J., Vrijens, B., Fissette, J., Albert, A., & Lamy, M. (1997). Psychological approaches during conscious sedation: Hypnosis versus stress reducing strategies: A prospective randomized study. *Pain, 73*, 361–367.

Frankel, F. H. (1976). *Hypnosis: Trance as a coping mechanism*. New York, NY: Plenum Press.

Fried, R. (1987). *The hyperventilation syndrome: Research and clinical treatment*. Baltimore, MD: Johns Hopkins University Press.

Gravitz, M. A. (1991). Early theories of hypnosis: A clinical perspective. In S. J. Lynn & J. W. Rhue (Eds.), *Theories of hypnosis: Current models and perspectives* (pp. 19–42). New York, NY: Guilford.

Gravitz, M. A. (1995). Hypnosis in the treatment of functional infertility. *American Journal of Clinical Hypnosis, 38*, 22–26.

Gravitz, M. A. (1997). First uses of "hypnotism" nomenclature: A historical record. *Hypnos, 24*, 42–46.

Gruzelier, J. H. (2000). Redefining hypnosis: Theory, methods, and integration. *Contemporary Hypnosis, 17*, 51–70.

Gwynne, P. H., Tosi, D. J., & Howard, L. (1978). Treatment of nonassertion through rational stage directed hypnotherapy (RSDH) and behavioral rehearsal. *American Journal of Clinical Hypnosis, 20*, 263–271.

Hammond, D. C. (1990). *Handbook of hypnotic suggestions and metaphors*. New York, NY: Norton.

Holroyd, J. (1987). How hypnosis may potentiate psychotherapy. *American Journal of Clinical Hypnosis, 29*, 194–200.

Jacobson, E. (1970). *Modern treatment of tense patients*. Springfield, IL: Charles C. Thomas.

Kirsch, I. (1996). Hypnotic enhancement of cognitive-behavioral weight loss treatments— another meta-reanalysis. *Journal of Consulting and Clinical Psychology, 64*, 517–519.

Kirsch, I., Montgomery, G., & Sapirstein, G. (1995). Hypnosis as an adjunct to cognitive-behavioral psychotherapy: A meta-analysis. *Journal of Consulting and Clinical Psychology, 63*, 214–220.

Lucas, O. (1975). The use of hypnosis in hemophilia dental care. *Annals of the New York Academy of Sciences, 240*, 263–266.

Moore, N. (1965). Behavior therapy in bronchial asthma: A controlled study. *Journal of Psychosomatic Research, 1*, 257–276.

Palan, B., & Chandwani, S. (1989). Coping with, examination stress through hypnosis: An experimental study. *American Journal of Clinical Hypnosis, 31*, 173–180.

Pekala, R. J., & Forbes, E. J. (1988). Hypnoidal effects associated with several stress management techniques. *Australian Journal of Clinical and Experimental Hypnosis, 16*, 121–132.

Pekala, R. J., & Forbes, E. J. (1990). Subjective effects of several stress management strategies: With reference to attention. *Behavioral Medicine, 16*, 39–43.

Pekala, R. J., Forbes, E. J., & Contrisciani, P. A. (1988). Assessing the phenomenological effects of several stress management strategies. *Imagination, Cognition and Personality, 8*, 265–281.

Raskin, M., Bali, L. R., & Peeke, H. V. (1980). Muscle biofeedback and transcendental meditation. *Archives of General Psychiatry, 37*, 93–97.

Rossi, E. R. (1986). *The psychobiology of mind–body healing*. New York: Norton.

Sapp, M. (1992). Relaxation and hypnosis in reducing anxiety and stress. *Australian Journal of Clinical Hypnotherapy and Hypnosis, 13*, 39–55.

Sarason, I. G. (1957). Effect of anxiety and two kinds of motivating instructions on verbal learning. *Journal of Abnormal and Social Psychology, 54*, 166–171.

Seif, B. B. (1982). Hypnosis in a man with fear of voiding in public facilities. *America Journal of Clinical Hypnosis, 24*, 288–289.

Selye, H. (1976). *Stress in health and disease*. Boston: Butterworth.

Smith, M. L., Glass, G. V., & Miller, T. I. (1980). *The benefits of psychotherapy*. Baltimore: Johns Hopkins University Press.

Speilberger, C. D. (1983). *State-Trait Anxiety*. Palo Alto, CA: Consulting Psychologists Press.

Soskis, D. A., Orne, E. C., Orne, M. T., & Dinges, D. F. (1989). Self-hypnosis and meditation for stress management: A brief communication. *International Journal of Clinical and Experimental Hypnosis, 37*, 285–289.

Stanton, H. E. (1989). Hypnosis and rational-emotive therapy—a de-stressing combination: A brief communication. *International Journal of Clinical and Experimental Hypnosis, 37*, 95–99.

Taylor, R. E. (1985). Imagery for the treatment of obsessional behavior: A case study. *American Journal of Clinical Hypnosis, 27*, 175–179.

Tosi, D. J. (1974). *Youth toward personal growth: A rational-emotive approach*. Columbus, OH: Charles Merrill.

Tosi, D., Howard, L., & Gwynne, P. H. (1982). The treatment of anxiety neurosis through rational stage directed hypnotherapy: A cognitive-experiential perspective. *Psychotherapy: Theory, Research and Practice, 191*, 95–101.

Whitehouse, W. G., Dinges, D. F., Orne, E. C., Keller, S. E., Bates, B. L., Bauer, N. K., Morahan, P., Haupt, B. A., Carlin, M. M., Bloom, P. B., Zaugg, L., & Orne, M. T. (1996). Psychosocial and immune effects of self-hypnosis training for stress management throughout the first semester of medical school. *Psychosomatic Medicine, 58*, 249–263.

Wolpe, J. (1958). *Psychotherapy by reciprocal inhibition*. Stanford, CA: Stanford University Press.

Wolpe, J., & Lazarus, A. A. (1966). *Behavior therapy techniques*. Elmsford, NY: Pergamon Press.

Chapter 14
Biofeedback in the Treatment of the Stress Response

The purpose of this chapter is to provide a basic introduction to biofeedback and to discuss how it relates to the treatment of excessive stress. Although being applied for more than 40 years, biofeedback may still be considered by some to be "high-technology" therapy that may be used to (1) engender a relaxation response, thus treating the stress response itself, or (2) alter target-organ activity, thus treating the symptoms of excessive stress arousal. Indeed, it can help to do this and possibly more by restoring and even enhancing balance and control to the systems involved.

Bios from the Greek for "life" and "feedback" defines the concept of providing focused information that enables performance enhancement. Biofeedback may, therefore, be conceptualized as a procedure in which data regarding an individual's biological activity are collected, processed, and conveyed back to the person so that he or she can modify that activity. In essence, biofeedback allows for the construction of a "feedback loop," which is illustrated in Fig. 14.1. Such feedback loops exist in almost all functions of the human body, from the rate-modifying feedback loops concerned with the most elementary biochemical reactions to the most complex human endeavors. Information regarding the result of any event is necessary at some level if it is to be modified.

Thus, the concept underlying biofeedback is fundamental in biology, and is widely employed in the therapeutic sciences. In the traditional medical model, the patient presents a physiological problem, data regarding his or her physiological functioning are collected by the clinician, then the clinician diagnoses the condition, and institutes appropriate interventions. The patient in this model has a basically passive role. This interaction, as shown in Fig. 14.2, represents an indirect closed loop of information, starting and ending with the patient and including information-gathering devices, the clinician, and therapeutic devices.

As can be seen in a comparison of Figs. 14.1 and 14.2, the principle on which biofeedback is based involves the active participation of the individual in the modification of his or her condition. Consider the case of a function such as breathing,

G.S. Everly and J.M. Lating, *A Clinical Guide to the Treatment of the Human Stress Response*, DOI 10.1007/978-1-4614-5538-7_14, © Springer Science+Business Media New York 2013

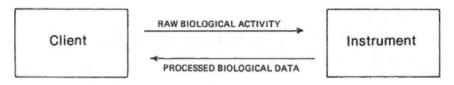

Fig. 14.1 "Feedback loop"

Fig. 14.2 Indirect closed
loop of information

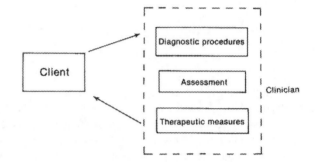

which is unique in the sense that we can control it voluntarily, but fortunately, occurs without conscious awareness. It is as if there are priorities for the human brain, with many functions occurring at subcortical levels—especially those that must be maintained in an ongoing fashion, such as heartbeat and biochemical reactions. Although this may be the most efficient way to function, it keeps the organism from being able to monitor many of its autonomic functions consciously and thus actively change them. This is what biofeedback provides for the individual—the potential to exert additional control over autonomic biological activity.

Given the information provided with biofeedback, we have repeatedly found that we can learn to alter bodily functions that were once thought to be inaccessible, including greater finite control over the activities of both the voluntary and the autonomic nervous systems. As will be discussed later in this chapter, the possible alterations that can be controlled range from voluntary muscle tension to more autonomic functions, such as blood flow and brain waves.

The purpose of this chapter is to expand the principles on which biofeedback is based and to describe how it may be beneficial in the treatment of the stress response. We also review some of the historical trends that have led to the present state of the art and then discuss some of the more traditional biofeedback modalities, as well as the more current trends in the field. Finally, we examine the role of the therapist in the biofeedback paradigm.

History

The term *biofeedback* was reportedly coined at the first annual meeting of the Biofeedback Research Society in 1969, as a shortened version of "biological feedback." Although the term itself may have been new, its foundations are not.

The historical development of biofeedback can be traced back to the early 1900s, and the work of Pavlov and Watson on the one hand and Thorndike on the other. Pavlov and Watson's research on classical conditioning of the autonomic nervous system (ANS) was thought to be discretely separate from the work of Thorndike on operant conditioning of the musculoskeletal system. Early researchers were convinced that conditioning that affected the ANS had to be accomplished through a classical conditioning paradigm (an S(stimulus)R(response) model involving conditioning on the basis of association rather than as a function of behavioral consequence as in an operant model). In fact, Kimble (1961), in his edited textbook *Conditioning and Learning,* stated unequivocally that autonomically mediated behavior could only be modified by classical, not operant conditioning.

However, in a discipline like psychology, assertions such as Kimble's often serve as challenges for others. For example, according to a review by Gatchel and Price (1979), case reports existed of individuals who reportedly could voluntarily alter autonomic functioning (see Lindsley & Sassaman, 1938; Luria, 1958; McClure, 1959; Ogden & Shock, 1939). Interestingly, Edmund Jacobson, the originator of progressive relaxation training (see Chap. 12), performed some of the earliest clinical biofeedback work in the 1930s using an oscilloscope to measure forearm tension in progressive relaxation trainees. However, since he used a raw electromyograph (EMG) signal, most people had difficulty understanding how to interpret the information, and Jacobson apparently discarded the method (Schneider, 1989). Following Kimble's published work, other researchers reported the use of operant conditioning of heart rate to avoid mild electrical shocks (Frazier, 1966; Shearn, 1962). Supporters of Kimble's may have argued, however, that these types of studies, in which changes in autonomically mediated responses (such as heart rate) were modified by responses under voluntary control (such as altered breathing), were actually consistent with a classical conditioning paradigm (Blanchard & Epstein, 1978).

Therefore, the animal studies of Miller (1969) and DiCara and Miller (1968a, 1968b, 1968c) in which laboratory rats were given injections of curare, a drug that produces complete muscle paralysis, provided additional and clearer support for the effect of operant conditioning of autonomic responses. These rats were kept alive via artificial respiration, and stimulation of an electrode implanted in the pleasure center of the hypothalamus served as a reinforcer. Using this research design, DiCara and Miller (1968a, 1968b, 1968c) successfully demonstrated operant conditioning of heart rate, blood pressure, and urine formation. Although later attempts to replicate these findings were not supported (Miller & Dworkin, 1974), this type of basic research, along with the pioneering work of other researchers such as Green, who built EMG, temperature, GSR, and EEG biofeedback equipment to assess self-control of the ANS (see Green & Green, 1977), helped to define and legitimize the field of biofeedback. In fact, in a review, Schwartz (1995) noted that "some professionals view biofeedback as essentially *instrumental* [italics added] conditioning of visceral responses" (p. 5).

Basmajian (1963), another originator in the field, reported on the ability of patients to control single motor-unit activity. In the late 1960s, Budzynski and Stoyva began utilizing behavioral therapy techniques to enhance efficacy of bio-feedback protocols for general relaxation and for the treatment of tension headaches [see Stoyva and Budzynski (1974), for an early review]. The early work of Kamiya (1969) and Brown (1977) in EEG biofeedback gained widespread attention for applications in relaxation and alteration of consciousness, although it was (Sterman, 1973; Sterman & Friar, 1972) work in clinical applications in the treatment of epilepsy that appeared to have the most clinical utility.

In recent years, biofeedback has shown potential applicability to a variety of clinical problems, including decubitus ulcers (pressure sores) (Verbunt & Bartneck, 2010), PTSD (Staples, Abdel Atti, & Gordon, 2011; Tan, Dao, Farmer, Sutherland, & Gevirtz, 2011; Wood, Wiederhold, & Spira, 2010), chronic pain disorders (Angoules et al., 2008; Caro & Winter, 2011; Hallman, Olsson, von Schéele, Melin, & Lyskov, 2011; Palermo, Eccleston, Lewandowski, Williams, & Morley; 2010), GI disorders (Chiarioni & Whitehead, 2008), epilepsy (Nagai, Goldstein, Fenwick, & Trimble, 2004; Sterman & Egner, 2006), stroke (Doğan-Aslan, Nakipoğlu-Yüzer, Doğan, Karabay, & Özgirgin, 2010; Drużbicki, Kwolek, Depa, & Przysada, 2010;Varoqui, Froger, Pélissier, &Bardy, 2011), attention-deficit disorders (Arns, de Ridder, Strehl, Breteler, &Coenen, 2009; Gevensleben, Moll, & Heinrich, 2010; Monastra, 2005), urinary incontinence (Imamura et al., 2010; Palmer, 2010), migraine headaches (McGrath, 1999; Reid & McGrath, 1996), and rehabilitation (Miller & Chang, 1999; Richards & Pohl, 1999).

As noted, biofeedback is not a new endeavor; the technology for its use has been available for decades. What is reasonably new, however, is the speed, precision, and range of applications available from today's computers in acquiring, storing, analyzing, and displaying data in virtual environments (Wong, 2008). The use of virtual reality, including the advances in dynamic three-dimensional (3D) technology, has been implemented with moderate success across a range of clinical applications, including generalize anxiety, balance in elderly patients who experienced traumatic brain injury (TBI), and PTSD (Bisson, Contant, Sveistrup, Lajoie, 2007; Gorini et al., 2010; Pallavicini, Algeri, Repetto, Gorini, & Riva, 2009; Repetto et al., 2009; Wiederhold & Rizzo, 2005; Wood et al., 2010). In addition to the potential uses of virtual reality environments to enhance therapeutic effects, collaborative and integrative approaches with primary care physicians may be a potentially burgeoning area where the implementation of biofeedback may address some of the aforementioned disorders and positively impact patient care (Gevirtz, 2006;Glick & Greco, 2010;Isler, 2006; Lynch, McGrady, Nagel, & Wahl, 2007; Ryan &Gevirtz, 2004).

Biofeedback Modalities

In this section, we briefly review several types of biofeedback, focusing on their nature and potential utility.

Electromyographic (EMG) Biofeedback

Description

The EMG instrument used in biofeedback detects minute electrical impulses through special sensors (electrodes), which are applied to the skin with electrode jelly used as a conducting medium. The strength of the electrical impulse is amplified, processed by the instrument and then fed back in ways that allow the data to be easily interpreted. This feedback incorporates a potential myriad of possible creative signals; numerical data, displays of lights, deflections of a meter, sounds, etc. that correlate with the magnitude of the signal, or any combination of these. Since measurement is of electrical correlates of muscle contraction, the numerical display of data in EMG biofeedback is expressed in volts, or more specifically, in microvolts, one-millionth of a volt. The displayed data serve as information to be processed by the client in order to modify function—in this case, muscle tension. The key here is that the data displayed are many times more sensitive than what a person can feel so that the instrument actually extends the person's awareness of minute changes that would otherwise be imperceptible.

The words *stress* and *tension* are often used interchangeably, and muscle tension itself is an obvious component of the fight-or-flight response. When a threat is perceived, any muscle throughout the body may tense; however, some do so in a characteristic way. For example, the muscles in the back of the neck characteristically become tense, as if in an effort to keep the head erect to aid in vigilance. Back, shoulder, and jaw muscles tense when the individual perceives him- or herself as being threatened, or when he or she is under stress. Other muscle tension is less obvious such as changes in intestinal motility or alterations in blood vessel diameter.

Because we are describing striated muscle, it would seem that control would be voluntary, and therefore easily responsive to learning. The difficulty arises when the contraction increases so slowly and imperceptibly that the individual is not aware of increased muscle tension until the muscles are already in spasm. The EMG apparatus allows the individual to become aware of small increments of change in muscle tension, thus allowing him or her to learn to relax the muscles involved. As noted by Basmajian (1967), the EMG signal indicates the status of the muscle as well as the status of the nervous system serving the muscle.

One can place the EMG sensors over virtually any striated muscle available to either skin or needle electrodes. Frontalis muscle biofeedback has traditionally been used for low-arousal training (Field, 2009; Stoyva & Budzynski, 1993). However, the effectiveness of frontalis placement for generalized relaxation has been questioned (Graham et al., 1986; Jones & Evans, 1981), and other evidence suggests that multiple- and reactive-site EMG biofeedback may be as effective as frontalis biofeedback in reducing sympathetic arousal (Mariela, Matt, &Burish, 1992). One of the other common EMG placements is the cervical paraspinal muscles (Donaldson, Donaldson, & Snelling, 2003).

Indications

For the purposes of this chapter, EMG biofeedback is used to treat the stress response in primarily two ways: first, it allows the patient to learn to relax a particular set of muscles (e.g., the masseter muscles in bruxism—teeth grinding), and second, it may be used to produce a more generalized state of relaxation and decreased arousal (e.g., frontalis or paraspinal muscle EMG biofeedback), thus affecting the stress response more centrally (see Donaldson et al., 2003; Mariela et al., 1992; Stoyva & Budzynski, 1993; see also Chap. 9).

Historically, two of the most commonly encountered, specific muscle contraction problems have been muscle tension-type headaches and bruxism. In a meta-analysis of 53 studies, results revealed that EMG biofeedback in combination with relaxation training yielded a large mean effect size (0.32) and was the most effective biofeedback modality in treating tension-type headaches (Nestoriuc, Rief, & Martin, 2008). In a subsequent comprehensive efficacy review, which incorporated the above meta-analysis along with a 2007 meta-analysis (Nestoriuc & Martin, 2007), Nestoriuc, Martin, Rief, and Andrasik (2008) reported a large effect size for EMG biofeedback that corresponded with a 69 % success rate for biofeedback compared with a 31 % improved rate in an untreated control group. In one of the studies used in these analyses, Rokicki and colleagues (1997) suggested that increase in self-efficacy as a result of EMG biofeedback training might be what accounts for the treatment's effectiveness.

Biondi and Picardi (1998) and Foster (2004) have reported on the benefits of biofeedback in the treatment of bruxism. In a meta-analysis, Crider and Glaros (1999) reported on the practical application of biofeedback to tempromandibular disorders (TMDs), disorders of the jaw muscles often related to bruxism. Jadidi, Castrillon, and Svensson (2008) have reported that "biofeedback with electrical pulses does not cause major disruption in sleep and is associated with pronounced reduction in temporalis EMG activity during sleep" (p. 181).

Sometimes the problem is loss of control or weakening of muscle function and EMG feedback can be used to strengthen muscle function. For instance, within the past two decades, the use of EMG biofeedback for the treatment of urinary incontinence has expanded. Using surface abdominal EMG, pelvic floor EMG, and rectal pressure, patients with urinary incontinence have been shown to learn successfully how to strengthen pelvic floor muscles and inhibit abdominal muscle contractions (Butler et al., 1999; McDowell et al., 1999; Weatherall, 1999). In a sample of 390 patients with stress or mixed urinary incontinence that was treated with EMG-biofeedback assisted pelvic floor muscle training (PFMT), Dannacker, Wolf, Raab, Hepp, and Anthuber (2005) reported an improvement in EMG potentials and self-report of incontinence symptoms, both short- and long term (avg. 2.8 years). In 2011, Huebner and colleagues reported on the benefits of PFMT using three different strategies of EMG biofeedback (PFMT with conventional and dynamic electrical stimulation, and no electrical stimulation). In a systematic review of the clinical effectiveness of non-surgical treatments for women with stress urinary incontinence, including survey, meta-analysis, and economic modeling (used to discern which combinations of treatments were most cost-effective) Imamura and colleagues (2010) reported that delivering PFMT more intensely, either through more sessions or augmented with biofeedback, appeared to be the most effective treatment. EMG biofeedback has also been shown to effectively treat urinary incontinence (e.g., secondary to dysfunctional voiding or giggling) in children (Palmer, 2010; Richardson & Palmer, 2009).

As noted in Chap. 5, and alluded to in this chapter, the frontalis muscles appear to have value in the treatment of the human stress response because of their potential ability to serve as an indicator of generalized arousal, for example, SNS arousal (Rubin, 1977), by virtue of what appears to be their dual neurological constituency, that is, alpha motor neuron innervation and sympathetic neural innervation (see Everly & Sobelman, 1987). When using the frontalis muscles as a means of engendering the relaxation response, it is important to keep in mind that it may first be necessary to have the patient learn to relax the frontalis specifically before expecting any generalizability to the ANS. That is to say, the frontalis muscles may serve as indicators of sympathetic activity only when they are in a relaxed state. Donaldson, Donaldson & Snelling (2003) and Hermens, Freriks, Disselhorst-Klug, & Rau (2000) note other issues related to skin preparation and instrument specifications in the use of EMG biofeedback. The EMG biofeedback paradigm has demonstrated its scientific integrity and clinical utility in the hands of competent, well-trained professionals (Schwartz & Montgomery, 2003) and should still be considered in the treatment of the human stress response (McKee, 2008; Sharpley& Rogers, 1984).

Temperature Biofeedback

Description

The use of temperature biofeedback is based on the fact that peripheral skin temperature is a function of vasodilatation and constriction. Thus, when the peripheral blood vessels are dilated and more blood flows through them, the skin is warmer. By measuring the temperature in the extremities, it is possible to get an indication of the amount of blood vessel constriction. Also, since constriction and dilation are controlled by the sympathetic portion of the ANS, one can get an indirect measurement of the amount of sympathetic activity (Peek, 2003).

The equipment used in thermal biofeedback has the same basic function as the EMG biofeedback equipment described earlier—that is, a sensor, a processor, and a display. The sensor is a thermistor, a small thermal sensor, or thermometer sensing device that is usually attached to the dorsal side of the finger. The thermistor and associated transducer transform the electrical signal, and amplify and processes it so that it can be presented as feedback though lights, sounds, or a change in meter reading show small increments of rising or lowering temperature in varying time intervals. Because skin temperature can be raised only to the theoretical high of core body temperature, 98.6 °F, there are practical limits to how much change can occur. Therefore, rather than set a specific temperature goal, more often the change in temperature is measured from the original or baseline reading and is used as a "change score from baseline" to gauge success of thermal biofeedback. For example, a patient with a baseline skin temperature of 75 °F will have a greater possible warming change than one with a baseline temperature of 94 °F. Response time, which indicates how rapidly a change in skin temperature occurs, absolute accuracy, or how closely the displayed temperature corresponds to the actual or "true" temperature, and resolution, which refers to the smallest temperature change that the thermistor may pick up and display, are other parameters of temperature biofeedback devices (Peek, 2003).

Indications

Temperature feedback has been useful for treating individuals with functional vascular disease or circulatory problems, such as Raynaud's disease (see Karavidas, Tsai, Yucha, McGrady, & Lehrer, 2006 for a comprehensive review), or advanced heart failure (Moser, Dracup, Woo, & Stevenson, 1997). It has also been used for patients with endocrine diseases, particularly diabetes (McGinnis, McGrady, Cox, & Grower-Dowling, 2005; McGrady, Graham, & Bailey, 1996; Rice, 2007), and in the treatment of migraine headaches in adults and children (Allen & Shriver, 1997; Biondi, 2005; Herman, Blanchard, & Flor, 1997; Holroyd & Penzien, 1994; Landy, 2004; Scharff et al. 2002), hypertension (Blanchard et al., 1996; Linden & Moseley, 2006), and in those instances when control over sympathetic activity is sought (e.g., asthma; Meany et al., 1988). Temperature biofeedback was also used as part of a comprehensive group treatment program for PTSD in 129 children in Gaza (Staples et al., 2011). Thermal biofeedback has also been used in psychotherapy to help determine areas of prominent sympathetic arousal and to address the issue of treatment resistance. As noted above, one minor difficulty involved in the interface between physiology and technology is the short but relevant delay of several seconds between the time of sympathetic discharge, vasoconstriction, and lowering of temperature in the extremity. This measurable reduction in temperature may be displayed several seconds after the event that caused the sympathetic discharge has passed. As a result, the measurements are often tracked and graphed over time to better display the type and rate of temperature change.

Temperature biofeedback has a clear role in the treatment of the stress response in that it is a good indicator of general SNS arousal. Therefore, it is a useful teaching tool for general relaxation, because individuals are instructed to try to raise their skin temperature. This mode of therapy may be used alone, alternatively with EMG, or in combination with it. See Lehrer and colleagues (1994) and Peek (2003) for a practical review of thermal biofeedback.

Electroencephalographic (EEG) Biofeedback

Description

The brain's electrical activity is continuous, most likely the result of discharges at synapses. In 1924, Hans Berger developed a graphic method for recording that electrical brain-wave activity. What appears to be recorded by the EEG are those synapses closest to the surface of the brain. There are many ascending pathways to the cortex; however, it is believed that the most highly represented area on the outermost surface of the cortex is the reticular activating system (Hall, 2011). These data are, however, difficult to analyze, because a single neuron may have as many as a thousand branchings in the cortex. Therefore, although data attained on the EEG are fairly nonspecific, it is generally agreed that various wave patterns do correlate with various states of consciousness and reflect activity, particularly in the reticular activating system.

Brain waves have been divided into four categories, depending on their predominant frequency and amplitude. The term *frequency* refers to the cycles/s, or per minute, and reflects the number of firings of neurons per unit of time. Brain-wave frequency on the surface of the scalp ranges from 1 every few seconds to 50 or more per second (Hall, 2011). The *amplitude refers* to the amount of electricity generated and reflects the number of neurons firing synchronously.

Brain waves are classified as alpha, beta, theta, and delta waves. Alpha waves are characterized by a frequency of 8–13 cycles/s and an amplitude of 20–100+μv. These rhythmic waves are related to an awake, relaxed state characterized by calmness and passive attention. Alpha waves do not occur when participants are asleep, or when they have their attention focused (Hall, 2011). Beta waves occur at a frequency of 14 or more cycles per second to as high as 80 cycles/s and have low amplitude. They are characteristic of an awake, attentive state when the subject is focusing his or her thoughts, or is aroused or have tense. Theta waves occur at a frequency of 4–7 cycles/s, with a usual amplitude of 20 μv or less. They are often considered part of the daydreaming state. Last, delta wave frequencies are from 0.5 to less than 4 cycles/s and are associated with deep sleep. Thus, when one is resting, dominant EEG activity is in the alpha and theta ranges; however, excitement shifts brain-wave activity toward the beta range. It is also of note that as we grow older, the relative proportion of beta-wave activity increases, whereas theta-wave activity decreases (Lubar, 1991).

Indications

Predicated on the work of Sterman and colleagues (Sterman, 1973; Sterman & Friar, 1972) involving sensorimotor rhythm (SMR) training, which is thought to capture activity of the sensorimotor cortex, one of the first areas investigated for use of EEG biofeedback training occurred in an attempt to manage epileptic seizures (Seifert & Lubar, 1975). This research expanded to include treatment of hyperkinetic children, in which EEG biofeedback was used to increase SMR production and inhibit theta-wave production (Lubar & Shouse, 1976; Shouse & Lubar, 1978). Lubar and colleagues (see Lubar, 1991; Lubar & Deering, 1981) later added enhanced beta-wave production via EEG biofeedback in the treatment of Attention Deficit Hyperactivity Disorder (ADHD). The premise behind the use of EEG biofeedback, which is also referred to as neurofeedback, neurotherapy, and alpha-theta feedback, is that ADHD is thought to be associated with neurological dysfunction at the cortical level, involving primarily the prefrontal lobes and central theta activity, which is marked by underarousal and decreased cortical activity (Chabot & Serfontein, 1996; El-Sayed, Larsson, Persson, & Rydelius, 2002; Lubar, 1995). The use of EEG neurofeedback is thought to normalize cortical function, which leads to normalization of behavior and overall academic and social adjustment (Lubar, 1995). More recently, the development of Quantitative EEG (QEEG) techniques has helped to more accurately assess EEG activity. QEEG is a computerized statistical procedure in which electrophysiological activity is rapidly and precisely measured and then converted using digital technology into forms that allow for more exact pattern recognition of amplitude, frequency, spectral plots, topographic maps, or functional connectivity maps (Kaiser, 2006). The QEEG information is in essence a helpful diagnostic adjunct that helps to facilitate more targeted sensor placement when using neurofeedback treatment techniques.

The clinical application of neurofeedback for the treatment of ADHD has flourished in the past decade (Holtmann & Stadler, 2006; Loo & Barkley, 2005); however, research support remains somewhat equivocal, due in part to the "scientific provincialism that is evident when new treatment paradigms are introduced" (Monastra, 2003, p. 438). To help address this issue, Arns and colleagues (2009) conducted a meta-analysis, which included randomized controlled trials, and concluded that neurofeedback for the treatment of ADHD is efficacious, and noted a high effect size for inattention and impulsivity and a medium effect size for hyperactivity.

QEEG-guided neurofeedback has been reported to be useful in the treatment of recurrent migraine headaches (Walker, 2011), children with histories of abuse and neglect (Huang-Storms, Bodenhamer-Davis, Davis, & Dunn, 2007), and in psychotherapy to treat patients diagnosed with antisocial personality disorder (Surmeli & Ertem, 2009) and schizophrenia (Monastra, 2003). Neurofeedback has also been used in the treatment of fibromyalgia (Kayiran, Dursun, Dursun, Ermutlu & Karamürsel, 2010), and in developing *peak alpha frequency* (PAF) (discrete frequency with the highest magnitude in the alpha range) in the elderly (Angelakis et al., 2007). Case studies also have shown EEG biofeedback to be effective in the treatment of Lyme disease (Packard & Ham, 1996), chronic fatigue syndrome (James & Folen, 1996), and depression (Baehr, Rosenfeld, & Baehr, 1997). Moreover, there has been use of alpha–theta EEG neurofeedback therapy and QEEG in the treatment of alcoholism and other addictive disorders [see Peniston and Kulkosky, (1999) and Sokhadze, Cannon, & Trudeau (2008) for reviews].

Particularly relevant to this text has been the use of topographic EEG mapping of Benson's relaxation response on 20 novice participants (Jacobs, Benson, & Friedman, 1996). Using a controlled, within-subjects design, the data revealed that elicitation of the relaxation response resulted in statistically significant reductions in frontal EEG beta activity, which reflects reduced cortical activation in anterior brain regions. EEG biofeedback has been shown to augment stress management training in helping to ameliorate aversive responses to infant crying (Tyson, 1996). EEG changes, including an increase in delta waves and a decrease in alpha and beta activity, as well as a shift toward left frontal activation (all are indicative of a relaxation response) have been observed in participants receiving moderate massage therapy (Diego, Field, Sanders, & Hernandez-Reif, 2004). There has also been a case study purporting the advantages of the innovative use of integrating imagery/video/EEG biofeedback (i.e., diaphragmatic breathing, coordination exercises, visual exercises to improve tracking, internal visual imagery, and video imagery) in mitigating anxiety and improving performance of a 21-year-old collegiate baseball player who suffered a fractured cheekbone and eye socket after being hit by a pitch (Davis & Sime, 2005).

Sensor placement in neurofeedback is usually standardized based on the International 10–20 System of electrode placement. For the neurotherapy systems typically in use, an experienced therapist requires only about 2 min to connect the sensors to the scalp. Training sessions include a baseline assessment to determine the average microvolt level of the brain waves being investigated. Reward criteria are then established by an amplitude "window," which sets high and low microvolt levels that are reinforced or inhibited. For example, in the beta–theta training used in treating ADHD, beta thresholds may be raised 1 μv higher, or theta levels may be set 1–2 μv lower (Lubar 1995; see Neumann Strehl & Birbaumer (2003) for a primer on EEG instrumentation). Rewards are typically auditory and visual, and given today's advancements in technology, the effects can be quite elaborate.

Electrodermal (EDR) Biofeedback

Description

Electrodermal is a generic term that refers to the electrical characteristics of the skin. There are numerous measurement options available when considering this type of biofeedback. The oldest and most commonly used is the galvanic skin response (GSR); the name attributed to Galvani's discovery of electrical activity in nerves and muscles. Generally, variation of the skin's electrical characteristics appears to be a function of sympathetic neural activity; therefore, when using EDR biofeedback, the patient appears to be training to affect sympathetic neural arousal. More specifically, what is being measured is the conductance and resistance of sweat gland activity and the units measured are micromhos or the newer term micro-siemens (Peek, 2003).

Indications

The major use for EDR is to reduce levels of sympathetic tone and reactivity. It has been used in conjunction with other biofeedback modalities in the treatment of hypertension (Khumar, Kaur, &Kaur, 1992; Patel & Marmot, 1988), asthma (Meany et al., 1988), epilepsy (Nagai, Critchley, Rothwell, Duncan, & Trimble, 2009), and Tourette syndrome (Nagai, Cavanna, & Critchley, 2009, and has also been used as an adjunct in psychotherapy. For example, EDR has been used for systematic desen-sitization, the theory being that relaxation and arousal cannot happen concurrently, and that phobias and anxiety would respond to this type of treatment. EDR has also been used as a tool for exploration in psychotherapy, and in "lie detector" equip-ment (Peek, 2003). The appeal of this modality is that the changes in response can be extremely rapid and relatively easy to measure.

Heart Rate Variability (HRV) Biofeedback

Within the past decade there has been enhanced development of clinical applica-tions of heart rate variability (HRV) biofeedback, a technique credited to Russian physiologist Evgney Vaschillo in the 1970s (Moss, 2008). Heart rate variability in essence means changes in the interval or distance between one beat of the heart and the next (i.e., interbeat interval or IBI) (Moss & Shaffer, 2009). In his work Vaschillo found that while participants could not consistently raise or lower heart rate using biofeedback, they could produce high-amplitude oscillations or variability. This variability, which was typically brought about by breathing controlled and slowly (i.e., diaphragmatically, see Chap. 11) around five to seven times per minute, is associated with improvement in a wide range of health and cognitive functioning. These improvements included athletic performance (Iellamo et al., 2002; Manzi et al., 2009), stress-related chronic pain (Hallman et al., 2011), ulcerative colitis (Maunder et al., 2012), asthma (Lehrer et al., 2006; Tsai, Lai, Chen, Jeng, 2011), trauma (Gevirtz & Dalenberg, 2008; Whitehouse & Heller, 2008), and depression (Karavidas et al., 2007). A more recent exploratory study did not find quantitative support for HRV biofeedback in the treatment of PTSD or depression in a sample of 49 active-duty military participants, even though many of them commented favor-ably on the biofeedback experience (Lande, Williams, Francis, Gragnani, & Morin, 2010). However, a recent pilot study suggests the benefit of incorporating HRV biofeedback in Acceptance and Commitment therapy (Kleen & Reitsma, 2011). Conversely, decreased heart rate variability has been associated with poor health outcomes (Gevirtz & Lehrer, 2003) including behavior problems in children (Calkins, Graziano, & Keane, 2007), depression in adults (Rechlin, Weis, Spitzer, & Kaschka, 1994), generalized anxiety in adults (Friedman, 2007), diabetes (Lindmark, Burén, & Eriksson, 2006), and alcoholism (Ingjaldsson, Laberg, & Thayer, 2003). Overall, and relative to one's age, abnormally low HRV is associated with all causes of mortality (Levy, Slade, Kunkel, & Kasl, 2002).

According to Lehrer and Vaschillo (2008), the mechanism surrounding HRV remains uncertain, due mostly to the complex nature of the autonomic nervous system, but theoretical and empirical support suggest that it is mediated more parasympathetically. What seems more important to these researchers regarding putative mechanisms associated with HRV is the resonance characteristics of the cardiovascular system, or the frequency at which heart rate variability is at its greatest. More specifically, the homeostatic balance of the sympathetic and parasympathetic branches of the ANS (see Chap. 2) produce an orderly increase and decrease in heart rate. The variations in heart rate produced SNS and PNS occur at different speeds or frequencies. Breathing air into the lungs temporarily shuts off the influence of the PNS on heart rate, and thus heart rate increases. When air is breathed out of the lungs, the parasympathetic influence occurs again and heart rate decreases. This oscillation in heart rate as a result of respiration is known as respiratory sinus arrhythmia. When we are experiencing acute stress, the SNS-driven response increases heart rate, but once the stress is over, the homeostatic increase in the PNS should rapidly bring heart rate to its normal slower rhythm. However, chronic stress, which is often exacerbated by negative thoughts and emotions, can overstimulate the SNS and render the PNS less effective in countering the SNS.

Furthermore, these autonomic branches are mediated by the sinoatrial (SA) node and atrioventicular (AV) nodes of the heart, also known as "pacemakers" in the heart. The SA node initiates an electrical signal that begins the cycle of the heart's pumping. This signal passes through the AV node that spreads the current through the ventricles. As noted above, there are factors, such as diaphragmatic breathing that affect specific rhythms in the heart. Other factors that increase the component rhythm of the heart include baroreceptors, which are pressure sensors in the arteries, thermal regulation, and emotional reactivity, such as anxious thinking (Moss & Shaffer, 2009). Thus, higher heart rate variability is indicative of optimal support between the two branches of the ANS, and is associated with physiological resiliency, behavioral flexibility, and increased capacity to adapt well to stress (Beauchaine, 2001). When the ANS is not working well together, the heart shows less stability in resting rate and more difficulty responding to changing body needs.

Current evidence supports the notion that an individual's "resonant frequency," when heart rate variability is at its greatest, can be measured by biofeedback instruments (Moss & Shaffer, 2009; Mueller, n.d.). The overarching goal of HRV biofeedback is to help facilitate physical and emotional well-being or coherence by learning to self-regulate emotional experience (McCraty, 2008) through (1) physical and emotional relaxation, (2) cognitive restructuring to reduce anxious thoughts and negative emotions, and (3) controlled, smooth, effortless diaphragmatic breathing (Moss & Shaffer, 2009). HRV biofeedback typically uses either an electrocardiogram (EKG) with sensors placed on a participant's wrists and torso to detect the electrical signal produced by the heart, or a photoplethysmogrpah (PPG) uses sensors placed on a finger (or in some cases the earlobe) to detect, amplify, and display real-time Interbeat Interval (IBI) so the user can visualize fluctuations in his or her pulse rate. Relaxed, diaphragmatic breathing helps facilitate having respiration and heart rate co-vary to produce a dominant HRV spike of around 0.1 Hz. Striefel (2008) has addressed the ethical issues of competence, informed consent, and home practice when using HRV biofeedback.

Biofeedback Precautions

Several adverse reactions can occur as a result of using biofeedback. The practitioner should be aware of the unfavorable conditions that may be produced or potentially exacerbated by its use (see Chap. 9, this volume; see also Schwartz and Andrasik, 2003). We briefly review several of these issues.

First is the case of patients taking medication for any purpose. Some patients may consider biofeedback a replacement for medication and prematurely or mistakenly stop taking medication they have received for some other purpose. Therefore, it is necessary to question patients closely regarding their medication history and also be willing to work closely with their physicians. The most dramatic example of this occurrence is diabetic patients who are taking insulin. In these cases, inducing relaxation may diminish the need for insulin, and the normal dosage that the patient had been taking may now precipitate a hypoglycemic coma. Changes in blood pressure as a result of efficacious biofeedback treatment are also an area of valid concern for patients taking medication for hyper- or hypotension and should be coordinated with his or her physician. In addition, seizures have occurred in patients undergoing biofeedback treatment for epilepsy.

Other problems may arise related to improper training of the patient by the therapist. An example might be treatment of bruxism with unilateral placement of EMG sensors, producing dislocation of the jaw through imbalance of the muscles. Muscle imbalance is also a potential precaution in the treatment of torticollis with biofeedback. All physical symptoms need to be evaluated medically prior to biofeedback treatment so that the cause of the symptom is not mistakenly ignored. For instance, headaches may result from injury, stroke, tumors, or other causes that require medical attention prior to biofeedback considerations.

Practitioners may also want to exercise caution in the selection of patients. For example, individuals experiencing psychosis, including hallucinations or delusions, and dissociative disorders are considered poor candidates for biofeedback training because they may misinterpret what is occurring, and they may have additional difficulty in controlling their cognitions or physiology.

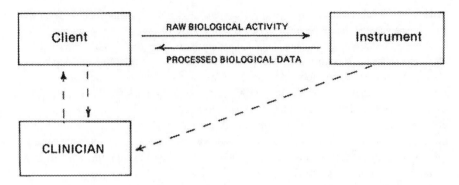

Fig. 14.3 Feeback loop incorporating clinician

Role of the Therapist and Other Factors

From the information covered thus far in this chapter, a reasonable conclusion may be that the major element in biofeedback is the instrument technology. However, it is how the instruments are used in the therapeutic relationship that determines the outcome. In fact, the clinician–patient dyad is by far the most important element in this form of therapy. More than many types of therapies, biofeedback requires that the therapist becomes in essence an effective coach and the patient becomes engaged, and motivated to learn to improve his or her performance, to practice between sessions and to transfer these skills to daily life. As noted, the relationship with the therapist is the foundation of the learning process.

A decisive factor in biofeedback success appears to be the extent to which cognitive restructuring helps patients recognize the ways in which the mind and body interact. Again, this occurrence is dependent on the patient's relationship with his or her clinician to facilitate the process. Within this context, biofeedback may be considered an adjunct to a more traditional psychotherapeutic relationship. It is comparable to hypnosis, relaxation therapy, and so on, in that it is a tool used to treat a symptom complex, but only within the context of the total therapeutic relationship and well thought out treatment plan. Thus, clinicians may be thought of as theatrical directors: They set the stage for change to occur by educating, giving useful hints, pointers, feedback, and encouragement. The actual change that occurs is the result of the patient's efforts. In this way the therapist becomes an instructor or coach who engages the patient's own abilities to help himself or herself and to do so with increasing probabilities of success. Our original diagram of the biofeedback encounter (Fig. 14.1) may now be modified as indicated in Fig. 14.3.

Thus, the clinician receives information regarding the patient's functioning from both the instrument and the patient, then provides information to the patient, allowing the patient better to use data acquired from the instrument. Again, the clinician, although not directly responsible for therapeutic change, plays an important role in the biofeedback loop. His or her empathetic skills, clinical demeanor, and effectiveness as a health educator interact with other factors, such as office setting, room temperature, and type of equipment, to affect the outcome of clinical feedback. It would be naive to believe that personality factors do not affect biofeedback skills acquisition. As noted in Chap. 6, individuals bring various strengths, vulnerabilities, and reservations to the clinical encounter. Also, as noted in Chap. 8, issues of mastery, self-control, and self-efficacy are quite germane to the biofeedback paradigm. Bandura (1982a, 1982b, 1997) has noted, however, that the perception of self-efficacy is even more salient than the degree of manifest self-efficacy. Once again, the clinician's function is paramount in assisting the patient to recognize meaningful acquisition in lieu of possible propensities for self-debasement, catastrophic ideation, or general pessimism.

In their reviews of the utilization and delivery of biofeedback within research and clinical applications, Striefel (2007, 2008), Shellenberger and Green (1986), and Schwartz & Andrasik (2003) discuss some of the most common errors, in addition to ways of ensuring competence. The following errors have particular relevance to the use of biofeedback in the treatment of excessive stress:

1. Failure of the clinician to receive proper training and experience in the use of applied biofeedback equipment and modalities.
2. Failure of the inexperienced clinician to ask for and use prudent supervision.
3. Failure to provide the patient with the appropriate number of training sessions. In biofeedback, which represents a form of learning, individual differences account for a large preponderance of the variation. In other words, no consistent rule governs the rate of skills acquisition. Nevertheless, it is apparent that most people cannot acquire useful biofeedback skills in only two or three sessions. Moreover, recall that 40–80 sessions may be required when using EEG biofeedback to treat ADHD.
4. Failure to provide the patient with homework exercises that reinforce and extend the skills acquired within the office or laboratory setting. Again, one of the primary goals of biofeedback is to generalize the response to settings outside of the office.
5. Failure of the clinician to recognize and facilitate the social–psychological and clinical aspects of biofeedback. Some clinicians erroneously believe that biofeedback is immune to the usual clinical variables that affect other aspects of clinical psychology and psychiatry. Therefore, it is often useful to conceptualize some forms of biofeedback as biofeedback-assisted psychotherapy.
6. Failure of the clinician to recognize that the patient's formation of a sense of control or self-efficacy serves as one of the most relevant clinical aspects or powerful therapeutic forces within the biofeedback paradigm.
7. Failure of the clinician to allow the patient ample time to adapt or habituate to the physiological assessment process. Biofeedback, in addition to being a therapeutic intervention, is also an exercise in physiological assessment. In any such paradigm, the participant must be allowed to adapt to the novel stimuli represented by the biofeedback training environment. Adaptation needs to occur within every training session.

8. Failure to take baseline measurements relevant to the biofeedback variables to be trained. In a sense, it is useful to consider the patient as the control within a single-subject research design and to structure the clinical paradigm with that in mind.
9. Failure of the clinician to train the clinical patient to mastery as opposed to initial skills acquisition. In other words, too many patients are prematurely terminated by biofeedback clinicians who lose sight of the need to have patients overlearn the acquired skills in self-regulation.

The Past and Future of Biofeedback

Similar to the previous editions of this text, we remain optimistic about the clinical utility and applications of various forms of biofeedback, although there seems to be some perception that its prominence in complementary and alternative medicine may have waned somewhat in recent years. However, publications such as *Applied Psychophysiology and Biofeedback, Journal of Evidence-Based Complementary & Alternative Medicine* and the *Journal of Neurotherapy* attest to the continued interest in biofeedback. There are also some recent reports that biofeedback devices (e.g., EEG, GSR) may interface with the video gaming industry, with exercise training, and with performance enhancement and recovery in athletes. For example, there are assisted telemetry systems that allow a person to workout, ride, shoot, or actually compete, and have data transmitted to monitors or coaches who are located distally (http://Heartmath.com; http://www.Thoughttechnology.com). It is relevant to note, however, that the field of biofeedback as a clinical technology has not always been universally accepted by clinicians and researchers. Past criticisms and scrutiny have focused on the soundness and rigor of some of the research design and methodology (Schwartz & Andrasik, 2003), as well as the apparently exaggerated claims of applied applications and successes made by some practitioners. For a good review of the epistemological issues that affect the conduct of inquiry as it pertains to the investigation of the clinical efficacy of biofeedback, the reader is referred to Shellenberger and Green (1986, 1987) and Lehrer et al. (1994). The increased technological sophistication and implementation of virtual reality devices appears to be a vibrant opportunity to enhance and expand the applications of biofeedback.

There are several professional organizations, such as the Association of Biofeedback and Psychophysiology (AAPB) and the International Society for Neurofeedback and Research (ISNR), that allow interested professionals to advance their understanding and use of biofeedback, applied psychophysiology and applied neuroscience. They promote education and research, as well as ways to help improve peoples' life functioning and well-being (AAPB, 2011; ISNR, 2011). Professionals who meet education and training standards can seek certification in general biofeedback, neurofeedback, and pelvic muscle dysfunction biofeedback through the Biofeedback Certification Institute of America (BCIA; http://www.bcia.org).

Summary

This chapter has explored biofeedback, the creation and clinical utilization of psychophysiological feedback loops for the purpose of treating excessive stress and/or its target-organ effects. Let us review the main points:

1. Biofeedback gives the recipient access to learning paradigms that involve physiological functions not previously accessible to conscious alteration.
2. Biofeedback can be used directly to modify the stress response itself, through the elicitation of the relaxation response or the alteration of target-organ activity.
3. EMG, temperature, EEG, which is also referred to as neurofeedback, and EDR biofeedback are commonly used forms of clinical biofeedback, but the use of Heart Rate Variability (HRV) has blossomed in the past decade.
4. The clinician's impact on the biofeedback paradigm can mean the difference between clinical success or failure. For this reason, the clinician should receive training in not only clinical psychophysiology but also the fundamentals of counseling or clinical psychology.
5. In understanding the process of therapeutic effect, one of the most important aspects of clinical biofeedback may be the creation of the perception of self-efficacy, as discussed by Bandura (1997) and supported by Rokicki and associates (1997) in the use of EMG biofeedback specifically.
6. For precautions that should be followed in using biofeedback, refer to Chap. 9.
7. Useful reviews of clinical biofeedback are found in Schwartz and Andrasik (2003), Shellenberger and Green (1986), and Basmajian (1989).

Acknowledgements We would like to thank Russ Hibler, PhD, ABPP, Affiliate Faculty Loyola University Maryland, for his early review of this chapter.

References

Allen, K. D., & Shriver, M. D. (1997). Enhanced performance feedback to strengthen biofeedback treatment outcome with childhood migraine. *Headache, 37*(3), 169–173.

Angelakis, E., Stathopoulou, S., Frymiare, J. L., Green, D. L., Lubar, J. F., & Kounios, J. (2007). EEG neurofeedback: A brief overview and an example of peak alpha frequency training for cognitive enhancement in the elderly. *The Clinical Neuropsychologist, 21*(1), 110–129.

Angoules, A. G., Balakatounis, K. C., Panagiotopoulou, K. A., Mavrogenis, A. F., Mitsiokapa, E. A., & Papagelopoulos, P. J. (2008). *Orthopedics, 31*(10), 980–984.

Arns, M., de Ridder, S., Strehl, U., Breteler, M., & Coenen, A. (2009). Efficacy of neurofeedback treatment in ADHD: The effects of inattention, impulsivity and hyperactivity: A meta-analysis. *Clinical EEG and Neuroscience, 40*(3), 180–189.

Association for Applied Psychophysiology & Biofeedback. (2011). About AAPB. Retrieved from: http://www.aapb.org/i4a/pages/index.cfm?pageid=3285

Baehr, E., Rosenfeld, J. P., & Baehr, R. (1997). The clinical use of an alpha asymmetry protocol in the neurofeedback treatment of depression: Two case studies. *Journal of Neurotherapy, 2*(3), 10–23.

Bandura, A. (1982a). Self-efficacy mechanism in human agency. *The American Psychologist, 37*, 122–147.

Bandura, A. (1982b). The self and mechanisms of agency. In J. Suls (Ed.), *Psychological perspectives on the self* (pp. 3–39). Hillsdale, NJ: Erlbaum.

Bandura, A. (1997). *Self-efficacy: The exercise of control.* New York, NY: Freeman.

Basmajian, J. V. (1963). Control and training of individual motor units. *Science, 141*, 440–441.

Basmajian, J. (1967). *Muscles alive. Their function revealed by electromyography* (2nd ed.). Baltimore, MD: Williams & Wilkins.

Basmajian, J. V. (1989). *Biofeedback: Principles and practice for clinicians* (3rd ed.). Baltimore, Maryland: Williams & Wilkins

Beauchaine, T. P. (2001). Vagal tone, development, and Gray's motivational theory: Toward an integrated model of autonomic nervous system functioning in psychopathology. *Development and Psychopathology, 13*, 183–214.

Biondi, D. M. (2005). Physical treatments for headache: A structured review. *Headache: The Journal of Head and Face Pain, 45*(6), 738–746.

Biondi, M., & Picardi, A. (1998). Temporomandibular joint pain–dysfunction syndrome and bruxism: Etiopathogenesis and treatment from a psychosomatic integrative viewpoint. In G. A. Fava & H. Freyberger (Eds.), *Handbook of psychosomatic medicine* (pp. 469–490). Madision, CT: International Universities Press.

Bisson, E., Contant, B., Sveistrup, H., & Lojoie, Y. (2007). Functional balance and dual-task reaction times in older adults are improved by virtual reality and biofeedback training. *Cyberpsychology and Behavior, 10*(1), 16–23.

Blanchard, E. B., Eisele, G., Vollmer, A., Payne, A., Gordon, M., Gornish, P., & Gilmore, L. (1996). Controlled evaluation of thermal biofeedback in treatment of elevated blood pressure in unmedicated mild hypertension. *Biofeedback and Self-Regulation, 21*(2), 167–190.

Blanchard, E. B., & Epstein, L. H. (1978). *A biofeedback primer.* Reading, MA: Addison-Wesley.

Brown, B. (1977). *Stress and the art of biofeedback.* New York, NY: Harper & Row.

Butler, R. N., Maby, J. I., Montela, J. M., & Young, G. P. (1999). Urinary incontinence: Primary care therapies for the older woman. *Geriatrics, 54*(11), 31–34, 39–40, 43–44.

Calkins, S. D., Graziano, P. A., & Keane, S. P. (2007). Cardiac vagal regulation differentiates among children at risk for behavior problems. *Biological Psychology, 74*(2), 144–153.

Caro, X. J., & Winter, E. F. (2011). EEG biofeedback treatment improves certain attention and somatic symptoms in fibromyalgia: A pilot study. *Applied Psychophysiology and Biofeedback, 36*(3), 193–200.

Chabot, R. J., & Serfontein, G. (1996). Quantitative electroencephalographic profiles in children with attention deficit disorder. *Biological Psychiatry, 40*, 951–963.

Chiarioni, G., & Whitehead, W. E. (2008). The role of biofeedback in the treatment of gastrointestinal disorders. *Nature Reviews Gastroenterology & Hepatology, 5*, 371–382.

Crider, A. B., & Glaros, A. G. (1999). A meta-analysis of EMG biofeedback treatment of temporomandibular disorders. *Journal of Orofacial Pain, 13*(1), 29–37.

Dannecker, C., Wolf, V., Raab, R., Hepp, H., & Anthuber, C. (2005). EMG-biofeedback assisted pelvic floor muscle training is an effective therapy of stress urinary or mixed incontinence: A 7-year experience with 390 patients. *Archives of Gynecology and Obstetrics, 273*, 93–97.

Davis, P. A., & Sime, W. E. (2005). Toward a psychophysiology of performance: Sport psychology principles dealing with anxiety. *International Journal of Stress Management, 12*(4), 363–378.

DiCara, L. V., & Miller, N. E. (1968a). Changes in heart rate instrumentally learned by curarized rats as avoidance responses. *Journal of Comparative Physiology and Psychology, 65*, 8–12.

DiCara, L. V., & Miller, N. E. (1968b). Instrumental learning of systolic blood pressure responses by curarized rats: Dissociation of cardiac and vascular changes. *Psychosomatic Medicine, 30*, 489–494.

DiCara, L. V., & Miller, N. E. (1968c). Instrumental learning of vasomotor responses by rats: Learning to respond differently in the two ears. *Science, 159*, 1485.

Diego, M. A., Field, T., Sanders, C., & Hernandez-Reif, M. (2004). Massage therapy of moderate and light pressure and vibrator effects on EEG and heart rate. *International Journal of Neuroscience, 114*, 31–45.

Doğan-Aslan, M., Nakipoğlu-Yüzer, G. F., Doğan, A., Karabay, İ., & Özgirgin, N. (2010). The effect of electromyographic biofeedback treatment in improving upper extremity functioning of patients with hemiplegic stroke. *Journal of Stroke and Cerebrovascular Diseases, 21*(3), 187–193.

Donaldson, S., Donaldson, M., & Snelling, L. (2003). SEMG Evaluations: An overview. *Applied Psychophysiology and Biofeedback, 28*(2), 121–127.

Druzbicki, M., Kwolek, A., Depa, A., & Przysada, G. (2010). The use of a treadmill with biofeedback function in assessment of relearning walking skills in post-stroke hemiplegic patcients – A preliminary report. *Neuologia i Neurochirurgia Polska, 44*(6), 567–573.

El-Sayed, E., Larsson, J. O., Persson, H. E., & Rydelius, P. A. (2002). Altered cortical activity in children with attention-deficit/hyperactivity disorder during attentional load task. *Journal of the American Academy of Child and Adolescent Psychiatry, 41*, 811–819.

Everly, G. S., Jr., & Sobelman, S. H. (1987). *The assessment of the human stress response: Neurological, biochemical, and psychological foundations.* New York, NY: American Management Systems Press.

Field, T. (2009). *Complementary and alternative therapies research.* Washington, DC: American Psychological Association.

Foster, P. S. (2004). Use of the Calmset 3 Biofeedback/Relaxation System in the assessment and treatment of chronic nocturnal bruxism. *Applied Psychophysiology and Biofeedback, 29*(2), 141–147.

Frazier, T. W. (1966). Avoidance conditioning of heart rate in humans. *Psychophysiology, 3*, 188–202.

Friedman, B. H. (2007). An autonomic flexibility-neurovisceral integration model of anxiety and cardiac vagal tone. *Biological Psychology, 74*, 185–199.

Gatchel, R., & Price, K. (1979). Biofeedback: An introduction and historical overview. In R. Gatchel & K. Price (Eds.), *Clinical applications of biofeedback: Appraisal and status.* Elmsford, NY: Pergamon Press.

Gevensleben, H., Moll, G. H., & Heinrich, H. (2010). Neurofeedback training in children with ADHD: Behavioral and neurophysiological effects. *Zeitschrift für Kinder – und Jugendpsychiatrie und psychotherapie, 38*(6), 409–419.

Gevirtz, R. (2006). Applied psychophysiology/biofeedback in primary care medicine. *Biofeedback, 34*(4), 145–147.

Gevirtz, R., & Dalenberg, C. (2008). Heart rate biofeedback in the treatment of trauma symptoms. *Biofeedback, 36*(1), 22–23.

Gevirtz, R. N., & Lehrer, P. (2003). Resonant frequency heart rate biofeedback. In M. S. Schwartz & F. Andrasik (Eds.), *Biofeedback: A practitioner's guide* (pp. 245–250). New York, NY: Guilford.

Glick, R. M., & Greco, C. M. (2010). Biofeedback and primary care. *Primary Care: Clinics in Office Practice, 37*(1), 91–103.

Gorini, A., Pallavincini, F., Algeri, D., Repetto, C., Gaggioli, A., & Giuseppe, R. (2010). Virtual reality in the treatment of generalized anxiety disorders. *Annual Review of CyberTherapy and Telemedicine, 8*, 31–35.

Graham, C., Cook, M. R., Cohen, H. D., Gerkovich, M. M., Phelps, J. W., & Fotopoulous, S. S. (1986). Effects of variation in physical effort on frontalis EMG activity. *Biofeedback and Self-Regulation, 11*(2), 135–141.

Green, E., & Green, A. (1977). *Beyond biofeedback.* San Francisco, CA: Delta.

Hall, J. E. (2011). *Guyton and Hall textbook of medical physiology* (12th ed.). Philadelphia, PA: Saunders Elsevier.

Hallman, D. M., Olsson, E. M., von Schéele, B., Melin, L., & Lyskov, E. (2011). Effects of heart rate variability biofeedback in subjects with stress-related chronic neck pain: A pilot study. *Applied Psychophysiology and Biofeedback, 36*(2), 71–80.

Herman, C., Blanchard, E. B., & Flor, H. (1997). Biofeedback treatment for pediatric migraine: Prediction of treatment outcome. *Journal of Consulting and Clinical Psychology, 65*(4), 611–616.

Hermens, H. J., Freriks, B., Disselhorst-Klug, C., & Rau, G. (2000). Development of recommendations for SEMG sensors and senor placement procedures. *Journal of Electromyography and Kinesiology, 10*, 361–374.

Holroyd, K. A., & Penzien, D. B. (1994). Psychosocial interventions in the management of recurrent headache disorders: I. *Overview and effectiveness. Behavioral Medicine, 20*(2), 53–63.

Holtmann, M., & Stadler, C. (2006). Electroencephalographic biofeedback for the treatment of attention-deficit hyperactivity disorder in childhood and adolescence. *Expert Review of Neurotherapeutics, 6*(4), 533–540.

Huang-Storms, L., Bodenhamer-Davis, E., Davis, R., & Dunn, J. (2007). QEEG-guided neurofeedback for children with histories of abuse and neglect: Neurodevelopmental rationale and pilot study. *Journal of Neurotherapy, 10*(4), 3–16.

Huebner, M., Riegel, K., Hinninghofen, H., Wallwiener, D., Tunn, R., & Reisenauer, C. (2011). Pelvic floor muscle training for stress urinary incontinence: A randomized, controlled trial comparing different conservative therapies *Physiotherapy Research International, 16*(3), 133–140.

Iellamo, F., Lagramant, J. M., Pigozzi, F., Spataro, A., Norbiato, G., Lucini, D., & Pagani, M. (2002). Conversion from vagal to sympathetic predominance with strenuous training in high-performance world class athletes. *Circulation, 105*, 2719–2724.

Imamura, M., Abrams, P., Bain, C., Buckley, B., Cardozo, L., Cody, J., & Vale, L. (2010). Systematic review and economic modelling of the effectiveness and cost-effectiveness of non-surgical treatments for women with stress urinary incontinence. *Health Technology Assessment, 14*(40), whole volume.

Ingjaldsson, J. T., Laberg, J. C., & Thayer, J. F. (2003). Reduced heart rate variability in chronic alcohol abuse: Relationship with negative mood, chronic thought suppression, and compulsive drinking. *Biological Psychiatry, 54*, 1427–1436.

International Society for Neurofeedback & Research. (2011). About ISNR. Retreived from: http://www.isnr.org/about-isnr/about-isnr.cfm

Isler, W. C. (2006). Collaborative approaches in primary care. *Biofeedback, 34*(4), 151–154.

Jacobs, G. D., Benson, H., & Friedman, R. (1996). Topographic EEG mapping of the relaxation response. *Biofeedback and Self-Regulation, 21*(2), 121–129.

Jadidi, F., Castrillon, E., & Svensson, P. (2008). Effect of conditioning electrical stimuli on temporalis electromyographic activity during sleep. *Journal of Oral Rehabilitation, 35*(3), 171–183.

James, L. C., & Folen, R. A. (1996). EEG biofeedback as a treatment for chronic fatigue syndrome: A controlled case report. *Behavioral Medicine, 22*(2), 77–81.

Jones, G. E., & Evans, P. A. (1981). Effectiveness of frontalis feedback training in producing general body relaxation. *Biological Psychology, 12*(4), 313–320.

Kaiser, D. A. (2006). What is quantitative EEG. *Journal of Neurotherapy, 10*(4), 37–52.

Kamiya, J. (1969). Operant control of the EEG alpha rhythm and some of its reported effects on consciousness. In C. T. Tart (Ed.), *Altered states of consciousness* (pp. 507–517). New York: Wiley.

Karavidas, M. K., Lehrer, P. M., Vaschillo, E., Vaschillo, B., Marin, H., Buyske, S., & Hassett, A. (2007). Preliminary results of an open label study of heart rate variability biofeedback for the treatment of major depression. *Applied Psychophysiology and Biofeedback, 32*, 19–30.

Karavidas, M. K., Tsai, P.-S., Yucha, C., McGrady, A., & Lehrer, P. M. (2006). Thermal biofeedback for primary Raynaud's phenomenon: A review of the literature. *Applied Psychophysiology and Biofeedback, 31*(3), 203–216.

Kayiran, S., Dursun, E., Dursun, N., Ermutlu, N., & Karamürsel, S. (2010). Neurofeedback intervention in fibromyalgia syndrome: A randomized, controlled, rater blind clinical trial. *Applied Psychopysiology and Biofeedback, 35*(4), 293–302.

Khumar, S. S., Kaur, P., & Kaur, J. (1992). A study of therapeutic effect of GSR biofeed-back on mild hypertension. *Journal of the Indian Academy of Applied Psychology, 18*(1–2), 23–28.

Kimble, G. A. (1961). *Hilgard and Marquis' conditioning and learning.* New York: Appleton–Century–Crofts.

Kleen, M., & Reitsma, B. (2011). Appliance of heart rate variability biofeedback in Acceptance and Commitment Therapy: A pilot study. *Journal of Neurotherapy: Investigations in Neuromodulation, Neurofeedback and Applied Neuroscience, 15*(2), 170–181.

Lande, R. G., Williams, L. B., Francis, J. L., Cragnani, C., & Morin, M. L. (2010). Efficacy of biofeedback for post-traumatic stress disorder. *Complementary Therapies in Medicine, 18,* 256–259.

Landy, S. (2004). Migraine throughout the life cycle: Treatment through the ages. *Neurology, 62* (5 suppl2)S2-S8

Lehrer, P. M., Carr, R., Sargunaraj, D., & Woolfolk, R. L. (1994). Stress management techniques: Are they all equivalent, or do they have specific effects? *Biofeedback and Self-Regulation, 19*(4), 353–401.

Lehrer, P., & Vaschillo, E. (2008). The future of heart rate variability biofeedback. *Biofeedback, 36*(1), 11–14.

Lehrer, P., Vaschillo, E., Lu, S.-E., Eckberg, D., Vaschillo, B., Scardella, A., & Habib, R. (2006). Heart rate variability biofeedback: Effects of age on heart rate variability, baroreflex gain, and asthma. *Chest, 129*(2), 278–284.

Levy, B. R., Slade, M. D., Kunkel, S. R., & Kasl, S. V. (2002). Longevity increased by positive self-perceptions of aging. *Journal of Personality and Social Psychology, 83*(2), 261–270.

Linden, W., & Moseley, J. V. (2006). The efficacy of behavioral treatments for hypertension. *Applied Psychophysiology and Biofeedback, 31*(1), 51–63.

Lindmark, S., Burén, J., & Eriksson, J. W. (2006). Insulin resistance, endocrine function and adipokines in type 2 diabetes patients at different glycaemic levels: Potential impact for glucotoxicity *in vivo. Clinical Endocrinology, 65,* 301–309.

Lindsley, D. B., & Sassaman, W. (1938). Autonomic activity and brain potentials associated with "voluntary" control of pilomotors. *Journal of Neurophysiology, 1,* 342–349.

Loo, S. K., & Barkley, R. A. (2005). Clinical utility of EEG in attention deficit hyperactivity disorder. *Applied Neuropsychology, 12*(2), 64–76.

Lubar, J. F. (1991). Discourse on the development of EEG diagnostics and biofeedback treatment for attention-deficit/hyperactivity disorders. *Biofeedback and Self-Regulation, 16,* 201–225.

Lubar, J. F. (1995). Neurofeedback for the management of attention-deficit/hyperactivity disorders. In M. Schwartz and Associates (Eds.), *Biofeedback: A practitioner's guide* (2nd ed., pp. 493–522). New York: Guilford.

Lubar, J. F., & Deering, W. M. (1981). *Behavioral approaches to neurology.* New York: Academic Press.

Lubar, J. F., & Shouse, M. N. (1976). EEG and behavioral changes in a hyperkinetic child concurrent with training of the sensorimotor rhythm (SMR): A preliminary report. *Biofeedback and Self-Regulation, 3,* 293–306.

Luria, A. R. (1958). *The mind of a mnemonist* (L. Solotaroff, trans.). New York: Basic Books.

Lynch, D. J., McGrady, A. V., Nagel, R. W., & Wahl, E. F. (2007). The patient-physician relationship and medical utilization. *The Primary Care Companion to the Journal of Clinical Psychiatry, 9*(4), 266–270.

Manzi, V., Castagna, C., Padua, E., Lombardo, M., D'Ottavio, S., Massaro, … Iellamo, F. (2009). Dose–response relationship of autonomic nervous system responses to individualized training impulse in marathon runners. *American Journal of Physiology-Heart and Circulatory Physiology, 296*(6), H1733-H1740

Mariela, S. C., Matt, D. A., & Burish, T. G. (1992). Comparison of frontalis, multiple muscle site, and reactive muscle site feedback in reducing arousal under stressful and nonstressful conditions. *Medical Psychotherapy: An International Journal, 5,* 133–148.

Maunder, R. G., Nolan, R. P., Hunter, J. J., Lancee, W. J., Steinhart, A. H., & Greenberg, G. R. (2012). Relationship between social support and autonomic function during a stress protocol in ulcerative colitis patients in remission. *Inflammatory Bowel Diseases, 18*(4), 732–742.

McClure, C. (1959). Cardiac arrest through volition. *California Medicine, 90,* 440–448.

McCraty, R. (2008). From depletion to renewal: Positive emotions and heart rhythm coherence feedback. *Biofeedback, 36*(1), 30–34.

McDowell, B. J., Engberg, S., Sereika, S., Donovan, N., Jubeck, M. E., Weber, E., & Engberg, R. (1999). Effectiveness of behavioral therapy to treat incontinence in homebound older adults. *Journal of the American Geriatric Society, 47*(3), 309–318.

McGinnis, R. A., McGrady, A., Cox, S. A., & Grower-Dowling, K. A. (2005). Biofeedback-assisted relaxation in Type 2 diabetes. *Diabetes Care, 28*(9), 2145–2149.

McGrady, A., Graham, G., & Bailey, B. (1996). Biofeedback-assisted relaxation in insulin-dependent diabetes: A replication and extension study. *Annals of Behavioral Medicine, 18*(3), 185–189.

McGrath, P. J. (1999). Clinical psychology issues in migraine headaches. *Canadian Journal of the Neurological Sciences, 26*(Suppl. 3), S33–S36.

McKee, M. G. (2008). Biofeedback: An overview in the context of heart-brain medicine. *Cleveland Clinic Journal of Medicine, 75*(Suppl. 2), S31–S34.

Meany, J., McNamara, M., Burks, V., Berger, T. W., & Sayle, D. M. (1988). Psychological treatment of an asthmatic patient in crisis: Dreams, biofeedback, and pain behavior modification. *Journal of Asthma, 25*(3), 141–151.

Miller, N. E. (1969). Learning of visceral and glandular responses. *Science, 163*, 434–445.

Miller, R. M., & Chang, M. W. (1999). Advances in the management of dysphagia caused by stroke. *Physical Medicine and Rehabilitation Clinics of North America, 10*(4), 925–941.

Miller, N. E., & Dworkin, B. R. (1974). Visceral learning: Recent difficulties with curarized rats and significant problems for human research. In P., A. Obrist, A. H. Black, J. Brener, & L. V. DiCara (Eds.), *Cardiovascular psychophysiology* (pp. 313–331). Chicago: Aldine.

Monastra, V. J. (2005). Electroencephalographic biofeedback (neurotherapy) as a treatment for attention deficit hyperactivity disorder: Rationale and empirical foundation. *Child and Adolescent Psychiatric Clinics of North America, 14*, 55–82.

Mosastra, V. J. (2003). Clinical applications of electroencephalographic biofeedback. In M. S. Schwartz, F. Andrasik (Eds.), *Biofeedback: A practitioner's guide* (pp.438-463). New York: Guilford.

Moser, D. K., Dracup, K., Woo, M. A., & Stevenson, L. W. (1997). Voluntary control of vascular tone by using skin-temperature biofeedback-relaxation in patients with advanced heart failure. *Alternative Therapies in Health and Medicine, 3*(1), 51–59.

Moss, D. (2008). Special Issue: The emergent science and practice of heart rate variability biofeedback. *Biofeedback, 36*(1), 1–4.

Moss, D. & Shaffer, F. (2009). Heart rate variability training. Retrieved from: http://www.bfe.org/articles/hrv.pdf

Mueller, H. (n.d.). Heart rate variability biofeedback. Learning to change heart rhythms. Retreived from: http://www.drmueller-healthpsychology.com/heart_rate_variability.html

Nagai, Y., Cavanna, A., & Critchley, H. D. (2009). Influence of sympathetic autonomic arousal on tics: Implications for a therapeutic behavioral intervention for Tourette syndrome. *Journal of Psychosomatic Research, 67*(6), 599–605.

Nagai, Y., Critchley, H. D., Rothwell, J. C., Duncan, J. S., & Trimble, M. R. (2009). Changes in cortical potential associated with modulation of peripheral sympathetic activity in patients with epilepsy. *Psychosomatic Medicine, 71*(1), 84–92.

Nagai, Y., Goldstein, L. H., Fenwick, P. B. C., & Trimble, M. R. (2004). Clinical efficacy of galvanic skin response biofeedback training in reducing seizures in adult epilepsy: A preliminary randomized controlled study. *Epilepsy & Behavior, 5*, 216–223.

Nestoriuc, Y., & Martin, A. (2007). Efficacy of biofeedback for migraine: A meta-analysis. *Pain, 128*, 111–127.

Nestoriuc, Y., Martin, A., Rief, W., & Andrasik, F. (2008). Biofeedback treatment for headache disorders: A comprehensive efficacy review. *Applied Psychophysiology and Biofeedback, 33*, 125–140.

Neuman, N., Strehl, U., & Birbaumer, N. (2003). A primer of electroencephalographic instrumentation. In M. S. Schwartz & F. Andrasik (Eds.), *Biofeedback: A practitioner's guide* (3rd ed., pp. 88–102). New York: Guilford Press.

Ogden, E., & Shock, N. (1939). Voluntary hypercirculation. *American Journal of the Medical Sciences, 98*, 329–342.

Packard, R. C., & Ham, L. P. (1996). EEG biofeedback in the treatment of Lyme disease: A case study. *Journal of Neurotherapy, 1*(3), 22–31.

Palermo, T. M., Eccleston, C., Lewandowski, A. S., Williams, A. C., & Morley, S. (2010). Randomized controlled trials of psychological therapies for management of chronic pain in childhood and adolescents: An updated meta-analytic review. *Pain, 148*(3), 387–397.

Pallavicini, F., Algeri, D., Repetto, C., Gorini, A., & Riva, G. (2009). Biofeedback, virtual reality and mobile phones in the treatment of generalized anxiety disorder (GAD): A phase-2 controlled clinical trial. *Journal of CyberTherapy & Rehabilitation, 2*(4), 315–327.

Palmer, L. S. (2010). Biofeedback in the management of urinary continence in children. *Current Urology Reports, 11*(2), 122–127.

Patel, C., & Marmot, M. (1988). Can general practitioners use training in relaxation and management of stress to reduce mild hypertension? *British Medical Journal, 296*, 21–24.

Peek, C. J. (2003). A primer of biofeedback instrumentation. In M. S. Schwartz, F. Andrasik (Eds.), *Biofeedback: A practitioner's guide* (pp.43-87). New York:Guilford

Peniston, E. G., & Kulkosky, P. J. (1999). Neurofeedback in the treatment of addictive disorders. In J. R. Evans (Ed.), *Introduction to quantitative EEG and neurofeedback* (pp. 157–179). San Diego: Academic Press.

Rechlin, T., Weis, M., Spitzer, A., & Kaschka, W. P. (1994). Are affective disorders associated with alterations of heart rate variability? *Journal of Affective Disorders, 32*, 271–275.

Reid, G. J., & McGrath, P. J. (1996). Psychological treatments for migraine. *Biomedical Pharmacotherapy, 50*(2), 58–63.

Repetto, C., Gorini, A., Algeri, D., Vigna, C., Gaggioli, A., & Riva, G. (2009). The use of biofeedback in clinical virtual reality: The intrepid project. *Studies in Health Technology and Informatics, 144*, 128–132.

Rice, B. I. (2007). Clinical benefits of training patients to voluntarily increase peripheral blood flow: The warm feet intervention. *The Diabetes Educator, 33*(3), 442–454.

Richards, L., & Pohl, P. (1999). Therapeutic interventions to improve upper extremity recovery and function. *Clinical Geriatric Medicine, 15*(4), 819–832.

Richardson, I., & Palmer, L. S. (2009). Successful treatment for giggle incontinence with biofeedback. *Journal of Urology, 182*(4 Suppl), 2062–2066.

Rokicki, L. A., Holroyd, K. A., France, C. R., Lipchik, G. L., France, J. L., & Kvaal, S. A. (1997). Change mechanisms associated with combined relaxation/EMG biofeedback training for chronic tension headache. *Applied Psychophysiology and Biofeedback, 22*(1), 21–41.

Rubin, L. R. (1977). *Reanimation of the paralyzed face*. St. Louis, MD: Mosby.

Ryan, M., & Gevirtz, R. (2004). Biofeedback-based psychophysiological treatment in a primary care setting: An initial feasibility study. *Applied Psychophysiology and Biofeedback, 29*(2), 79–93.

Scharff, L., Marcus, D. A., & Masek, B. J. (2002). A controlled study of minimal-contact thermal biofeedback treatment in children with migraine. *Journal of Pediatric Psychology, 27*(2), 109–119.

Schneider, C. J. (1989). A brief history of biofeedback. *Biofeedback, 17*(1), 4–7.

Schwartz, M. S. (1995). *Biofeedback: A practitioner's guide* (2nd ed.). New York: Guilford.

Schwartz, M. S., & Andrasik, F. (2003). *Biofeedback: A practitioner's guide* (3rd ed.). New York: Guilford.

Schwartz, M. S., & Montgomery, D. D. (2003). Entering the field and assuring competence. In M. Schwartz & F. Andrasik (Eds.), *Biofeedback: A practitoner's guide* (3rd ed., pp. 20–26). New York: Guilford.

Seifert, A. R., & Lubar, J. F. (1975). Reduction of epileptic seizures through EEG biofeedback training. *Biological Psychology, 3*, 157–184.

Sharpley, C. F., & Rogers, H. (1984). A meta-analysis of frontal EMG levels with biofeedback and alternative procedures. *Biofeedback and Self-Regulation, 9*, 385–393.

Shearn, D. W. (1962). Operant conditioning of heart rate. *Science, 137*, 530–531.

Shellenberger, R., & Green, J. (1986). *From the ghost in the box to successful biofeedback training.* Greeley, CO: Health Psychology.

Shellenberger, R., & Green, J. (1987). Specific effects of biofeedback versus biofeedback-assisted self-regulation training. *Biofeedback and Self-Regulation, 12*(3), 185–209.

Shouse, M. N., & Lubar, J. F. (1978). Physiological bases of hyperkinesis treated with methylphenidate. *Pediatrics, 62,* 343–351.

Sokhadze, T. M., Cannon, R. L., & Trudeau, D. L. (2008). EEG biofeedback as a treatment for substance use disorders: Review, rating of efficacy, and recommendations for further research. *Applied Psychophysiology and Biofeedback, 33*(1), 1–28.

Staples, J. K., Abdel Atti, J. A., & Gordon, J. S. (2011). Mind-body skills groups for posttraumatic stress disorder and depression symptoms in Palestinian children and adolescents in Gaza. *International Journal of Stress Management, 18*(3), 246–262.

Sterman, M. B. (1973). Neurophysiological and clinical studies in an epileptic following sensorimotor EEG biofeedback training: Some effects on epilepsy. In L. Birk (Ed.), *Biofeedback: Behavioral medicine.* New York: Grune & Stratton.

Sterman, M. B., & Egner, T. (2006). Foundation and practice of neurofeedback for the treatment of epilepsy. *Applied Psychophysiology and Biofeedback, 31*(1), 21–35.

Sterman, M. B., & Friar, L. (1972). Suppression of seizures in an epileptic following sensorimotor EEG feedback training. *Electroencephalography and Clinical Neurophysiology, 33,* 89–95.

Stoyva, J. M., & Budzynski, T. H. (1974). Cultivated low-arousal: An anti-stress response? In L. DiCara (Ed.), *Recent advances in limbic and autonomic nervous systems research* (pp. 369–394). New York: Plenum Press.

Stoyva, J. M., & Budzynski, T. H. (1993). Biofeedback methods in the treatment of anxiety and stress disorders. In P. Lehrer & R. Woolfolk (Eds.), *Principles and practice of stress management* (2nd ed., pp. 263–300). New York: Guilford.

Striefel, S. (2007). Ethical and legal electromyography. *Biofeedback, 35,* 3–7.

Striefel, S. (2008). Ethical issues in heart rate variability biofeedback. *Biofeedback, 36,* 5–8.

Surmeli, T., & Ertem, A. (2009). QEEG guided neurofeedback therapy in personality disorders: 13 case studies. *Clinical EEG and Neuroscience, 40*(1), 5–10.

Tan, G., Dao, T. K., Sutherland, R. J., & Gevirtz, R. (2011). Heart rate variability (HRV) and posttraumatic stress disorder (PTSD): A pilot study. *Applied Psychophysiology and Biofeedback, 36*(1), 27–35.

Tsai, Y.-S., Lai, F.-C., Chen, S.-R., & Jeng, C. (2011). The influence of physical activity level on heart rate variability among asthmatic adults. *Journal of Clinical Nursing, 20*(1–2), 111–118.

Tyson, P. D. (1996). Biodesensitization: biofeedback-controlled systematic desensitization of the stress response to infant crying. *Biofeedback & Self Regulation, 21*(3), 273–290.

Varoqui, D., Froger, J., Pélissier, J.-Y., & Bardy, B. G. (2011). Effect of coordination biofeedback on (re)learning preferred postural patterns in post-stroke patients. *Motor Control, 15,* 187–205.

Verbunt, M., & Bartneck, C. (2010). Sensing senses: Tactile feedback for the prevention of decubitus ulcers. *Applied Psychophysiology and Biofeedback, 35,* 243–250.

Walker, J. E. (2011). QEEG-guided neurofeedback for recurrent migraine headaches. *Clinical EEG and Neuroscience, 42*(1), 59–61.

Weatherall, M. (1999). Biofeedback or pelvic floor muscle exercises for female genuine stress incontinence: A meta-analysis of trials identified in a systematic review. *BJU International, 83,* 1015–1016.

Whitehouse, B., & Heller, D. P. (2008). Heart rate in trauma: Patterns found in somatic experiencing and trauma resolution. *Biofeedback, 36*(1), 24–29.

Wiederhold, B. K., & Rizzo, A. (2005). Virtual reality and applied psychophysiology. *Applied Psychophysiology and Biofeedback, 30*(3), 183–185.

Wong, Y. M. (2008). Early-generation biofeedback instruments and modern computers. *Biofeedback, 36*(3), 116–117.

Wood, D. P., Wiederhold, B. K., & Spira, J. (2010). Lessons learned from 350 virtual-reality sessions with warriors diagnosed with combat-related posttraumatic stress disorder. *Cyberpsychology, Behavior, and Social Networking, 13*(1), 3–11.

Chapter 15
Physical Exercise and the Human Stress Response

It has been suggested (Chavat, Dell, & Folkow, 1964; Kraus & Rabb, 1961; Nesse, Bhatnagar, & Young, 2007) that the "wisdom of the body" dictates that the human stress response should lead to physical exertion or exercise. Indeed, physical exercise appears to be the most effective way of ventilating, or expressing, the stress response in a health-promoting manner, once it has been engendered.

Having reviewed the psychophysiological nature of human stress in Part I, it seems reasonable to conclude that stress represents a psychophysiological process that prepares the body for physical action. The increased blood supply to the heart and skeletal muscles, coupled with increased neuromuscular tension, circulating free fatty acids and glucose, as well as the diminished blood flow to the GI system, all lead to the conclusion that the stress response prepares the organism for action (Benson, 1975; Cannon, 1914, 1929; Chavat, Dell, & Folkow, 1964; Kraus & Rabb, 1961; Smith, 2002).

It also seems feasible to assume that, thousands of years ago, the highly active lifestyle of primitive humans afforded ample opportunity to express physically the arousal that resulted from the frustrations and dangers they encountered on a daily basis. Similarly, there was likely sufficient opportunity for our ancestors to develop many of the positive physical and psychological advantages known to accrue from regular physical exercise. Yet in developing from "physical beings" to "thinking beings," humans have fewer chances to ventilate frustrations, failures, and challenges in healthful physical expression. This need to ventilate and refresh our minds and bodies through exercise is apparently so important that some have suggested (Chavat et al., 1964; Greenberg, Dintiman, & Myers-Oakes, 1998; Kraus & Rabb, 1961; Smith, 2002) that the lack of physically active somatomotor expression may lead to an increased risk of disease and dysfunction. In a narrative review by Warbuton, Nicol and Bredin (2006), they conclude, "there is incontrovertible evidence that regular physical activity contributes to the primary and secondary prevention of several chronic diseases and is associated with a reduced risk of premature death" (p. 807).

G.S. Everly and J.M. Lating, *A Clinical Guide to the Treatment of the Human Stress Response*, DOI 10.1007/978-1-4614-5538-7_15,
© Springer Science+Business Media New York 2013

Predicated on information from the World Health Organization (WHO), Chavat et al. (1964) concluded that when the body is aroused for physical action, but that physical expression is suppressed, a condition of strain or psychophysiological overload may be created. They note: "When in civilized man ... [stress] reactions are produced, the... [physically motivating] component is usually more or less suppressed.... What is obvious is that often repeated incidents of... [suppressed somatomotor activity] must imply an increased load on heart and blood vessels" (pp. 130–131).

Similarly, Kraus and Raab (1961) proposed that suppressed physical expression has a preeminent role in the etiology of a variety of anxiety- and stress-related diseases, which they referred to as "hypokinetic diseases." This concept is said to have influenced President John F. Kennedy to promote physical fitness as a major national priority during the early 1960s. In 2010, President Barack Obama announced the establishment of an interagency task force on childhood obesity to develop and implement strategies to reduce the childhood obesity rate to 5% by 2030. First Lady Michelle Obama, as part of this ambitious effort, unveiled her nationwide physical activity campaign "Let's Move" to help achieve the goal of having children born today reach adulthood at a healthy weight. These initiatives seem particularly timely and relevant, considering that the WHO (2012) recently noted that globally, around 31% of adults aged 15 years and older were insufficiently active in 2008. Moreover, they suggested that approximately 3.2 million deaths each year are attributable to inadequate physical activity (WHO).

If, indeed, we have accurately interpreted the "wisdom of the body" as intending that the stress response be consummated in some form of physical somatomotor expression, then a rationale quickly emerges for the consideration of physical exercise as a powerful therapeutic tool in prevention, treatment, and rehabilitation programs for stress-related disease and dysfunction.

History of Therapeutic Exercise

It seems reasonable to assume that our ancient ancestors suffered from few stress-related "hypokinetic" diseases because of their physically demanding lifestyles. It also appears that ancient Greeks, at least for a period of time, had an appreciation of the need to create a balance between physical and intellectual ventures. Plato [as cited in Simon and Levisohn (1987, p. 50)] claimed that "physical exercise is not merely necessary to the health and development of the body, but to balance and correct intellectual pursuits as well.... The right education must tune the strings of the body and mind to perfect spiritual harmony." Physical exercise likely gained the potential for therapeutic application when our physically active culture evolved into a more sedentary one.

Perhaps the earliest use of exercise in a therapeutic capacity, according to Ryan (1974), was in the fifth century B.C. It was during this time that the Greek physician Herodicus prescribed gymnastics for various diseases. In the second century B.C.,

Asclepiades prescribed walking and running in conjunction with diet and massage for disease, as well as for the ills of an "opulent" society.

In 16th-century Europe, Joseph Duchesne is thought to have been the first to use swimming as a therapeutic tool. He is said to have used such physical activity to strengthen the heart and lungs. As a result, exercise gained great popularity in Europe for its therapeutic and preventive applications.

In 1829, the *Journal of Health,* a monthly magazine published in Philadelphia and intended for the general population as well as the medical profession, covered topics such as the health effects of food, drink, atmospheric variables, minerals, hygiene, and exercise. Edward Hitchcock, a professor of chemistry and natural history at Amherst College, and the first professor of physical education in the USA, was a strong supporter of the journal. The publication advocated regular exercise, and Hitchcock considered walking the very best exercise for retaining health (Green, 1986). However, it was not until after the Civil War that exercise and fitness expanded to include all age groups in America.

Following World War I, therapeutic exercise and the study of exercise physiology gained momentum in the USA. According to Miller and Allen (1995), Hans Selye contended that regular exercise would better prepare someone to resist other stressors, and that stressful situations would not be as perilous to a physically fit individual compared with someone who has led a sedentary lifestyle. Physical fitness came into vogue for the lay public with the advent of the President's Council on Physical Fitness in 1956, and the urging of President Kennedy in the 1960s.

As more and more individuals began exercising, more data became available regarding its nature and effects. Physical fitness was promoted in occupational settings with the founding of organizations such as the American Association of Fitness Directors in Business and Industry, which actively and vigorously promoted the "Good health is good business" philosophy to millions at the job site.

Also in the 1960s, America experienced the advent of the urban "health spa." These urban/suburban facilities were centers for the promotion of a health-oriented culture; however, they were typically segregated by gender. The 1970s and the 1980s witnessed two revolutions in the pursuit of exercise that changed the gender separation. The first was the invention of exercise equipment, such as Nautilus, which made weightlifting easier, safer, and more efficient. Moreover, when practiced using the recommended protocol, it actually yielded the potential to facilitate skeletomuscular development while concurrently improving the efficiency of the cardiorespiratory system, thus achieving what exercise enthusiasts at the time considered the best of both worlds. Equipment, such as Cybex®, Hammer Strength®, Precor®, Life Fitness®, and Technogym®, has continued to refine this type of training.

The second revolution involved the image of physical exercise. As noted earlier, there existed two different psychologies of exercise, one for women and one for men. Under the influence of writers such as Kenneth Cooper (*The Aerobics Way: New Data on the World's Most Popular Exercise Program,* 1977) and Jimm Fixx (*The Complete Book of Running,* 1977), as well as the marketing and development of sophisticated exercise facilities that fostered social support, the social barriers to physical exercise fell. For the first time in American history, exercise became a social as well as physical activity that both men and women could pursue and enjoy together.

The 1980s also produced an escalation of scientific research interest in how exercise may be related to mental health (Rejeski & Thompson, 1993). Moreover, the 1980s, with stores such as the General Nutrition Center (GNC), proliferated the current multibillion dollar a year supplement industry that sold products claiming to provide sundry functions such as adding muscle, reducing fat, and accelerating metabolism. The 1980s also spawned the advent of step aerobics, which continues even today in some fitness facilities. The decades of the 1990s and 2000s saw the increase in mind–body therapeutic techniques in fitness facilities, such as yoga, including hot yoga studios, and pilates. Recent trends in the USA such as cycling classes, sports performance training, and muscle confusion and plyometric-style training (e.g., P90X), supercharged workouts and kettle bells (a cast-iron weight resembling a cannonball with a handle) or BOSU® balls (an inflated rubber hemisphere attached to a rigid platform) have demonstrated the cross-training interplay between cardiorespiratory, resistance, and flexibility to create a total body workout. In addition, many facilities are including fitness and nutrition consultations to foster members exercising outside the gym. The introduction of the Nintendo Wii in 2006 changed how video games are played and even how we exercise. The interactivity of the controllers and the ability to track body movements provide a novel approach to exercising, and a host of fitness games like Wii Fit, Wii Fit Plus, EA Sports Active, and EA Sports Active: More Workouts have been created.

Exercise continues to enjoy tremendous popularity in the USA and, as noted earlier, remains a viable area of pursuit for health care professionals. This chapter examines exercise as a therapeutic tool for the treatment of excessive stress.

Mechanisms of Action

Exercise itself represents an intense form of stress response, yet it differs greatly from the stress response implicated in the onset of psychosomatic disease. Why then is the stress of exercise health promoting, in most instances, and the emotionally related stress of living in a competitive urban environment, for example, health eroding? We now examine the mechanisms that may answer this question.

Three therapeutic mechanisms of action serve to explain the clinical effectiveness of exercise in the treatment of excessive stress.

1. Mechanisms active during exercise.
2. Mechanisms active shortly after exercise.
3. Long-term mechanisms.

The therapeutic mechanisms at work during the acute process of exercising are manifest in the propensity for such physical activity healthfully to utilize the potentially harmful constituents of the stress response. The stress-responsive gluconeogenic hormones (primarily cortisol) begin to break down adipose tissue for energy during the stress response. In this process, a form of fat, called *free fatty acid* (FFA), is released into the bloodstream (Ganong, 2005; Laugero et al. 2011). During the stress of physical exercise, FFA levels actually decline, because the FFA is utilized for energy by the active muscles. In contrast, however, during emotionally related stress, FFA is not utilized as rapidly because of the sedentary nature of this type of stress. The FFA persists in the bloodstream and is converted to triglycerides and, ultimately, to low-density lipoproteins (LDLs). LDLs are considered a major source of atherosclerotic plaque associated with premature coronary artery disease (Greco et al., 2010; Olgac et al. 2011; Sarafino & Smith, 2011).

A second factor to consider during the stress response is the significant demand placed on the cardiovascular and cardiorespiratory systems. Cardiac output (heart rate × stroke volume), blood pressure, and resistance to peripheral blood flow all increase. Also, breathing rate increases and bronchial tubes dilate during the stress response. By the use of moderate physical activity, however, these factors are utilized in a healthful form. Although cardiac output must increase, the rhythmic use of the striated muscles actually assists the return of blood to the heart (increase of venous return). Moreover, physical training allows the body to redistribute blood from less active tissues, such as digestive organs and kidneys, to active muscles, and even to the skin for heat dissipation (Sharkey, 1990; Wilmore, Costill, & Kenney, 2008). Blood pressure must increase during exercise as well, but not so dramatically as is seen when one remains inactive when stressed (e.g., as when sitting in a traffic jam). Regarding respiratory and O_2 transport, physical activity and training improve the efficiency of breathing muscles, allowing greater lung capacity. Thus, a moderately active individual uses fewer breaths to move the same amount of air, which improves diffusion of O_2 into the lungs.

Third, during the stress response, the hormones epinephrine and norepinephrine are released. Research (Dimsdale & Moss, 1980; Fibiger & Singer, 1984; Hoch, Werle, & Weicker, 1988; Lundberg, 2005; Wilmore et al., 2008) has shown that during the stress of exercise, norepinephrine is preferentially released, whereas during emotion-related stress, epinephrine is preferentially released. Circulating epinephrine represents the greatest risk to the integrity of the heart muscle, because the ventricles are maximally responsive to epinephrine, not norepinephrine, so in an individual suffering from heart ischemia, high levels of epinephrine could induce a lethal arrhythmia (Krantz, Quiqley, & O'Callahan, 2001; Lovallo, 2005; McCabe & Schneiderman, 1984). Also, during the stress response, the resistance of blood flow to the skin and other peripheral aspects increases. During the stress of exercise, resistance of blood flow in the skin actually decreases, which has implications for cooling the body and lowering blood pressure [(Duncker & Bache, 2008); also see Ganong (2005), for a discussion of cardiovascular dynamics). Overall, exercise seems to fine-tune the body's secretions and response to hormones, leading to a more efficient use of energy sources (Sharkey, 1990; Wilmore et al. 2008).

The preceding examples are indicative of the different ways the body responds to the stress of exercise in contrast to the stress response that we undergo if we remain static or inactive. Clearly, the acute strain on the body is quite different if one undergoes a stress response in an active rather than inactive state. Although physical activity is capable of using the constituents of the stress response in a constructive manner, the therapeutic reactions may persist beyond the acute period of exercise.

The short-term therapeutic mechanisms associated with exercise entail the initiation of a state of relaxation following the physical activity. In most circumstances, plasma catecholamines return to resting levels within minutes of acute exercise (Mastorakos, Pavlatou, Diamanti-Kandarakis, & Chrousos, 2005). Clearly, exercise itself represents a powerful ergotropic response mediated by the SNS; however, according to Balog (1978), on completion of exercise, the organism may undergo psychophysiological recovery by initiating a trophotropic response mediated by the PNS. According to de Vries (1966), gamma motor neural discharge may also be inhibited during recovery from physical activity. The gamma motor system is a complementary connection from the cerebral cortex to the striated musculature. The result of such inhibition is said to be striated muscle relaxation.

The muscle-relaxant qualities of exercise have important implications for short-term declines in diffuse anxiety and ergotropic tone in autonomic as well as striated muscles. It has been demonstrated that striated muscle tension contributes to diffuse anxiety and arousal in striated and autonomic musculature through a complex feedback system (Gellhorn, 1964a, 1967; Jacobson, 1978). This system involves afferent (incoming) proprioceptive stimulation from striated muscles to the limbic emotional centers, the hypothalamus and cerebral cortex. Therefore, reduction in striated muscle tension should lead to a generalized decrease in ergotropic tone throughout the body, as well as a decrease in diffuse anxiety levels. These results have been demonstrated empirically by Gellhorn (1958a), and de Vries (1968, 1981), and the notion that exercise leads to decreased skeletal muscle tension now appears readily accepted (Foss & Keteyian, 1998; McGuigan & Lehrer, 2007).

Several theoretical rationales have been generated to explain the physiological benefits of physical exercise in reducing stress and anxiety. These include the endorphin hypothesis, which suggests that it is the release and binding of morphine-like endogenous opioids, such as beta endorphin, that affect feelings such as euphoria that have been associated with the anecdotal reports of a runner's high (Cox, 2002; Dishman & O'Connor, 2009). Another hypothesis is the monoamine neurotransmitter theory, or norepinephrine hypothesis, which suggests that the affective benefits of exercise may derive from increased levels of norepinephrine. The thermogenic hypothesis contends that the elevation in body temperature that occurs during exercise leads to decreased stress (Tuson & Sinyor, 1993; Craft & Perna, 2004). Although these theories are readily accepted in this field of study, it is worth noting that none has received conclusive empirical support.

The most significant long-term mechanisms of health promotion inherent in exercise appear to emerge when exercise is aerobic and practiced for a minimum of at least 1 month. One of the areas most positively affected is the ability to use O_2 more efficiently. Exercise training of an aerobic nature increases maximum ventilatory O_2 uptake by increasing both maximum cardiac output (the volume of blood ejected by the heart per minute, which determines the amount of blood delivered to the exercising muscles) and the ability of muscles to extract and use O_2 from blood (Banerjee, Mandal, Chanda, & Chakraborti, 2003; Fletcher et al., 1996). In addition to reduced cardiovascular responses to stress, which lead to long-term, reduced risk of clinical manifestations of coronary heart disease (CHD), recent data suggest that physical activity may help in the prevention and treatment of osteoporosis and certain cancers, most notably colon cancer (Courneya et al., 2007; Fletcher et al.; Knols, Aaronson, Uebelhart, Fransen, & Aufdemkampe, 2005; Mutrie et al., 2007; Valenti et al., 2008). There has been a recent study (Bouchard et al., 2012), however, involving 1,687 exercising participants, in which 10% experienced adverse metabolic responses on at least one measure related to heart disease (blood pressure, levels of insulin, HDL cholesterol, or triglycerides) and 7% experienced adverse metabolic responses to at least two measures. Clearly more research is needed in this area.

Researchers have also continued to investigate the effects of exercise on improved psychological functioning in the areas of anxiety, self-esteem, and most notably depression. DiLorenzo and associates (1999) reported that exercise-induced increases in aerobic fitness using a stationary bicycle resulted in improved short- and long-term effects on the psychological variables of anxiety, depression, self-concept, and vigor. Furthermore, Ekeland, Heian, and Hagen (2005) have shown that exercise interventions can improve self-esteem in children and young people.

Blumenthal and associates (2005), in a randomized control trial of 134 patients with stable ischemic heart disease (IHD) and exercises-induced myocardial ischemia, who were assigned to either a stress management group (16 weeks of 1.5 h/week of a cognitive-social learning model) plus usual care (routine medical care), an exercise group (35 min three times/week for 16 weeks of stationary biking, walking and jogging) plus usual care, or just a usual care group, reported that the exercise training group and stress management training group "exhibited greater improvements in psychosocial functioning, including less emotional distress and lower levels of depression compared with usual control groups" (p. 1632). Other studies specifically assessing anxiety sensitivity, or the belief that anxiety-related sensations can have negative consequences (e.g., lead to panic attacks), have demonstrated the efficacy of brief aerobic exercise regimens in lowering anxiety sensitivity scores compared with non-exercisers or waitlist controls (Broman-Fulks & Storey, 2008; Smits et al., 2008; Smits, Tart, Rosenfield, & Zvolensky, 2011). In a recent review of different treatment approaches to pain-related fear associated with chronic musculoskeletal pain, De Peuter and colleagues (2009) suggested that patients might benefit from graded activity (GA), which is an intervention based on learning principles in which selected behaviors or exercises are shaped through positive reinforcement, combined with education about fear avoidance and challenging irrational beliefs (e.g., catastrophizing).

While efficacy studies related to exercise and anxiety are expanding, the preponderance of intervention studies has investigated the relation between exercise and depression. Herman and colleagues (2002) randomly assigned 156 participants aged 50 years and older who were diagnosed with depression into one of three conditions (medication only, exercise only, and combination of exercise and medication). Their results showed that participants who rated themselves as high on state anxiety or low on life satisfaction were more likely to drop out of treatment prematurely, or if they stayed in the treatment condition, they did not experience amelioration of their depressive symptoms. It was additionally noteworthy that these results were observed across all three of the conditions.

A 2009 Cochrane review of 144 potential studies resulting in a sample of 28 randomized controlled trials (25 of which provided suitable data for meta-analysis) evaluated the effect of exercise (aerobic, resistance, or a mixture of the two) compared with no exercise, CBT, pharmacotherapy and light therapy on symptoms of depression (Mead et al., 2009). For the 23 trials (907 participants) that compared exercise to no treatment or a control condition, the pooled analysis found that exercise had a large clinical treatment effect in reducing depression. However, Meade and colleagues noted that most of the studies analyzed had notable methodological weaknesses. Additional subgroup analyses within the same Cochrane Review revealed that resistance exercise and mixed exercise reduced symptoms of depression more than aerobic exercise alone. Moreover, one study ($N = 23$) included in the Review noted increased improvement in Beck Depression Inventory scores in patients who exercised 3–5 times a week for 30-min sessions compared with patients who only exercised once a week (Legrand & Heuze, 2007). The notion of higher-dose exercising being more effective in alleviating symptoms of depression than lower-dose exercising was further supported in a recent randomized control study (Trivedi et al., 2011).

Despite the noted methodological uncertainties and limitations addressed in the Cochrane Review, exercise is considered to reduce symptoms of depression as effectively as CBT and pharmacotherapy, and should be considered a viable treatment option for patients with symptoms of mild, as compared to moderate-to-severe, depression (Blumenthal et al., 2007; Blumenthal & Ong, 2009; Dinas, Koutedakis, & Flouris, 2011; Gill, Womack, & Safranek, 2010; Hoffman et al., 2010). Blumenthal and Ong (2009) recommend the future use of well-standardized mulitcenter clinical trials to assess the efficacy of exercise on depression, and a more recent meta-analysis has suggested the inclusion of quality of life (QoL) measures to assess further the impact of exercise on symptoms of depression (Schuch, Vasconcelos-Moreno, & Fleck, 2011).

In a systematic meta-analytic review of intervention studies designed to alleviate concomitant depression in elderly patients with osteoarthritis (OA), Yohannes and Caton (2010) reported that four of the seven exercise program studies reviewed evidenced significantly reduced depressive symptoms. One of the studies by Penninx and colleagues (2002) demonstrated that aerobic exercise had a more beneficial clinical effect on depression than did resistance exercise. Yohannes and Caton concluded that future studies should explore the benefits of community-based exercise programs to increase social support, as well as assessing the sustainable effects of exercise programs on depression in OA patients. More recently, Shahidi and colleagues (2011) in a randomized trial of 60 women aged 60 years or older noted the comparable benefits of exercise and Laughter Yoga, which combines yoga breathing, stretching, and laughter, in alleviating depression.

Collectively, it may well be that the long-term physiological and psychological mechanisms of action that support the use of exercise in the treatment and prevention of stress-related disease represent a higher level of physical and psychological fitness and, therefore, a higher level of stress resistance. This higher level of fitness may then aid the individual, both psychologically and physically, in withstanding the potentially injurious effects of excessive stress. One might consider such a level of fitness as a buffer to excessive stress reactivity (Rejeski & Thompson, 1993). Based upon the work of Sime (1984), Weller and Everly (1985), Sharkey (1990), Seraganian (1993), Weyerer and Kupfer (1994), Haskell (1995), Mokdad et al. (2004), and Vuori (2010), we suggest that the stress-resistant aspects of sustained, chronic exercise include the following:

1. Improved cardiorespiratory efficiency.
2. Improved glucose utilization.
3. Reduced body fat.
4. Reduced resting blood pressure.
5. Reduced resting muscle tension.
6. Decreased ANS reactivity.
7. Increased steroid reserves to counter stress.
8. Reduced trait anxiety.
9. Improved self-concept.
10. Improved sense of self-efficacy, physical self-concept, and self-control.

All of these potential alterations are relevant in that they contribute to the individual's ability to tolerate high levels of stress, and, therefore, decrease the likelihood of developing stress-related pathology.

Research Supporting Therapeutic Exercise for Stress

A review of the following current and past literature on the clinical use of exercise in the treatment of excessive stress and stress-related disease provides ample support and rationale for the application of exercise:

1. Full-time employment for men, even in sedentary occupations, is positively associated with measured physical activity compared with men not working (Van Domelen et al., 2011).
2. Promoting physical activity is a common target of worksite health promotion programs for women (Janer & Kogevinas, 2008).
3. Exercise-based cardiac rehabilitation programs are associated with higher return to work rates and improved job satisfaction (Yonezawa et al., 2009).
4. It is estimated that more than 30% of coronary heart disease worldwide is due to physical inactivity, defined as less than 2.5 h/week of moderate exercise or 1 h/week of vigorous exercise (WHO, 2009).
5. In a review by Blair and colleagues (1996), moderately fit male non-smokers had a 41% lower all-cause death rate than those in the corresponding low fit category. Also, moderately fit female non-smokers had a 55% lower all-cause death rate than those who were low fit. Moreover, high fit men with two or three

other risk-factor predictors had a 15% lower death rate than did low fit men with none of the predictors. High fit women with two or three other risk factors had a 50% lower death rate than did low fit women with none of the predictors.

6. Graded exercise therapy (GET), provided alone or in combination with cognitive behavioral therapy (CBT), has been shown to improve physical and emotional functioning in patients with chronic fatigue syndrome (Castell, Kazantis, & Moss-Morris, 2011; Schreurs, Veehof, Passade, & Vollenbroek-Hutten, 2011).

7. Poor fitness is a diagnostic marker in patients with type 2 diabetes, and a meta-analysis of 266 patients who exercised for at least three times/week for 49 min/session for a minimum of 8 weeks (the mean was 20 weeks of exercise) showed an 11.8% increase in peak oxygen uptake (VO_2max) compared with a 1% decrease in the control group (Boule, Kenny, Haddad, Wells, & Sigal, 2003).

8. In a randomized-control trail of 309 patients with rheumatoid arthritis, a two-year intensive exercise program (consisting of cycling, strength training, and volleyball, basketball, football, or badminton two times/week lasting 75 mins) resulted in improved functional ability, emotional status, and a decreased loss of bone minerals (de Jong et al. 2003, 2004) compared with a usual care group.

9. A meta-analysis of 25 randomized controlled trials yielding a total of 1,404 participants revealed that aerobic exercise (of an estimated average of 120 min/ week) resulted in a significant increase in HDL-C level, and that exercise was more effective in patients who exercised for a longer duration, had higher initial total cholesterol levels, and were less obese (BMI < 28) (Kodama et al., 2007).

10. Approximately 15.2% of all deaths in the USA are attributable to poor diet and lack of regular physical activity (Mokdad, Marks, Stroup, & Gerberding, 2005), and in Finland, physical inactivity, smoking, and limited consumption of vegetables were the most important lifestyle behaviors explaining relative educational level differences in cardiovascular and all-cause mortality for men and women (Laaksonen et al., 2008).

11. Engaging in exercise five or more times/week compared with rarely or no exercising was associated with reduced risk of colon cancer among men, whereas sedentary behavior (e.g., watching television) was positively associated with colon cancer (Howard et al., 2008).

12. A cost effectiveness study that assessed physical activity and disease incidence showed that physical activity interventions, compared with no interventions, reduced disease incidence and were cost effective, with dollars per quality-adjusted life year (QALY) gained ratios ranging from $14,000 to $69,000 (Roux et al., 2008).

This section on research may be summarized cogently by the conclusion drawn by Sime (1984) close to 30 years ago: "If stress is defined in the traditional fight-or-flight terminology, then exercise is a classic method of stress management through its active, dynamic release of physiological preparedness" (p. 502).

Exercise Guidelines

Once the decision to exercise has been made, the issue of how much exercise is enough to promote health and better cope with stress needs to be addressed. An acronym often used to account for the ingredients of exercise prescription is FITT, which stands for *F*requency, *I*ntensity, *T*ime (duration), and *T*ype (Foss & Keteyian, 1998). Before beginning an exercise program, it is wise to consider some type of screening or medical evaluation that includes a comprehensive history; a physical exam, including a measure of resting heart rate and blood pressure; blood analysis for fasting blood sugar and cholesterol levels; a measurement of expired gases; a 12-lead resting electrocardiogram (ECG); and an exercise tolerance or stress test with ECG monitoring (American College of Sports Medicine, 2010). Exercise tolerance tests include the Harvard Step Test, the Cooper 12-Minute Test, the Rockport One-Mile Fitness Walking Test, the YMCA protocol, and the Astrand–Ryhming test. These evaluations are useful in determining fitness levels, target heart rates, and maximal aerobic power, and screening for latent abnormalities that may only be evident during physical exertion (Table 15.1).

Returning to the question of how much exercise is enough, the American College of Sports Medicine (ACSM) has been providing minimum guidelines for enhancing cardiorespiratory efficiency since 1975. These recommendations have been based on data on dose–response improvements in performance capacity, especially in maximal aerobic power (maximum O_2 consumption) for otherwise healthy adults of all ages, and apply to adults with chronic diseases or disabilities when evaluated and followed by a health-care professional.

Table 15.1 Estimated Maximum Heart Rates and Exercise Training Heart Rates by Age for Normal Persons

Age	Maximum	Percent		
		70	60	50
21–30	195	159	147	135
31–40	185	152	141	130
41–50	175	145	135	125
51–60	165	138	129	120
61–70	155	131	123	115

Values are listed in beats/minute (bpm), computer using a heart rate of 75 bpm (adapted from Foss & Keteyian, 1998; Topend Sports Network, 2012).

Following these guidelines, Garber and colleagues (2011) from the ACSM, in a special communication in *Medicine & Science in Sports & Exercise,* an official journal of the ACSM, provide the following evidence-based physical exercise recommendations for enhanced cardiorespiratory fitness.

For adults, 150 min of moderate–intensity exercise (65% maximal oxygen uptake; VO_2max) per week that can be met through 30–60 min 5 days/week or 20–60 min of more vigorous-intensity exercise (80% maximal oxygen uptake VO_2max) 3 days/week. Multiple shorter exercise sessions (at least 10 min worth) or one continuous session are both considered adequate to meet the desired amount of daily exercise. Even for those who cannot adhere to these minimum standards, they can still benefit from some form of activity. Increased adherence and decreased injury risk are related to gradual progression of exercise duration, frequency, and intensity.

Exercise sessions for enhancing cardiorespiratory fitness efficiency should be structured using a format that contains a warm-up phase, an exercise phase, and a cool-down phase. Although there is some controversy about whether warming up and cooling down after exercising offers health benefits (Mayo Clinic, 2011), including reducing the number of injuries sustained during physical activity (Fradkin, Gabbe, & Cameron, 2006), since they pose minimal risks, if time allows, it seems worthwhile to implement them. The benefits of the warm-up phase, according to Ribisl (1984), Foss and Keteyian (1998) and Wilmore et al., 2008 include the following:

1. Facilitation of enzymatic activity due to an increase in body and muscle temperature.
2. Increased metabolic activity.
3. Improved blood flow and oxygen delivery.
4. Decreased peripheral resistance.
5. Increased speed of nerve conduction.

Another important component of the warm-up phase is not to begin by immediately stretching a cold muscle. Time should first be taken to do the sport activity at a slow, mild pace for 4–5 min. Foss and Keteyian (1998) suggest that this provides the most physiological benefits and minimizes muscle injuries, such as tears.

The actual aerobic activity itself may include walking, jogging, dance or step aerobics, rollerblading, cycling, and swimming, among others. If these exercise activities are performed according to appropriately prescribed FITT standards, then improved cardiorespiratory efficiency and increased resistance to stress should result. It is important to emphasize that to gauge intensity, standards should be based on heart rate instead of the myth that one must experience pain in order to receive the benefits of training.

The cool-down phase, especially for adults, facilitates venous return. This prevents pooling of blood in the extremities, which reduces the possibility of muscle soreness and cardiovascular strain, and the likelihood of becoming dizzy. The cool-down phase also enhances the removal of lactic acid and other metabolic waste products. This phase, which is the one most likely to be forgotten, is just as important as the two preceding phases for healthful, safe exercising.

Again, these recommendations are for aerobic fitness training, the type of exercise training most often associated with improved cardiovascular health. However, the components of muscular strength, most often associated with anaerobic fitness or resistance training, should also be considered for their potential health benefits. Exercises such as weightlifting, speed skating, and rapid sprinting that require short bursts of "all-out" effort are examples of anaerobic activities. During these types of activities, the body demands more O_2 than can be supplied by the vascular system. Therefore, anaerobic exercises (without O_2), which rely on energy being generated within the muscle by adenosine triphosphate (ATP), creatine phosphate, and the lactic acid (anaerobic glycolysis) system (Greenberg, Dintiman, & Myers-Oakes, 1998), cannot be performed indefinitely.

Although anaerobic activities rely on intensity, frequency, and duration of effort to achieve benefits, intensity (how hard one exercises) is considered the most important factor. Anaerobic performance enhancement typically relies on a process known as interval training, which incorporates the concept of the overload principle. As the name implies, the overload principle requires near maximal intensity in the performance of a series of repeated exercises known as work intervals or sets (e.g., rate, distance, number of repetitions) alternated with periods of relief (e.g., amount of time at rest between intervals, or the performance of some sort of light activity between sets). The number of intervals and periods of relief vary depending on the type of anaerobic activity and the goal of training; however, Garber and colleagues (2011), for general and overall muscular fitness, recommend training each major muscle group (chest, shoulders, back, hips, legs, trunk, and arms) 2 or 3 days each week using a variety of equipment and exercises. Most adults will respond favorably (e.g., hypertrophy and strength gains) to two to four sets of resistance exercises (for each exercise 8–12 repetitions to improve strength and power, 10–15 repetitions to improve strength in middle-aged and older persons just beginning a resistance program, and 15–20 repetitions to improve muscular endurance) per muscle group incorporating 2–3 min rest intervals between each set of exercises. A rest period of 48–72 h between exercise sessions is advisable to promote the cellular/molecular adaptations that foster strength and increased muscle size. Also worth noting is that most aerobic activities can be performed anaerobically by increasing the intensity of effort to approximately 85% or more of the heart rate reserve (Miller & Allen, 1995).

There are many notable benefits to enhancing muscular fitness, including lower risk of all-cause mortality (FitzGerald et al., 2004; Gale, Martyn, Cooper, & Sayer, 2007), improved body composition and image (Greenberg et al., 1998; Sillanpää et al., 2009), improved blood glucose levels (Castaneda, Layne, & Castaneda, 2006; Sigal et al., 2007), improved blood pressure in pre-hypertensive patients (Collier et al., 2008), increased bone density and strength (Kohrt, Bloomfield, Little, Nelson, & Yingling, 2004; Suominen, 2006), and increased energy (Puetz, 2006). These collective benefits serve to enhance an individual's self-concept and increase resistance to stress.

In addition to cardiorespiratory and muscular fitness training recommendations, Garber and her colleagues (2011) provide evidence-based exercise recommendations for the components of flexibility exercise and neuromotor exercise training, and note, as does Wilmore and his colleagues (2008), how all these exercise components can provide valuable health benefits, whether practiced independently or in combination. Even though joint flexibility decreases with age, it is important to incorporate flexibility exercises that have the goal of developing range of motion in the major muscle-tendon groups (shoulder, girdle, chest, neck, trunk, lower back, hips, posterior and anterior legs, and ankles), and to enhance postural stability and balance (particularly when combined with resistance exercises). Garber and colleagues (2011) encourage that flexibility exercises (e.g., static stretching, ballistic or "bouncing" stretching, dynamic stretching or proprioceptive neuromuscular facilitation (PNF)) be done at least 2 or 3 days each week, and should be done when the muscle is warm (either through light aerobic activity or external sources, such as heat packs or taking a hot bath). For static stretching (that may be either active or passive), each stretch should be held for 10–30 s until there is tightness or slight discomfort (there is little benefit from holding for longer durations) and repeated two to four times with the goal of 60s' total time per flexibility exercise.

According to Garber and associates (2011) neuromotor exercise training incorporates motor skills (e.g., balance), coordination, agility, gait, and proprioceptive training, and data show that it has been beneficial in reducing the risk of falls in older adults (Bird, Hill, Ball, Hetherington, & Williams, 2011; Jahnke, Larkey, Rogers, Etnier, & Lin, 2010; Li, Devault, & Van Oteghen, 2007). Examples of neuromuscular training include tai chi, certain forms of yoga, and qigong, which in essence, combine neuromotor exercise, resistance exercise, and flexibility exercise. Studies that have successfully employed neuromotor training incorporated it 2–3 days/week for 20–30 min duration each session. Garber and her colleagues (2011) suggest, however, that more research is needed before making definite recommendations regarding its use.

An additional consideration in developing exercise guidelines concerns adherence issues. Obviously, just providing a fitness program is not enough. The availability of the most modern exercise facilities does not significantly improve exercise adherence. Buckworth and Dishman (2007) have noted some of the major factors affecting exercise adherence:

1. Access to facilities.
2. Perceived availability of time.
3. Social support or reinforcement.
4. Exercise intensity.
5. Self-motivation.
6. History of lack of adherence.

This variety of different factors clearly suggests the multidimensional nature of physical activity determinants in establishing and sustaining exercise adherence.

In their 1995 article, Pate and his colleagues provided a formal and distinctly separate statement regarding *physical activity* and *health*. It is important to note that most exercise regimens have traditionally focused primarily on exercise recommendations and prescriptions for fitness (i.e., cardiorespiratory or muscular). These prescriptive guidelines for improved *general health* were updated in 2007 by the ACSM and the American Heart Association, and Haskell and his colleagues (2007) in this document state that "to promote and maintain health, all healthy adults aged 18–65 years need moderate–intensity aerobic physical activity for a minimum of 30 min on 5 days each week or vigorous-intensity aerobic activity for a minimum of 20 min on 3 days each week. Also, combinations of moderate- and vigorous-intensity activity can be performed to meet this recommendation" (p. 1083). The authors give the example of walking briskly for 30 min two times during the week (moderate intensity) and then jogging for 20 min (vigorous intensity) on two other days of the week as one way to meet the suggested guideline. In addition to these aerobic recommendations, muscle-strengthening activities (lifting weights, weight bearing calisthenics) for a minimum of 2 days each week have been added to the 2007 guidelines. For the estimated 49% of Americans who met neither the aerobic activity nor muscle-strengthening guidelines (National Center for Health Statistics, 2011), it is worth noting that moderate to vigorous routine daily life activities (gardening, carpentry, briskly walking to work) can count toward the recommendations, but they need to occur for at least 10 min.

These guidelines on physical activity for improved health are not meant to detract from the previous exercise recommendations reviewed for fitness. Rather, these current suggestions, based on a comprehensive review of the literature, expand the opportunity for Americans simply to be more active solely for health purposes.

Exercise for Stress Management

It seems that exercise designed for stress management should:

1. Generally be a combination of aerobic and anaerobic training.
2. Exercise should contain rhythmic, coordinated movements rather than random, uncoordinated movements that might place excessive strain on joints or connective tissue.
3. Exercise, from a psychological perspective, should entail a sense of being ego-less; that is, it should either avoid competitive paradigms or allow one to win on every occasion. Part of a stress management strategy may include helping the individual define what winning means. Ideally, exercise for stress management should be exercise for the sake of exercise. Its goals should be intrinsic — self-improvement, ventilation, long-range improvement in somatomotor coordination and motoric skill. Whenever exercise and self-evaluation or self-esteem become intertwined, the healthful characteristics of exercise become more equivocal.

Additional Caveats about Physical Exercise

In this chapter, physical exercise has been discussed as a tool in assisting in stress management. The guidelines are offered *not* as an exercise prescription, but as a model to demonstrate to the clinician the therapeutic considerations associated with exercise. Readers interested primarily in exercise prescription should refer to the American College of Sports Medicine (2010), Garber and colleagues (2011), and Haskell et al. (2007). However, we still offer the following considerations.

- Physical exercise is a potent stressor. Intense exercise stresses both the cardio-respiratory and the musculoskeletal systems.
- Physical exercise has the potential to evoke a greater stress response than any imaginable psychosocial stressor. Although physical exertion does appear to divert most of the potential pathogenic qualities associated with psychophysiolog-ical arousal, the abrupt quantity of arousal during physical exercise can be over-whelming to the cardiorespiratory system. There are many documented cases of individuals who die from cardiac failure while exercising for their health.
- The musculoskeletal system is also vulnerable to the strain of physical exercise. Numerous joint and connective-tissue problems are related to excessive physical exercise. Therefore, it is recommended that persons use only proper equipment and technique when exercising.
- Exercise is an individualistic, unique activity; what works for some may not be right for others. It is always a reasonable idea to have a family physician assess an individual's physiological readiness to participate in an exercise program and then suggest appropriate guidelines.
- The success of an exercise program depends on its consistent utilization. Therefore, the question of motivation arises. It is important for the participant to find an exercise program that is not aversive. A common mistake is that eager individuals overdo an exercise program. The results are, typically, soreness, inju-ries, or the realization that the program too lofty a time commitment. Therefore, people should engage in programs that they will continue. Emphasis should be placed on patience and the need to integrate the exercise program into one's life-style. It may help to locate an exercise partner, one with whom the person can exercise, not compete.
- The cardiovascular, pulmonary, and weight-reducing aspects of an exercise pro-gram will become manifest within several weeks. The therapeutic psychological effects will likely take longer to realize. Therefore, patience is again required.

Summary

In this chapter, the use of physical exercise has been considered for its utility as an instrument in the treatment of excessive stress and its pathological correlates. Let us review the main points:

1. There is ample evidence to suggest that the stress response is nature's way of preparing the human species for muscular exertion. Physical exercise may then represent nature's prescription for how to ventilate healthfully and utilize the initiated stress response.

2. There is also evidence that suppression of the intrinsic need for somatomotor expression that accompanies the stress response may well be pathogenic itself, hence the concept of hypokinetic diseases and related concepts.
3. The idea that exercise can be therapeutic dates back to the fifth century B.C. and the Greek physician Herodicus.
4. In American society, regular exercise is now accepted as a regular part of the lifestyle.
5. Regular exercise appears to be therapeutic by virtue of: for the following reasons:
   - During exercise, constituents of the stress response such as lactic acid, free fatty acid, and epinephrine are utilized in a healthful manner.
   - Upon short-term cessation of exercise, a rebound relaxation effect occurs, which results in feelings of reduced muscle tension and increased feelings of tranquility.
   - Exercise promotes the development of physical and psychological character-istics that appear to facilitate a certain degree of stress resistance, for exam-ple, reduced adipose tissue, electrical stabilization of the myocardium, an improved lipoprotein profile, and improved myocardial strength and physi-cal self-concept.
6. Several theoretical rationales have been proposed to explain the physiological benefits of exercise in reducing stress and anxiety, including the endorphin hypothesis, the epinephrine hypothesis, and the thermogenic hypothesis.
7. The major criteria in designing exercise protocols to enhance fitness involve the acronym FITT—Frequency, Intensity, Time, and Type. Generally accepted, minimum exercise guidelines to achieve fitness for normal healthy adults include performing moderate–intensity exercise at a minimum of 65% of maxi-mum heart rate for at least 150 min/week,
8. Actual exercise sessions should contain warm-up, exercise, and cool-down periods. If exercise is not convenient, supported, and perceived as reinforcing, it will most likely not be sustained.
9. Anaerobic activities may also have stress-resistant benefits.
10. The American College of Sports Medicine and the American Heart Association have issued statements suggesting that health benefits can be attained from the accumulation of 30 or more minutes of moderate–intensity exercise 5 days/week or 20 min of vigorous-intensity activity 3 days/week daily, moderate intensity exercise.

In summary, there is ample research evidence to conclude that physical exercise can promote psychological and physical alterations that are antithetical to the patho-genic processes of excessive stress. It may well be that physical exercise activates a form of coping mechanism unlike that of any other stress management intervention—ventilation/utilization of the stress response before it leads to disease, as depicted in the introduction to Part II.

References

American College of Sports Medicine. (2010). *ACSM's guidelines for exercise testing and prescription* (8th ed.). Philadelphia, PA: Lippincott Williams & Wilkins.

Balog, L. F. (1978). *The effects of exercise on muscle tension and subsequent muscle relaxation.* Unpublished doctoral dissertation, University of Maryland, College Park.

Banerjee, A. K., Mandal, A., Chanda, D., & Chakraborti, S. (2003). Oxidant, antioxidant and physical exercise. *Molecular and Cellular Biochemistry, 253*(1–2), 307–312.

Benson, H. (1975). *The relaxation response.* New York, NY: Morrow.

Bird, M., Hill, K. D., Ball, M., Hetherington, S., & Williams, A. D. (2011). The long-term benefits of a multi-component exercise intervention to balance and mobility in healthy older adults. *Archives of Gerontology and Geriatrics, 52*(2), 211–216.

Blair, S. N., Kampert, J. B., Kohl, H. W., Barlow, C. E., Macera, C. A., Paffenberger, R. S., & Gibbons, L. W. (1996). Influences of cardiorespiratory fitness and other precursors on cardiovascular disease and all-cause mortality in men and women. *Journal of the American Medical Association, 276*(3), 205–210.

Blumenthal, J. A., Babyak, M. A., Doraiswamy, M., Watkins, L., Hoffman, B. M., Barbour, K. A., Herman, S., Craighead, W. E., Brosse, A. L., Waugh, R., Hinderliter, A., & Sherwood, A. (2007). Exercise and pharmacotherapy in the treatment of major depressive disorder. *Psychosomatic Medicine, 69,* 587–596.

Blumenthal, J. A., & Ong, L. (2009). A commentary on "Exercise and Depression" (Mead et al., 2008): And the verdict is…. *Mental Health and Physical Activity, 2*(2), 97–99.

Blumenthal, J. A., Sherwood, A., Babyak, M. A., Watkins, L. L., Waugh, R., Georgiades, A.& Hinderliter, A. (2005). Effects of exercise and stress management training on markers of cardiovascular risk in patients with ischemic heart disease. *Journal of the American Medical Association, 293*(13), 1626–1634.

Bouchard, C., Blair, S. N., Church, T. S., Earnest, C. P., Hagbert, J. M., Häkkinen, K., Rankinen, T. (2012). Adverse metabolic response to regular exercise: Is it a rare or common occurrence? *PLoS One, 7*(5), e37887.

Boule, N. G., Kenny, G. P., Haddad, E., Wells, G. A., & Sigal, R. J. (2003). Meta-analysis of the effect of structured exercise training on cardiorespiratory fitness in Type 2 diabetes mellitus. *Diabetologia, 46,* 1071–1081.

Broman-Fulks, J. J., & Storey, K. M. (2008). Evaluation of a brief aerobic exercise intervention for high anxiety sensitivity. *Anxiety Stress Coping, 21*(2), 117–128.

Buckworth, J., & Dishman, R. K. (2007). Exercise adherence. In G. Tenenbaum & R. C. Eklund (Eds.), *Handbook of sport psychology* (3rd ed., pp. 509–536). Hoboken, NJ: John Wiley & Sons.

Cannon, W. B. (1914). The emergency function of the adrenal medulla in pain and in the major emotions. *American Journal of Physiology, 33,* 356–372.

Cannon, W. B. (1929). *Bodily changes in pain, fear, hunger, and rage.* New York, NY: Appleton.

Castaneda, F., Layne, J. E., & Castaneda, C. (2006). Skeletal muscle sodium glucose co-transporters in older adults with type 2 diabetes undergoing resistance training. *International Journal of Medical Sciences, 3*(3), 84–91.

Castell, B. D., Kazantzis, K., & Moss-Morris, R. E. (2011). Cognitive behavioral therapy and graded exercise for chronic fatigue syndrome: A meta-analysis. *Clinical Psychology: Science and Practice, 18*(4), 311–324.

Chavat, J., Dell, P., & Folkow, B. (1964). Mental factors and cardiovascular disorders. *Cardiologia, 44,* 124–141.

Collier, S. R., Kanaley, J. A., Carhart, R., Jr., Frechette, V., Tobin, M. M., Bennett, N., Fernhall, B. (2008). Cardiac autonomic function and baroreflex changes following 4 weeks of resistance versus aerobic training in individuals with pre-hypertension. *Acta Physiologica, 195*(3), 339–348.

Cooper, K. H. (1977). *The aerobics way: New data on the world's most popular exercise program.* New York, NY: M. Evans.

Courneya, K. S., Segal, R. J., Mackey, J. R., Gelmon, K., Reid, R. D., Friedenreich, C. M., & Kenzie, D. C. (2007). Effects of aerobic and resistance exercise in breast cancer patients receiving adjuvant chemotherapy: A multicenter randomized controlled trial. *Journal of Clinical Oncology, 25*(28), 4396–4404.

Cox, R. H. (2002). *Sport psychology: Concepts and applications.* St. Louis, MO: McGraw-Hill Publishers.

Craft, L. L., & Perna, F. M. (2004). The benefits of exercise of the clinically depressed. *The Primary Care Companion to the Journal of Clinical Psychiatry, 6*(3), 104–111.

de Jong, Z., Munneke, M., Lems, W. F., Zwinderman, A. H., Kroon, H. M., Pauwels, K. J., Hazes, J. M. W. (2004). Slowing of bone loss in pateitns with rheumatoid arthirisi by long-term high-intensity exercise. Results of a randomized, controlled trial. *Arthritis & Rheumatism, 50*(4), 1066–1076.

de Jong, Z., Munneke, M., Zwinderman, A. H., Kroon, H. M., Jansen, A., Ronday, K. H., Hazes, J. M. (2003). Is a long-term high-intensity exercise program effective and safe in patients with rheumatoid arthritis? Results of a randomized controlled trial. *Arthritis & Rheumatism, 48,* 2415–2424.

De Peuter, S., de Jong, J., Crombez, G., & Vlaeyen, J. W. S. (2009). The nature and treatment of pain-related fear in chronic musculoskeletal pain. *Journal of Cognitive Psychotherapy: An International Quarterly, 23*(1), 85–103.

de Vries, H. (1966). *Physiology of exercise.* Dubuque, IA: Brown.

de Vries, H. (1968). Immediate and long-term effects of exercise upon resting muscle action potential level. *Journal of Sports Medicine and Physical Fitness, 8,* 1–11.

de Vries, H. (1981). Tranquilizer effect of exercise. *America's Journal of Physical Medicine, 60,* 57–66.

DiLorenzo, T. M., Bargman, E. P., Stucky-Ropp, R., Brassington, G. S., Frensch, P. A., & LaFontaine, T. (1999). Long-term effects of aerobic exercise on psychological outcomes. *Preventive Medicine, 28,* 75–85.

Dimsdale, J. E., & Moss, J. (1980). Plasma catecholamines in stress and exercise. *Journal of the American Medical Association, 243,* 340–342.

Dinas, P. C., Koutedakis, Y., & Flouris, A. D. (2011). Effects of exercise and physical activity on depression. *Irish Journal of Medical Science, 180,* 319–325.

Dishman, R. K., & O'Commor, J. P. (2009). Lessons in exercise neurobiology: The case of endorphins. *Mental Health Physical Activity, 2*(1), 4–9.

Duncker, D. J., & Bache, R. J. (2008). Regulation of coronary blood flow during exercise. *Physiological Reviews, 88*(3), 1009–1086.

Ekeland, E., Heian, F., & Hagen, K. B. (2005). Can exercise improve self esteem in children and young people? A systematic review of randomized controlled trials. *British Journal of Sports Medicine, 39,* 792–798.

Fibiger, W., & Singer, G. (1984). Physiological changes during physical and psychological stress. *Australian Journal of Psychology, 36,* 317–326.

FitzGerald, S. J., Barlow, C. E., Kampert, J. B., Morrow, J. R., Jackson, A. W., & Blair, S. N. (2004). Muscular fitness and all-cause mortality: Prospective observations. *Journal of Physical Activity and Health, 1,* 7–18.

Fixx, J. F. (1977). *The complete book of running.* New York, NY: Random House.

Fletcher, G. F., Balady, G., Blair, S. N., Blumenthal, J., Caspersen, C., & Chaitman, B., Pollock, M. L. (1996). Statement on exercise: Benefits and recommendations for physical activity programs for all Americans: A statement for health professionals by the committee on exercise and cardiac rehabilitation of the Council on Clinical Cardiology, American Heart Association. *Circulation, 94,* 857–862.

Foss, M. L., & Keteyian, S. J. (1998). *Fox's physiological basis for exercise and sport* (6th ed.). Boston, MA: McGraw-Hill.

Fradkin, A. J., Gabbe, B. J., & Cameron, P. A. (2006). Does warming up prevent injury in sport?:The evidence from randomised controlled trials? *Journal of Science and Medicine in Sport, 9*(3), 214–220.

Gale, C. R., Martyn, C. N., Cooper, C., & Sayer, A. A. (2007). Grip strength, body composition, and mortality. *International Journal of Epidemiology, 36*(1), 228–235.

Ganong, W. F. (2005). *Review of medical physiology* (22nd ed.). New York, NY: McGraw-Hill.

Garber, C. E., Blissmer, B., Deschernes, M. R., Franklin, B. A., Lamonte, M. J., Lee, I.-M., & Swain, D. P. (2011). Quantity and quality of exercise for developing and maintaining cardio-respiratory, musculoskeletal, and neuromotor fitness in apparently healthy adults: Guidance for prescribing exercise. *Medicine & Science in Sports & Exercise, 43*(7), 1334–1359.

Gellhorn, E. (1958a). The physiological basis of neuromuscular relaxation. *Archives of Internal Medicine, 102*, 392–399.

Gellhorn, E. (1964a). Motion and emotion. *Psychological Review, 71*, 457–472.

Gellhorn, E. (1967). *Principles of autonomic-somatic integrations.* Minneapolis, MN: University of Minnesota Press.

Gill, A., Womack, R., & Safranek, S. (2010). Does exercise alleviate symptoms of depression? *The Journal of Family Practice, 59*(9), 530–531.

Greco, T. P., Conti-Kelly, A. M., Anthony, J. R., Greco, T., Jr., Doyle, R., & Boisen, M., Lopez, L. R., (2010). Oxidized-LDL/β_2-Glycoprotein I complexes are ssociated with disease severity and increased risk for adverse outcomes in patients with acute coronary syndromes. *American Journal of Clinical Pathology, 133*, 737–743.

Green, H. (1986). *Fit for America: Health, fitness, sport, and American society.* New York, NY: Pantheon Books.

Greenberg, J. S., Dintiman, G. B., & Myers-Oakes, B. (1998). *Physical fitness and wellness* (2nd ed.). Boston, MA: Allyn & Bacon.

Haskell, W. L. (1995). Physical activity in the prevention and management of coronary heart disease. *Physical Activity and Fitness Research Digest, 2*, 1–8.

Haskell, W. L., Lee, I.-M, Pate, R. P., Powell, K. E., Blair, S. N., Franklin, B. A., & Bauman, A. (2007). Physical activity and public health: Updated recommendations for adults from the American College of Sports Medicine and the American Heart Association. *Circulation, 116*, 1081–1093.

Herman, S., Blumenthal, J. A., Babyak, M., Khatri, P., Craighead, W. E., Krishnan, K. R. & Doraiswamy, P. M. (2002). Exercise therapy for depression in middle-aged and older adults: Predictors of early dropout and treatment failure. *Health Psychology, 21*, 553–563.

Hoch, F., Werle, E., & Weicker, H. (1988). Sympathoadrenergic regulation in elite fencers in training and competition. *International Journal of Sports Medicine, 9*, 141–145.

Hoffman, B. M., Babyak, M. A., Craighead, W. E., Sherwood, A., Doraiswamy, P. M., Coons, M. J., & Blumenthal, J. A. (2010). Exercise and pharmacotherapy in patients with major depression: One-year follow-up of the SMILE study. *Psychosomatic Medicine, 73*, 127–133.

Howard, R. A., Freedman, D. M., Park, Y., Hollenbeck, A., Schatzkin, A., & Letizman, M. F. (2008). Physical activity, sedentary behavior, and the risk of colon and rectal cancer in the NIH-AARP Diet and Health Study. *Cancer Causes & Control, 19*(9), 939–953.

Jacobson, E. (1978). *You must relax.* New York, NY: McGraw-Hill.

Jahnke, R., Larkey, L., Rogers, C., Etnier, J., & Lin, F. (2010). A comprehensive review of health benefits of qigong and tai chi. *American Journal of Health Promotion, 52*(2), 211–216.

Janer, G., & Kogevinas, M. (2008). Promoting physical activity and a healthy diet among working women. In A. Linos & K. Wilhem (Eds.), *Promoting health for working women* (pp. 319–332). New York, NY: Springer Science + Business Media.

Knols, R., Aaronson, N. K., Uebelhart, D., Fransen, J., & Aufdemkampe. (2005). Physical exercise in cancer patients during and after medical treatment: A systematic review of randomized and controlled trials. *Journal of Clinical Oncology, 23*(6), 3830–3842

Kodama, S., Tanaka, S., Saito, K., Shu, M., Sone, Y., Onitake, F., Sone, H. (2007). Effect of aerobic exercise training on serum levels of high-density lipoprotein cholesterol. *Archives of Internal Medicine, 167*(10), 999–1008.

Kohrt, W. M., Bloomfield, S. A., Little, K. D., Nelson, M. E., & Uingling, V. R. (2004). American College of Sports Medicine. Position Stand: Physical activity and bone health. *Medical Science and Sports Exercise, 36*(11), 1985–1996.

Krantz, D. S., Quigley, J. F., & O'Callahan, M. (2001). Mental stress as a trigger of acute cardiac events: The role of laboratory studies. *Italian Heart Journal: Official Journal of the Italian Federation of Cardiology, 2*(12), 895–899.

Kraus, H., & Raab, W. (1961). *Hypokinetic disease.* Springfield, IL: Charles C. Thomas.

Laaksonen, M., Talala, K., Martelin, T., Rahkonen, O., Roos, E., Helakorpi, S., … Prättälä, R. (2008). Health behaviors as explanations for educational level differences in cardiovascular and all-cause mortality: A follow-up of 60,000 men and women over 23 years. *The European Joural of Public Health, 18*(1), 38–43

Laugero, K. D., Smilowitz, J. T., German, J. B., Jarcho, M. R., Mendoza, S. P., & Bales, K. L. (2011). Plasma omega 3 polyunsaturated fatty acid status and monounsaturated fatty acids are altered by chronic social stress and predict endocrine responses to acute stress in titi monkeys. *Prostaglandins, Leukotrienes and Essential Fatty Acides, 84*, 71–78.

Legrand, F., & Heuze, J. P. (2007). Antidepressant effects associated with different exercise conditions in participants with depression: A pilot study. *Journal of Sport and Exercise Psychology, 29*, 348–364.

Let's Move! (n.d.). *Learn the facts.* Retrieved from http://www.letsmove.gov/learn-facts/epidemic-childhood-obesity

Li, Y., Devault, C. N., & Van Oteghen, S. (2007). Effects of extended tai chi intervention on balance and selected motor functions of the elderly. *The American Journal of Chinese Medicine, 35*(3), 383–391.

Lovallo, W. R. (2005). *Stress & health: Biological and psychological interactions* (2nd ed.). Thousand Oaks, CA: Sage Publications.

Lundberg, U. (2005). Stress hormones in health and illness: The roles of work and gender. *Psychoneuroendocrinology, 30*(10), 1017–1021.

Mastorakos, G., Pavlatou, M., Diamanti-Kandarakis, E., & Chrousos, G. P. (2005). Exercise and the stress system. *Hormones, 4*(2), 73–89.

Mayo Clinic Staff. (n.d.). Aerobic exercise: How to warm up and cool down. http://www.mayoclinic.com/health/exercise/SM00067. Retrieved June 8, 2011

McCabe, P., & Schneiderman, N. (1984). Psychophysiologic reactions to stress. In N. Schneiderman & J. Tapp (Eds.), *Behavioral medicine* (pp. 3–32). Hillsdale, NJ: Erlbaum.

McGuigan, F. J., & Lehrer, P. M. (2007). Progressive relaxation: Origins, principles, and clinical applications. In P. M. Lehrer, R. L. Woolfolk, & W. E. Sime (Eds.), *Principles and practices of stress management* (3rd ed., pp. 57–87). New York: Guilford.

Mead, G. E., Morley, W., Campbell, P., Greig, C. A., McMurdo, M., & Lawlor, D. A. (2009). Exercise for depression. *Cochrane Database of Systematic Reviews.* Issue 3. Art. No.:CD004366.

Miller, D. K., & Allen, T. E. (1995). *Fitness: A lifetime commitment* (5th ed.). Boston: Allyn & Bacon.

Mokdad, A. H., Marks, J. S., Stroup, D. F., & Gerberding, J. L. (2004). Actual causes of death in the United States, 2000. *Journal of the American Medical Association, 291*, 1238–1245.

Mokdad, A. H., Marks, J. S., Stroup, D. F., & Gerberding, J. L. (2005). Correction: Actual Causes of Death in the United States, 2000. *Journal of the American Medical Association, 293*(3), 293–294.

Mutrie, N., Campbell, A. M., Whyte, F., McConnachie, A., Emslie, C., Lee, L., … Ritchie, D. (2007). Benefits of supervised programme for women being treated for early stage breast cancer: Pragmatic randomized controlled trial. *BMJ, 334,* 517

National Center for Health Statistics. (2011). Health, United States, 2011: With special feature on socioeconomic and health. Hyattsville, MD

Nesse, R. M., Bhatnager, S., & Young E. A. (2007). Evolutionary origins and functions of the stress response. *Encyclopedia of Stress* (2nd ed.), *1*, 965–970

Olgac, U., Knight, K., Poulikakos, D., Saur, S. C., Alkadhi, H., Desbiolles, L. M., Cattin, P. C., & Kurtcuoglu, V. (2011). Computed high concentrations of low-density lipoprotein correlate with plaque locations in human coronary arteries. *Journal of Biomechanics, 44*(13), 2466–2471.

Pate, R. R., Pratt, M., Blair, S. N., Haskell, W. L., Macera, C. A., Bouchard, C., Buchner, D., Ettinger, W., Heath, G. W., King, A. C., Kriska, A., Leon, A. S., Marcus, B. H., Morris, J., Paffenbarger, R. S., Partrick, K., Pollock, M. L., Rippe, J. M., Sallis, J., & Wilmore, J. H. (1995). Physical activity and public health: A recommendation from the centers for disease control and prevention and the American College of Sports Medicine. *Journal of the American Medical Association, 273*, 402–407.

Penninx, B. W., Rejeski, W. J., Pandya, J., Miller, M. E., Di Bari, M., Appelgate, W. B., & Pahor, M. (2002). Exercise and depressive symptoms: A comparison of aerobic and resistance exercise effects on emotional and physical function in older persons with high and low depressive symptomatology. *Journal of Gerontology: Psychological Sciences, 57B*(2), P124–P132.

Puetz, T. W. (2006). Physical activity and feelings of energy and fatigue: Epidemiological evidence. *Sports Medicince, 36*(9), 767–780.

Rejeski, W. J., & Thompson, A. (1993). Historical and conceptual roots of exercise psychology. In P. Seraganian (Ed.), *Exercise psychology: The influence of physical exercise on psychological processes* (pp. 3–35). New York: Wiley.

Ribisl, P. (1984). Developing an exercise prescription for health. In N. Miller, J. D. Matarazzo, S. W. Weiss, A. J. Herd, & S. M. Weiss (Eds.), *Behavioral health* (pp. 448–466). New York: Wiley.

Roux, L., Pratt, M., Tnegs, T. O., Yore, M. M., Yanagawa, T. L., Van Den Bos, J., ... Buchner, D. M. (2008). Cost effectiveness of community-based physical activity interventions. *American Journal of Preventive Medicine, 35*(6), 578–588

Ryan, A. (1974). A history of sports medicine. In A. Ryan & F. Allman (Eds.), *Sports medicine* (pp. 1–3). New York: Academic Press.

Sarafino, E. P., & Smith, T. W. (2011). *Health psychology: Biopsychosocial interactions* (7th ed.). Hoboken, NJ: Wiley.

Schreurs, K. M. G., Veehof, M. M., Passade, L., & Vollenbroek-Hutten, M. M. R. (2011). *Behavior Research and Therapy, 49*(12), 908–913.

Schuch, F. B., Vasconcelos-Moreno, M. P., & Fleck, M. P. (2011). The impact of exercise on quality of life within exercise and depression trials: A systematic review. *Mental Health and Physical Activity, 4*(2), 43–48.

Seraganian, P. (1993). *Exercise psychology: The influence of physical exercise on psychological processes.* New York: Wiley.

Shahidi, M., Mojtahed, A., Modabbernia, A., Motjahed, M., Shafiabady, A., Delavar, A., & Honari, H. (2011). Laughter Yoga versus group exercise program in elderly depressed women: A randomized controlled trial. *International Journal of Geriatric Psychiatry, 26*, 322–327.

Sharkey, B. J. (1990). *Physiology of fitness* (3rd ed.). Champaign, IL: Human Kinetics.

Sigal, R. J., Kenny, G. P., Boulé, N. G., Wells, G. A., Prud'homme, D., Fortier, M., ... Jaffey, J. (2007). Effects of aerobic training, resistance training, or both on glycemic control in type 2 diabetes: A randomized trial. *Annals of Internal Medicine, 147*(6), 357–369

Sillanpää, E., Laaksonen, D. E., Häkkinen, A., Karavirta, L., Jensen, B., Kraemer, W. J., ... Häkkinen, K. (2009). Body composition, fitness, and metabolic health during strength and endurance training and their combination in middle-aged and older women. *European Journal of Applied Physiology, 106*(2), 285–296

Sime, W. (1984). Psychological benefits of exercise training in the healthy individual. In J. Matarazzo, S. Weiss, J. Heid, N. Miller, & S. Weiss (Eds.), *Behavioral health* (pp. 488–508). New York: Wiley.

Simon, H. B., & Levisohn, S. R. (1987). *The athlete within: A personal guide to total fitness.* Boston: Little, Brown.

Smith, J. C. (2002). *Stress management: A comprehensive handbook of techniques and strategies.* New York, NY: Springer Publishing Company.

Smits, J. A., Berry, A. C., Rosenfield, D., Powers, M. B., Behar, E., & Ott, M. W. (2008). Reducing anxiety sensitivity with exercise. *Depression and Anxiety, 25*, 689–699.

Smits, J. A., Tart, C. D., Rosenfield, D., & Zvolensky, M. J. (2011). The interplay between physical activity and anxiety sensitivity in fearful responding to carbon dioxide challenge. *Psychosomatic Medicine, 73*(6), 498–503.

Suominen, H. (2006). Muscle training for bone strength. *Aging Clinical and Experimental Research, 18*(2), 85–93.

Topend Sports Network. (2012): http://www.topendsports.com/fitness/heartrate-range.htm

Trivedi, M. H., Greer, T. L., Church, T. S., Carmody, T. J., Grannemann, B. D., Galper, D. I., … Blair, S. N. (2011). Exercise as an augmentation treatment for nonremitted major depression disorder: A randomized, parallel dose comparison. *Journal of Clinical Psychiatry, 72*(5), 677–684

Tuson, K. M., & Sinyor, D. (1993). On the affective benefits of acute exercise: Taking stock after twenty years of research. In P. Seraganian (Ed.), *Exercise psychology: The influence of physical exercise on psychological processes* (pp. 80–121). New York: Wiley.

Valenti, M., Porzio, G., Ailli, F., Verna, L., Cannita, K., Manno, R., … Ficorella, C. (2008). Physical exercise and quality of life in breast cancer survivors. *International Journal of Medical Sciences, 5*(1), 24–28

Van Domelen, D. R., Koster, A., Caserotti, P., Brychta, R. J., Chen, K. Y., McClain, J. J., & Harris, T. B. (2011). Employment and physical activity in the U.S. *American Journal of Preventive Medicine, 41*(2), 136–145

Vuori, I. (2010). Physical activity and cardiovascular disease prevention in Europe: An update. *Kinesiology, 42*(1), 5–15.

Warburton, D. E. R., Nicol, C. W., & Bredin, S. S. D. (2006). Health benefits of physical activity: The evidence. *Canadian Medical Association Journal, 174*(6), 801–809.

Weller, D., & Everly, G. S., Jr. (1985). Occupational health through physical fitness programming. In G. S. Everly & R. Feldman (Eds.), *Occupational health promotion* (pp. 127–146). New York: Macmillan.

Weyerer, S., & Kupfer, B. (1994). Physical exercise and psychological health. *Sports Medicine, 17*, 108–116.

White House Task Force on Childhood Obesity. (2010, May). *Solving the problem of childhood obesity within a generation: White House task force on childhood obesity report to the President.* Available from http://www.letsmove.gov/sites/letsmove.gov/files/TaskForce_on_Childhood_Obesity_May2010_FullReport.pdf

Wilmore, J. H., Costill, D. L., & Kenney, W. L. (2008). *Physiology of sport and exercise* (4th ed.). Champaign, IL: Human Kinetics.

World Health Organization (WHO). (2009). *Global health risks: Mortality and burden of disease attributable to selected major risks.* Genenva: World Health Organization.

World Health Organization (WHO). (2012). Physical inactivity: A global public health problem. Retrieved from http://www.who.int/dietphysicalactivity/factsheet_inactivity/en/index.html

Yohannes, A. M., & Caton, S. (2010). Management of depression in older people with osteoarthritis: A systematic review. *Aging & Mental Health, 14*(6), 637–651.

Yonezawa, R., Masuda, T., Matsunaga, A., Takahashi, Y., Saitoh, M., Ishii, A., … Izumi, T. (2009). Effects of phase II cardiac rehabilitation on job stress and health-related quality of life after return to work in middle-aged patients with acute myocardial infarction. *International Heart Journal, 50*, 279–290.

Chapter 16
The Pharmacological Management of Stress Reactions

Jason M. Noel
University of Maryland School of Pharmacy, 655 West Baltimore Street, Baltimore, MD 21201, USA

Judy L. Curtis
Sunovion Pharmaceuticals, 2542 Quarry Lake Drive, Baltimore, MD 21209, USA

The use of drug therapies in the management of acute stress reactions and chronic stress-related disorders has emerged as understanding of the pathophysiology of these conditions has become better understood. The general approach to treatment has evolved from the use of predominantly rapid-acting sedative agents for the treatment of acute anxiety attacks, to the more frequent use of agents to control the underlying anxiety disorder.

With most psychiatric conditions, conservative strategies for treatment should be employed before more restrictive interventions, such as drug therapies, are used. In the case of stress arousal, relaxation therapies that promote the development of the client's own response mechanisms should be attempted if his or her condition is responsive to such techniques. Cognitive-behavioral therapies, structured breathing, neuromuscular relaxation, and clinical hypnosis (see Chaps. 8, 11, 12, and 13) are generally preferred over drug therapy in situations where clients respond to these treatments, because these methods avoid the potential dependency problems and adverse effects of pharmacological agents.

However, there are instances in which drug therapy is appropriate for treatment of excessive stress. Drug therapy is a useful adjunct for the treatment of panic attacks associated with panic disorder and social phobia, increased arousal and traumatic recall associated with PTSD, and anxiety and compulsive behaviors associated with obsessive–compulsive disorder (OCD).

The present chapter reviews the major classes of pharmacological agents used in the treatment of pathological stress arousal states. Indications and target symptoms (i.e., the undesired physiological states that may be reversible with treatment) are discussed, along with potential problems associated with these agents—adverse effects, dependency liabilities, and drug interactions. We begin with a basic discussion of psychotropic drug pharmacology.

G.S. Everly and J.M. Lating, *A Clinical Guide to the Treatment* 317
of the Human Stress Response, DOI 10.1007/978-1-4614-5538-7_16,
© Springer Science+Business Media New York 2013

Pharmacology

Psychotropic drugs exert various effects in the CNS. Most currently available psychotropic medications modulate the activity of neurotransmitters in the brain. Neurotransmitters are small molecules or peptides that carry signals between neurons, i.e., across synapses, the gaps between adjacent nerve cells. Receptors located on pre- and postsynaptic neuronal membranes are the targets for the activity of neurotransmitters and certain drugs.

Norepinephrine (NE), for example, is a monoamine neurotransmitter that has important functions in both the central and peripheral nervous systems. In the brain, several noradrenergic neuronal tracts have been identified, most of which originate in the locus ceruleus. These noradrenergic pathways modulate mood, attention, energy, motor movements, and autonomic functions such as blood pressure control and perspiration. Peripherally, norepinephrine plays a major role in the somatic manifestations of the acute stress response. Elevations in heart rate and urinary retention are mediated by noradrenergic projections from the spinal cord.

Serotonin (5-HT) is an abundant neurotransmitter derived from the dietary amino acid tryptophan. Cell bodies for the serotonergic neurons in the brain are concentrated in the raphe nuclei. Projections from the raphe nuclei are involved in the regulation of mood, motor activity, appetite, sleep, and sexual functioning. Anxiety and panic are also regulated by CNS serotonergic projections. Serotonin release is controlled, in part, by its interactions with norepinephrine, which can either enhance or inhibit serotonin release through interconnecting pathways in the brain stem and the cortex.

Gamma-aminobutyric acid (GABA) is an amino acid derivative that serves as the major inhibitory neurotransmitter in the CNS. It has several functions associated with CNS inhibition, including anxiolytic activity, anticonvulsant activity, sleep promotion, and muscle relaxation. Upon ligand signaling to the GABA-ergic neuron, a very rapid neuronal inhibition is produced. The operation of this mechanism may play an important role in mediating the sensation of anxiety and the initiation of the relaxation response.

Many specific biochemical abnormalities have been identified in psychiatric illnesses. For example, an excess of dopamine neurotransmission in the mesolimbic tract has been correlated with the presence of positive symptoms (e.g., hallucinations and delusions) in patients with schizophrenia. Major depression is felt to be due, in part, to a relative deficiency of serotonin, norepinephrine, and dopamine. Similarly, anxiety states have been associated with an excess of norepinephrine discharge in the locus ceruleus and a relative deficiency of GABA neurotransmission. It is important to note, however, that the identification of these neurotransmitter abnormalities does not necessarily suggest any underlying pathology. In fact, most mental illnesses develop as a result of a combination of genetic, neurodevelopmental, environmental, and social factors.

Current drug therapy, while not always addressing the underlying causes for these mental illnesses, can symptomatically treat these disorders through its effects on the various neurotransmitter systems. There are several mechanisms by which drugs can modulate neurotransmission in the CNS:

- Direct agonist activity at pre- and postsynaptic receptors.
- Facilitation of the release of stored neurotransmitters.
- Inhibition of presynaptic neurotransmitter reuptake.
- Inhibition of enzymatic neurotransmitter degradation.
- Inhibition of neurotransmitter synthesis and storage.
- Alteration of feedback mechanisms modulating neurotransmitter release.
- Alteration of receptor or ion channel binding sites, leading to facilitation or inhibition of neurotransmission.

With the exception of the sedatives–hypnotics, and stimulant treatments used for attention deficit/hyperactivity disorder, therapeutic effects of psychotropic drug therapy generally occur after several weeks of continuous dosing. Changes in synaptic neurotransmitter concentration tend to lead to altered sensitivity and concentrations of the postsynaptic receptors. These changes occur over the course of several weeks, resulting in the delay in clinical response. Since adverse effects of psychotropic agents are usually most severe at the onset of therapy, a delayed therapeutic response significantly compromises patient adherence to treatment. This is an especially significant consideration when dealing with manifestations of excessive stress, when the patient needs immediate relief from the discomfort associated with the disorder and has little tolerance for side effects. Fortunately, there are many agents available, and while not being optimal for long-term treatment, they can provide a faster onset of symptom resolution.

Many CNS depressants, including sedatives–hypnotics, have a more direct mechanism of action, leading to a more immediate therapeutic effect. While this type of pharmacological profile maybe more desirable to patients, problems with dependence and adverse effects associated with CNS depression make the agents most useful for short-term intervention.

The following sections of this chapter review the classes of drugs used in the treatment of disorders characterized by excessive stress. The mechanisms of action, indications, adverse effects, expected therapeutic outcomes, and relevant drug interactions are described. Our objective is to provide a basic familiarity with the concepts and the role of drug treatment for stress.

Benzodiazepines

The benzodiazepines are a widely used class of medications for the treatment of anxiety disorders and stress reactions. This class of drugs includes diazepam (Valium®), lorazepam (Ativan®), oxazepam (Serax®), alprazolam (Xanax®), clorazepate (Tranxene®), and chlordiazepoxide (Librium®).

Other drugs in this class that are used primarily for sleep disturbances include triazolam (Halcion®), flurazepam (Dalmane®), estazolam (ProSom®), and temazepam

Table 16.1 Comparative characteristics of benzodiazepines

Drug	Dosage range (mg/day)	Duration of action ($t_{1/2}$) in hours	Onset of action (oral absorption)
Alprazolam (Xanax®)	0.25–4.0	12–15	Intermediate
Clonazepam (Klonopin®)	0.5–12.0	18–50	Intermediate
Clorazepate (Tranxene®)	7.5–60.0	Metabolite-dependent Desmethyldiazepam (30–200) Oxazepam (3–21)	Fast
Chlordiazepoxide (Librium®)	10–100	5–30 Demoxepam (14–95) Desmethylchlordiazepoxide (18)	Intermediate
Diazepam (Valium®)	5–60	20–50 Desmethyldiazepam (30–200) 3-Hydroxydiazepam (5–20) Oxazepam (3–21)	Fastest
Lorazepam (Ativan®)	2–16	10–20	Intermediate
Oxazepam (Serax®)	15–60	3–21	Intermediate

(Restoril®). Other related sedative anxiolytic drugs, including the barbituates, meprobamate, chloral hydrate, gluthethimide and ethchlorvynol, are older agents with significant toxicity profiles that are no longer widely used.

The benzodiazepines are all identical in their mechanism of action, and the only differences among them lie in their pharmacokinetic properties (absorption, metabolism, and elimination half-life) (Grimsley, 1995). Table 16.1 lists pharmacokinetic differences and usual therapeutic doses. The benzodiazepines work by enhancing GABA in the brain. These agents have four therapeutic effects—antianxiety, sedative–hypnotic, muscle relaxant, and anticonvulsant. Typically, sedative effects are seen at lower doses. Anxiolytic, muscle relaxant, and anticonvulsant effects are seen at moderate doses. At high doses, benzodiazepines can be used to induce sleep.

In the treatment of anxiety, benzodiazepines are most appropriately used for the treatment of acute panic attacks and to treat residual symptoms not controlled with other agents, such as antidepressants (American Psychiatric Association, 2004, 2009). Certain longer acting benzodiazepines (e.g., clonazepam, diazepam) are approved for long-term use in the prevention of anxiety symptoms such as those seen in panic disorder and generalized anxiety disorder. However, chronic use may lead to tolerance, the phenomenon whereby a certain fixed dose loses its effectiveness over time. Patients may try to counteract this by increasing their own dose, potentially leading to physical dependence, addiction, and abuse. Continued use of the drugs may also result in more difficult withdrawal (discussed below).

Choice of agents depends on the clinical state of the individual for whom they are prescribed. Benzodiazepines with shorter half-lives, such as lorazepam, alprazolam, and oxazepam, may be most useful for persons requiring limited treatment for acute anxiety due to a stressful situation. Those with longer half-lives, such as diazepam, clonazepam, clorazepate, and chlordiazepoxide, may be better for persons requiring longer therapy for chronic anxiety. Shorter-acting agents may also be preferred for the elderly or those with impaired liver function. These individuals would be more prone to adverse effects from drug accumulation, such as over sedation (American Geriatrics Society, 2012; Hamilton, Gallagher, Ryan, Byrne, & O'Mahony, 2011).

Side effects of the benzodiazepines include sedation, confusion, amnesia, unsteady gait, and lethargy. They are relatively safe on overdose except when combined with other CNS-depressant drugs such as alcohol or other sedatives–hypnotics. The most serious problem with benzodiazepine therapy can be serious withdrawal reactions, the result of physical dependence. Physical dependence may occur after 4–6 months with usual doses or more rapidly, 2–3 weeks, with high doses (Brown, Rakel, Wells, Downs, & Akiskal, 1993). Withdrawal symptoms are frequently the opposite of the usual therapeutic effects of the benzodiazepines. Psychological symptoms include irritability, insomnia, feelings of apprehension, and dysphoria. Physical symptoms may include tremor, palpitations, dizziness, muscle spasm, and sweating. Perceptual symptoms include hypersensitivity to sound, light, and touch, and depersonalization. In severe situations, seizures may occur. Withdrawal symptoms can be minimized by using a slow taper (i.e., a gradual dose reduction over 4–16 weeks, depending on the starting dose and duration of therapy). Adjunctive therapy may be needed, such as beta-blocking agents or sedating antidepressants. Benzodiazepines should never be discontinued abruptly unless serious side effects warrant the risk of withdrawal.

Antidepressants

Antidepressant agents are so named because drugs possessing the common pharmacology of these agents are traditionally used in the treatment of depressive disorders. All currently available antidepressants facilitate neurotransmission of serotonin, norepinephrine, and/or dopamine. However, the exact neuronal targets (e.g., enzymes, reuptake pumps, and autoreceptors) differ from class to class. It is interesting to note, however, that despite the wide array of mechanisms of action of the antidepressants, no agent or class of drugs has been shown to be more consistently efficacious in the treatment of depression. Drug choice is based on presenting symptoms and adverse effect profile, among other clinical factors. However, in the treatment of anxiety states, the pharmacological profiles of the agents determine the spectrum of disorders for which the drugs are likely to be effective.

Antidepressant-associated increases in serotonin (5-HT) and norepinephrine (NE) neurotransmission may have effects other than their direct benefits in affective and somatic manifestations of depression and anxiety. Increasing evidence suggests that by increasing NE and 5-HT neurotransmission in the neurons of the hippocampus, the nerve damage induced by chronic stress can be reversed. The expression of neurotrophic factors that serve to promote neuronal survival and growth in the CNS is decreased during stress. Antidepressant treatment may reverse these changes by upregulating neurotrophic-factor expression (Duman, Malberg, & Thome, 1999; Hellweg, Ziegenhorn, Heuser, & Deuschle, 2008).

The antidepressant drugs are classified by pharmacological mechanism or chemical structure (see Table 16.2). The monoamine oxidase inhibitors (MAOIs) and the tricyclics were the first classes of antidepressants developed. The selective serotonin reuptake inhibitors (SSRIs) and various other agents with novel mechanisms of action were later introduced to address the tolerability issues of the earlier drugs, and have supplanted the older agents as the drugs of choice for stress-related conditions.

Monoamine Oxidase Inhibitors (MAOIs)

Phenylzine (Nardil®) and tranylcypromine (Parnate®) work by irreversibly inhibiting the enzyme that degrades monoamine neurotransmitters. As a result, the concentration of NE and other catecholamines is increased in the synaptic cleft, thereby facilitating neurotransmission.

The benefits of MAOI therapy in the treatment of depression and stress-related disorders are significant. These agents are considered to be very effective in the prevention of panic attacks associated with panic and social anxiety disorder. In clinical trials, 60–70% of patients with panic and social anxiety disorder show significant decreases in the frequency of panic attacks after 8–12 weeks of MAOI therapy (Spiegel, Wiegel, Baker, & Greene, 2000).

However, due to significant food and drug interactions associated with treatment, MAOIs are not currently employed as first- or second-line agents. By irreversibly inhibiting monoamine oxidase, MAOIs subject the patient to a prolonged inability to metabolize tyramine, an amino acid found in aged cheeses, red wines, and cured meats. Elevated levels of tyramine can cause a life-threatening syndrome of elevated blood pressure, palpitations, and hyperthermia. These effects may be avoided by adopting a diet with very low levels of tyramine and avoiding the use of drugs with sympathomimetic effects (e.g., over-the-counter decongestants); however, most clinicians prefer to first use drugs with a better safety profile, avoiding these concerns, unless absolutely necessary.

Tricyclic Antidepressants (TCAs)

The TCAs are a fairly large group of structurally and pharmacologically similar drugs. The therapeutic effects of these agents are thought to be due to their activity as inhibitors of presynaptic NE and 5-HT reuptake. A variety of other receptor effects that differ from drug to drug impact clinical utility and adverse effect profiles.

The TCAs have been found to be consistently effective for panic disorder and generalized anxiety disorder. Imipramine (Tofranil®) has been shown to have efficacy comparable to that of alprazolam in suppressing panic attacks associated with panic disorder. In generalized anxiety disorder, imipramine has been shown to

Table 16.2 Trade name, usual dosage, and indicated uses of antidepressants

Generic name	Trade name	Usual daily dosage (in mg)	Indications	
MAO inhibitors				
Phenelzine	Nardil	45–90	MDD, PD	Used only as last-line agents due to drug interactions
Tranylcypromine	Parnate	20–50	MDD, PD	
TCAs and related agents				
Amitriptyline	Elavil	100–300	MDD, PD, pain	May have severe anticholinergic and cardiovascular side effects
Amoxapine	Asendin	200–600	Insomnia, enuresis	
Desipramine	Norpramin	100–300		
Doxepin	Sunequan	100–300		
Imipramine	Tofranil	100–300		
Maprtiline	Ludiomil	150–225		
Nortriptyline	Pamelor	50–200		
Protriptyline	Vivactil	20–60		
Trimipramine	Surmontil	100–300		
Clomipramine	Anafranil	100–250	OCD	Higher risk of seizures
SSRIs				
Citalopram	Celexa	20–40	MDD	Lower doses effective for
Fluoxetine	Prozac	Oct-80	MDD, PD, OCD	Depressive disorders; higher
Fluvoxamine	Luvox	100–300	OCD, SP	Doses generally needed for
Paroxetine	Paxil	20–60	MDD, OCD, GAD, PD, PTSD, SP	Anxiety disorders
Sertraline	Zoloft	50–200	MDD, OCD, PD, SP, PTSD	
Escitalopram	Lexapro	5–20	MDD, GAD	
Others				
Mirtazapine	Remeron	15–45	MDD	Sedating effects only at lower doses
Nefazodone	Serzone	300–600	MDD	
Trazodone	Desyrel	200–600	MDD	Used primarily as a hypnotic
Venlafaxine	Effexor	75–375	MDD, GAD, PD	

Note: MDD major depressive disorder, *PD* panic disorder, *OCD* obsessive compulsive disorder, *SP* social phobia, *PTSD* posttraumatic stress disorder, *GAD* generalized anxiety disorder significantly improve symptoms in 60–70% of patients, again, comparable to the response seen with benzodiazepines (Spiegel et al., 2000). However, for all disorders, the effects may only be seen after 3–4 weeks of continuous treatment and tend to disappear after drug discontinuation. Clomipramine (Anafranil®), nortriptyline (Pamelor®), desipramine (Norpramin®), and other agents in this class may produce similar effects at therapeutic doses.

In the treatment of OCD, clomipramine has a level of efficacy not seen with other TCAs. This is thought to be due to this agent's more potent effects in inhibiting serotonin reuptake. About half of clomipramine-treated patients demonstrate moderate improvement (35% reduction in symptoms) in obsessive thoughts and compulsive behaviors (Spiegel et al., 2000).

Several significant liabilities with TCA therapy severely limit their utility. They are associated with anticholinergic side effects such as constipation, urinary retention, and blurred vision. Many of these agents are very sedating due to antihistamine effects. Small doses of amitriptyline (Elavil®) and doxepin (Sinequan®) are used as adjuncts for sleep disorders.

TCAs may cause cardiovascular effects such as arrhythmias and postural hypotension. There are also the risks of seizures, weight gain, light sensitivity, and cognitive impairment associated with TCA therapy. Because of these effects, these agents are usually an alternative to the newer, safer drugs for nonresponders.

Selective Serotonin Reuptake Inhibitors (SSRIs)

The selective serotonin reuptake inhibitors, fluoxetine (Prozac®), fluvoxamine (Luvox®), citalopram (Celexa®), paroxetine (Paxil®), sertraline (Zoloft®), and escitalopram (Lexapro®) are a structurally heterogeneous group of compounds that primarily exert their effects as inhibitors of presynaptic serotonin reuptake. Their relative lack of noradrenergic activity does not seem to reduce their antidepressant efficacy significantly. However, these agents have significant advantages in that their relative absence of anticholinergic and antihistaminic effects provides improved tolerability profiles.

The SSRIs have been shown to have a broad spectrum of activity in the treatment of anxiety disorders and other psychiatric conditions (Kent, Coplan, & Gorman, 1998). Drugs in this class have been approved for use in panic disorder, social phobia, OCD, and PTSD. In most cases, the SSRIs are considered the drugs of choice for these disorders (American Psychiatric Association, 2004, 2009). In panic disorder and social phobia, the SSRIs have shown consistent reductions in frequency of panic attacks after 10–12 weeks of treatment. As with clomipramine, SSRI therapy can reduce the symptoms of obsessions and compulsions associated with OCD. In PTSD, SSRIs have displayed benefits in reducing avoidance, arousal, and depressive symptoms. These agents have also been used to treat eating disorders, impulse control disorders, and premenstrual dysphoric disorder.

It appears that the efficacy for the treatment of anxiety disorders may be similar for all SSRIs. However, there are subtle differences between them. When choosing from among the SSRIs the clinician should consider the drugs' CNS-activating properties and the potential for drug interactions. Side effects include jitteriness (a significant problem for people with anxiety disorders), GI discomfort, sexual dysfunction, tremors, and headaches. Fluvoxamine and fluoxetine tend to have a high rate of CNS-activating effects. Paroxetine, less activating than the other agents in the class, does exhibit mild anticholinergic effects not seen with the other SSRIs. Fluvoxamine and fluoxetine exert potent inhibitory effects on the liver metabolism of many drugs, including many benzodiazepines. Citalopram and escitalopram appear to be relatively free of liver enzyme inhibitory effects.

Other Antidepressants

Venlafaxine (Effexor®) an inhibitor of NE, 5-HT, and dopamine reuptake, is an accepted treatment for generalized anxiety disorder. It can reduce the constant symptoms of anxiety associated with this disorder within the first few weeks of treatment. It is associated with dose-related increases in blood pressure, GI discomfort, and sexual dysfunction.

Nefazodone (Serozone®), a 5-HT–NE reuptake inhibitor, may be useful in the treatment of some anxiety disorders due to its antagonist activity at serotonin 5-HT2 receptors. Antagonism of this receptor subtype confers advantages not seen with other serotonin reuptake inhibitors. Nefazodone is associated with fewer acute anxiety symptoms and less sexual dysfunction than the SSRIs and venlafaxine. Typical side effects include sedation and postural hypotension. Less frequently, it has been associated with liver toxicity, which has caused the use of this drug to decline significantly.

Mirtazapine (Remeron®) is a facilitator of NE and serotonin neurotransmission that shares the 5-HT2 blockade profile with nefazodone. This agent has been found in small studies to be effective for phobic anxiety and post-traumatic stress. Mirtazapine may cause excessive sedation, weight gain, and postural hypotension.

Buspirone

Buspirone (BuSpar®), an anxiolytic, is structurally unrelated to benzodiazepines and antidepressants. It functions as a treatment for generalized anxiety in certain patients but is largely ineffective for most anxiety disorder subtypes, including panic disorders. It is a partial agonist at serotonin type 5-HT1A receptors. Anxiolytic effects of this agent are thought to be due to long-term adaptations that take place with neurotransmitter receptors (Stahl, 2000). Buspirone therefore requires continuous therapy for several weeks to achieve complete resolution of generalized anxiety.

As a chronic therapy, buspirone has advantages over traditional sedatives–hypnotics that clinicians may find useful. Unlike the benzodiazepines, buspirone is not associated with CNS depression, dependence, and withdrawal symptoms upon discontinuation. This profile may make buspirone useful for the elderly and for individuals with a substance abuse history. However, anxiety sufferers may not be able to tolerate the 2- to 4-week latency to clinical effect. Indeed, patients with generalized anxiety disorder who have a history with benzodiazepine treatment tend not to be affected by buspirone therapy (Schweitzer, Rickels, & Lucky, 1986). Adverse effects of buspirone are mild and include headache, nausea, dizziness, and insomnia.

Antipsychotic Medications

Antipsychotic medications are primarily used for individuals that suffer from psychotic syndromes such as schizophrenia. Many of the newer (second-generation antipsychotic agents) also carry indications for bipolar disorder, both manic and depressed state, irritability associated with autism and other disorders. First-generation antipsychotics include agents such as haloperidol, thioridazine, chlorpromazine, thiothixene mesoridazine, and others. Newer or second-generation (sometimes also called "atypical") antipsychotic medications include risperidone (Risperdal®), olanzapine (Zyprexa®), clozapine (Clozaril®), quetiapine (Seroquel®), ziprasidone (Geodon®), aripiprazole (Abilify®), paliperidone (Invega®), iloperidone (Fanapt®), asenapine (Saphris®), and lurasidone (Latuda®). The older antipsychotic agents are largely ineffective in treating anxiety- or stress-related disorders (Grimsley, 1995). Their use is discouraged for treatment of anxiety disorders due to potentially serious side effects, such as tardive dyskinesia, sedation, cognitive difficulties, blood problems (clozapine), decreased blood pressure, and extrapyramidal symptoms (parkinsonian symptoms).

Several of the second-generation antipsychotics have been studied in clinical trials. Randomized controlled trials have been performed with quietiapine, risperidone, and olanzapine (Lorenz, Jackson, & Saitz, 2010). Open-label trials have been conducted with aripiprazole and ziprasidone. In a placebo-controlled trial, people receiving olanzapine added to a fluoxetine regimen showed a greater reduction in anxiety scores than those that received placebo. The results suggest there may be a therapeutic effect; however, the patients on olanzapine gained more than 10 pounds on average in 6 weeks. Quietiapine has also been systematically studied in anxiety, and positive results occurred in two studies. There are data to support the use of quietiapine in patients with anxiety disorders, particularly those with severe or treatment refractory anxiety. Studies with risperidone showed some improvement in patients with treatment refractory generalized anxiety. However, more work needs to be done to establish its place in therapy. The open-label trials with aripiprazole showed improvement in anxiety rating scales for the treatment of refractory generalized anxiety. These trials had significant limitations in that they had a small number of patients and were not placebo controlled. Further study is warranted (Lorenz 2010).

Atypical antipsychotic medications may be useful in patients with treatment refractory generalized anxiety or those with comorbid psychotic disorders.

They remain second- or third-line agents and should be reserved for those patients for whom other treatments have failed. These agents may also cause significant adverse such as weight gain, hyperglycemia, and hyperlipidemia.

Miscellaneous Agents

Beta-Adrenergic Blocking Agents

This group of medications includes popranolol (Inderal®), metoprolol (Lopressor®), nadolol (Corgard®), and atenolol (Tenormin®). By directly counteracting the increased adrenergic tone seen with stress, these agents are used to treat physical manifestations such as tremor and increased heart rate. They are not as effective as the benzodiazepines at treating anxiety. Beta-adrenergic blocking agents are effective in treating the acute physical reactions to a stressful event such as stage fright and public speaking. These drugs do not alter consciousness.

Beta-adrenergic agents should be used with caution in people who have asthma, since they can exacerbate the disorder. They should also be avoided in people with diabetes, since they can mask a hypoglycemic event. Side effects of the beta-adrenergic blocking agents include lethargy, sedation, low blood pressure, decreased heart rate, dizziness, tiredness, insomnia, and depression in susceptible individuals with chronic use (Grimsley, 1995).

Antihistamines

Antihistamines have also been used. The most commonly used antihistamines are dephenhydramine (Benadryl®) and hydroxyzine (Vistaril, Atarax®). These agents do not have anxiolytic effects and both possess significant sedative properties. There is no evidence that they are useful in primary anxiety disorders, but they may be useful in periodic and short-term use for insomnia. These agents also have potent anticholinergic effects and can cause side effects such as confusion, constipation, cognitive impairment, and nausea. Elderly patients, especially those who have dementia or are medically ill, are particularly susceptible to these side effects (American Geriatrics Society, 2012).

Barbiturates and Non-barbiturate Sedative–Hypnotics

Barbiturates such as phenobarbital should be used very sparingly, if at all, due to their side effects and abuse potential. These drugs are profoundly sedating and cause cognitive difficulty. They are also potentially lethal in overdose. Non-barbiturates include meprobamate (Miltown®, Equanil), glutethimide (Doriden®), and ethchlorvynol (Placidyl®). The primary effect of these drugs is also sedation, and these agents are potentially lethal in overdose and may be no more effective than placebo in treating anxiety due to stressful events.

Summary

The armamentarium of available pharmacological agents for the treatment of stress-related syndromes and anxiety disorders is evolving as safer alternatives to the CNS-depressant drugs become available. Let us review some of the main points covered in this chapter:

- Symptomatic improvement of the symptoms of acute stress can be addressed with a short-term course of CNS depressants, such as benzodiazepines. Use of benzodiazepines for longer term therapy has the liabilities of development of tolerance, dependence, and withdrawal symptoms. However, the benzodiazepines do represent a significant improvement in drug safety over barbiturates and non-barbiturate sedative–hypnotics.
- Situational anxiety may respond to as-needed treatment with beta-adrenergic blocking agents. These drugs directly antagonize the NE-mediated peripheral manifestations of the stress response.
- Antihistamines may also be used episodically for sedation.
- Over the long term, most anxiety disorders are most appropriately treated with antidepressant drugs. Because these agents work by inducing long-term alterations in neurotransmitter receptor function and sensitivity, response may take several weeks of continuous treatment. However, improvements in the safety profiles of the newer antidepressants make these agents viable choices in the treatment of anxiety disorders.

References

American Psychiatric Association. (2004). *Practice guideline for the treatment of patients with acute stress disorder and posttraumatic stress disorder*. Arlington, VA: American Psychiatric Association. Available online at: http://psychiatryonline.org/guidelines.aspx.

American Psychiatric Association. (2009). *Treatment of patients with panic disorder*. Arlington, VA: American Psychiatric Association. Available online at: http://psychiatryonline.org/guidelines.aspx.

Brown, C., Rakel, R., Wells, B., Downs, J., & Akiskal, H. (1993). A practical update on anxiety disorders and their pharmacologic treatment. *Archives of Internal Medicine, 151*, 873–884.

Duman, R. S., Malberg, J., & Thome, J. (1999). Neural plasticity to stress and antidepressant treatment. *Biological Psychiatry, 46*, 1181–1191.

Grimsley, S. R. (1995). Anxietydisorders. In L. Y. Young, M. A. Koda-Kimble, W. A. Kradjan, & B. J. Guglielmo (Eds.), *Applied therapeutics: The clinical use of drugs* (6th ed., pp. 73-1–73-31). Vancouver, WA: Applied Therapeutics.

Hamilton, H., Gallagher, P., Ryan, C., Byrne, S., & O'Mahony, D. (2011). Potentially Inappropriate Medications Defined by STOPP Criteria and the Risk of Adverse Drug Events in Older Hospitalized Patients. *Archives of Internal Medicine, 171*, 1013–1019.

Hellweg, R., Ziegenhorn, A., Heuser, I., & Deuschle, M. (2008). Serum concentrations of nerve growth factor and brain-derived neurotrophic factor in depressed patients before and after anti-depressant treatment. *Pharmacopsychiatry, 41*(2), 66–71.

Kent, J. M., Coplan, J. D., & Gorman, J. M. (1998). Clinical utility of the selective serotonin reuptake inhibitors in the spectrum of anxiety. *Biological Psychiatry, 44*, 812–824.

Lorenz, R., Jackson, C. W., & Saitz, M. (2010). Adjunctive use of atypical antipsychotics for treatment-resistant generalized anxiety disorder. *Pharmacotherapy, 30*(9), 942–951.

Schweizer, E., Rickels, K., & Lucky, I. (1986). Resistance to the anti-anxiety effect of buspirone in patients with a history of benzodiazepine use. *New England Journal of Medicine, 314*, 719–720.

Spiegel, D. A., Wiegel, M., Baker, S. L., & Greene, K. A. I. (2000). Pharmacological management of anxiety disorders. In D. I. Mostofsky & D. H. Barlow (Eds.), *The management of stress and anxiety in medical disorders* (pp. 36–65). Needham Heights, MA: Allyn & Bacon.

Stahl, S. M. (2000). *Essential psychopharmacotogy* (2nd ed.). New York: Cambridge University Press.

The American Geriatrics Society. (2012) Beers Criteria Update Expert Panel. American Geriatrics Society Updated Beers Criteria for Potentially Inappropriate Medication Use in Older Adults. *Journal of the American Geriatrics Society* Available online at: http://www.americangeriatrics.org/files/documents/beers/2012BeersCriteria_JAGS.pdf

Part III
Special Topics and the Human Stress Response

Special Topics and the Human Stress Response Part III is the last of three major sections in this book. It is dedicated to the presentation of "special topics" relevant to the phenomenology and treatment of human stress. Chapter 17 introduces the notion of spirituality and religion and the roles they may play in the prevention and treatment of pathogenic stress.

It is been said we are what we eat. In Chap. 18 we examine this notion as it pertains to the stress. Certain foods have been shown to increase stress, while others may actually decrease stress. There is recent great interest in antioxidants, organic foods, and energy drinks. We review the implications for each.

No book on stress would be complete without a discussion of sleep. It seems certain that sleep can heal, yet its absence can prove pathogenic. In Chap. 19 we look at this critical, yet much neglected human experience and its relation to stress.

Chapter 20 examines grief and loss. This age-old topic is dramatically updated with the latest information on phenomenology and treatment. There is also a brief discussion of children and grief.

Chapter 21 examines a topic of great current relevance "Posttraumatic Stress Disorder." Especially because of issues such as war and disaster, PTSD remains an important topic within any volume dedicated to human stress. Analysis of both phenomenology as well as clinical outcome reveals PTSD to be the most severe form of human stress arousal. Within this chapter we review both biological and psychological foundations. Furthermore, we make suggestions on a neurocognitive approach to intervention.

Chapter 22 reviews the field of crisis intervention with a special emphasis upon psychological first aid (PFA). PFA has been widely embraced as the standard of care in acute psychological intervention.

Chapter 23 offers a historical account of the father of the stress concept Dr Hans Selye. This highly unique perspective is provided by one of Selye's colleagues, Dr Paul Rosch.

Chapter 17
Religion, Spirituality, and Stress

Science without religion is lame; religion without science is blind.

Albert Einstein (1879–1955)

In Chap. 10, we reviewed the process of meditation as a treatment for human stress. The reader will recall that the history of meditation is grounded firmly in religion. We will now take a closer look at religion and spirituality, over and above their meditative components, as tools for the reduction or amelioration of stress and disease.

A relevant and actively debated cursory question on this topic involves whether or not religion is beneficial to one's health. Within the past 20 years, objective empirical data have explored the relationship between spiritual and religious involvement and physical and emotional health. Even with the accumulation of methodologically sound data, the debate over religion's role in health is far from resolved. The purpose of this chapter is to provide a brief review of some of the pertinent literature in this area, particularly relative to stress.

Before addressing some of the possible mechanisms of action and the research literature, it may be helpful to define and clarify the terms *spiritual* and *religious*. Not surprisingly, the terms are interrelated; however, Josephson and Peteet (2004) have differentiated them in the following way: "…*spirituality* refers to one's connection to realities larger than oneself or larger than the material universe. It is an umbrella concept under which the specific category of *religion* is subsumed. … Religions formalize what the spiritual individual experiences" (p. 16), and as Richards and Bergin (1997) note, "It is possible to be religious without being spiritual and spiritual without being religious" (p. 13).

Mechanisms of Action

Herbert Benson, the originator of "the relaxation response," has investigated and written extensively on how beliefs and expectancies, including religious beliefs, have a positive impact on one's physical and emotional health. He introduced the term *remem-*

G.S. Everly and J.M. Lating, *A Clinical Guide to the Treatment*
of the Human Stress Response, DOI 10.1007/978-1-4614-5538-7_17,
© Springer Science+Business Media New York 2013

bered wellness in an attempt to replace the term *placebo effect*, which he felt had a rather negative connotation. *Remembered wellness* is a term designed to capture the powerful healing and empowering force of individual beliefs in promoting and enhancing treatment and curative effects. Benson (1996) further described the combination of the physiological powers of the relaxation response and the construct of remembered wellness as the "faith factor." He provides an example of this combination by suggesting that the influence of religious rituals practiced in childhood may actually have the potential to regenerate neural pathways that are related to faith and well-being in later adulthood. Chang, Casey, Dusek, & Benson (2010) have more recently reported that an increase in the relaxation response was associated with enhanced spiritual well-being and improved measures of psychological outcomes like depression, anxiety, hostility, and the global severity index in cardiac rehabilitation patients.

Benson (1996) further suggests that belief in God, in whatever transcendent form an individual chooses to manifest it, may serve as an influential source of strength and healing. For example, Van der Merwe, Van Eeden and Van Deventer (2010) suggest that a belief in God in Christians of African descent provides a contribution to their sense of meaning and psychological well-being. Benson further acknowledges that worship services may possess certain therapeutic effects, including the chance to listen to soothing music in a pleasant environment, to be distracted from daily psychosocial stressors and socialize with others, to perform comfortable and familiar rituals, and to reflect, pray, and learn. Scheiman, Bierman, & Ellison (2010) found that praying was indirectly associated with an increased "sense of mattering" among older adults (age 65 years and older) through divine control beliefs, which combine personal empowerment with divine involvement. To elaborate, Koenig (1997) notes that religious beliefs can provide a sense of control over one's destiny when a person puts his or her complete trust in a personal God and asks for forgiveness. Moreover, he suggests how this relief may occur:

> There is no sin or mistake in life that cannot be confessed and forgiven. Thus, no matter what a person has done in the past, he or she can start fresh again by recommitting one's life to God. Guilt, which religion itself can provoke, is erased by the simple act of asking for forgiveness. Not surprisingly, such beliefs may have powerful psychological consequences, and may indeed bring comfort to those who are lonely anxious, discouraged, or feeling out of control. (p. 68)

From 1997 to 2004, the number of studies related to forgiveness quadrupled (Worthington & Scherer 2004), and the topic continues to garner considerable research attention. Worthington (2005) has broadly defined forgiveness as a process of mitigating inter-related negative resentment-based emotions, motivations, and cognition, and separates it into two types: a decision to control one's behaviors (i.e., decisional forgiveness) and one that involves changes in cognitions, emotions and motivations (i.e., emotional forgiveness). Forgiveness is broadly conceived, therefore, as a reduction in unforgiveness, along with promotion of more positive emotion and understanding (Baetz & Toews, 2009). Unforgiveness has been associated with increased stress response reactions such as higher EMG change scores, higher change scores in skin conductance levels (SCLs), greater heart rate increases and significantly increased mean arterial pressure (Witvliet, Ludwig, & Vander Laan, 2001). The authors concluded that chronic unforgiving "may contribute to adverse health outcomes by perpetuating anger and heightening SNS arousal and cardiovascular reactivity" (Witvliet et al., p. 122). Conversely, studies have demonstrated the positive effects of forgiveness on chronic pain (Carson, et al., 2005; Rippentrop, Altmaier, Chen, Found, & Keffala, 2005), hypertension (Buck, Williams, Musick, & Sternthal, 2009; Tibbits, Ellis, Piramelli, Luskin, & Lukman, 2006), substance abuse (Lin, 2010; Webb, Robinson, & Brower, 2011), and PTSD (Solomon, Dekel, & Zerach, 2009; Witvliet, Phipps, Feldman, & Beckham, 2004). Jankowski and Sandage (2011) have more recently advanced a theoretical model in which meditative prayer increases hope which leads to feelings of attachment and security which leads to enhanced forgiveness. Implementing a randomized controlled 6-week group-based forgiveness training program that incorporated psychoeducation, cognitive restructuring, visualization, and heart-focused meditation, Harris and colleagues (2006) reported that the program was two to three times more effective in reducing negative thoughts, anger and stress, and produced significant increases in positive thoughts, forgiveness self-efficacy, and forgiveness in novel situations than a control condition.

Research

It is notable that both lay and professional interest in complementary and alternative medicine (CAM) treatments for illness has increased tremendously in the past decade. Even more relevant are the data in the USA that prayer for self (43%) and prayer for others (24.4%) are the two most noted alternative medicine procedures (Barnes, Powell-Griner, McFann, & Nahin, 2002). In a national survey of 726 critical care nurses, Tracy et al. (2005) determined that 73% used prayer in their practices, 81% had recommended its use to patients, and 79% had been requested by patients or families to pray on their behalf. It is also worth noting that around 67% of accredited medical schools offer courses on spirituality in medicine (Fortin & Barnett, 2004). Despite the common practice of prayer, there are many challenges associated with empirically studying aspects of spirituality, including the perception that it is too "subjective" and "invisible" or that there are residual professorate biases against graduate students studying domains that are not naturalistic or secular (Richards & Bergin, 2005). In fact, a review by Galek, Flannelly, & Porter (2008) of the studies included in the *Handbook of Religion and Health* (Koenig et al., 2001) revealed that only about 10% of studies on mental health studies and 5% of studies on physical health measured religious beliefs. These perceived biases and limited measures of religious beliefs appear to be ameliorating, and there appears to be a growing empirical literature on spirituality and religion.

Emotional Health

Available data are generally supportive of the benefits of religious beliefs relative to many outcome measures of emotional and social adjustment. In a meta-analysis of 49 studies assessing the relationship between religious coping and psychological adjustment to stress, Ano and Vasconcelles (2005) concluded that "individuals who used religious coping strategies such as benevolent religious reappraisals, collaborative religious coping, seeking spiritual support, etc. typically experienced more stress-related growth, spiritual growth, positive effect, and had higher self-esteem, etc." (p. 473). Conversely, they found that negative religious coping strategies (e.g., spiritual discontent, reappraisal of God's powers as punishing) were associated with poorer psychological adjustment, and increased depression, anxiety, and distress). Magyar-Russell and colleagues (2007) examined the impact of religious beliefs and spirituality in a sample of 87 burn survivors, and reported that positive religious coping was related to better physical functioning, whereas negative religious coping was related to poor sleep, body image dissatisfaction and symptoms of PTSD after discharge. In a more recent study of 103 women who were part of a perinatal loss project and who were assessed for severity of grief for at least one year following their loss, religious struggle and negative religious coping were associated with more severe grief (Cowchock, Lasker, Toedter, Skumanich, & Koenig, 2010).

Donahue (1985) noted that people who use religion as an end in itself (i.e., the intrinsically religious) seem to do better emotionally than those who use religion as a means to achieving some other end (i.e., the extrinsically religious). More recently, Ardelt and Koenig (2006, 2007) noted that older individuals near death have a better subjective sense of well-being if they have an intrinsic religious orientation compared to one that is extrinsic. Intrinsic religiosity has been associated with higher distress shortly after a traumatic event, but lower severity of PTSD symptoms over time, and increased posttraumatic growth eight months or more after the trauma (Schaefer, Blazer, & Koenig, 2008). Other studies have shown that frequency of prayer (Byrd, Hageman, & Isle, 2007) and the social support that occurs from membership in a religious organization (Byrd, Lear, & Schwenka, 2000) are associated with psychological well-being. Adherence and belief in religious traditions have been linked with greater self-esteem and less stress (Yakushko, 2005), greater emotional support (Krause & Wulff, 2005), and less depressive symptoms (Eliassen, Taylor, & Lloyd, 2005; Keyes & Reitzes, 2007).

Religious factors have been associated with reduced alcohol, cigarette, and drug use, as well as improved quality-of-life measures for patients suffering from cancer (Larson & Larson, 2003; Matthews, Larson, & Barry, 1993; Menagi, Harrell, & June, 2008; Nagel & Sgoutas-Emch, 2007; Sekulic, Kostic, Rodek, Damjanovic, & Ostojic, 2009; VonDras, Schmitt, & Marx, 2007). Religious messages and religious-based social mechanisms also have been associated with decreased obesity in Korean women living in the USA (Ayers et al., 2010). Moreover, religious involvement has been associated with more frequent exercise, better sleep quality, better diet, and even more regular seat belt usage (Hill, Burdette, Ellison, & Musick, 2006; Hill, Ellison, Burdette, & Musick, 2007).

Koenig and his colleagues have done much of the seminal work examining the general health benefits of religion. For example, in a sample of 298 patients admitted consecutively to the general medical services at Duke University Medical Center, 40% ranked religion as the most important factor that enabled them to cope with the stress of their illness (Koenig, 1997). Moreover, Koenig and associates (1995) reported that higher religious beliefs as assessed by the Religious Coping Index (RCI) were associated with lower cognitive symptoms (anhedonia, boredom, social withdrawal, and feeling sad, blue, or hopeless), but not necessarily fewer somatic symptoms (weight loss, sleep disturbance, fatigue, loss of energy, psycho-motor retardation) of depression in a sample of 832 men, with an average age of 70 years, admitted to a VA hospital. Frazier, Mintz, and Mobley (2005) found in a sample of 86 elderly (mean age 68.7 years), urban, African Americans (50 women and 36 men) living in different parts of New York City that more religious involve-ment, whether organizational, nonorganizational or subjective, was associated with psychological well-being. More recently, Krause, Shaw, and Liang (2011) found that older African American adults, but not older whites, who identify with their congregation adopt healthier lifestyles when encouraged by their fellow church members.

A recent cross-sectional retrospective study of 608 bereaved participants (reported the loss of a family member, colleague, or friend associated with attacks on World Trade Center, Pentagon, or aboard the airplanes) 2.5 to 3.5 years after the attacks of September 11, 2001 (Seirmarco et al., (2012) assessed the impact of changes in religious beliefs and their association with complicated grief (see Chap. 20), PTSD (see Chap. 21), and major depressive disorder. Results revealed that 78% of participants reported no change in importance of religion after 9/11, 11% reported that religion became more important, and 10% reported that their religion was less important. Religious beliefs became less important for participants who lost a child as compared to other personal loss, and also for those who watched the attacks live on television. Compared to those who reported no change in reli-gious beliefs, participants who reported decreased religious importance were close to three times more likely to screen positive for Complicated Grief, 2.5 times more likely to screen for major depressive disorder and almost two times more likely to report probable PTSD.

Additional treatment outcome data regarding religion have been gathered when accepted psychotherapeutic interventions have been modified to include a spiritual component. Efficacy studies have also compared spiritually focused cognitive-behavioral therapy (CBT) with standard CBT. In one of the earlier well-controlled of these investigations, Propst, Ostrom, Watkins, Dean, and Mashburn (1992) reported that Christian participants who received CBT with religious content had significantly less depression at the end of treatment com-pared to participants in the regular CBT group or a wait-list control group. More recent models of integrating spirituality and CBT have shown effectiveness with older adults (Snodgrass, 2009), and Walker and colleagues (2010) have devised a model that integrates religion with trauma-focused cognitive behavior therapy as relating to children and adolescent victims of sexual and physical abuse. The flourishing of mindfulness-based treatment strategies (see Chap. 8), referred to as the third-wave of CBT traditions, is relevant to this topic since they emerged and are grounded in spiritual and religious foundations (Hathaway & Tan, 2009; Hayes, 2002).

Physical Health

Interest on the relation between spirituality, religion, and physical health has become increasingly prevalent in the past two decades, as both professional journals and the popular press have offered substantial coverage. Several of these studies have assessed the effect of religious or spiritual involvement on cardiac and heart surgery patients. Saudia, Kinney, Brown, and Young-Ward (1991) reported that 96 of 100 coronary artery bypass grafting (CABG) patients reported using prayer as a means to cope with the stress of impending surgery, and 70 of the participants gave prayer the highest rating of effectiveness. Oxman, Freeman, and Manheimer (1995), who investigated mortality rates after elective, open-heart surgery for coronary artery disease or aortic valvular stenosis in 232 patients over the age of 55 years, reported that "patients receiving no strength and comfort from religion were over three times more likely to die after heart surgery" (p. 10). These results occurred even after controlling for history of previous surgery, functional impairment prior to surgery, and age. In a convenience sample of 142 patients, Contrada and colleagues (2004) reported that stronger religious beliefs were associated with fewer surgical compli-cations and shorter hospital stays, with the effect on complications mediating the effect on length of stay. However, they also found that more frequent attendance to religious services was related to longer hospital stays, not shorter ones, and that frequency of prayer had no effect on recovery. In a more recent study of 92,395 postmenopausal women involved in the Women's Health Initiative (WHI) who were followed for an average of 7.7 years, Schnall and colleagues (2010) reported that, after controlling for demographic, socioeconomic, and prior health factors, reli-gious-related variables (i.e., self-report of religious affiliation, frequent religious service attendance, and religious strength and comfort) were not associated with reduced risk of CHD morbidity and mortality. However, they reported that these religion-related variables were associated with a reduction of all-cause mortality.

A large-scale epidemiological study and a levels-of-evidence methodological approach have shown that church service attendance is related to lower mortality rates (Koenig et al., 1999; Powell, Shahabi, & Thoresen, 2003), although a more recent longitudinal study assessing church attendance and health over the lifespan (Koenig & Vaillant, 2009) found little direct association between mortality and church attendance. When other variables, such as past health, smoking, alcohol abuse/dependence and mood were included in the regression model, the direct effect of church attendance on objective and physical health was not significant. There was, however, direct support for an association between church attendance and reported well-being. Other studies have demonstrated the beneficial effects of religious and spiritual beliefs and interventions (e.g., prayer) on oncology patients (Kaplar, Wachholtz, & O'Brien, 2004), postsurgical patients (Contrada et al., 2004), chronic pain patients (Wacholtz & Pearce, 2007), spinal cord injury patients (Brillhart, 2005), and stroke, traumatic brain injury, and other rehabilitation patients (Giaquinto, Spiridigliozzi, & Caracciolo, 2007; Kalpakjian, Lam, Toussaint, & Hansen Merbitz, 2004; Pargament, Magyar-Russell, & Murray-Swank, 2005). In a nationally repre-sentative sample of 2,262 men and women with a history of cancer, 68.5% used prayer for health and 88% had prayed during the past year (Ross, Hall, Fairley, Taylor, & Howard, 2008). Moreover, the authors found that being older, female, married, non-Hispanic black, and living outside the West were relevant indicators of praying for one's health. There are studies suggesting that higher levels of religious involvement are associated with lower blood pressure and decreased chances of hypertension (Koenig, McCullough, & Larson, 2001; Seeman, Dubin, & Seeman, 2003); however, Fitchett and Powell (2009) did not find that higher scores on the Daily Spiritual Experiences Scale (DSES) affected the systolic blood pressure or hypertension in a sample of 1,060 Caucasian and 598 African-American midlife women participating in Study of Women's Health Across the Nation (SWAN).

Dean Ornish (1990) received considerable attention for well-designed research demonstrating that the progression of coronary atherosclerosis could be stopped or reversed in patients without the use of lipid-lowering drugs. Instead of medications, patients in the experimental group were prescribed an intensive lifestyle component that included diet, exercise, smoking cessation, and stress management. Also included in this program, and a factor that Ornish considered essential for success, was a spiritual component designed to help patients seek communion with God or a Higher Power. Ornish and his colleagues (1998) reported on the continued improvement and success of the patients with heart disease who incorporated and adhered to these lifestyle changes for 5 years. Ornish and his colleagues (2005) have reported similar success in implementing lifestyle changes to positively affect the progression of prostate cancer. Schnall and colleagues (2010) found that stronger religious beliefs and practices were related to lower all-cause mortality rates, but not related to risk of coronary heart disease.

When the last edition of this text was published there was accumulating lay interest and growing discourse on the intriguing, yet controversial empirical studies demonstrating the beneficial effects of intercessory prayer (IP; praying for the benefits of others, also known as "distant prayer"). In one of these studies, Byrd (1988) investigated the effects of intercessory prayer on 393 patients admitted to the coronary care unit at San Francisco General Hospital over a 10-month period. In this double-blind study, patients were randomly assigned to either the intercessory prayer group or a nonprayer group, and three to seven active, "devotional" Christians were randomly assigned to pray for the 192 patients in the intercessory prayer group.

The results of the study revealed that members of the prayer group did significantly better than the nonprayer group on a number of health-related measures (e.g., congestive heart failure, diuretic use, cardiopulmonary arrest, pneumonia, antibiotic use, and need for intubation/ventilation) during the course of their hospitalizations. Byrd acknowledged that he did not attempt to limit the amount of prayer that the control group received from outside persons not associated with the study, or the amount of individual prayer or religiosity held by the participants.

Harris and colleagues (1999) replicated Byrd's (1988) work in a sample of 990 patients admitted to the coronary care unit (CCU). Using a randomized, controlled, double-blind procedure, in which the 466 patients in the IP group were prayed for daily for four weeks, compared to usual care for 524 patients, the IP group had lower CCU scores (a weighted and summed scoring system that resulted in a continuous variable from 1 to 10 that described patient outcomes from excellent to catastrophic). More specifically, there was an 11% reduction in scores in the prayer group compared with the usual care group.

Sicher, Targ, Moore, and Smith (1998) used intercessory prayer in a randomized trial of 40 patients diagnosed with advanced AIDS and matched by age, CD4+ count, and number of AIDS-defining diseases (ADDs). At the 6-month study endpoint, the prayer group experienced significantly fewer outpatient visits, hospitalizations (and days in the hospital), and ADDs, and higher ratings of improved mood compared to the nonprayer group. Sicher and associates (1998) offer several possible secular explanations for their results but also recognize that these provocative data cannot be completely dismissed without considering other possible benefits of intercessory prayer.

Shealy, Smith, Liss, and Borgmeyer (2000) reported on the alteration of EEG brain maps (see Chap. 14) on 110 volunteers who received distant or absent "healing." In all instances, notable changes in EEG activity occurred within the first 5 min of receiving healing energy at distances ranging from 100 feet to 160 miles. Sometimes, however, the EEG alterations appeared most dramatically 20 min post-intervention.

Since the publication of the last edition of this text, there has been considerable empirical interest in systematically assessing the efficacy of intercessory prayer. In a meta-analytic review of 14 studies using a random effects model, Masters, Spielmans, & Goodson (2006) concluded that "the most parsimonious statement to be made from this literature is that there is no scientifically discernable effect that differentiates that status of individuals who are recipients of IP from those who are not" (p. 24). Howard and colleagues (2009), using techniques of meta-analysis and Bayesian analysis of IP studies on cardiac care patients, concluded that "our data suggest that remote intercessory prayer is not a real phenomenon. Further, the research literature is likely due to an excessive number of Type I errors mixed with a few non-significant results" (p.162).

These rather discouraging conclusions of the empirical data should not, however, keep people from practicing intercessory prayer. In a 2005 review of the theological and theoretical foundations of IP published prior to his meta-analytic study noted above, Masters aptly notes that "the results of scientific experimentation are never normative of behavior, they are only statements of observations given certain conditions. Christians should continue, as they always have, to offer up prayers on the basis of their belief and understanding that a sovereign God hears and answers according to God's will" (p. 275).

Incorporating Spiritual and Religious Beliefs into Practice and Therapy

Interest in the relation between counseling and religion has grown and prospered substantially over the past decade. For example, as of 2011, the American Association of Christian Counselors (AACC) had more than 50,000 active members (http://www.aacc.net); it had 2,000 members in 1993 (Worthington, Kurusu, McCullough, & Sandage, 2007).

The use of spiritual themes and religion in intervention and counseling is not new. For example, 12-step programs or fellowships, most notably, Alcoholics Anonymous (AA), which has an estimated membership of about two million worldwide with 115,773 groups registered as of January 2010, have as their base the relevance of spiritual processes in clinical outcomes. The emphasis of the AA model is that success requires surrendering to a Higher Power, along with an acknowledgment of the need for God's assistance. Given the success of the AA model, other spiritually based, 12-step programs have been developed (e.g., Gamblers Anonymous and Narcotics Anonymous). Galanter (2007) offers a model based on empirical psychological research to help define the diagnosis of addiction, and criteria, such as social networks, attributing meaning to experiences and positive psychology as mechanisms involved in the spiritual 12-step programs.

Within the psychotherapeutic setting, individuals often present with concerns related to life perspectives, deep personal and relationship values, and well-being (Martinez, Smith, & Barlow, 2007). It is worth noting that religious issues frequently relate to these concerns and therefore, should be addressed (Smith & Richards, 2005), In fact, psychologists have an ethical obligation to provide services that address client context, including religious contexts (American Psychological Association [APA], 2002), and should be sensitive to the dilemmas that may arise, including informed consent (Hawkins & Bullock, 1995), dual relationships (Sonne, 1994), boundaries (Richards & Bergin, 2005), and therapist competence (Barnett & Fiorentino, 2000). Interventions, such as praying (including with clients in certain settings and certain conditions; Richards & Bergin, 2005), discussion of religious writings or sacred texts, spiritual meditation, and forgiveness have, however, been shown to enhance therapeutic effectiveness for some disorders, including those stress and anxiety-related (Smith, Bartz, & Richards, 2007).

Richards and Bergin (2005) have suggested a number of religious and spiritual factors that they consider relevant for success within an integrative, multidimensional, psychotherapeutic approach. For clients willing to pursue this strategy, they define the following approaches that therapists may employ:

1. Helping clients experience and affirm their spiritual identity and divine worth.
2. Assisting clients in seeking guidance and strength from God to assist them in coping, healing, and growing.
3. Obtaining support (i.e., social, emotional, and material) from religious community.
4. Modifying religious and spiritual beliefs and practices that are dysfunctional.
5. Using a more spiritual perspective to understand problems.
6. Working through religious and spiritual doubts.
7. Being able to forgive and heal.
8. Accepting responsibility for their harmful and selfish behaviors.
9. Helping to grow in faith, commitment and religious and spiritual beliefs.

Ellis (2000) has suggested his own set of spiritual goals that he believes therapists should consider, including:

1. Acquiring an outstanding meaning or purpose in life.
2. Unconditional self-acceptance combined with unconditional other acceptance.

3. Having unusual social interest and compassion for other people.
4. Being one's authentic self, even if others do no like it.

Summary

This chapter has provided a general overview of the relation between stress and spirituality. Let us review the main points of this chapter:

1. We began with a differentiation of the terms *religious*, which is considered to be external, denomination, and public, and *spiritual* which is thought to be ecumenical, internal, and private.
2. Various mechanisms of action regarding the potential psychological benefits of religion were then proposed. Herbert Benson's more recent work on the "faith factor" and therapeutic benefits of worship services was covered, as well as other psychological benefits, such as increased sense of meaning and control, self-esteem, and forgiveness.
3. Potential physical benefits of religion include perceiving the body as a "temple of the Holy Spirit" (Koenig, 1997), increased medical adherence and coping, fewer post-surgical complications, and reduced mortality rates.
4. Research has shown a positive relation between forgiveness and emotional and physical health.
5. Spiritual themes have been used in interventions such as Alcoholics Anonymous, Gamblers Anonymous, and Narcotics Anonymous.
6. Finally, Richards and Bergin (2005) suggest a number of religious and spiritual factors that may be incorporated during psychotherapy.

References

American Psychological Association (2002). *Ethical principles of psychologists and code of conduct.* Washington, DC: Author

Ano, G. G., & Vasconcelles, E. B. (2005). Religious coping and psychological adjustment to stress: A meta-analysis. *Journal of Clinical Psychology, 61*(4), 461–480.

Ardelt, M., & Koenig, C. S. (2006). The role of religion for hospice patients and relatively healthy older adults. *Research on Aging, 28,* 184–215.

Ardelt, M., & Koenig, C. S. (2007). The importance of religious orientation and purpose in life for dying well: Evidence from three case studies. *Journal of Religion, Spirituality and Aging, 19*(4), 61–79.

Ayers, J. W., Hofstetter, C. R., Irvin, V. L., Song, Y., Park, H. R, Paik, H. Y., & Hovell, M. F. (2010). Can religion help prevent obesity? Religious messages and the prevalence of being overweight or obese among Korean women in California. *Journal for the Scientific Study of Religion, 49,* 536–549.

Baetz, M., & Toews, J. (2009). Clinical implications of research on religion, spirituality, and mental health. *Canadian Journal of Psychiatry, 54*(5), 292–301.

Barnes, P., Powell-Griner, E., McFann, K., & Nahin, R. (2002). *CDC advance data report #343: Complementary and alternative medicine use among adults: United States, 2002.* Washington, DC: U.S. Government.

Barnett, J. E., & Fiorentino, N. (2000). Spirituality and religion: Clinical and ethical issues for psychotherapists. Part II. *Psychological Bulletin, 35*, 32–35.

Benson, H. (1996). *Timeless healing: The power and biology of belief.* New York, NY: Scribner.

Brillhart, B. (2005). A study of spirituality and life satisfaction among persons with spinal cord injury. *Rehabilitation Nursing, 30*(1), 31–34.

Buck, A. C., Williams, D. R., Musick, M. A., & Sternthal, M. J. (2009). An examination of the relationship between multiple dimensions of religiosity, blood pressure, and hypertension. *Social Science and Medicine, 68*(2), 314–322.

Byrd, R. B. (1988). Positive therapeutic effects of intercessory prayer in a coronary care unit population. *Southern Medical Journal, 81*, 826–829.

Byrd, K. R., Hageman, A., & Belle Isle, D. (2007). Intrinsic motivation andsubjective well-being: The unique contribution of intrinsic religious motivation. *The International Journal for the Psychology of Religion, 17*(2), 141–156.

Byrd, K. R., Lear, D., & Schwenka, S. (2000). Mysticism as a predictor of subjective well-being. *The International Journal for the Psychology of Religion, 10*(4), 259–269.

Carson, J. W., Keefe, F. J., Goli, V., Fras, A. M., Lynch, T. R., Thorp, S. R., & Buechler, J. L. (2005). Forgiveness and chronic low back pain: A preliminary student examining the relationship of forgiveness to pain, anger, and psychological distress. *The Journal of Pain, 6*(2), 84–91.

Chang, B., Casey, A., Dusek, J. A., & Benson, H. (2010). Relaxation response and spirituality: Pathways to improve psychological outcomes in cardiac rehabilitation. *Journal of Psychosomatic Research, 69*, 93–100.

Contrada, R. J., Goyal, T. M., Cather, C., Ragalson, L., Idler, E. L., & Krause, T. J. (2004). Psychosocial factors in outcomes of heart surgery: The impact of religious involvement and depressive symptoms. *Health Psychology, 23*(3), 227–238.

Cowchock, F. S., Lasker, J. N., Toedter, L. J., Skumanich, S. A., & Koenig, H. G. (2010). Religious beliefs affect grieving after pregnancy loss. *Journal of Religion and Health, 49*(4), 485–497.

Donahue, M. J. (1985). Intrinsic and extrinsic religiousness: Review and meta-analysis. *Journal of Personality and Social Psychology, 48*, 400–419.

Eliassen, A. H., Taylor, J., & Lloyd, D. A. (2005). Subjective religiosity and depression in the transition to adulthood. *Journal for the Scientific Study of Religion, 44*(2), 187–199.

Ellis, A. (2000). Spiritual goals and spirited values in psychotherapy. *The Journal of Individual Psychology, 56*(3), 277–284.

Fitchett, G., & Powell, L. H. (2009). Daily spiritual experiences, systolic blood pressure, and hypertension among midlife women in SWAN. *Annals of Behavioral Medicine, 37*(3), 257–267.

Fortin, A. H., VI, & Barnett, K. G. (2004). Medical school curricula in spirituality and medicine. *Journal of the American Medical Association, 291*(23), 2883.

Frazier, C., Mintz, L. B., & Mobley, M. (2005). A multidimensional look at religious involvement and psychological well-being among urban elderly African Americans. *Journal of Counseling Psychology, 52*(4), 583–590.

Galanter, M. (2007). Spirituality and recovery in 12-Step programs: An empirical model. *Journal of Substance Abuse Treatment, 33*, 265–272.

Galek, K., Flannelly, K. J., & Porter, M. (2008). *The importance of cognitions in measuring spirituality and religion: The case for personal theological beliefs.* Paper presented at the annual meeting of the Society for Spirituality, Theology, and Health.

Giaquinto, S., Spiridigliozzi, C., & Caracciolo, B. (2007). Can faith protect from emotional distress after stroke? *Stroke, 38*, 993–997.

Harris, A. H. S., Luskin, F., Norman, S. B., Standard, S., Bruning, J., & Evans, S., et al. (2006). Effects of a group forgiveness intervention on forgiveness, perceived stress, and trait-anger. *Journal of Clinical Psychology, 62*(6), 715–733.

Harris, A. H. S., Thoresen, C. E., McCullough, M. E., & Larson, D. B. (1999). Spirituality and religiously oriented health interventions. *Journal of Health Psychology, 4*(3), 413–433.

Hathaway, W., & Tan, E. (2009). Religiously oriented mindfulness-based cognitive therapy. *Journal of Clinical Psychology, 65*(2), 158–171.

Hawkins, I. A., & Bullock, S. L. (1995). Informed consent and religious values: A neglected area of diversity. *Psychotherapy: Theory, Research, Practice, Training, 32*(2), 293–300.

Hayes, S. C. (2002). Buddhism and acceptance and commitment therapy. *Cognitive and Behavioral Practice, 9*, 58–66.

Hill, T. D., Burdette, A. M., Ellison, C. G., & Musick, M. A. (2006). Religious attendance and health behaviors of Texas adults. *Preventative Medicine, 42*, 309–312.

Hill, T. D., Ellison, C. G., Burdette, A. M., & Musick, M. A. (2007). Religiousinvolvement and healthy lifestyles: Evidence from the survey of Texas adults. *Annals of Behavioral Medicine, 34*, 217–222.

Howard, G. S., Hill, T. L., Maxwell, S. E., Baptista, T. M., Farias, M. H., Coelho, C., & Coulter-Kern, R. (2009). What's wrong with research literatures? And how to make them right. *Review of General Psychology, 13*(2), 146–166.

Jankowski, P. J., & Sandage, S. J. (2011). Meditative prayer, hope, adult attachment, and forgiveness: A proposed model. *Psychology of Religion and Spirituality, 3*(2), 115–131.

Josephson, A. M., & Peteet, J. R. (Eds.). (2004). *Handbook of Spirituality and Worldview in Clinical Practice*. Arlington, VA: American Psychiatric Publishing.

Kalpakjian, C. Z., Lam, C. S., Toussaint, L. L., & Hansen Merbitz, N. K. (2004). Describing quality of life and psychosocial outcomes after traumatic brain injury. *American Journal of Physical Medicine and Rehabilitation, 83*(4), 255–265.

Kaplar, M. E., Wachholtz, A. B., & O'Brien, W. H. (2004). The effect of religious and spiritual interventions on the biological, psychological, and spiritual outcomes of oncology patients. *Journal of Psychosocial Oncology, 22*(1), 39–49.

Keyes, C. L. M., & Reitzes, D. C. (2007). The role of religious identity in the mental health of older working and retired adults. *Aging and Mental Health, 11*(4), 434–443.

Koenig, H. G. (1997). *Is religion good for your health? The effects of religion on physical and mental health*. New York: Hayworth Pastoral Press.

Koenig, H. G., Cohen, J. J., Blazer, D. G., & Krishnan, K. R. R. (1995). Religious coping and cognitive symptoms of depression in elderly medical patients. *Psychosomatics, 36*, 369–375.

Koenig, H. G., Hays, J. C., Larson, D. B., George, L. K., Cohen, H. J., McCullough, M. E., Meador, K. G., & Blazer, D. G. (1999). Does religious attendance prolong survival? A six-year follow-up study of 3,968 older adults. *Journal of Gerontology, 54A*, M370–M376.

Koenig, H. G., McCollough, M. E., & Larson, D. B. (2001). *Handbook of religion and health*. New York, NY: Oxford University Press.

Koenig, L. B., & Valiant, G. E. (2009). A prospective study of church attendance and health over the lifespan. *Health Psychology, 28*(1), 117–124.

Krause, N., Shaw, B., & Liang, J. (2011). Social relationships in religious institutions and healthy lifestyles. *Health Education and Behavior, 38*(1), 25–38.

Krause, N., & Wulff, K. M. (2005). Research: "Church-based social ties, a sense of belonging in a congregation, and physical health status. *International Journal for the Psychology of Religion, 15*(1), 73–93.

Larson, D. B., & Larson, S. S. (2003). Spirituality's potential relevance to physical and emotional health: A brief review of quantitative research. *Journal of Psychology and Theology, 31*(1), 37–51.

Lin, W. F. (2010). The treatment of substance abuse disorders by the psychological forgiveness. *Bulletin of Educational Psychology, 41*(4), 859–883.

Magyar-Russell, G., Bresnick, M. G., McKibben, J., Arceneaux, L., Fauerbach, J. A., & Pargament, K. I. (2007). Religious and spiritual coping among burn patients: Implications for mental and physical health. *Journal of Burn Care & Research, 28*(2), S67.

Martinez, J. S., Smith, T. B., & Barlow, S. H. (2007). Spiritual interventions in psychotherapy: Evaluations by highly religious clients. *Journal of Clinical Psychology, 63*(10), 943–960.

Masters, K. S. (2005). Research on the healing power of distant intercessory prayer: Disconnect between science and faith. *Journal of Psychology and Theology, 33*(4), 268–277.

Masters, K. S., Spielmans, G. I., & Goodson, J. T. (2006). Are there demonstrable effects of distant intercessory prayer? A meta-analytic review. *Annals of Behavioral Medicine, 32*(1), 21–26.

Matthews, D. A., Larson, D. B., & Barry, C. P. (1993). *The faith factor: An annotated bibliography of clinical research on spiritual subjects* (Vol. 1). John Templeton Foundation.

Menagi, F. S., Harrell, Z. A. T., & June, L. N. (2008). Religiousness and college student alcohol use: Examining the role of social support. *Journal of Religion and Health, 47*(2), 217–226.

Nagel, E., & Sgoutas-Emch, S. (2007). The relationship between spirituality, health beliefs, and health behaviors in college students. *Journal of Religion and Health, 46*(1), 141–154.

Ornish, D. (1990). *Dr. Dean Ornish's program for reversing heart disease.* New York: Ballantine.

Ornish, D., Schwerwitz, L. W., Billings, J. H., Gould, L., Merritt, T. A., Sparler, S., Armstrong, W. T., Ports, T. A., Kirkeeide, R. L., Hogeboom, C., & Brand, R. J. (1998). Intensive lifestyle changes for reversal of coronary heart disease. *Journal of the American Medical Association, 280,* 2001–2007.

Ornish, D., Weidner, G., Fair, W. R., Marlin, R., Pettengill, E. B., Raisin, C. J., … Carroll, P. R. (2005). Intensive lifestyle changes may affect the progression of prostate cancer. *The Journal of Urology, 174,* 1065–1070.

Ornstein, R. (1972). *The psychology of consciousness.* San Francisco: Freeman.

Oxman, T. E., Freeman, D. H., & Manheimer, E. D. (1995). Lack of social participation or religious strength and comfort as risk factors for death after cardiac surgery in the elderly. *Psychosomatic Medicine, 57,* 5–15.

Pargament, K. I., Magyar-Russell, G. M., & Murray-Swank, N. A. (2005). The sacred and the search for significance: Religion as a unique process. *Journal of Social Issues, 61*(4), 665–687.

Powell, L. H., Shahabi, L., & Thorensen, C. E. (2003). Religion and spirituality: Linkages to physical health. *American Psychologist, 58*(1), 36–52.

Propst, L. R., Ostrom, R., Watkins, P., Dean, T., & Mashburn, D. (1992). Comparative efficacy of religious and nonreligious cognitive-behavioral therapy for the treatment of clinical depression in religious individuals. *Journal of Consulting and Clinical Psychology, 60,* 94–103.

Richards, P. S., & Bergin, A. E. (1997). *A spiritual strategy for counseling and psychotherapy.* Washington, DC: American Psychological Association.

Richards, P. S., & Bergin, A. E. (2005). *A spiritual strategy for counseling and psychotherapy* (2nd ed.). Washington, DC: American Psychological Association.

Rippentrop, A. E., Altmaier, E. M., Chen, J. J., Found, E. M., & Keffala, V. J. (2005). The relationship between religion/spirituality and physical health, mental health, and pain in a chronic pain population. *Pain, 116*(3), 311–321.

Ross, L. E., Hall, I. J., Fairley, T. L., Taylor, Y. J., & Howard, D. L. (2008). Prayer and self-reported health among cancer survivors in the United States, national health interview survey, 2002. *The Journal of Alternative and Complementary Medicine, 14*(8), 931–938.

Saudia, T. L., Kinney, M. R., Brown, K. C., & Young-Ward, L. (1991). Health locus of control and helpfulness of prayer. *Heart & Lung, 20*(1), 60–65.

Schaefer, F. C., Blazer, D. G., & Koenig, H. G. (2008). Religious and spiritual factors and the consequences of trauma: A review and model of the interrelationship. *International Journal of Psychiatry in Medicine, 38*(4).

Schieman, S., Bierman, A., & Ellison, C. G. (2010). Religious involvement, beliefs about God, and the sense of mattering among older adults. *Journal for the Scientific Study of Religion, 49*(3), 517–535.

Schnall, E., Wassertheil–Smoller, S., Swencionis, C., Zemon, V., Tinker, L., O'Sullivan, M. J., … Goodwin, M. (2010). The relationship between religion and cardiovascular outcomes and all-cause mortality in the women's health initiative observational study. *Psychology and Health, 25*(2), 249–263.

Seeman, T. E., Dubin, L. F., & Seeman, M. (2003). Religiosity/spirituality and health: A critical review of the evidence for biological pathways. *American Psychologist, 58*(1), 53–63.

Seirmarco, G., Neria, Y., Insel, B., Kiper, D., Doruk, A. Gross, R., & Litz, B. (2012). Religiosity and mental health: Changes in religious beliefs, complicated grief, posttraumatic stress disorder, and major depression following the September 11, 2011 attacks. *Psychology of Religion and Spirituality, 4*(1), 10–18.

Sekulic, D., Kostic, R., Rodek, J., Damjanovic, V., & Ostojic, Z. (2009). Religiousness as a protective factor for substance use in dance sport. *Journal of Religion and Health, 48*(3), 269–277.

Shealy, C. N., Smith, T., Liss, S., & Borgmeyer, V. (2000, November). *EEG alterations during absent "healing."* Paper presented at the meeting of the American Institute of Stress, Kohala Coast, Hawaii.

Sicher, F., Targ, E., Moore, D., & Smith, H. (1998). A randomized double-blind study of the effect of distant healing in an advanced AIDS population. *Western Journal of Medicine, 169*, 356–363.

Smith, T. B., Bartz, J., & Richards, P. S. (2007). Outcomes of religious and spiritual adaptations to psychotherapy: A meta-analytic review. *Psychotherapy Research, 17*(6), 643–655.

Smith, J. E., Richardson, J., Hoffman, C., & Pilkington, K. (2005). Mindfulness-based stress reduction as supportive therapy in cancer care: Systematic review. *Journal of Advanced Nursing, 52*, 315–327.

Snodgrass, J. (2009). Toward holistic care: Integrating spirituality and cognitive behavioral therapy for older adults. *Journal of Religion, Spirituality and Aging, 21*(3), 219–236.

Solomon, Z., Dekel, R., & Zerach, G. (2009). Posttraumatic stress disorder and marital adjustment: The mediating role of forgiveness. *Family Process, 48*(4), 546–558.

Sonne, J. (1994). Multiple relationships: does the new ethics code answer the right questions? *Professional Psychology: Research and Practice, 25*(4), 336–343.

Tibbits, D., Ellis, G., Piramelli, C., Luskin, F., & Lukman, R. (2006). Hypertension reduction through forgiveness training. *Journal of Pastoral Care and Counseling, 60*(1–2), 27–34.

Tracy, M. F., Lindquist, R., Savik, K., Watanuki, S., Sendelback, S., Kreitzer, M. J., & Berman, B. (2005). Use of complementary and alternative therapies: A national survey of critical care nurses. *American Journal of Critical Care, 14*, 404–415.

Van der Merwe, E. K., Van Eeden, C., & Van Deventer, H. J. M. (2010). A psychological perspective on god-belief as a course of well-being and meaning. *HTS Teologiese Studies/Theological Studies, 66*(1), 1–10.

VonDras, D. D., Schmitt, R. R., & Marx, D. (2007). Associations between aspects of spiritual well-being, alcohol use, and related social-cognitions in female college students. *Journal of Religion and Health, 46*(4), 500–515.

Wachholtz, A. B., Pearce, M. J., & Koenig, H. (2007). Exploring the relationship between spirituality, coping and pain. *Journal of Behavioral Medicine, 30*, 311–318.

Walker, D., Reese, J. B., Hughes, J. P., & Troskie, M. (2010). Addressing religious and spiritual issues in trauma-focused cognitive behavior therapy for children and adolescents. *Professional Psychology, Research and Practice, 41*, 174–180.

Webb, J. R., Robinson, E. A. R., & Brower, K. J. (2011). Mental health, not social support, mediates the forgiveness-alcohol outcome relationship. *Psychology of Addictive Behaviors, 25*(3), 462–473.

Witvliet, C. V. O., Ludwig, T. E., & Vander Laan, K. L. (2001). Granting forgiveness or harboring grudges: Implications for emotion, physiology, and health. *Psychological Science, 12*(2), 117–123.

Witvliet, C. V. O., Phipps, K. A., Feldman, M. E., & Beckham, J. C. (2004). Posttraumatic mental and physical health correlates of forgiveness and religious coping in military veterans. *Journal of Traumatic Stress, 17*(3), 269–273.

Worthington, E. L., Kurusu, T. A., McCullough, M. E., & Sandage, S. J. (1996). Empirical research on religion and psychotherapeutic processes and outcomes: A 10-year review and research prospectus. *Psychological Bulletin, 119*, 448–487.

Worthington, E. L. Jr. (2005). More questions about forgiveness: Research agenda for 2005–2015. In E.L. Worthington Jr. (Ed.), *Handbook of forgiveness* (pp. 557–574). New York: Brunner – Routledge.

Worthington, E. L. & Scherer, M. (2004). Forgiveness is an emotion-focused coping strategy that can reduce health risks and promote health resilience: Theory, review, and hypothesis. *Psychology and Health, 19*(3), 385–405.

Worthington, E. L., Jr., Witvliet, C. V. O., Pietrini, P., & Miller, A. J. (2007). Forgiveness, health, and well-being: A review of evidence for emotional versus decisional forgiveness, dispositional forgivingness, and reduced unforgiveness. *Journal of Behavioral Medicine, 30*, 291–302.

Yakushko, O. (2005). Influence of social support, existential well-being, and stress over sexual orientation on self-esteem of gay, lesbian, and bisexual individuals. *International Journal for the Advancement of Counselling, 27*(1), 131–143.

Chapter 18
Nutrition and Stress

Rich Blake and Jeffery M. Lating
Loyola University Maryland

George S. Everly, Jr.
The Johns Hopkins University School of Medicine
The Johns Hopkins Bloomberg School of Public Health

This text has emphasized the body's adaptive mechanisms that attempt to maintain homeostasis in response to physical and psychosocial stressors (see Chap. 2 for a detailed explanation). However, as we have noted, intense stress can deplete and weaken the body, including, for example, the SNS response to inhibit digestion. As Whitney, Hamilton, and Rolfes (1990) note, "Much of the disability imposed by prolonged stress is nutritional" (p. 13). The purpose of this chapter is to briefly review how some of the basics of nutrition are involved in the stress response, including fatty acids, antioxidants, and serotonin, and will conclude with an introduction of future directions for dietary intervention.

It has been suggested that the mental health of entire nations may be linked to diet, and that the deleterious effects of excessive caloric intake in wealthy countries rivals those from malnutrition in poor ones (Gómez-Pinilla, 2008). The importance of nutrition is apparent when examining the impact of specific foods or diets on disease. For example, the Mediterranean diet, characterized by breads, pastas, legumes, vegetables, fruits, olive oil, ocean fish, and the moderate consumption of red wine, has been associated with lower incidence of Alzheimer's disease and Parkinson's disease (Sofi, Cesari, Abbate, Gensini, & Casini, 2008). Similarly, it has been suggested that a lower incidence of Alzheimer's disease in India may be attributed to the antioxidant-rich curcumin, a medicinal herb found in curry (Frautschy et al., 2001).

Nutrients and Energy

Nutrients are diverse and complex substances that provide energy for body functions such as growth, metabolism, respiration, and circulation. The type of nutrients and their proportion to others we consume appears to be nearly as important as having

G.S. Everly and J.M. Lating, *A Clinical Guide to the Treatment of the Human Stress Response*, DOI 10.1007/978-1-4614-5538-7_18, © Springer Science+Business Media New York 2013

enough food. When responding to stress, our bodies rely on the energy-yielding macronutrients of carbohydrates, proteins, and fats (Charrondiere, Chevassus-Agnes, Marroni, & Burlingame, 2004). Alcohol is the only other source of energy in the diet, but unlike the other macronutrients it is not needed for survival. Both carbohydrates and proteins contain 4 calories per gram, whereas alcohol contains 7 calories per gram, and fat contains 9 calories per gram. To maintain health and regulate weight, energy expenditure should match energy (caloric) intake, or should exceed it to reduce weight (Institute of Medicine [IOM], 2005).

Carbohydrates

It is recommended that 45–65% of the human diet consist of carbohydrates (United States Department of Agriculture; (USDA), 2010). Carbohydrates, the body's main source of energy, exist in substantial amounts in grains, potatoes, fruits, and milk, and in lesser concentration in vegetables and legumes. There are two general types of carbohydrates: simple and complex. Simple carbohydrates or sugars (monosaccharides and disaccharides) come from fruits and vegetables (e.g., glucose, fructose, maltose, and sucrose) and from milk or milk products (lactose and galactose). Simple carbohydrates are especially concentrated in sweeteners such as table sugar, confectioner's sugar, brown sugar, honey, and molasses. Complex carbohydrates, which are mainly starches, include oligosaccharides and polysaccharides and are found in grains such as rice, wheat, rye, barley, and oats. Another important source of starch is legumes such as peanuts, beans, peas, and soybeans. Potatoes, yams, and cassava, a tropical American plant with a starchy root from which tapioca is derived, are other sources of starches. Complex carbohydrates are metabolized more slowly than simple carbohydrates and serve as our major source of vitamins (except B12) and minerals.

Fiber is the indigestible portion of complex carbohydrates (Greenberg, Dintiman, & Myers-Oakes, 1998). Although it is not considered a nutrient because it is not used in metabolism, fiber facilitates digestion and elimination, and certain viscous fibers may delay the movement of food from the stomach to the intestine, creating a sensation of fullness. Fiber can also impact the absorption of fat and cholesterol (IOM, 2005; USDA, 2010). Increased intake of dietary fiber has been associated with a decreased risk for heart disease, stroke, diabetes, hypertension, obesity, hemorrhoids, acid reflux, constipation, and other gastrointestinal conditions (Anderson et al., 2009).

Dietary sugar intake has been a source of considerable debate for years. Despite popular opinion that sugar is related to hyperactivity in children, a meta-analysis of 23 studies indicated that sugar intake does not affect behavior or cognitive performance (Wolraich, Wilson, & White, 1995). A more recent review of a decade of evidence suggests that high-quality studies do not reveal a positive correlation between sugar intake and body mass index (BMI), and no consistent evidence links sugar consumption with attention deficit/hyperactivity disorder (ADHD), dementia, or depression (Ruxton, Gardner, & McNulty, 2010).

Proteins

The USDA (2010) recommends that 10–35% of the human diet consist of proteins. Proteins, which are used to rebuild, repair, and replace the body's cells, are found in meats, poultry, fish, dairy products, nuts, and legumes, and in smaller amounts in starchy foods and vegetables. Proteins are necessary for tissue growth, retaining lean muscle, generating hormones and enzymes, immune functions, and also as a source of energy in the absence of carbohydrates. Amino acids are the building blocks of proteins. Isoleucine, leucine, lysine, methionine, phenylalanine, threonine, tryptophan, valine, and histidine are considered essential dietary amino acids because the body cannot synthesize them. Recently, other amino acids such as tyrosine have been classified as indispensable under certain conditions (IOM, 2005; USDA, 2010). Serotonin, which is formed from the essential amino acid tryptophan, will be reviewed later.

Fats

Despite continuing to receive considerable, albeit understandable, "bad press" in current dieting literature, it is recommended that 20–35% of the human diet consist of fats (USDA, 2010). The body's fat (adipose) cells contain large stores of triglycerides that meet ongoing energy needs. When we are resting, our muscles expend little energy; therefore, it is not necessary to produce adenosine triphosphate (ATP) rapidly. Instead, the body's oxygen system, which uses carbohydrates, fats, and proteins as energy sources, provides required ATP for the resting physiological processes (Williams, 2007). More specifically, carbohydrates and fats combine with oxygen in the cells to provide major sources of energy during rest (Williams, 2007). In fact, in a normal diet fat supplies about 60% of the body's resting energy requirement (Eschelman, 1996; Groff, Gropper, & Hunt, 1995). However, during periods of potential food deprivation, such as those occurring during prolonged stress, fat stores are likely to contribute an even higher percentage of energy needs (Whitney & Rolfes, 2011). Red meats, whole milk, cheeses, peanut butter, ice cream, butter, bacon, avocados, chocolate, and nuts are examples of foods containing an appreciable quantity of fat. Although fat provides the body with a concentrated source of energy, unused fat from the food we eat is also easily converted to body fat, or adipose tissue, which has an essentially unrestricted storage capacity (Whitney & Rolfes, 2011). Consider, for example, that "the energy liberated from each gram of carbohydrate as it is oxidized to carbon dioxide and water is 4.1 Calories... and that liberated from fat is 9.3 Calories" (Hall, 2011, p. 843). Therefore, it is worth noting that even though fat may be helpful during periods of prolonged stress, a small amount of fat in the body typically goes a long way, particularly during periods of low stress or limited energy expenditure.

Fat is necessary for growth, cushioning of the organs, maintenance of cell membranes, and the absorption of carotenoids and the fat-soluble vitamins A, D, E, and

K. Saturated fat, monounsaturated fat, and cholesterol (a fat steroid) are adequately synthesized by the body and thus unnecessary in the diet. Saturated fat and trans fat, an unsaturated fat with an E-isomer, have been associated with heart disease. Polyunsaturated fats are essential fats that our body needs yet cannot produce. Examples of polyunsaturated fats include omega-6 and omega-3, which play a crucial role in brain function and normal growth and development. Therefore, despite the popular view that consumption of fat should be minimized, recent research suggests that the type of fat consumed is nearly as important as the amount in affecting the body's functions (IOM, 2005; USDA, 2010). Excessive fat intake is a well-known health risk, but fat deficiencies are also associated with poor outcomes including the dysregulation of chronobiological activity and cognitive function (Yehuda, Rabinovitz, & Mostofsky, 1997). We will now explore the relation between fatty acids and stress.

Fatty Acids and Stress

As noted, essential fatty acids (EFA) must be provided by diet, and are involved in many vital processes including energy production, air-to-blood oxygen transfer, hemoglobin manufacturing, and the transmission of nerve impulses. There are two types of EFAs. The omega-6 EFAs consist of linoleic and arachidonic acids, and the omega-3 EFAs consist of linolenic, eicosapentanoic, and docosahexaneoic acids (Wertz, 2009; Yehuda, Rabinovitz, & Mostofsky, 2006). Vegetables, vegetable oils, and ocean fish are important sources of EFAs, whereas wild fresh water fish are not. Simopoulos (2006) suggested that, based on a study of diets in early humans, the ratio of omega-6 to omega-3 EFAs for optimal functioning would be 1:1. The ratio in the current Western diet is as high as 20:1, and Simopoulos credits this imbalance to pathologies such as cardiovascular disease, cancer, depression, and autoimmune diseases.

Simopoulos (2001) compared consumers of the Mediterranean diet in France and Greece to examine the effects of the EFA ratio variants. The EFA ratio in the Greeks was 1:1, while it was 6:1 for the French. The difference in EFAs was accounted for by the Greek diet which consists mostly of ocean fish, as compared to the French diet where they eat more fresh water fish, higher vegetable consumption in Greece, and differences in methods of egg production. It is notable in this study that the Greeks exhibit lower rates of disease and higher life expectancy. The balance of EFAs appears important, but it is also important to avoid excessive EFA consumption as it is associated with health risks such as degenerative diseases, cardiovascular disease, cancer, and diabetes (Yehuda et al., 2006).

Omega-3 diet supplementation has been suggested as a treatment for many disorders associated with the EFA imbalance. Of particular relevance are studies noted by Yehuda et al. (2006) that reported EFA supplementation resulting in improved cardiac response to stress (Rosetti, Seiler, DeLuca, Laposata, & Zurier, 1997), and other studies noting that EFAs can decrease the stress response (Hamazaki et al., 1999;

Sawazaki, Hamazaki, Yazawa, & Kobyashi, 1999). Benefits of supplementation have been reported for many groups including individuals following heart attack (GISSI Prevensione Investigators, 1999), those diagnosed with bipolar disorder (Stoll et al., 1999), elderly depression (Tajalizadekhoob et al., 2011), and animal models of Parkinson's disease (Bousquet et al., 2011). Moreover, omega-3 supplementation has been associated with a decrease in cognitive deficits in children with developmental disorders (Richardson & Montgomery, 2005). However, other studies in individuals with bipolar disorder (Keck et al., 2006), Alzheimer's disease (Boston, Bennett, Horrobin, & Bennett, 2004), and ADHD (Hirayama, Hamazaki, & Terasawa, 2004; Voigt et al., 2001) reported no effect. In a recent systematic review of the role of fatty acids in health and disease, Riediger, Othman, Suh, and Moghadasian (2009) concluded that the beneficial effects of omega-3s have been demonstrated to the degree that their consumption should be increased.

Energy Sources and Stress

Previously, we addressed the percentage of fat used as an energy source within the body. However, an additional consideration is the energy potential or energy value of food itself. According to Eschelman (1996), in a typical American diet, "the energy value of food is 48% from carbohydrate, 35% from fat, and 14% to 18% from protein" (p. 123). Particularly relevant for the purposes of this chapter are that under low or mildly stressful conditions, the body gives preference to carbohydrates first and then fats as an energy source. In fact, carbohydrates and fats are often referred to as "protein sparers." However, during periods of severe, excessive stress, when hunger may be suppressed and digestion may be inefficient, the body may begin to consume protein stores rapidly for energy, often at six to seven times the typical rate, once carbohydrates and fats have been depleted. When this process occurs, dietary protein, along with lean muscle tissue throughout the body (including major organs such as the heart), is converted to glucose to supply energy for the nervous system. Obviously, if this process, known as ketosis, occurs for prolonged periods, then it may seriously jeopardize health.

Therefore, if you are able to eat during a period of stress, do so, of course. You may discover, however, that it is prudent to limit your caloric intake per meal, although you may try to eat more frequently. Also, the body, which conserves fluids during stress, will excrete what it does not need. Therefore, drink fluids, especially water (our most essential nutrient), which will enable your kidneys to help reestablish homeostasis. Although we do not obtain energy directly from water, vitamins, such as A, B, C, D, E, and K, which are organic chemicals, or minerals, such as calcium, iron, phosphorous, potassium, zinc, copper, iodine, magnesium, and fluoride, which are inorganic substances, "provide important components for the metabolic processes that produce the energy required for growth, development, and all life functions" (Brehm, 1998, p. 186). In converting nutrients to energy, vitamins may also produce hormones and break down waste products and toxins. It is also worth noting that the best way to obtain necessary vitamins and minerals is from the diet, not from supplements.

It also is important to note that when excessive stress begins to subside and homeostasis is being reestablished, we should take the opportunity to replenish ourselves with a healthy balance of foods and exercise (see Chap. 15) to restore both lean and fat tissue. Also, it may be helpful during times of recuperation to recognize the difference between hunger and appetite. When we are physically hungry, our bodies crave the nutrients found in the calories, vitamins, and minerals of food. Appetite, which is often described as "psychological hunger," is associated with a desire for specific foods. Fortunately, for most of us, the episodes of sustained, intense, debilitating, stress described earlier occur infrequently. Instead, we are generally accustomed to coping with recurrent episodes of mild to moderate psychosocial stressors on a regular basis.

As most of us are aware, mild to moderate and sometimes even high psychosocial stressors can trigger appetites. When this occurs, we may crave and then consume energy dense, sweet and starchy foods, as both our stress level and coping abilities dictate when and how much food we eat (Macht, 1996; Torres & Nowson, 2007). Polivy and Herman (1999) suggest that people disguise their life-related distress by overeating in order to associate their stress with binge eating rather than with the more uncontrollable areas of their lives. When we overeat, we blame ourselves for being weak and lacking self-control, but research suggests that overeating is not necessarily an issue of willpower. According to Wurtman and Suffes (1997), the hunger we experience when under notable levels of psychosocial stressors is biologically rooted, and this is why our cravings generally do not subside until sated and intensify when denied.

Macht (1996) discusses the possible relation between stress and the consumption of low-energy foods heavy in fat, salt, and sugar. He concludes that a person's emotional stress level heightens when he or she eats food that provide little energy, and this increase in anxiety can then lead to an increase in his or her desire to eat. Low-energy foods such as cheese, potato chips, and cookies are generally deficient in the natural chemicals that moderate stress, whereas a diet that includes high-energy foods such as cereals, beans, raw vegetables, and fruit is helpful in mitigating the stress and cravings we experience.

Serotonin and Stress

Stress and serotonin levels are thought to play an integral role in mood disorders (Maes & Meltzer, 1995), but the direct impact of diet on mood is difficult to quantify because so many complex systems are involved. Serotonin is a monoamine neurotransmitter that is found in carbohydrates and involved in the regulation of mood, sleep, and appetite. Increased serotonin activity in the brain improves the body's ability to cope with acute stress (Anisman & Zacharko, 1992; Chaouloff, Berton, & Mormède, 1999). However, chronic exposure to stress may lead to the continuous increase of serotonin activity resulting in an overloaded system and serotonin deficiency. Thus, one's vulnerability and reaction to stressors are important factors in determining serotonin activity (Markus et al., 1998, 2000).

When serotonin levels are low, the brain sends signals to notify the body that serotonin is needed, and this is when we have an impulse to eat. When the food we eat, particularly carbohydrates, are digested, insulin is secreted from the pancreas into the bloodstream, which delivers glucose to the cells to be used as an energy source. Because serotonin from carbohydrates is not activated until about 30 min after digestion, we may tend to overeat because we generally consume food quickly and do not stop until we feel full. If our bodies lack adequate amounts of serotonin, then the food cravings we experience are intense. We may then binge on fatty, salty and sweet food until we feel comfortable. A diet that includes carbohydrates with every meal should maintain our serotonin levels, decreasing impulses to eat unhealthy food (see Wurtman & Suffes, 1997, for additional details).

A diet rich in carbohydrates and low in proteins increases the brain's uptake of the large neutral amino acid (LNAA) tryptophan, the precursor to serotonin. Carbohydrates do not contain tryptophan, but they elevate glucose levels causing insulin secretion, which modifies the ratio of tryptophan to other LNAAs. Insulin has little impact on tryptophan levels, but it significantly decreases the level of other LNAAs such as valine, tyrosine, and leucine (Tadeka et al., 2004). Though proteins contain tryptophan, a diet high in proteins and low in carbohydrates decreases tryptophan availability because proteins possess higher levels of the other amino acids that are competing for access across the blood–brain barrier.

Increasing the uptake of carbohydrates may increase the ratio of tryptophan to other LNAAs by as much as 25%, but the effects on altering mood and coping are limited (Markus, Panhuysen, Jonkman, & Bachman, 1999). However, supplementing food with alpha-lactalbumin (ALAC), a whey-derived protein with high levels of tryptophan, has been shown to increase the plasma concentration of tryptophan (measured as a ratio of tryptophan to the sum of other neutral amino acids) by 50–130% and has been related to improved brain serotonin function, mood, and concentration (Booij, Merens, Markus, & Van der Does, 2006; Markus et al., 2000, 2005). More recently, the administration of hydrolyzed protein has yielded greater increases in plasma concentration of tryptophan and longer-lasting effects on improved mood when compared to the administration of alpha-lactalbumin and pure tryptophan in healthy participants (Markus, Firk, Gerhardt, Klock, & Smolders, 2008).

Though it has been established that tryptophan availability increases serotonin and that serotonin is involved in adaptation to stress, the mechanisms by which this occurs remains poorly understood. According to Soh and Walter (2011), there is little evidence to suggest that diet modification can elevate mood as is frequently reported in the popular media. For example, studies in humans often measure tryptophan levels in blood plasma which does not translate to a corresponding level in the brain. There remains great potential to find further dietary implications for serotonin activity and coping, and we await further research.

Antioxidants and Stress

Antioxidants, which play a prominent role in maintaining physiological well-being, are another group of neurochemicals associated with diet and stress, and continue to be popular as supplements. Substances that act as antioxidants defend our bodies from an imbalance in the production of free radicals, which are capable of damaging cells and genetic material. Free radicals, which come in various sizes, shapes and chemical configurations, occur from many sources. The body produces free radicals as a byproduct of active aerobic metabolism (turning food into energy), but they are also in the food we eat, the air we breathe, and result from exposure to sunlight (Harvard School of Public Health, (n.d.), http://www.hsph.harvard.edu/nutritionsource/what-should-you-eat/antioxidants/). For the purpose of this chapter, since all cells in the human body use O_2 to break down the energy sources of carbohydrates, fats, and proteins, free radicals are formed when O_2 molecules lose an electron during this metabolic process. The free radicals, technically O_2 molecules now with a missing electron, will then attempt to stabilize themselves by indiscreetly stealing, or scavenging, an electron from any nearby molecule, whether the molecule is a protein, fat, or another chemical, such as nucleic acids. Unfortunately, free radicals may attach to and subsequently damage these chemicals in their stabilization quest.

An excess of free radicals, along with its damaging effects, has been referred to as oxidative stress (Sies, 1993), and is enhanced with aging (Knight, 2000). To defend against free radicals and to repair the damage caused by them, the body's cells produce antioxidants, which "donate" electrons to free radicals without turning into free radicals, or electron scavengers, themselves (Lobo, Patil, Phatak, & Chandra, 2010). This in essence may delay or halt the oxidation of other substances. There are likely thousands of substances that can act as antioxidants, but the most familiar ones are vitamin E, vitamin C, selenium, beta-carotene, lycopene, and other carotenoids (Valko et al., 2007).

The use of antioxidants as a means to counter the deleterious effects of free radicals or oxidative stress flourished in the 1990s, when data began to accumulate about the association among free radical damage and degenerative diseases (Harvard School of Public Health, n. d.). Some researchers noted that activation of the sympathetic nervous system increases the number of free radicals and is associated with contributing to heart failure (Belch, Bridges, Scott, & Chopra, 1991; McMurray, Chopra, Abdullah, Smith, & Dargie, 1993). Other studies have suggested the involvement of free radicals in other degenerative diseases, such as cancer, Alzheimer's disease, cognitive impairment, cataracts, and macular degeneration (Asian & Ozben, 2004; Meyer & Sekundo, 2005; Ryan-Harshman & Aldoori, 2005; Valko, Izakovic, Mazur, Rhodes, & Telser, 2004). Moreover, psychiatric illnesses, including autism, dementia, and schizophrenia, as well as anxiety, mood, sleeping and eating disorders have been associated with oxidative stress (Tsaluchidu, Cocchi, Tonello, & Puri, 2008).

In response to these, and other similar findings regarding the effects of oxidative stress, there has been a tremendous push in the past 15 years to increase the consumption of foods rich in antioxidants, and to assess their health benefits empirically. The rationale behind this surge is that if free radicals are contributing to chronic degenerative diseases, then substances with antioxidant properties should ameliorate the problem. More than 250 selected foods were evaluated for their Oxygen Radical Absorbance Capacity (ORAC), a measure of antioxidant success, and results revealed that fruits such as blueberries, acai berries, apples, plums, cranberries, and raspberries, vegetables such as artichokes, spinach, broccoli and sweet potatoes, beans such as kidney and pinto, nuts such as pecans, walnuts, pistachios, hazelnuts, and almonds, herbs such as cinnamon, oregano, cloves, and ginger, beverages such as green tea, red wine, coffee and fruit juices (e.g., pomegranate), and finally dark chocolate for dessert, are among the best sources of antioxidants (Bliss, 2007; Hensrud, 2009).

In 2000, the Food and Nutrition Board of the Institute of Medicine provided recommendations for antioxidant intake for healthy people. The recommended Daily Allowance (RDA) for vitamin E was 15 mg/day, for vitamin C it was 90 mg/day for adult men and 75 mg/day for adult women, with a recommended additional 35 mg/day for cigarette smokers because smoking increases oxidative stress and metabolic turnover of vitamin C, for selenium it was 55 µg/day, and for beta-carotene it was 3–6 mg/day. As part of its 2010 dietary guidelines, the USDA recommends that the average American eat approximately 4–5 cups of produce per day (2.5 cups of vegetables and 2 cups of fruit), or more simply, for every meal or eating occasion, make sure half of your plate contains fruits and vegetables. Obviously, many of the fruits and vegetables chosen are likely to have antioxidant properties. This rationale of fruit and vegetable consumption at every meal seems particularly prudent since the more antioxidants one has circulating in the body, the more free radicals are debilitated. Moreover, since the life cycle of most antioxidants in the diet is relatively brief (http://www.organic-center.org), replenishing them every 4–6 h provides the more continual effects (Breakstone, n.d.). However, antioxidants at higher concentrations may adversely impact lipids, proteins, and DNA (Valko et al., 2007).

In addition to the antioxidants found in natural food sources, there is a $500 million dollar and growing antioxidant supplement industry (Harvard School of Public Health) that has proliferated in response to the touted benefits of antioxidants. In fact, a 2009 study assessing the use of antioxidant supplements reported that they accounted for 54% of vitamin C, 64% of vitamin E, 14% of carotenes, 11% of selenium, and 2% of flavonoid use for US adults (Chun et al., 2009). Despite these relatively high percentages for vitamins C and E, the use of antioxidant supplements may not be as effective as food in providing your body with maximum antioxidant benefits. Unlike supplements that often contain a single or maybe several types of antioxidants, foods contain thousands of types of antioxidants, and it may be this combination of substances in foods that interact with our body's cellular and genetic constituencies to produce a more-noted effect (Hensrud, 2009).

The benefits of antioxidants, whether in dietary or supplement form, have garnered almost panacea-like impact in the media and in consumer products for promoting health or preventing disease. Despite these rather lofty claims, the current empirical evidence suggests that the mechanisms of antioxidant action are reasonably complex, and randomized controlled trials offer little support that taking antioxidants provides substantial protection against chronic conditions such as heart disease or cancer (Cook et al., 2007; Hennekens et al., 1996; Lee et al., 2005; Lonn et al., 2005).

Success in the treatment of neurological disorders through the administration of antioxidants has been demonstrated in animal models, but not in humans, possibly due to human research being mostly observational. Moreover, studies often examine the association of reduced incidence of disease to consumption of foods rich in antioxidants, but fail to demonstrate that it is the antioxidants that are actually responsible for lowered risk (Krauss et al., 2000). It has been suggested that there is a need to more clearly define antioxidants for research purposes because many substances exhibit antioxidant qualities in vitro, but fail to do so in vivo (Kamat et al., 2008).

The current evidence in support of taking antioxidant supplements is less promising than its use in dietary form. A Cochrane Review, consisting of a comprehensive meta-analytic review of 67 randomized clinical trials of more than 230,000 participants assessing antioxidant supplements (beta-carotene, vitamin A, vitamin C, vitamin E and selenium) versus placebo concluded overall that the antioxidant supplements had no significant effect on mortality or on primary or secondary prevention and that beta-carotene, vitamin E and vitamin A are potentially harmful (Bjelakovic, Nikolova, Gluud, Simonetti, & Gluud, 2008). Although many experts have questioned the Cochrane Review's findings, an updated review of 78 randomized trials of close to 300,000 participants once again reached similar conclusions (Bjelakovic, Nikolova, Gluud, Simonetti, & Gluud, 2012). In light of the current inability to confirm direct links between antioxidants, stress, and ensuing pathologies, future intervention trials are needed to determine further the putative mechanisms involved and the recommended dietary intakes and benefits or adverse effects of supplemental intakes.

Stress and Appetite

By the turn of this century in America, one-third of adults and one-sixth of children and adolescents were obese (Baskin, Ard, Franklin, & Allison, 2005). Obesity, defined as meeting or exceeding a body mass index (BMI) of 30 (National Institutes of Health, 2011), has been associated with daily stressors including job strain (Brunner, Chandola, & Marmot, 2007) and lower socioeconomic status (Kanjilal et al., 2006). From a neurochemical perspective, corticotrophin-releasing hormone has an appetite-suppressing effect during acute stress, whereas the residual cortisol following stress has an appetite-stimulating effect. In addition, disturbances in HPA-axis functioning have been related to visceral fat accumulation (Rutters, Nieuwenhuizen, Lemmens, Born, & Westerterp-Plantenga, 2010), and cortisol levels have been associated with eating disorders (Lawson et al., 2011).

Stress in daily living has been associated with a preference for high calorie foods (Zellner et al., 2006). In fact, Rutters, Nieuwenhuizen, Lemmens, Born and Westerterp-Plantenga (2008) studied the effects of psychological stress on food intake and food preference in normal and overweight men and women, and reported that stress conditions were associated with food intake even in the absence of hunger and with a preference for sweet fatty foods. In a review of 22 studies, Adams, Minogue, and Lucock (2010) concluded that mental health problems are associated with poor dietary practices, including frequent consumption of saturated fat and refined sugar, and lower consumption of omega-3.

Caffeinated Energy Drinks

The USA leads the world in the total volume sales of energy drinks, with world-wide consumption of these beverages reaching 906 million gallons in 2006 (Reissig, Strain, & Griffiths, 2009). Self-reports indicate that energy drinks are consumed by 30–50% of adolescents and young adults (Seifert, Schachter, Hershorin & Lipshultz, 2011), and in a sample of college students, those who used energy drinks reported they consumed them for insufficient sleep (67%) to increase energy (65%) and to use in conjunction with alcohol (54%) (Malinauskas, Aeby, Overton, Carpenter-Aeby, & Barber-Heidal, 2007). Although energy drinks contain natural products such as ginseng, taruine, and guarana, their quantity is typically well below what would be expected to produce either therapeutic benefits or adverse effects (Clauson, Shields, McQueen, & Persad, 2008). Caffeine, on the other hand, is the primary active ingredient in energy drinks, and while its content in a six ounce cup of coffee typically ranges between 77 and 150 mg, caffeinated energy drinks can reach 505 mg (Griffiths, Juliano, & Chausmer, 2003). Caffeine, which is a central nervous system stimulant, is considered safe in healthy adults at intake levels of less than 400 mg/day (Cannon, Cooke & McCarthy, 2001; Seifert et al.). Potential performance-enhancing effects of energy drink consumption have been suggested such as their beneficial use when given to sleepy drivers (Horne & Reyner, 2001) or their significant effects on task performance and self-rated mood (Smit & Rogers, 2002).

However, the frequently higher levels of caffeine intake in energy drinks may result in caffeine intoxication, which is recognized as a clinical disorder in both the Diagnostic and Statistical Manual of Mental Disorders (American Psychiatric Association, 2004) and the International Classification of Diseases (World Health Organization, 2008). Symptoms of caffeine intoxication include insomnia, anxiety, headache, tachycardia, psychomotor agitation, gastrointestinal irritation, increased blood pressure tremors, diabetes, mood disturbance, behavioral disorder, and in rare cases death (Clauson et al., 2008; O'Brien, McCoy, Rhodes, Wagoner, & Wolfson, 2008; Rogers, 2007; Scholey & Kennedy, 2004; Seifert et al., 2011; Whelton et al., 2002). These numerous adverse effects have in part led Seifert and her colleagues (2011) to conclude that, "energy drinks have no therapeutic benefit" (p. 522). Despite Seifert and colleagues claim, the consumer market for and use of energy drinks does not appear to be diminishing anytime soon. Therefore, it seems that additional controlled studies are needed to further assess the use and effects of energy drinks.

Future Directions

In a recent article in the *American Psychologist*, Walsh (2011) suggested that health professionals have significantly underestimated the importance of nutrition and other lifestyle factors for mental health as well as the potential therapeutic benefits of proper nutrition in the treatment of psychopathology. He addressed the efficacy of various therapeutic lifestyle changes including diet modification, and included an evolutionary perspective. For example, he noted that just as ADHD may be a result of modern children developing in environments far different than those of our ancestors (Bjorklund & Pelligrini, 2002), the shift to a diet radically different than our ancestors likely contributes to many current pathologies. Moreover, some studies suggest that the impact of diet on mental health can be epigenetically transmitted across generations (Gómez-Pinilla, 2008).

Another of the recent trends in the past decade has been the surge of organic foods. In fact, organic food sales in the USA were 26.7 billion in 2010 (Organic Trade Association's 2011 Organic Industry Survey). Organic foods are grown and produced without the use of synthetic pesticides, artificial fertilizers, genetic engineering or ionizing radiation (used to kill bacteria), and the USDA has established requirements that all foods labeled as organic meet stringent government standards (Health & Nutrition, 2006). The absence of pesticides and fertilizers is thought to provide higher nutritional value than conventional food, and there are some data linking the use of pesticides with increasing the stress response and producing oxidative stress in bacterial cells and fish (Miller, Rasmussen, Palace, & Hontela, 2009; Özcan Oruc & Usta, 2007; Pham, Min, & Gu, 2004). However, a critical review of the literature on the safety of organic foods concluded that there are currently limited empirical data "to support or refute claims that organic food is safer and thus, healthier, than conventional food, or vice versa" (Magkos, Arvaniti, & Zampelsa, 2006, p. 47). Regardless, organic foods are infused in our mainstream culture and their popularity continues to grow dramatically. Additional longitudinal research will be helpful in determining their safety, and if they do, indeed, possess superior nutritional composition compared to conventional food production.

There also has been a recent increase in the production of designer foods, which have been commonly referred to in the literature as nutraceuticals or functional foods. Neutraceutical has been defined as any food, part of a food, supplement, genetically engineered food or diet that provides health benefits (DeFelice, 1992). Tadeka et al. (2004) described a functional food as having a tertiary function beyond nutritional necessities for survival and sensory satisfaction. Specifically, they described some tertiary functions as biorhythm regulation, immune and body defense, and as contributions to psychological life components. Many of these nutraceuticals or functional foods, such as omega-3 or antioxidant supplements were discussed in this chapter. As stated earlier, direct effects of supplemental interventions have not been reliably demonstrated.

One of the most promising fields of study to address these difficulties is that of nutrigenomics. Nutrigenomics is the study of the effects of nutrition at the genetic level (Ardekani & Jabbari, 2009). More specifically, it is the study of how nutrition influences homeostasis, and attempts to identify genes that are associated with risk of nutrition-related pathology. It is thought that with new developments in the genome map that optimal diets can be identified and individualized.

The potential for nutrigenomics is apparent in recent studies. For example, Bakker et al. (2010) demonstrated the modulation of inflammation, oxidative stress, and metabolism in overweight subjects utilizing an analysis of gene expression, proteins, and metabolites following the supplementation of diet with products including vitamin C and omega-3s. Sun, Morris, and Zemel (2008) utilized nutrigenomic methods to demonstrate that calcitrol regulates fat cell gene expression and cortisol production in fat cells, and that dietary calcium intake inhibits visceral fatty tissue gene expression. In studies of mice and humans, they identified a calcitrol/cortisol interaction in obesity suggesting that there is potential for dietary interventions to reduce fatty tissue through calcitrol suppression.

Conclusion

The nutrients we consume, their proportion to other nutrients, and genetic predispositions influence how our body copes with stress. Many nutrients have been identified as particularly relevant to the regulatory systems of the stress response. These include antioxidants which exist in high levels in many plant-based foods, tryptophan which synthesizes into serotonin, and essential fatty acids such as omega-3s. Because our systems and pathways of metabolizing these nutrients are interactive and complex, as well as methodological challenging when conducting human research, it has been difficult to identify causal links of nutrients to specific pathologies. However, the associations between nutrition and physical and mental health are convincing. Pescovegetarian diets, such as the Mediterranean diet, are frequently associated with better health outcomes and are recommended throughout the literature. The recent research advances in the developing field of nutrigenomics shows promise in identifying effective dietary interventions.

Summary

This chapter presents a brief overview of how diet and nutrition are associated with the human stress response. The main points are:

1. Many health outcomes including physical and psychological pathologies have been associated with diet.
2. According to the USDA (2010), it is recommended that 45–65% of the human diet consists of carbohydrates, 10–35% consists of proteins, and 20–35% consists of fats. Our bodies rely on these energy sources when responding to stress.
3. Of the two general types of carbohydrates, simple and complex, simple carbohydrates (monosaccharides and disaccharides), or sugars come primarily from fruits, vegetables, and milk (or milk products), and are found in many different sweeteners (e.g., table sugar, honey, molasses). Complex carbohydrates (polysaccharides) are found in grains (e.g., rice, wheat, rye, barley, and oats), legumes (e.g., peanuts, peas, beans), and potatoes.
4. Proteins, composed of amino acids, are used to repair, rebuild, and replace cells. Eggs, milk, beef, fish, and soybeans are foods high in protein.
5. Fat provides the body with a concentrated energy source that may be especially relevant during periods of intense stress. Red meats, whole milk, cheeses, butter, bacon, chocolate, and nuts provide a large quantity of fat.
6. Excessive and deficient fat consumption are both associated with health risk. Omega-6 and omega-3 are two types of essential fatty acids, and an even consumption has been suggested for optimal functioning. Western diets significantly favor omega-6 EFAs, and this imbalance facilitates disease. Omega-3s are found in vegetables, vegetable oils, and saltwater fish.
7. During periods of excessive stress, the body, which usually conserves protein as its energy source, may begin to consume protein stores rapidly when carbohydrates and fats are depleted.
8. Serotonin influences sleep, mood, and appetite. Tryptophan, the precursor to serotonin, is found in proteins among many other large neutral amino acids. Though carbohydrates do not contain tryptophan, a diet rich in carbohydrates and low in protein enhances tryptophan uptake in the brain by modifying the ratio of tryptophan to competing amino acids.
9. Oxidative stress is the imbalance of the oxidant–antioxidant ratio in favor of the oxidants, or free radicals. Antioxidants inhibit or delay oxidation. Oxidative stress has been associated with many physical and mental disorders, and, even though the data are equivocal, there has been a proliferation in the use of dietary antioxidants and supplement antioxidants to try and mitigate the impact of

oxidative stress. Appetite is an important trigger during psychosocial stressors. Stress has been associated with eating in the absence of hunger and a preference for sweet, calorie-dense foods.

10. Nutrition has been associated with pathology known to have a stress component, but direct causal links among nutrients and disease have not been conclusively demonstrated.

11. Caffeinated energy drinks have been associated to date with adverse effects including tachycardia, anxiety, seizures, mood disturbance, and tremors, and more controlled studies are needed to further assess these claims.

12. The surge in organic food consumption in the USA is expected to continue, and more empirical efficacy studies should be conducted.

13. Nutrigenomics holds promise to identify and individualize optimum diets in light of one's genetic predisposition to disease. In the meantime, a pescovegetarian diet such as the Mediterranean diet has been consistently associated with positive health outcomes.

Acknowledgment We would like to thank Stephen F. Bono, Ph.D., Clinical Pain Psychologist, Kernans Orthopaedics and Rehabilitation, University of Maryland Medical System, for his early review of this chapter.

References

Adams, K., Minogue, V., & Lucock, M. (2010). Nutrition and mental health recovery. *Mental Health and Learning Disabilities Research and Practice, 7*(1), 43–57.

American Psychiatric Association. (2004). *Practice guideline for the treatment of patients with acute stress disorder and posttraumatic stress disorder*. Arlington, VA: American Psychiatric Association. Available online at: http://psychiatryonline.org/guidelines.aspx.

Anderson, J. W., Baird, P., Davis, R. H., Ferreri, S., Knudtson, M., Koraym, A., & Williams, C. L. (2009). Health benefits of dietary fiber. *Nutrition Reviews, 67,* 188–205.

Anisman, H., & Zacharko, R. M. (1992). Depression as a consequence of inadequate neurochemical adaptation in response to stressors. *The British Journal of Psychiatry, 160,* 36–43.

Ardekani, A. M., & Jabbari, M. (2009). Nutrigenomics and cancer. *Avicenna Journal of Medical Biotechnology, 1*(1), 9–17.

Asian, M., & Ozben, T. (2004). Reactive oxygen and nitrogen species in Alzheimer's disease. *Current Alzheimer Research, 1,* 111–119.

Bakker, G. C. M., van Erk, M. J., Pellis, L., Wopereis, S., Rubingh, C. M., Cnubben, N. H. P., & Hendriks, H. F. J. (2010). An antiinflammatory dietary mix modulates inflammation and oxidative and metabolic stress in overweight men: A nutrigenomics approach. *The American Journal of Clinical Nutrition, 91,* 1044–1059.

Baskin, M. L., Ard, J., Franklin, F., & Allison, D. B. (2005). Prevalence of obesity in the United States. *Obesity Reviews, 6,* 5–7.

Belch, J. J., Bridges, A. B., Scott, N., & Chopra, M. (1991). Oxygen free radicals and congestive heart failure. *British Heart Journal, 65,* 245–248.

Bjelakovic, G., Nikolova, D., Gluud, L. L., Simonetti, R. G., & Gluud, C. (2008). Antioxidant supplements for prevention of mortality in healthy participants and patients with various diseases. *Cochrane Database of Systematic Reviews, 2,* CD007176.

Bjelakovic, G., Nikolova, D., Gluud, L. L., Simonetti, R. G., & Gluud, C. (2012). Antioxidant supplements for prevention of mortality in healthy participants and patients with various diseases. *Cochrane Database of Systematic Reviews, 3,* CD007176.

Bjorklund, D. F., & Pelligrini, A. D. (2002). *The origins of human nature.* Washington, DC: American Psychological Association.

Bliss, R. M. (2007). *Data on food antioxidants aid research.* United States Department of Agriculture. Retrieved June 16, 2012, from http://www.ars.usda.gov/is/pr/2007/071106.htm

Booij, L., Merens, W., Markus, C. R., & Van der Does, A. J. (2006). Diet rich in {alpha}-lactalbumin improves memory in unmedicated recovered depressed patients and matched controls. *Journal of Psychopharmacology, 20,* 526–535.

Boston, P. F., Bennett, A., Horrobin, D. F., & Bennett, C. N. (2004). Ethyl-EPA in Alzheimer's disease – A pilot study. *Prostaglandins, Leukotrienes, and Essential Fatty Acids, 71,* 341–346.

Bousquet, M., Gue, K., Emond, V., Julien, P., Kang, J. X., Cicchetti, F., & Calon, F. (2011). Transgenic conversion of omega-6 into omega-3 fatty acids in a mouse model of Parkinson's Disease. *Journal of Lipid Research, 52,* 263–271.

Breakstone, S. (n.d.). Eat to live longer. Shed unwanted pounds and slow aging with 6 tops diet tips. *Prevention.* Available online: http://www.prevention.com/eattolivelonger/index.shtml

Brehm, B. A. (1998). *Stress management: Increasing your stress resistance.* New York, NY: Longman.

Brunner, E. J., Chandola, T., & Marmot, M. G. (2007). Prospective effect of job strain on general and central obesity in the Whitehall II study. *American Journal of Epidemiology, 165,* 828–837.

Cannon, M. E., Cooke, C. T., & McCarthy, J. S. (2001). Caffeine-induced cardiac arrhythmia: An unrecognised danger of healthfood products. *Medical Journal of Australia, 174*(10), 520–521.

Carlsen, M. H., Halvorsen, B. L., Holte, K., Bohn, S. K., Dragland, S., Sampson, L., … Blomhoff, R. (2010). The total antioxidant content of more than 3100 foods beverages, spices, herbs and supplements worldwide. *Nutrition Journal, 9.* Retrieved from http://www.nutritionj.com/content/9/1/3

Chaouloff, F., Berton, O., & Mormède, P. (1999). Serotonin and stress. *Neuropsychopharmacology, 21,* 28S–32S.

Charrondiere, U. R., Chevassus-Agnes, S., Marroni, S., & Burlingame, B. (2004). Impact of different macronutrient definitions and energy conversion factors on energy supply estimations. *Journal of Food Composition and Analysis, 17,* 339–360.

Chun, O. K., Floegel, A., Chung, S.-J., Chung, C. E., Song, W. O., & Koo, S. I. (2009). Estimation of antioxidant intakes from diet and supplements in U.S. adults. *The Journal of Nutrition, 140,* 317–324.

Clauson, K. A., Shields, K. M., McQueen, C. E., & Persad, N. (2008). Safety issues associated with commercially available energy drinks. *Pharmacy Today, 14*(5), 52–64.

Cook, N. R., Albert, C. M., Gaziano, J. M., Zaharris, E., MacFadyen, J., Danielson, E., Manson, J. E. (2007). A randomized factorial trial of vitamins C and E and beta carotene in the secondary prevention of cardiovascular events in women: Results from the Women's Antioxidant Cardiovascular Study. *Archives of Internal Medicine, 167*(15), 1610–1618.

DeFlice, S. L. (1992). The nutraceutical initiative: a recommendation for U.S. economic and regulatory reforms. *Genetic Engineering News, 12,* 13–15.

Eschelman, M. M. (1996). *Introductory nutrition and nutrition therapy* (3rd ed.). Philadelphia, PA: Lippincott.

Food and Nutrition Board Institute of Medicine. (2000). *Dietary reference intakes far vitamin C, vitamin E, selenium, and carotenoids (A Report of the Panel on Dietary Antioxidants and Related Compounds, Subcommittees on Upper Reference Levels of Nutrients and Interpretation and Uses of Dietary Reference Intakes, and the Standing Committee on the Scientific Evaluation of Dietary Reference Intakes).* Washington, DC: National Academy Press.

Frautschy, S. A., Hu, W., Kim, P., Miller, S. A., Chu, T., Harris-White, M. E., & Cole, G. M. (2001). Phenolic anti-inflammatory antioxidant reversal of Aβ induced cognitive deficits and neuropathology. *Neurobiology of Aging, 22,* 993–1005.

GISSI Prevensione Investigators. (1999). Dietary supplementation with n-3 polyunsaturated fatty acids and vitamin E after myocardial infarction: Results of the GISSI-Prevenzione trial. Gruppo Italiano per lo Studio della Soprawivenza nell'Infarto miocardico. *Lancet, 354*, 447–455.

Gómez-Pinilla, F. (2008). Brain foods: The effects of nutrients on brain function. *Nature Reviews Neuroscience, 9*, 568–578.

Greenberg, J. S., Dintiman, G. B., & Myers-Oakes, B. (1998). *Physical fitness and wellness* (2nd ed.). Boston, MA: Allyn & Bacon.

Griffiths, R. R., Juliano, L. M., & Chausmer, A. L. (2003). Caffeine: Pharmacology and clinical effects. In A. W. Graham, T. K. Schultz, M. F. Mayo-Smith, R. K. Ries, & B. B. Wilford (Eds.), *Principles of addiction medicine* (3rd ed., pp. 193–224). Chevy Chase, MD: American Society of Addiction.

Groff, J., Cropper, S., & Hunt, S. M. (1995). *Advanced nutrition and human metabolism* (2nd ed.). Minneapolis, St. Paul: West.

Hall, J. E. (2011). *Guyton and Hall Textbook of Medical Physiology* (12th ed.). Philadelphia, PA: Saunders Elsevier.

Hamazaki, T., Sawazaki, S., Nagasawa, T., Nagao, Y., Kanagawa, Y., & Yazawa, K. (1999). Administration of docosahexaenoic acid influence behavior and plasma catecholamine levels at times of psychological stress. *Lipids, 34*, S33–S37.

Harvard School of Public Health (n.d.). The nutrition source. Antioxidants Beyond the hype. Retrevied from: http://www.hsph.harvard.edu/nutritionsource/what-should-you-eat/antioxidants/

Health & Nutrition (2006). *Get the facts about organic foods*. http://cleveland.ces.ncsu.edu/index.php?page=news&ci=HEAL+4. Retrieved June 19, 2012.

Hennekens, C. H., Buring, J. E., Manson, J. E., Stampfer, M., Rosner, B., Cook, N. R., & Peto, R. (1996). Lack of effect of long-term supplementation with beta carotene on the incidence of malignant neoplasms and cardiovascular disease. *New England Journal of Medicine, 334*(18), 1145–1149.

Hensrud, D. (2009). Food sources the best choice for antioxidants. Medical Edge Newspaper Column. Mayo Clinic. www.mayoclinic.org/medical-edge-newspaper-2009/jun-05b.htm. Retrieved June 16, 2012

Hirayama, S., Hamazaki, T., & Terasawa, K. (2004). Effect of docosahexaenoic acid-containing food administration on symptoms of attention deficit/hyperactivity disorder – a placebo-controlled double-blind study. *European Journal of Clinical Nutrition, 58*, 467–473.

Horne, J. A., & Reyner, L. A. (2001). Beneficial effects of an "energy drink" given to sleepy drivers. *Amino Acids, 20*, 83–89.

Institute of Medicine. (2005). *Dietary reference intakes for energy, carbohydrate, fiber, fat, fatty acids, cholesterol, protein, and amino acids (macronutrients)*. Washington DC: National Academies Press.

Kamat, C. D., Gadal, S., Mhatre, M., Williamson, K. S., Pye, Q. N., & Hensley, K. (2008). Antioxidants in central nervous system diseases: Preclinical promise and translational challenges. *Journal of Alzheimer's Disease, 15*, 473–493.

Kanjilal, S., Gregg, E. W., Cheng, Y. J., Zhang, P., Nelson, D. E., & Mensah, G., et al. (2006). Socioeconomic status and trends in disparities in 4 major risk factors for cardiovascular disease among US adults, 1971–2002. *Archives of Internal Medicine, 166*, 2348–2355.

Keck, P. E., Mintz, J., McElroy, S. L., Freeman, M. P., Suppes, T., Frye, M. A., & Post, R. M. (2006). Double-blind, randomized, placebo-controlled trials of ethyl-eicosapentanoate in the treatment of bipolar depression and rapid cycling bipolar disorder. *Biological Psychiatry, 60*, 1020–1022

Knight, J. A. (2000). The biochemistry of aging. *Advances in Clinical Chemistry, 35*, 1–62.

Krauss, R. M., Eckel, R. H., Howard, B., Appel, L. J., Daniels, S. R., Deckelbaum, R. J., … Bazzarre, T. L. (2000). Revision 2000: A statement for healthcare professionals from the nutrition committee of the American Heart Association. *Circulation, 102*, 2284–2289

Lawson, E. A., Eddy, K. T., Donoho, D., Misra, M., Miller, K. K., Meenaghan, E., … Klibanski, A. (2011). Appetite-regulating hormones cortisol and peptide YY are associated with disordered eating psychopathology, independent of body mass index. *European Journal of Endocrinology, 164,* 253–261.

Lee, I. M., Cook, N. R., Gaziano, J. M., Gordon, D., Ridker, P. M., Manson, J. E., ... Buring, J. E. (2005). Vitamin E in the primary prevention of cardiovascular disease and cancer: The Women's Health Study: A randomized controlled trial. *Journal of the American Medical Association, 294*(1), 56–65

Lobo, V., Patil, A., Phatak, A., & Chandra, N. (2010). Free radicals, antioxidants, and functional foods: Impact on human health. *Pharmacognosy Review, 4,* 118–126.

Lonn, E., Bosch, J., Yusuf, S., Sheridan, P., Pogue, J., Arnold, J. M. ... HOPE and HOPE-TOO Trial Investigators (2005). Effects of long-term vitamin E supplementation on cardiovascular events and cancer: A randomized controlled trial. *Journal of the American Medical Association, 293*(11), 1338–1347

Maes, M., & Meltzer, H. (1995). The serotonin hypothesis of major depression. In F. E. Bloom & D. J. Kupfer (Eds.), Psychopharmacology: *The fourth generation of progress* (pp. 933–934). New York: Raven Press.

Macht, M. (1996). Effects of high-and low-energy meals on hunger, physiological processes and reactions to emotional stress. *Appetite, 26*(1), 71–88.

Magkos, R., Arvaniti, F., & Zampelas, A. (2006). Organic food: Buying more safety or just peace of mind? A critical review of the literature. *Critical Reviews in Food Science and Nutrition, 46,* 23–56.

Malinauskas, B. M., Aeby, V. G., Overton, R. F., Carpenter-Aeby, T., & Barber-Heidal, K. (2007). A survey of energy drink consumption patterns among college students. Nutrition Journal, 6(35), 1–7; Available online: http://www.biomedcentral.com/content/pdf/1475-2891-6-35.pdf

Markus, C. R., Firk, C., Gerhardt, C., Klock, J., & Smolders, G. F. (2008). Effect of different tryptophan sources on amino acids availability to the brain and mood in health volunteers. *Psychopharmacology, 201,* 107–114.

Markus, C. R., Jonkman, L. M., Lammers, J. H., Deutz, N. E., Messer, M. H., & Rigtering, M. (2005). Evening intake of alpha-lactalbumin increases plasma tryptophan availability and improves morning alertness and brain measures of attention. *American Journal of Clinical Nutrition, 81,* 1026–1033.

Markus, C. R., Olivier, G., Paynhuysen, G., Van der Gugten, J., Alles, M. S., Tuiten, A., ... de Hann, E. (2000). The bovine protein α-Lactalbumin increases the plasma ratio of tryptophan to the other large neutral amino acids, and in vulnerable subjects raises brain serotonin activity, reduces cortisol concentration, and improves mood under stress. *American Journal of Clinical Nutrition, 71,* 1536–1544.

Markus, C. R., Panhuysen, G., Jonkman, L. M., & Bachman, M. (1999). Carbohydrate intake improves cognitive performance of stressprone individuals under controllable laboratory stress. *British Journal of Nutrition, 82,* 457–467.

Markus, C. R., Panhuysen, G., Tuiten, A., Koppenschaar, H., Fekkes, D., & Peters, M. L. (1998). Does carbohydrate-rich, protein-poor food prevent a deterioration of mood and cognitive performance of stress-prone subjects when subjected to a stressful task? *Appetite, 31,* 49–65.

McMurray, J., Chopra, M., Abdullah, I., Smith, W. E., & Dargie, H. J. (1993). Evidence of oxidative stress in chronic heart failure in humans. *European Heart Journal, 14,* 1493–1498.

Meyer, C. H., & Sekundo, W. (2005). Nutritional supplementation to prevent cataract formation. *Developmental Opthalmology, 38,* 103–119.

Miller, L. L., Rasmussen, J. B., Palace, V. P., & Hontela, A. (2009). Physiological stress response in white suckers from agricultural drain waters containing pesticides and selenium. *Ecotoxicology and Environmental Safety, 72,* 1249–1256.

National Institutes of Health. (2011). *Overweight.* Retrieved from http://www.nlm.nih.gov/medlineplus/ency/article/003101.htm

O'Brien, M. C., McCoy, T., Rhodes, S. D., Wagoner, A., & Wolfson, M. (2008). Caffeinated cocktails: Get wired, get drunk, get injured. *Academy of Emergency Medicine, 15,* 453–460.

Organic Trade Association. (2011). *Industry statistics and projected growth.* http://www.ota.com/organic/mt/business.html. Retrieved June 19, 2012

Özcan Oruc, E., & Usta, D. (2007). Evaluation of oxidative stress responses and neurotoxicity potential of diazinon in different tissues of *Cyprinus carpo. Environmental Toxicology and Pharmacology, 23*, 48–55.

Pham, C. H., Min, J., & Gu, M. B. (2004). Pesticide induced toxicity and stress response in bacterial cells. *Bulletin of Environmental Contamination and Toxicology, 72*, 380–386.

Polivy, J., & Herman, C. P. (1999). Distress and eating: Why do dieters overeat? *International Journal of Stress Management, 5*(1), 57–75.

Reissig, C. J., Strain, E. C., & Griffiths, R. R. (2009). Caffeinated energy drinks – A growing problem. *Drug and Alcohol Dependence, 99*(1), 1–10.

Richardson, A. J., & Montgomery, P. (2005). The Oxford-Durham Study: A randomized, controlled trial of dietary supplementation with fatty acids in children with developmental co-ordination disorder. *Child: Care, Health, and Development, 31*, 629–630.

Riediger, N. D., Othman, R. A., Suh, M., & Moghadasian, M. H. (2009). A systematic review of n-3 fatty acids in health and disease. *Journal of the American Dietetic Association, 109*, 668–679.

Rogers, P. J. (2007). Caffeine, mood and mental performance in everyday life. *Nutrition Bulletin, 32*(suppl 1), 84–89.

Rosetti, R. G., Seiler, C. M., Deluca, P., Laposata, M., & Zurier, R. B. (1997). Oral administration of unsaturated fatty acids: Effects on human peripheral blood T lymphocyte proliferation. *Journal of Leukocyte Biology, 62*, 438–443.

Rutters, F., Nieuwenhuizen, A. G., Lemmens, S. G. T., Born, J. M., & Westerterp-Plantenga, M. S. (2008). Acute stress-related changes in eating in the absence of hunger. *Obesity, 17*, 72–77.

Rutters, F., Nieuwenhuizen, A. G., Lemmens, S. G. T., Born, J. M., & Westerterp-Plantenga, M. S. (2010). Hypothalamic-pituitary-adrenal (HPA) axis functioning in relation to body fat distribution. *Clinical Endocrinology, 72*, 738–743.

Ruxton, C. H. S., Gardner, E. J., & McNulty, H. M. (2010). Is sugar consumption detrimental to health? A review of the evidence 1995–2006. *Critical Reviews in Food Science and Nutrition, 50*(1), 1–19.

Ryan-Harshman, M., & Aldoori, W. (2005). The relevance of selenium to immunity, cancer, and infectious/inflammatory diseases. *Canadian Journal of Dietetic Practice and Research, 66*, 98–102.

Sawazaki, S., Hamazaki, T., Yazawa, K., & Kobyashi, M. (1999). The effect of docosahexoanoic acid on plasma catecholamine concentrations and glucose tolerance during long-lasting psychological stress: A double blind placebo-controlled study. *Journal of Nutritional Science and Vitaminology, 45*, 655–665.

Scholey, A. B., & Kennedy, D. O. (2004). Cognitive and physiological effects of an "energy drink": An evaluation of the whole drink and of glucose, caffeine and herbal flavouring fractions. *Psychopharmacology, 176*(3–4), 320–330.

Seifert, S. M., Schachter, J. L., Hershorin, E. R., & Lipshulz, S. E. (2011). Health effects of energy drinks on children, adolescents, and young adults. *Pediatrics, 127*, 511–528.

Sies, H. (1993). Strategies of antioxidant defense. *European Journal of Biochemistry, 215*, 213–219.

Simopoulos, A. P. (2001). The Mediterranean diets: What is so special about the diet of Greece? The scientific evidence. *Journal of Nutrition, 131*, 3065S–3073S.

Simopoulos, A. P. (2006). Evolutionary aspects of diet, the omega-6/omega-3 ratio and genetic variation: nutritional implications for chronic diseases. *Biomedicine & Pharmacotherapy, 60*, 502–507.

Smit, H. J., & Rogers, P. J. (2002). Effects of "energy" drinks on mood and mental performance: Critical methodology. *Food Quality and Preference, 13*(5), 317–326.

Sofi, F., Cesari, F., Abbate, R., Gensini, F., & Casini, A. (2008). Adherence to Mediterranean diet and health status: Meta-analysis. *British Medical Journal.* Available Online: http://www.ncbi. nlm.nih.gov/pmc/articles/PMC2533524/pdf/bmj.a1344.pdf

Soh, N. L., & Walter, G. (2011). Tryptophan and depression: Can diet alone be the answer? *Acta Neuropsychiatrica, 23,* 3–11.

Stoll, A. L., Locke, C. A., Marangell, L. B., & Severus, W. E. (1999). Omega-3 fatty acids and bipolar disorder: A review. *Prostaglandins, Leukotrienes and Essential Fatty Acids, 60*(5–6), 329–337.

Sun, X., Morris, K. L., & Zemel, M. B. (2008). Role of calcitriol and cortisol on human adipocyte proliferation and oxidative and inflammatory stress: a microarray study. *Journal of Nutrigenetics and Nutrigenomics, 1*(1–2), 30–48.

Tadeka, E., Terao, J., Nakaya, Y., Miyamoto, K., Baba, Y., Chuman, H., & Rokutan, K. (2004). Stress control and human nutrition. *The Journal of Medical Investigation, 51,* 139–145.

Tajalizadekhoob, Y., Sharifi, F., Fakhrzadeh, H., Mirarefin, M., Ghaderpanahi, M., Badamchizade, Z., & Azimipour, S. (2011). The effect of low-dose omega 3 fatty acids on the treatment of mild to moderate depression in the elderly: a double-blind, randomized, placebo-controlled study. *European Archives of Psychiatry and Clinical Neuroscience.* Advance Online Publication. Available from http://www.ncbi.nlm.nig.gov/pubmed/

Torres, S., & Nowson, C. (2007). Relationship between stress, eating behavior and obesity. *Nutrition, 23*(11–12), 887–894.

Tsaluchidu, S., Cocchi, M., Tonello, L., & Puri, B. (2008). Fatty acids and oxidative stress in psychiatric disorders. *BMC Psychiatry, 8,* S1–S5.

U.S. Department of Veterans Affairs, Veterans Health Administration, Office of Public Health and Environmental Hazards. (2010). Analysis of VA health care utilization among U.S. Global War of Terrorism (GWOT) veterans. Unpublished quarterly report (cumulative through 4th quarter FY 2009). Washington, DC: Author.

United States Department of Agriculture. (2010). *Report of the Dietary Guidelines Advisory Committee on the Dietary Guidelines for Americans.* Retrieved from http://www.cnpp.usda. gov/Publications/DietaryGuidelines/2010/DGAC/Report/2010DGACReport-camera-ready-Jan11-11.pdf

Valko, M., Izakovic, M., Mazur, M., Rhodes, C. J., & Telser, J. (2004). Role of oxygen radicals in DNA damage and cancer incidence. *Molecular Cell, 266,* 37–57.

Valko, M., Leibfritz, D., Moncol, J., Cronin, M., Mazur, M., & Telser, J. (2007). Free radicals and antioxidants in physiological functions and human disease. *The International Journal of Biochemistry & Cell Biology, 39,* 44–84.

Voigt, R. G., Llorente, A. M., Jensen, C. L., Fraley, J. K., Berretta, M. C., & Heird, W. C. (2001). A randomized, double-blind, placebo-controlled trial of docosahexaenoic acid supplemenation in children with attention deficit/hyperactivity disorder. *The Journal of Pediatrics, 139,* 189–196.

Walsh, R. (2011). Lifestyle and mental health. *American Psychologist, 66*(7), 579–592.

Wertz, P. W. (2009). Essenetial fatty acids and dietary stress. *Toxicology and Industrial Health, 25,* 279–283.

Whelton, P. K., He, J., Appel, L. J., Cutler, J. A., Havas, S., Kotchen, T. A., … Karimbakas, J. (2002). Primary prevention of hyptertension: Clinical and public health agency advisory from the National High Blood Pressure Education Program. *Journal of the American Medical Association, 288*(15), 1882–1888.

Whitney, E. N., Hamilton, E. M., & Rolfes, S. R. (1990). *Understanding nutrition* (5th ed.). St. Paul, MN: West.

Whitney, E., & Rolfes, S. R. (2011). *Understanding nutrition* (12th ed.). Belmont, CA: Wadsworth.

Williams, M. H. (2007). *Nutrition for health, fitness, and sport* (8th ed.). Boston: McGraw-Hill.

Wolraich, M. L., Wilson, D. B., & White, J. W. (1995). The effect of sugar on behavior or cognition in children. A meta-analysis. *Journal of the American Medical Association, 274,* 1617–1621.

World Health Organization. (2008). *ICD-10: International statistical classification of diseases and related health problems* (10 Revth ed.). New York, NY: Author.

Wurtman, J., & Suffes, S. (1997). *The serotonin solution: To achieve permanent weight control.* New York: Ballentine Books.

Yehuda, S., Rabinovitz, S., & Mostofsky, D. I. (1997). Effects of essential fatty acids preparation (SR-3) on brain biochemistry and on behavioral and cognitive functions. In S. Yehuda & D. I. Mostofsky (Eds.), *Handbook of essential fatty acids biology: Biochemistry physiology and behavioral neurobiology* (pp. 427–452). Totawa, NJ: Humana.

Yehuda, S., Rabinovitz, S., & Mostofsky, D. I. (2006). Essential fatty acids and stress. In S. Yehuda & D. I. Mostofsky (Eds.), *Nutrients, stress, and medical disorders* (pp. 99–110). Totawa, NJ: Humana.

Zellner, D. A., Loaiza, S., Gonzalez, Z., Pita, J., Morales, J., Pecora, D., & Wolf, A. (2006). Food selection changes under stress. *Physiological Behavior, 87*, 789–793.

Chapter 19
Sleep and Stress

"The effect is too much, sleep is winning, my whole body
argues dully that nothing, nothing life can attain is quite so
desirable as sleep. My mind is losing resolution and control.

Charles Lindbergh regarding his 1927 transatlantic flight

Sleep is the best cure for waking troubles.

Miguel de Cervantes

We spend roughly one-third of our lives craving, pursuing, forgoing, and savoring sleep. While it is apparent that sleep, which is considered a "complex amalgam of physiologic and behavioral processes" (Carskadon & Dement, 2011, p. 16) is universal and has vital life-preserving functions, its essential purpose remains unknown (Goldsmith & Casola, 2006; Hirshkowitz, Moore, & Minhoto, 1997; Horne, 2006). Theories suggest that sleep restores homeostasis in the central nervous system, conserves energy, regulates heat, or allows for processing of affective information (Goldsmith & Casola, 2006; Schwartz & Roth, 2008). While none of these theories have been supported definitively, what is accepted is that sleep is an intricate and active process involving many parts of the brain and is associated with health and personal well-being (Horne, 2006; National Institute of Neurological Disorders and Stroke, NINDS, 2008). For example, sleep loss has been associated with compromising the immune system, including reducing lymphocyte count and Natural Killer cell activity, making people with decreased sleep more vulnerable to infection (Kendall-Tackett, 2009). Before discussing more of the specifics the impact of stress on sleep, it seems prudent to provide a brief overview of the basic constructs of sleep.

Basics of Sleep

The normal pattern of sleep has traditionally followed five phases or stages (Carskadon & Dement 2000): stages 1, 2, 3, 4, and rapid eye movement (REM) sleep, which entails dreaming. The different stages of sleep are categorized

G.S. Everly and J.M. Lating, *A Clinical Guide to the Treatment of the Human Stress Response*, DOI 10.1007/978-1-4614-5538-7_19,
© Springer Science+Business Media New York 2013

primarily by electroencephalographic (EEG) brain-wave activity that is not only assessed by sensors attached to the scalp but also may be assessed and categorized by electrooculographic (eye movement) and submental electromyographic (chin muscle) movement (Hirshkowitz et al., 1997). Stage 1 sleep, associated with drowsiness, is relatively short lived (around 10–15% of sleep or 1–7 min at the onset of sleep) (Carskadon & Dement, 2011) and occurs when we drift in and out of sleep and can be awakened easily (Horne, 2006). Eyes move slowly as does muscle activity; however, there may be instances of sudden muscle contractions, known as *hypnic myoclonia*, the sensation that makes us "jump" because we feel as if we are falling (National Institute of Neurological Disorders and Stroke; NINDS, 2008). During stage 2 sleep, which constitutes about half of all sleep, eye movements cease, and brain waves alternate between occasional single patterns that are slower and typical of deeper sleep, known as "K complexes" and occasional bursts of rapid waves called *sleep spindles* (Horne; NINDS, 2008). Stage 1 and stage 2 sleep combine to form what is known as light sleep. Stage 3 sleep is characterized by the development of extremely slow brain waves, known as delta waves, which account for between 20 and 50% of the EEG activity during a recording period, and is interspersed with smaller, faster, waves, and lasts only a few minutes in the first cycle of sleep (Carskadon & Dement, 2011). Stage 4 sleep is comparable to stage 3 sleep, except that the brain produces more than 50% of delta waves during a recording period and usually lasts about 20–40 min during the first sleep cycle (Carskadon & Dement, 2011; NINDS, 2008; Rechtschaffen & Kales, 1968). Stage 3 and stage 4 sleep, in which there is no eye movement or muscle activity, combine to what is referred to as deep sleep, delta sleep or slow-wave sleep (SWS). Adults spend approximately 20% of their sleeping time in SWS. Stages 1–4 are often grouped together and referred to as non-REM (NREM) sleep.

In 2007, the American Academy of Sleep Medicine (AASM) restructured NREM sleep as occurring in the following three stages, instead of the four stages just noted: Stage N1 sleep—the transition from wakefulness to sleep (the lightest stage of sleep in which some may not even perceive being asleep); Stage N2 sleep—a true sleep state, and accounts for 40–50% of time asleep; and Stage N3 sleep—referred to as deep sleep, delta sleep, or slow wave sleep, and accounts for 20% of sleep (Iber, Ancoli-Israel, Chesson, & Quan, 2007). Despite these new delineations, some experts continue to use the traditional terminology and definitions, since most of the influential descriptive research has been based on the four-stage classification (Carskadon & Dement, 2011).

REM sleep, or stage 5, which occurs about 20–25% of sleep time, is characterized by rapid, irregular and shallow breathing, abrupt and episodic bursts of eye movements, temporary limb paralysis, increased heart rate, and most notably, vivid dream recall (Dement & Kleitman, 1957; NINDS, 2008). REM sleep, which is usually not divided into stages, is distinct in that brain activity is consistent with wakefulness, and thus, is often referred as paradoxical sleep. Moreover, evidence suggests that the eye movements noted in REM sleep are likely not associated specifically with dream imagery, since dreams are created in the cortex and REM sleep occurs subcortically in regions that cannot dream (Horne, 2006).

As noted previously, the stages of sleep progress in cyclic patterns throughout the night, with the most obvious being the alteration between non-REM and REM sleep. After progressing through the first four stages of sleep, the first REM sleep period usually occurs about 70–100 min after sleep and lasts for about 1–5 min (Carskadon & Dement, 2011). NREM and REM sleep alternate through the night in cyclic fashion, with 4–5 cycles occurring during each night's sleep (National Sleep Foundation, 2001b). The average length of the second and later sleep cycles is about 90–120 min. Most SWS occurs in the first one-third of the night, whereas REM sleep occurs more in the second half of the night (Carskadon & Dement, 2011). By the morning, most people spend all their sleep time in stages 1, 2, and REM (NINDS, 2008).

Length of Sleep

The length of sleep depends on a number of factors, including lifestyle, health determinants (such as waking to an alarm, staying up late, drinking alcohol or caffeine, being diabetic, or being overweight) and genetics (Karacan & Moore, 1979; Rupp, Acebo, Van Reen, & Carskadon, 2007; Van Reen, Jenni, & Carskadon, 2006).

Other factors impact sleep as well, the most prominent being age, in particular the marked decrease in SWS with advanced age. Prior sleep history, body temperature (Williams, Karacan, & Hursch, 1974) and sleep disorders, including sleep apnea, in which pauses in breathing or showing breaths occur while sleeping, and narcolepsy, a disorder that causes extreme daytime sleepiness and possibly muscle weakness, also affect sleep. Individuals also differ on what is known as *basal sleep need*—or the amount of sleep our bodies need on a regular basis to perform optimally, and *sleep debt*—the accumulated lost sleep that occurs due to factors such as poor sleep habits, being ill, waking up due to environmental reasons (National Sleep Foundation, 2011b).

Another factor affecting sleep length is circadian (Latin for "around a day") rhythms, which are generally considered regular changes in mental and physical features that occur during a day (NINDS, 2008). Most circadian rhythms are controlled by the body's biological clock, a "timekeeper" located in the suprachiasmatic nucleus (SCN) of the hypothalamus that is active for internal 24-h rhythms (Howard, Rosekind, Katz, & Berry, 2002; Lydic, Schoene, Czeisler, & Moore-Ede, 1980). Light is the most prominent factor in coordinating the SCN, while melatonin, a neurohormone derived from serotonin and secreted by the pineal gland, serves as a complementary synchronizer of the SCN (Guardiola-Lemaître & Quera-Salva, 2011; Howard et al., 2002). Melatonin levels, which are inhibited by light, are low during the day, begin to increase just after darkness, reach their peak levels at mid darkness, and then decease late at night to return to their low daytime levels shortly before light occurs (Guardiola-Lamaître & Quera-Salva, 2011). The increase in melatonin after darkness is what helps make people feel drowsy, and accounts for its popular use as a supplement to assist in sleeping.

Given the number of factors involved in nocturnal sleep, including, as noted, the impact of age, it is challenging to definitively classify what constitutes a

Table 19.1 Suggested amounts of sleep

Age	Suggested amount of sleep
Newborns (up to 2 months)	12–18 h per day
Infants (3–11 months)	14–15 h per day
Toddlers (1–3 years)	12–14 h per day
Preschool-aged (3–5 years)	11–12 h per day
School-aged (5–10 years)	10–11 h per day
Adolescents (10–17 years)	9–10 h per day
Adults (including the elderly)	7–9 h per day

Adapted from National Sleep Foundation (2011b) and National Heart Lung and Blood Institute (2012)

"normal" amount of sleep. Table 19.1 provides the following suggested amounts of sleep for various ages:

Stress and Sleep

Stress is considered to be the primary factor in enduring psychophysiological insomnia (Morin, Rodrigue, & Ivers, 2003), and people with disturbed sleep often have comparable physiological changes as those under stress, including increased levels of cortisol, body temperature, heart rate, and oxygen consumption (Åkerstedt, 2006; Bonnet & Arand, 1996). However, according to Åkerstedt, Perski, and Kecklund (2011), systematic longitudinal data supporting these contentions are limited. In the few studies that have assessed stress and sleep longitudinally, the results suggest that work demands, poor psychosocial environment, and nighttime ruminations most likely predicted sleep disturbance (Åkerstedt, Kecklund, & Axelsson, 2007; Jansson & Linton, 2006; Linton, 2004). The putative connection between stress and sleep is that the heightened physiological activation associated with stress directly counters the "requirement of physiologic deactivation during sleep" (Åkerstedt et al., 2007, p. 101). For example, Sadeh (1996) proposed two possible sleep-related reactions to stress, depending on the type of stressor. Acute stress or trauma will lead to vigilance and difficulty falling asleep, while chronic exposure to stress or trauma will result in deep and prolonged sleep in an effort to escape or avoid what has occurred.

There are a number of studies that purport to establish the epidemiological link between stress and sleep, many of them investigating more common life stressors, such as studying for exams (Holdstock & Verschoor, 1974), living in an inner city, or doing shift work. Caldwell and Redeker (2009), for instance, reported that 115 women living in inner cities acknowledged high levels of life stress, self-reported sleep pattern disturbance and psychological distress.

Regarding the challenges associated with shift work, Åkerstedt (1998) reported that more than 75% of shift workers reported that their sleep is adversely affected, and data show sleep loss occurring primarily because of decreases in stage 2 sleep and REM sleep (stages 3 and 4 do not seem to be affected; Åkerstedt, 2006). Ambulatory EEG recordings in a sample of night-shift workers provide data to support that they fell asleep while at work (Torsvall, Åkerstedt, Gillander, & Knutsson, 1989). In the same study, 25% of train engineers and truck drivers have shown incidents of repeated bursts of alpha and theta EEG activity, closed eyes, and slow rolling eye movements (all indicators of attempts to resist sleep) while driving at night.

According to the American Academy of Sleep Medicine (n.d.), there are more than 250,000 sleep-related traffic accidents each year. Moreover, 20% of serious traffic accidents are sleep related, and 1,500 of these resulted in fatalities. Parenthetically, it is worth noting that 17–19 h without sleep has been shown to produce motor performance impairment comparable with a blood alcohol level (BAL) of 0.05%, and after 20–25 h without sleep impaired task performance was equivalent to that of a BAL of 0.1% (Williamson & Feyer, 2000). To help remedy this situation in fatigued drivers, a 10-min nap, in a semi-recumbent position, has been suggested as a means to improve driving ability for 1–2 h (Hayashi & Abe, 2008; Tietzel & Lack, 2002).

When performing long hours or shift work, particularly in settings that require "24/7" coverage, it seems relevant to consider the expectations and experiences of medical residents and physicians. There are numerous examples of health care tragedies occurring because of fatigue. One, in particular, was the March 4, 1984 death of 18-year-old Libby Zion, who died of cardiac arrest at a New York hospital after being admitted with fever and unexplained jerking movements. Although the malpractice trial ultimately assigned equal blame to the hospital and Libby, for supposedly concealing her past cocaine use, the real legacy of the case was the attention placed on work hours and supervision of resident physicians. In late 1989, the state of New York adopted the recommendations of a panel of experts regarding the number of hours and need for supervision of residents, and in 2003, the Accreditation Council for Graduate Medical Education (ACGME) mandated that all residency programs duty hours be fewer than 80 per week. Several studies have investigated whether this reduction in hours has improved safety (Howard et al., 2004; Fletcher et al., 2004), with one outcome noting that residents reported work-related stress (a composite of fatigue, excessive workload, stress, minimal time, and distractions) as the factor contributing most to medical errors, not the number of hours worked. In a study from the Mayo Clinic assessing fatigue and distress, both independently and concurrently, on perceived medical errors among 380 internal medicine resident physicians (West, Tan, Habermann, Sloan, & Shanafelt, 2009), results revealed that higher levels of fatigue and distress are independently associated with errors. These results collectively suggest that it may be important to focus on the variety of factors related to stress, and not just fatigue, in trying to mitigate the impact of medical errors.

DSM-IV Sleep Disorders

DSM-IV-TR (2000) includes diagnostic subtype of a Circadian Rhythm Sleep Disorder known as shift-work type that is associated with disruption because "they force sleep and wakefulness into aberrant circadian positions and prevent any consistent adjustment" (p. 623). Drake, Roehrs, Richardson, Walsh, and Roth (2004) estimate that this disorder occurs in around 14–32% of night-shift workers and 8–26% of rotating-shift workers. In the same study, shift workers who experienced either insomnia or excessive sleeplessness reported higher rates of ulcers, depression, sleepiness-related accidents, and missed worked days compared to those without sleep problems. Treatments used to address shift work difficulties include use of light therapy (in general, every hour of properly timed exposure to bright light will result in a 0.5-h shift in internal biological time) with properly timed exogenous melatonin, exercise, napping, caffeine, improved sleep hygiene and monitored use of benzodiazepines (Barger, Wright, Hughes, & Czeisler, 2004; Burgess, Sharkey, & Eastman, 2002; Burgess, Revell, & Eastman, 2008; Czeisler et al., 1990; Gooley, 2008; Leger et al., 2009; Smith & Eastman, 2008; Schweitzer, Randazzo, Stone, Erman, & Walsh, 2006; Thorpy, 2010; Walsh et al., 1991).

Another DSM-IV-R diagnostic subtype of a Circadian Rhythm Sleep Disorder, and one like shift work that is frequently associated with stress, is jet lag type (DSM-IV-TR, 2000). The impetus for jet lag is the body's inability to resynchronize its circadian rhythms rapidly after sudden shifts in the timing of the light–dark cycle (Reilly, 2009; Waterhouse, Reilly, Atkinson, & Edwards, 2007; Zisapel, 2001). The signs of jet lag include fatigue, irritability, loss of sleep, headaches, decreased psychomotor coordination, decreased cognitive skills and general malaise, and severity is related to the number of time zones crossed (Drake & Wright, 2011; Waterhouse et al., 2005; Zisapel, 2001). Eastward travel, which shortens the day and thus advances sleep–wake hours, is usually more challenging to tolerate than westward travel, which lengthens the day and thus delays sleep–wake hours (DSM-IV-TR, 2000). There are several treatment strategies used to treat jet lag, including use of melatonin, use of eyeshades and earplugs if traveling eastward at night, adapting to the new bed time and awakening times of the new time zone, preadaptation (i.e., going to bed and waking up earlier for 1–2 days before an eastward flight or going to bed and waking up later before westward flight), proper use of bright light exposure therapy, exercise, and monitored use of benzodiazepines (Arendt, Skene, Middleton, Lockley, & Deacon, 1997; Burgess, Crowley, Gazda, Fogg, & Eastman, 2003; Eastman, Gazada, Burgess, Crowley, & Fogg, 2005; Jamieson, Zammit, Rosenberg, Davis, & Walsh, 2001; Sack, 2010; Shiota, Sudou, & Ohshima, 1996).

The Effects of Fatigue and Lack of Sleep on the Occurrence of Critical Incidents

Several of the most highly publicized industrial accidents in the past several decades have been associated with sleep deficits. For example, the National Transportation Safety Board investigation of the March 24, 1989 Exxon Valdez oil tanker accident, in which 250,000 barrels of oil were spilled into Alaska's Prince William Sound, determined that fatigue associated with long work hours was one of the probable causes (National Transportation Safety Board, 1990). Similarly, the nuclear reactor accident at Three Mile Island, which occurred near Harrisburg Pennsylvania at 4:00 am on March 28, 1979, and the nuclear plant meltdown at Chernobyl, which occurred in the Ukraine on April 25, 1986, were both thought to have circadian factors that contributed in the disasters (Mitler et al., 1988; Moss & Sills, 1981). Additionally, fatigue was acknowledged as an important factor in the flawed decision making that contributed to the January 28, 1986 *Challenger* space shuttle accident (Report of the Presidential Commission on the Space Shuttle Challenger Accident, 1986, U. S. Government Printing Office).

Fatigue in the form of sleep irregularities, extended days, early starts to the day and night flying has also been a contributor to numerous other aviation accidents (Caldwell, 2005; Graeber, 1988; Petrilli, Roach, Dawson, & Lamond, 2006). A 2003 survey of 739 pilots reported that fatigue for international pilots was caused primarily by night flights (59%) and jet lag (45%) (Bourgeois-Bougrine, Carbon, Gounelle, Mollard, & Coblentz, 2003). In the May 22, 2010 Air India jet crash that killed 158 people after the jet overran the runway and went off a cliff, the captain was heard on a cockpit recorder snoring (Levin, 2010). Investigators concluded that he was suffering from "sleep inertia" which is defined as a "period of time immediately on awakening during which alertness and performance are impaired" (Silva & Duffy, 2008; p. 928). Also, in the February 12, 2009 commuter Colgan Air plane, operating as a Continental connection flight, that crashed on its way to Buffalo-Niagara International Airport and killed 50 people, fatigue was listed as contribution factor (NTSB, 2010a). It is notable that in her remarks before the National Sleep Foundation in 2010, Deborah Hersman, Chairperson of the National Transportation Safety Board, noted that "the Board has issued 34 separate recommendations concerning fatigue spanning all modes of transportation: aviation, highway, marine, railroad, and pipeline" (NTSB, 2010b).

Sleep, Dreams, and Stress

Dreaming was initially regarded as a transitory interruption of a dormant state that may have had its impetus from internal stimulation from the digestive tract or some other internal source (Dement, 2011). Freud's psychoanalytic theory, in which dream interpretation was a central part of his therapeutic approach, dominated the field of psychology during the middle part of the twentieth century. Within the past decade, the impact of psychosocial stressors (e.g., academic, occupational, experimental stressors) on dreams and dream content has been studied (Duke & Davidson, 2002). These studies have led some researchers to suggest that dream content may be related to stress adaptation attempts in certain circumstances (Mellman & Pigeon, 2011). For those diagnosed with PTSD, in which "recurrent distressing dreams of the event" is one of the re-experiencing symptoms, dreams appear more likely to be similar to the memory of the actual event, and are associated with increased sympathetic/noradrenergic activity during REM sleep (Mellman & Hipolito, 2006).

No single traumatic event in the past dozen years has impacted the USA more than the September 11, 2001 terrorist attacks. In a longitudinal study with a nationally representative sample of 560 US adults at time 1 (September 14–16, 2001) and 395 adults at time 2 (November 9–28, 2001), 13% of the sample reported substantial stress (defined as an answer "quite a bit" or "extremely" on a five-point Likert-type scale) in response to the question, "Have you been bothered by trouble falling or staying asleep" at time 1, and 7% of the sample reported substantial sleep distress at time 2 (Stein et al., 2004). Although not specifically addressed in this study, it seems probable that dreams may have been impacted in these participants.

Traumatic events have been thought to impact dreams by producing scenarios of what occurred (David & Mellman, 1997; Mellman, David, Bustamante, Torres, & Fins, 2001), related themes, characters, locations or objects (Esposito, Benitez, Barza, & Mellman, 1999; Opalic & Psihijatrija, 2000) or unpleasant emotions (Kroth, Thompson, Jackson, Pascali, & Ferreira, 2002). In a repeated measures design of 324 dream reports from 16 individuals 1 month before and 1 month after the events of September 11, Hartmann and Basile (2003) reported an increase in intensity of dream images, more fear emotions, and a trend toward more attack images. Propper, Strickgold, Keely, and Christman (2007) expanded on these findings by also assessing the relation between exposure to media coverage and subsequent dream content. Previous studies have reported that the amount of disturbing content watched on television on September 11 was positively correlated with the incidence of PTSD (Marshall & Galea, 2004; Schuster et al., 2001).

Propper et al. (2007) investigated 150 dream reports from 11 participants who were enrolled in a course on sleep and dreaming and recorded their dreams both before and after the September 11 attacks. Dreams were scored by three independent judges for specific references to September 11, general threats, themes related to the attacks, and the valence of emotions. Compared with dreams before September 11, dreams after the attacks were twice as likely to contain specific references to September 11, four times more likely to be classified as threatening, and although not statistically significant, to increase negative emotional valence. Moreover, "every hour of television watching resulted in a significant 5–6% increase in the proportion of post-September 11 dreams containing features related to the attacks" (Propper et al., 2007; p. 339). Also of note in this study was the finding that talking about the events with friends or relatives was not associated with dream references to September 11. In a study summarizing many of the claims associated with contemporary dream research and the attacks of September 11, Bulkeley and Kahan (2008) reported that the terrorist attacks had a tangible impact on the content of dreams but not the cognitive process of their dreaming (i.e., what they dreamed about, but not the way they dreamed).

The preponderance of previous research on dreaming has been done with adults. However, in a qualitative study assessing 104 children ages 5 years or younger who lived close to Ground Zero and experienced the sensory responses associated with September 11 (Klein, Devoe, Miranda-Julian, & Linas, 2009), parents described that many of their children slept deeply during the disaster, subsequent evacuation, and morning following the attacks. But in the months after the attacks, parents described many more nighttime sleep problems, including difficulty going to sleep, refusal to sleep alone, frequent night wakening, crying out during sleep and nightmares in their children. Overall, these studies provide data on the compelling association among sleep, dreams and traumatic events.

Methods to Enhance Sleep

Worry, rumination and anticipation are inconsistent with optimal sleep (McEwen, 1998; Tang & Harvey, 2004), and cortical arousal is often the pathoneumonic feature of insomnia (Perlis, Giles, Mendelson, Bootzin, & Wyatt, 1997). Currently insomnia is generally defined as an insufficient amount or compromised quality of sleep, and its prevalence in the general population ranges from 10 to 30% (Dikeos & Soldatos, 2005). More than 30 years ago, sleep laboratory documentation of diminished sleep quantity was necessary for the diagnosis of insomnia (Association of Sleep Disorders Centres, 1979). However, according to DSM-IV-TR (2000) and ICD-10, insomnia may now be diagnosed entirely on an individual's subjective report of unsatisfactory sleep quantity and quality at least three times per week for at least 1 month and is associated with distress and functional impairment (World Health Organization, 2011). Insomnia is conceptualized in terms of chronicity (acute or chronic), type (i.e., forms, such as idiopathic, psychophysiologic, inadequate sleep hygiene, comorbid with medical conditions), and subtype (i.e., phenotype, initial, middle, late or mixed) (Perlis, Shaw, Cano, & Espie, 2011).

Treatment options for insomnia can be divided into three broad classes of interventions including psychological and behavioral therapies, pharmacotherapy (see Chap. 16), and complementary and alternative therapies (Morin, 2011). We will focus primarily on suggestions consistent with psychological and behavioral therapies, which include cognitive therapy (see Chap. 8), relaxation training (see Chaps. 10, 11, and 12), hypnosis (see Chap. 13) as well as the following restrictive (curtailing time spent in bed), stimulus control (reinforcing the association between bed, bedroom, and sleep), sleep hygiene education (general guidelines about health practices, including diet and sleep, and environmental factors), and complementary perspectives accrued from a variety of resources (Edinger, Means, Carney, & Manber, 2011; Spielman, Saskin, & Thorpy, 1987; Morin, 2011; National Sleep Foundation, 2011a; Nursing Online Education Database, 2008). The following are some of the purported strategies for enhancing sleep:

- Maintain a regular schedule of when you go to bed and get out of bed.
- Associate your bed with sleeping (i.e., avoid using your bed for other activities like watching television, eating, or doing chores).
- Sleep in a dark room. Avoid having the television on or a computer screen.
- Avoid staying awake in bed too long. If you are not asleep in 20 min, get up and doing something boring until you feel sleepy again.

- Cover your alarm clock or turn it in the other direction. Staring contests with alarm clocks are a prescription for frustration.
- Do not hit the snooze button in the mornings. In order not to lose valuable moments of quality sleep, set your alarm clock later and get up right away.
- Reduce caffeine. Given the half-life of caffeine (which can cause sleep problems up to 12 h after drinking it), consider eliminating it after lunch or cutting back your overall intake.
- Avoid alcohol before bed. While it may help you get to sleep faster, alcohol reduces sleep quality.
- Drink something warm about 20 min before going to bed to raise your body's temperature (which will help to induce sleep). Warm milk has the added advantage of containing tryptophan (an essential amino acid), which serves as a precursor for serotonin, a neurotransmitter that helps regulate sleep.
- Employing a similar rationale, take a warm bath or shower about 45 min before going to bed.
- Avoid drinking too much of any beverage before attempting to go to sleep to avoid awakenings because of the need to urinate during the night.
- Do not try to sleep on a particularly full stomach. Digestion will disrupt your sleep.
- Conversely, do not go to bed hungry. Recognize, however, that some foods are more conducive for a better night's sleep. Carbohydrate-rich foods complement dairy foods by increasing levels of tryptophan, so good late-night snacks include a bowl of cereal and milk, bread, yogurt, crackers, rice, pretzels, or jelly beans.
- Some anecdotal data suggest the combined use of celery and honey as an herbal remedy to relax.
- Exercise. Not only regularly but also at the right time for you. Exercising too close to bedtime for some people has been associated with alertness and sleep disruption. Exercise, however, has been shown to promote and improve sleep in adults, the elderly, cardiac patients, and shift workers, all suffering with insomnia (Paparrigopoulos, Tsavara, Theleritis, Soldatos, & Tountas, 2010; Passos et al., 2010; Reid et al., 2010; Thorpy, 2010).
- While some experts suggest avoiding daytime napping (Morin, 2011), others note that napping, ideally for 10–20 min, even for individuals who get the sleep they need on a nightly basis, may lead to improved mood, alertness, and cognitive performance (Hayashi & Hori, 1998; Hayashi, Ito, & Hori, 1999; Tietzel & Lack, 2002).
- Use sleep diaries to help quantify your sleep patterns

Summary

This chapter provided a brief overview of the effects of sleep and stress.

1. The chapter began with a description of the basic stages of non-REM and REM sleep, as well as factors affecting the length of sleep.

2. Their role of psychosocial stressors, including occupational stressors such as shift work and prolonged work hours, and their impact on sleep in occupations such as truck drivers and physicians, were discussed.
3. DSM-IV-TR subtype criteria for Circadian Rhythm Sleep Disorder (i.e., shift work and jet lag) were reviewed, along with supporting empirical data on ways to potentially mitigate its impact.
4. The purported impact of fatigue and sleep deprivation on industrial accidents, such as the Exxon Valdez, Three Mile Island, and Chernobyl, and aviation accidents, such as the Challenger, were reviewed.
5. The theoretical and empirical data on the association between traumatic events, for example September 11, and dreaming suggest that this event impacted the intensity of dreams and evoked more fear emotions in adults and children.
6. Several practical intervention options for sleep enhancement were provided.

References

Accreditation Council for Graduate Medical Education. (2003). *ACGME duty hours standards fact sheet*. Retreived, from http://www.acgme.org/acWebsite/newsRoom/newsRm_dutyHours.asp

Åkerstedt, T. (1998). Shift work and disturbed sleep/wakefulness. *Sleep Medicine Review, 2*, 117–128.

Åkerstedt, T. (2006). Psychosocial stress and impaired sleep. *Scandinavian Journal of Work and Environmental Health, 32*(6), 493–501.

Åkerstedt, T., Kecklund, G., & Axelsson, G. (2007). Impaired sleep after bedtime stress and worries. *Biological Psychology, 76*, 170–173.

Åkerstedt, T., Perski, A., & Kecklund, G. (2011). Sleep, stress, and burnout. In M. H. Kryger, T. Roth, & W. C. Dement (Eds.), *Principles and practice of sleep medicine* (5th ed., pp. 814–821). St. Louis: Elsevier Saunders.

American Academy of Sleep Medicine, (n.d). Retreived, from http://www.aasmnet.org/resources/factsheets/drowsydriving.pdf

American Psychiatric Association. (2000). *Diagnostic and statistical manual of mental disorders, 4th Edition, Text revision*. Washington, DC: Author.

Arendt, J., Skene, D., Middleton, B., Lockley, S. W., & Deacon, S. (1997). Efficacy of melatonin treatment in jet lag, shift work, and blindness. *Journal of Biological Rhythms, 12*(6), 604–617.

Association of Sleep Disorders Centres. (1979). Diagnostic classification of sleep and arousal disorders. *Sleep, 2*, 1–137.

Barger, L. K., Wright, K. P., Jr., Hughes, R. J., & Czeisler, C. A. (2004). Daily exercise facilitates phase delays of circadian rhythm in very dim light. *American Journal of Physiology – Regulatory, Integrative and Comparative Physiology, 286*(6), R1077–R1084.

Bonnet, M. H., & Arand, D. L. (1996). Metabolic rate and the restorative function of sleep. *Physiology and Behavior, 59*, 777–782.

Bourgeois-Bougrine, S., Carbon, P., Gounelle, C., Mollard, R., & Coblentz, A. (2003). Perceived fatigue for short-and long-haul flights: A survey of 739 airline pilots. *Aviation, Space, and Environmental Medicine, 74*(10), 1072–1077.

Bulkeley, K., & Kahan, T. L. (2008). The impact of September 11 on dreaming. *Consciousness and Cognition, 17*(4), 1248–1256.

Burgess, H. J., Crowley, S. J., Gazda, C. J., Fogg, L. F., & Eastman, C. I. (2003). Preflight adjustment to eastward travel: 3 days of advancing sleep with and without morning bright light. *Journal of Biological Rhythms, 18*(4), 318–328.

Burgess, H. J., Revell, V. L., & Eastman, C. I. (2008). A three pulse phase response curve to three milligrams of melatonin in humans. *The Journal of Physiology, 586*, 639–647.

Burgess, H. J., Sharkey, K. M., & Eastman, C. I. (2002). Bright light, dark and melatonin can promote circadian adaptation in night shift workers. *Sleep Medicine Review, 6*, 407–420.

Caldwell, J. A. (2005). Fatigue in aviation. *Travel Medicine and Infectious Disease, 3*(2), 85–96.

Caldwell, B. A., & Redeker, N. S. (2009). Sleep patterns and psychological distress in women living in and inner city. *Research in Nursing and Health, 32*(2), 177–190.

Carskadon, M. A., & Dement, W. C. (2000). Normal human sleep: An overview. In M. H. Kryger, T. Roth, & W. C. Dement (Eds.), *Principles and practice of sleep medicine* (3rd ed., pp. 134–154). Philadelphia, PA: W.B. Saunders Company.

Carskadon, M. A., & Dement, W. C. (2011). Normal human sleep: An overview. In M. H. Kryger, T. Roth, & W. C. Dement (Eds.), *Principles and practice of sleep medicine* (5th ed., pp. 16–26). St. Louis, MO: Elsevier Saunders.

Czeisler, C. A., Johnson, M. P., Duffy, J. F., Brown, E. N., Ronda, J. M., & Kronauer, R. E. (1990). Exposure to bright light and darkness to treat physiologic maladaptation to night work. *The New England Journal of Medicine, 322*, 1253–1259.

David, D., & Mellman, T. A. (1997). Dreams following hurricane Andrew. *Dreaming, 7*, 209–214.

Dement, W. C. (2011). History of sleep physiology and medicine. In M. H. Kyger, T. Roth, & W. C. Dement (Eds.), *Principles and practice of sleep medicine* (5th ed., pp. 3–15). St. Louis, Missouri: Elsevier Saunders.

Dement, W., & Kleitman, N. (1957). The relation of eye movements during sleep to dream activity: An objective method for the study of dreaming. *Journal of Experimental Psychology, 53*, 339–346.

Dikeos, D. G., & Soldatos, C. R. (2005). The condition of insomnia: Etiopathogenetic considerations and their impact on treatment practices. *International Review of Psychiatry, 17*(4), 255–262.

Drake, C. L., Roehrs, T., Richardson, G., Walsh, J. K., & Roth, T. (2004). Shift work sleep disorder: Prevalence and consequences beyond that of symptomatic day workers. *Sleep, 27*(8), 1453–1462.

Drake, C. L., & Wright, K. P., Jr. (2011). Shift work, shift-work disorder, and jet lag. In M. H. Kryger, T. Roth, & W. C. Dement (Eds.), *Principles and practice of sleep medicine* (5th ed., pp. 784–798). Philadelphia, PA: W.B. Saunders Company.

Duke, T., & Davidson, J. (2002). Ordinary and recurrent dream recall of active, past and non-recurrent dreamers during and after academic stress. *Dreaming, 12*, 185–197.

Eastman, C. I., Gazda, C. J., Burgess, H. J., Crowley, S. J., & Fogg, L. F. (2005). Advancing circadian rhythms before eastward flight: A strategy to prevent or reduce jet lag. *Sleep, 28*(1), 33–44.

Edinger, J. D., Means, M. K., Carney, C. E., & Manber, R. (2011). Psychological and behavioral treatments for insomnia II: Implementation and specific populations. In M. H. Kryger, T. Roth, & W. C. Dement (Eds.), *Principles and practice of sleep medicine* (5th ed., pp. 884–904). Philadelphia, PA: W.B. Saunders Company.

Esposito, K., Benitez, A., Barza, L., & Mellman, T. (1999). Evaluation of dream content in combat-related PTSD. *Journal of Traumatic Stress, 12*, 681–687.

Fletcher, K. E., Underwood, W., III, Davis, S. Q., Mangrulkar, R. S., McMohan, L. F., Jr., & Saint, S. (2004). Systematic review: Effects of resident work hours on patient safety. *Annals of Internal Medicine, 141*(11), 851–857.

Goldsmith, J. R., & Casola, P. G. (2006). The basics for psychiatrists: An overview of sleep, sleep disorders, and psychiatric medications' effects on sleep. *Psychiatric Annals, 36*(12), 833–840.

Gooley, J. J. (2008). Treatment of circadian rhythm sleep disorders with light. *Annals Academy of Medicine Singapore, 37*(8), 669–676.

Graeber, R. C. (1988). Fatigue and circadian rhythmicity. In E. L. Weiner & D. C. Nagel (Eds.), *Aircrew fatigue and circadian rhythmicity* (pp. 305–344). New York, NY: Academic Press.

Guardiola-Lema tre, B., & Quera-Salva, M. A. (2011). Melatonin and the regulation of sleep and circadian rhythms. In M. H. Kryger, T. Roth, & W. C. Dement (Eds.), *Principles and practice of sleep medicine* (5th ed., pp. 420–430). Philadelphia, PA: W.B. Saunders Company.

Hartmann, E., & Basile, R. (2003). Dream imagery becomes more intense after 9/11/01. *Dreaming, 13*, 61–66.

Hayashi, M., & Abe, A. (2008). Short daytime naps in a car seat to counteract daytime sleepiness: The effect of backrest angle. *Sleep and Biological Rhythms, 6,* 34–41.

Hayashi, M., & Hori, T. (1998). The effects of a 20-min nap before post-lunch dip. *Psychiatry & Clinical Neuroscience, 52*(2), 203–204.

Hayashi, M., Ito, S., & Hori, T. (1999). The effects of a 20-min nap at noon on sleepiness, performance and EEG activity. *International Journal of Psychophysiology, 32,* 173–180.

Hirshkowitz, M., Moore, C. A., & Minhoto, G. (1997). Understanding sleep: The evaluation and treatment of sleep disorders. In R. Mark & W. C. Orr (Eds.), *Application and practice in health psychology* (pp. 11–34). Washington, DC: American Psychological Association Press.

Holdstock, T. L. & Verschoor, G. J. (1974). Student sleep patterns before, during and after an examination period. *South African Journal of Psychology, 4,* 16–24.

Horne, J. (2006). *Sleepfaring: A journey through the science of sleep.* New York, NY: Oxford University Press.

Howard, S. K., Rosekind, M. R., Katz, J. D., & Berry, A. J. (2002). Fatigue in anesthesia: Implications and strategies for patient and provider safety. *Anesthesiology, 97,* 1281–1294.

Howard, D., Silber, J., & Jobes, D. (2004). Do regulations limiting resident's work hours affect patient mortality? *Journal of General Internal Medicine, 19,* 1–7.

Iber, C., Ancoli-Israel, S., Chesson, A., & Quan, S. F. (2007). *The AASM manual for the scoring of sleep and associated events: Rules, terminology, and technical specifications.* Westchester, IL: American Academy of Sleep Medicine. Retreived from: http://www.nswo.nl/userfiles/files/AASM%20-%20Manual%20for%20the%20Scoring%20ofSleep%20and%20Associted%20Events%20-%2005-2007_2.pdf

Jamieson, A. O., Zammit, G. K., Rosenberg, R. S., Davis, J. R., & Walsh, J. K. (2001). Zolpidem reduces the sleep disturbance of jet lag. *Sleep Medicine, 2*(5), 423–430.

Jansson, M. & Linton, S. J. (2006). Psychosocial work stressors in the development and maintenance of insomnia: A prospective study. *Journal of Occupational Health Psychology, 11*(3), 241–248.

Karacan, I., & Moore, C. A. (1979). Genetics and human sleep. *Psychiatric Annals, 9,* 11–23.

Kendall-Tackett, K. (2009). Psychological trauma and physical health: A psychoneuroimmunology approach to etiology of negative health effects and possible interventions. *Psychological Trauma: Theory, Research, Practice, and Policy, 1,* 35–48.

Klein, T. P., Devoe, E. R., Miranda-Julian, C., & Linas, K. (2009). Young children's responses to September 11th: The New York City experience. *Infant Mental Health Journal, 30*(1), 1–22.

Kroth, J., Thompson, L., Jackson, J., Pascali, L., & Ferreira, M. (2002). Dream characteristics of stock brokers after a major market downturn. *Psychological Reports, 90,* 1097–1100.

Leger D., Philip, P., Jarriault, P., Metlaine, A., & Choudat, D. (2009). Effects of a combination of napping and bright light pulses on shift workers' sleepiness at the wheel: A pilot study. *Journal of Sleep Research, 18*(4), 472–479.

Levin, A. (2010). Air India pilot's "sleep inertia" caused crash. *USA Today,* Available online: http://www.usatoday.com/news/world/2010-11-18-airindia18_ST_N.htm

Linton, S. J. (2004). Does work stress predict insomnia? A prospective study. British *Journal of Health Psychology, 9,* 127–136.

Lydic, R., Schoene, W. C., Czeisler, C. A., & Moore-Ede, M. C. (1980). Suprachiasmatic region of the human hypothalamus: Homolog to the primate circadian pacemaker? *Sleep, 2,* 355–361.

Marshall, R. D., & Galea, S. (2004). Science for the community. Assessing mental health after 9/11. *The Journal of Clinical Psychiatry, 65,* 37–43.

McEwen, B. S. (1998). Protective and damaging effects of stress mediators. *New England Journal of Medicine, 338,* 171–179.

Mellman, T. A., David, D., Bustamante, V., Torres, J., & Fins, A. (2001). Dreams in the acute aftermath of trauma and their relationship to PTSD. *Journal of Traumatic Stress, 14,* 241–247.

Mellman, T. A., & Hipolito, M. M. (2006). Sleep disturbances in the aftermath of trauma and posttraumatic stress disorder. *CNS Spectrums, 11,* 611–615.

Mellman, T. A., & Pigeon, W. R. (2011). Dreams and nightmares in posttraumatic stress disorder. In M. H. Kryger, T. Roth, & W. C. Dement (Eds.), *Principles and practice of sleep medicine* (5th ed., pp. 613–619). Philadelphia, PA: W.B. Saunders Company.

Mitler, M. M., Carskadon, M. A., Czeisler, C. A., Dement, W. C., Dinges, D. F., & Graeber, R. C. (1988). Catastrophes, sleep and public policy: Consensus Report. *Sleep, 11*(1), 100–109.

Morin, C. M. (2011). Psychological and behavioral treatments for insomnia I: Approaches and efficacy. In M. H. Kryger, T. Roth, & W. C. Dement (Eds.), *Principles and practice of sleep medicine* (5th ed., pp. 866–883). Philadelphia, PA: W.B. Saunders Company.

Morin, C. M., Rodrique, S., & Ivers, H. (2003). Role of stress, arousal, and coping skills in primary insomnia. *Psychosomatic Medicine, 65*, 259–267.

Moss, T. H., & Sills, D. L. (Eds.) (1981). *The Three Mile Island nuclear accident: Lessons and implications*. New York. New York Academy of Sciences.

National Heart Lung & Blood Institute. (2012). How much sleep is enough? Retreived from: http://www.nhlbi.nih.gov/health/health-topics/topics/sdd/howmuch.html.

National Institute of Neurological Disorders and Stroke. (2008). Brain basics-understanding sleep. Retreived from: http://www.ninds.nih.gov/education/brochures/Brain-Basics-Sleep-6-10-08-pdf-508.pdf (6/10/08).

National Sleep Foundation. (2011a). Can't sleep? What to know about insomnia. Retreived from: http://www.sleepfoundation.org/article/sleep-related-problems/insomnia-and-sleep.

National Sleep Foundation. (2011b). How much sleep do we really need? Retreived from: http://www.sleepfoundation.org/article/how-sleep-works/how-much-sleep-do-we-really-need.

National Transportation Safety Board (1990). Grounding of US tankship Exxon Valdez on Bligh Reef, Prince William Sound near Valdez, AK, March 24, 1989. Washington, DC: National Transportation Safety Board.

National Transportation Safety Board. (2010a). Loss of control on approach Colgan Air, Inc. Operating as Continental connection flight 3407 Bombardier DHC-8-400, N200WQ Clarence Center, New York February 12, 2009. Accident report. Retreived from: http://www.ntsb.gov/doclib/reports/2010/aar1001.pdf.

National Transportation Safety Board. (2010b). Remarks of Honorable Deborah A. P. Hersman, Chairman, NTSB before the National Sleep Foundation. Washington, D.C., March 5, 2010. Retreived from: http://www.ntsb.gov/news/speeches/hersman/daph100305.html.

Nursing Online Education Database. (2008). 50 ways to boost your energy without caffeine. Retreived from: http://noedb.org/library/features/50_ways_to_boost_your_energy_without_caffeine.

Opalic, P., & Psihijatrija, D. (2000). Research of the dreams of traumatized subjects. *Psihijatrija Danas, 32*, 129–147.

Paparrigopoulos, T., Tsavara, C., Theleritis, C., Soldatos, C., & Tountas, Y. (2010). Physical activity may promote sleep in cardiac patients suffering from insomnia. *International Journal of Cardiology, 143*(2), 209–211.

Passos, G. S., Poyares, D., Santana, M. G., Garbuio, S. A., Tufik, S., & Mello, M. T. (2010). Effect of acute physical exercise on patients with chronic primary insomnia. *Journal of Clinical Sleep Medicine, 6*(3), 270–275.

Perlis, M. L., Giles, D. E., Mendelson, W. B., Bootzin, R. R., & Wyatt, J. K. (1997). Psychophysiological insomnia: The behavioural model and a neurocognitive perspective. *Journal of Sleep Research, 6*, 179–188.

Perlis, M., Shaw, P. J., Cano, G., & Espie, C. A. (2011). Models of insomnia. In M. H. Kryger, T. Roth, & W. C. Dement (Eds.), *Principles and practice of sleep medicine* (5th ed., pp. 850–865). Philadelphia, PA: W.B. Saunders Company.

Petrilli, R. M., Roach, G. D., Dawson, D., & Lamond, N. (2006). The sleep, subjective fatigue, and sustained attention of commercial airline pilots during an international pattern. *Chronobiology International, 23*(6), 1347–1362.

Propper, R. E., Stickgold, R., Keeley, R., & Christman, S. D. (2007). Is television traumatic? Dreams, stess and media exposure in the aftermath of September 11, 2011. *Psychological Science, 18*(4), 334–340.

Rechtschaffen, A. & Kales, A. (1968). *A manual of standardized terminology, techniques, and scoring system for sleep stages of human subjects* (National Institutes of Health Publication No. 204). Washington, D. C.: U. S. Government Printing Office.

Reid, K. J., Baron, K. G., Lu, B., Naylor, E., Wolfe, L., & Zee, P. C. (2010). Aerobic exercise improves self-reported sleep and quality of life in older adults with insomnia. *Sleep Medicine, 11*(9), 934–940.

Reilly, T. (2009). How can travelling athletes deal with jet-lag? *Kinesiology, 41*(2), 128–135.

Report of the Presidential Commission on the Space Shuttle Challenger Accident. II. (1986). Washington, DC: U.S. Government Printing Office.

Rupp, T. L., Acebo, C., Van Reen, E., & Carskadon, M. A. (2007). Effects of a moderate evening alcohol dose. I: Sleepiness. *Alcoholism: Clinical & Experimental Research, 31*, 1358–1364.

Sack, R. L. (2010). Jet lag. *The New England Journal of Medicine, 362*, 440–447.

Sadeh, A. (1996). Stress, trauma, and sleep in children. *Child and Adolescent Psychiatric Clinics of North America, 5*(3), 685–700.

Schuster, M. A., Stein, B. D., Jaycox, L. H., Collins, R. L., Marshall, G. N., Elliott, M. N., & Berry, S. H. (2001). A national survey of stress reactions after the September 11, 2001, terrorist attacks. *The New England Journal of Medicine, 345*(20), 1507–1512

Schwartz, J. R. L., & Roth, T. (2008). Neurophysiology of sleep and wakefulness: Basic science and clinical implications. *Current Neuropharmacology, 6*(4), 367–378.

Schweitzer, P. K., Randazzo, A. C., Stone, K., Erman, M., & Walsh, J. K. (2006). Laboratory and field studies of naps and caffeine as practical countermeasures for sleep-wake problems associated with night work. *Sleep, 29*(1), 39–50.

Shiota, M., Sudou, M., & Ohshima, M. (1996). Using outdoor exercise to decrease jet lag in airline crew members. *Aviation, Space and Environmental Medicine, 67*, 1155–1160.

Silva, E. J., & Duffy, J. F. (2008). Sleep inertia varies with circadian phase and sleep stage in older adults. *Behavioral Neuroscience, 122*(4), 928–935.

Smith, M. R., & Eastman, C. I. (2008). Night shift performance is improved by a compromise circadian phase position: Study 3. Circadian phase after 7 nights shifts with an intervening weekend off. *Sleep, 31*(12), 1639–1645.

Spielman, A. J., Saskin, P., & Thorpy, M. J. (1987). Treatment of chronic insomnia by restriction of time in bed. *Sleep, 10*, 45–56.

Stein, B. D., Elliott, M. N., Jaycox, L. H., Collins, R. L., Barry, S. H., Klein, D. J., & Schuster, M. A. (2004). A national longitudinal study of the psychological consequences of the September 11, 2001 terrorist attacks: Reactions, impairment, and help-seeking. *Psychiatry: Interpersonal and Biological Processes, 67*(2), 105–117.

Tang, N. K. Y., & Harvey, A. G. (2004). Effects of cognitive arousal and physiological arousal on sleep perception. *Sleep, 27*, 69–78.

Thorpy, M. J. (2010). Managing the patient with shift-work disorder. *Journal of Family Practice, 59*, S24–31.

Tietzel, A., & Lack, L. C. (2002). The recuperative value of brief and ultra-brief naps on alertness and cognitive performance. *Journal of Sleep Research, 11*(3), 213–218.

Torsvall, L., Åkerstedt, T., Gillander, K., & Knutsson, A. (1989). Sleep on the night shift: 24-hour EEG monitoring of spontaneous sleep/wake behavior. *Psychophysiology, 3*, 352–358.

Van Reen, E., Jenni, O., & Carskadon, M. A. (2006). Effects of alcohol on sleep and the sleep electroencephalogram in healthy young women. *Alcoholism: Clinical & Experimental Research, 30*(6), 974–981.

Walsh, J. K., Schweitzer, P. K., Anch, A. M., Muehlbach, M. J., Jenkins, N. A., & Dickins, Q. S. (1991). Sleepiness/alertness on a simulated night shift following sleep at home with triazolam. *Sleep, 14*(2), 140–146.

Waterhouse, J., Nevill, A., Finnegan, J., Williams, P., Edwards, B., Kao, S.-Y., & Reilly, T. (2005). Further assessments of the relationship between jet lab and some of its symptoms. *Chronobiology International, 22*(1), 121–136.

Waterhouse, J., Reilly, T., Atkinson, G., & Edwards, B. (2007). Jet lag: Trends and coping strategies. *The Lancet, 369*, 1117–1129.

West, C. P., Tan, A. D., Habermann, T. M., Sloan, J. A., & Shanafelt, T. A. (2009). Association of resident fatigue and distress with perceived medical errors. *Journal of the American Medical Association, 302*(12), 1294–1300.

Williams, R. L., Karacan, I., & Hursch, C. J. (1974). *EEG of human sleep: Clinical applications.* New York: John Wiley & Sons.

Williamson, A. M., & Feyer, A. M. (2000). Moderate sleep deprivation produces impairments in cognitive and motor performance equivalent to legally prescribed levels of alcohol intoxication. *Occupational and Environmental Medicine, 57*, 649–655.

World Health Organization. (2011). The ICD-1- classification of mental and behavioral disorders. Geneva: Author. Retreived from: http://homeofinsomniac.blogspot.com/2011/05/icd-10-diagnostic-criteria-for-non.html

Zisapel, N. (2001). Circadian rhythm sleep disorders: Pathophysiology and potential approaches to management. *CNS Drugs, 15*(4), 311–328.

Chapter 20
Grief, Loss, and Stress

Everyone can master grief but he who has it

Shakespeare

Death is the unavoidable endpoint of a terminal life. Since death is inevitable, grief is not only predictable but also likely to occur repeatedly during the course of someone's life. Despite being ubiquitous, grief is also mercurial, and may evince its qualities uniquely and at various times. For example, grief may begin at the thought of someone's death, it may occur well after someone has died, or it may occur for losses other than the loss of life. According to Holmes and Rahe (1967), who developed the Life Stress Inventory, the death of a spouse is the highest weighted life change event (i.e., stressful event) that an individual can experience. The purpose of this chapter is to review the terms associated with grief, the classic stage-based theories related to grief, the construct of prolonged or complicated grief, stress-related symptoms and prolonged grief, and intervention considerations for grief and loss with adults and children.

Definition of Terms

There are generally accepted definitions and fundamental concepts associated with grief, bereavement, and mourning. Bereavement, is the "term used to denote the objective situation of having lost someone significant through death" (Stroebe, Hansson, Schut, & Stroebe, 2008 p. 4). Understandably, bereavement is associated with considerable distress and is influenced by social and cultural norms (Jeffreys, 2005). Grief is the term generally applied to the internal emotional or affective reaction to loss, most typically of a loved one through death, but it could be from other tangible, symbolic or psychosocial losses, or even threats of losses (DeSpelder & Strickland, 2005; Jeffreys, 2005; Stroebe, Hansson, Schut, & Stroebe, 2008). Grief

G.S. Everly and J.M. Lating, *A Clinical Guide to the Treatment*
of the Human Stress Response, DOI 10.1007/978-1-4614-5538-7_20,
© Springer Science+Business Media New York 2013

is a complex process with myriad reactions (e.g., loneliness, anger, frustration) that is often classified in terms of stages and has been considered to be something to be worked through (Bonanno, 2001; Bowlby, 1980; Goodkin et al., 2001; Shuchter & Zisook, 1993). Mourning, which is often differentiated from grief, refers "to the public display of grief, the social expressions or acts expressive of grief that are shaped by the (often religious) beliefs and practices of a given society or cultural group" (Stroebe et al., 2008, p. 5). It is generally accepted, however, that grief and mourning may equally influence each other. Before exploring the relation between these constructs and stress, the prominent theories of grief will be reviewed briefly.

Grief Theories

There have been several notable theories to explore the grieving process. Erich Lindemann, one of the seminal figures in social psychiatry and community mental health, and Chief of Psychiatry at Massachusetts General Hospital in the 1940s did some of the earliest empirical work on the process of grieving. After a tragic fire at the Cocoanut Grove Night Club in Boston on November 28, 1942, in which 492 people died, Lindemann found that many of the 101 family members he worked with had similar reactions after the loss (Lindemann, 1944). These reactions included somatic distress, preoccupation with thoughts or images of the deceased, guilt regarding the circumstances responsible for the death, hostility, or anger, and decreased functioning that were not present before the event. In his article, he suggested that eight to ten sessions over a month and a half would help to mitigate the impact of the loss and asserted that the tasks of grief entailed: emancipation from bondage to the deceased; readjustment to the environment in which the deceased is missing; and formation of new relationships (Lindemann, 1944). Lindemann's work was very influential, but his setting a proposed time frame of 4–6 weeks as a marker to mitigate ensuing grief may have inadvertently created a "normative" time standard, and that those who took longer to recover from their grief reactions may have been considered maladjusted (Simos, 1979).

Elisabeth Kübler-Ross, a psychiatrist who was born in Zurich, Switzerland, and became a US citizen in 1961, published her seminal text *On Death and Dying: What the Dying Have to Teach Doctors, Nurses, Clergy and Their Own Families* in 1969, in which, based on interviews with more than 200 dying cancer patients and their families, she described her now classically regarded five stages of grief. The following stages of Denial and Isolation, Anger, Bargaining, Depression, and Acceptance, imply a framework or model, but were not necessarily intended to be a rigid series or uniform progression through bereavement. The first stage, denial was originally conceptualized by Kübler-Ross as a time when the person diagnosed would "doctor shop" to ensure that the terminal diagnosis was correct. Many counselors have misinterpreted this stage as "resistance" and something to be confronted and worked through (Walter & McCoyd, 2009). Kübler-Ross considered it, however, to a "healthy way of dealing with the uncomfortable and painful situation with which these patients have to live for a long time" (1969, p. 39). Denial and isolation are thought to help us pace our feelings of grief and enable us to survive. Anger, which can be manifested at oneself or others (often caregivers), including doctors and sometimes God, is thought to provide a bridge or structure for underlying expression of pain and abandonment. Bargaining for those terminally ill seems intuitive (e.g., "If I pray more or make amends with others, maybe I will improve") to alleviate pain or emotional discomfort, whereas for those bereaved due to the loss, they may attempt to bargain or negotiate to mitigate the pain of the loss. Depression for those preparing to die may include withdrawing from others in an effort to conserve energy, reflect upon their lives, and explore spiritual meaning (Jeffreys, 2005). It is naturally associated with feelings of sadness, fear, uncertainty, regret, and a certain amount of acceptance. For those bereaving the loss, it may feel as if it will never remit, but the sadness and pain may be seen as an appropriate response. Acceptance, which should not be mistaken for happiness, is often when the pain for the person dying has subsided, his or her interests have diminished and he or she often prefers to be left alone (Kübler-Ross, 1969). For those bereaving, it is learning to live with the loss, having more good days than bad ones, listening to uncomfortable feelings, and eventually reaching out to others.

John Bowlby, a psychiatrist noted for his research on attachment and child development, studied children separated from their parents in World War II, widows, and a few widowers, to develop his four phases of grief. According to Bowlby (1980), the four phases of grief are: (1) numbness, which occurs immediately following a loss, is associated with feelings of shock and intense distress that may last up to a week and serve as a protective defense that allows the person to survive emotionally; (2) yearning and searching, which may last for months and sometimes years, involves a pining for the deceased, a longing for his or her return and is associated with anxiety, anger, confusion, weeping and guilt; (3) disorganization and despair is associated with less yearning as the loss becomes more "real", more apathy, and an attempt to reorganize the loss; and (4) reorganization, the final phase, occurs when the grieving person begins to accept a new condition of "normal". During this phase grief does not end, but thoughts of sadness and despair diminish and are replaced with positive memories of the deceased.

With the past 5 years, William Worden (2008), a psychologist who has been studying life-threatening illness and life-threatening behavior for more than 40 years, has developed a task-based grief theory, partly in response to the stage-based models presented above. According to Worden, four tasks of mourning, which are intended to help the bereaved come to a better understanding of his or her loss, are (1) accept the reality of the loss, (2) work through the pain (both physically and emotionally), (3) adjusting to the new environment in which the deceased is missing (i.e., accepting new identity as a widow or widower), and (4) emotionally relocate the deceased and move on (e.g., not to forget the relationship with the deceased, but letting go of attachments so new relationships can form). Worden does not necessarily believe that the tasks need to occur in this particular order, and he did not set a specific time for how long these tasks should take. However, they are usually experienced over months and years as compared to days or weeks.

Complicated Grief

As noted, grief in response to loss is a normal experience of emotional reactions couched in cultural norms that is often mitigated by social support and personal resources and most often does not require professional intervention (Kyrouz, Humphreys, & Loomis, 2002; Malkinson, Rubin, & Witztum, 2005). It is clear that people grieve in different ways, for various durations, and with painful and disruptive symptoms that range from depression to anger to limited functioning. About 80–90% of people are thought to cope with the grieving process in a normal, uncomplicated manner (Barry, Kasl, & Prigerson, 2001; Boelen, van den Bout, & de Keijser, 2003; Bonanno, 2004; Latham & Prigerson, 2004). According to Prigerson (2004), by 6 months post-loss most bereaved individuals attain some sense of acceptance, are able to work productively, feel increasingly optimistic about the future, find meaning and purpose in their lives, maintain supportive relationships, cultivate new relationships and find pleasure in their spare time. In addition, self-esteem and sense of accomplishment remain intact in those experiencing more normal grief reactions.

There are, however, a minority of individuals, with estimates ranging from 15 to 20% (Bonanno, Wortman, & Neese, 2004; Prigerson, Frank, et al., 1995), who do not experience what may be considered normal grief reactions. For these individuals, signs and symptoms consistent with major depressive disorder (MDD), PTSD, or suicidal thoughts and gestures occur that preclude the individual from functioning adequately and may last for a prolonged period of time (Howarth, 2011; Prigerson, Vanderwerker, & Maciejewski, 2008). Individuals bereaved through deaths that are violent, unexpected, or untimely are at a heightened risk for these experiences (Lichtenthal, Cruess, & Prigerson, 2004; Stroebe, Schut, & Stroebe, 2007). Many terms have been used to describe these atypical grief reactions, with the two most prevalent being complicated grief (CG) and prolonged grief (PG). Prigerson and colleagues (2008) have worked to clarify the terms and provide compelling rationale to use the term prolonged grief to denote the elevated symptoms associated with the challenging adjustment to loss. The authors are quick to note that the word prolonged is an encompassing term for the distress associated with the disorder and not simply to imply that duration is the sole indicator of the pathological nature of grief. Moreover, Prigerson et al. (2008) note that the term complicated grief may be readily confused with the term complicated bereavement, used in the *DSM-IV* to describe symptoms of major depression secondary to bereavement. Despite these efforts to refine these constructs, the current literature continues to use both terms, often interchangeably.

Currently, PG or CG is not considered a mental disorder, and the construct of bereavement, which is limited to a single paragraph in *DSM-IV*, is mostly used as a potential exclusion criterion for other disorders, such as MDD or an adjustment disorder (*DSM-IV-TR;* American Psychiatric Association, 2000) and is classified in *DSM-IV-TR* as a "V" code, or one of "additional conditions that may be a focus of clinical attention" (p. 739). Prigerson et al. (2008, 2009) note distinctive phenomenology, etiology, and course associated with PG that results in substantial distress and disability and warrants inclusion as a separate mental disorder.

In a field trial designed specifically to develop diagnostic criteria of PGD, Prigerson et al. (2009) propose the following: Criterion A: Bereavement following the loss of a significant other is the event; Criterion B: Separation Distress defined as yearning (e.g., craving, pining, or longing for the deceased; suffering (both emotional and physical) by not being able to be reunited with deceased) daily or to a disabling degree; Criterion C: Cognitive, emotional, and behavioral symptoms; specifically five or more of the following nine symptoms (1) confusion about one's life role or diminished sense of self (i.e., feeling as if a part of oneself has died); (2) trouble accepting the loss; (3) avoidance of reminders of the deceased, (4) difficulty trusting others; (5) feelings of bitterness or anger related to the loss; (6) difficulty in moving on with life (i.e., cultivating interests, making new friends); (7) emotional numbness; (8) a perception of life as empty or meaningless, and (9) feeling stunned, dazed, or shocked by the loss; Criterion D: Timing, proposed diagnosis not made until after 6 months have passed since the loss; Criterion E: Impairment, in the form of clinically significant distress in social, occupational, or even domestic functioning; Criterion F: Relation to other mental disorders, meaning that the disturbance is not better accounted for by substance use, a general medial condition or MDD, generalized anxiety disorder, or PTSD. For this last criterion, studies have shown that symptoms such as yearning, emptiness, bitterness, and disbelief about the death are indicators that separate PGD from MDD (Boelen, van den Bout, & de Keijser, 2003; Prigerson et al., 1996, 1997; Prigerson, Frank, et al., 1995; Prigerson, Maciejewski, et al., 1995). Moreover, in contrasting PGD from PTSD (Prigerson et al., 2000; Shear & Mulhare, 2008), distress for the former is triggered by the loss of a close attachment while in PTSD it is triggered by a real or perceived physical threat. The two differ in the primary emotion expressed, with fear, along with hyperarousal, being more prevalent in PTSD, while sadness is the primary emotion in PGD. The two also differ in the type of avoidance displayed, with trauma victims experiencing more of a phobic avoidance of reminders of events as a compensatory strategy to mitigate arousal, whereas with PGD, there is more of an avoidance of accepting the loss as real, avoidance of moving on with one's life, and general difficulty accepting the loss. Also, separation distress, with symptoms such as yearning for the deceased, is not seen in PTSD.

Confirmatory factor analytic procedures on 456 bereaved adults were conducted to assess whether normal grief, CG, as well as the revised criteria of CG that make up PGD, differed (Dillen, Fontaine, & Verhofstadt-Denève, 2008). The factor analytic procedures suggested that CG/PGD symptoms are by nature distinguishable from NG, except for "strong yearning" which loaded on both factors. The authors noted, however, the Dutch translation of yearning may have accounted for this effect, so they were reluctant to imply that "intense yearning" does not distinguish between NC and CG/PGD. Overall, the findings support the contention that CG/PGD is separate and distinct from normal grief reactions and warrants consideration as a DSM 5 diagnoses. A more recent confirmatory factor analysis on 292 elderly participants (mean age 70 years; SD=3.47) noted, however, a large overlap between PGD and PTSD, especially the intrusive component of PTSD (O'Connor, Lasgaard, Shevlin, & Guldin, 2010). The authors noted, however, the nonclinical nature of their sample and the low frequencies of CG (9%) and PTSD (6%). There was also an average of 13.5 months for the most significant losses chosen with a SD of 13.1 and a range from 0 to 63 years. Clearly, more empirical research is needed on this important topic.

At the time of the writing of this chapter, the DSM 5 is still in development, but the condition, persistent complex bereavement-related disorder is being recommended for further study. Therefore, since comments are still being received and considered for possible diagnostic criteria, it would be imprudent at this time to convey anything more than a cursory summary of the APA workgroups' current document   (http://www.dsm5.org/ProposedRevision/Pages/proposedrevision. aspx?rid=577). The current working criteria proposed for this condition overlap in many ways with Prigerson and colleagues' (2008, 2009) proposed criteria for PGD presented previously, with both placing an emphasis on symptoms of yearning, sorrow, and preoccupation with the deceased. The current draft of the proposed DSM 5 criteria of persistent complex bereavement-related disorder also structure additional symptoms into the categories of reactive distress to the death (e.g., bitterness, avoidance, maladaptive appraisals) and social/identity disruption (e.g., trust issues, confusion, detachment). The current APA proposed criteria also are more definitive regarding the timing of the loss (the individual experienced the death of a close family member or friend at least 12 months ago; however, in the case of a bereaved child, this death may have occurred at least 6 months ago). Both PGD and the upcoming DSM 5 offer proposed criteria-related functional impairment. It also is worth noting that in addition to persistent complex bereavement-related disorder being recommended for further study, the proposed DSM 5 updated criteria for MDD, single episode, currently includes the stipulation that the normal and expected response to a significant loss such as bereavement may resemble the symptoms of a depressive episode.

Complicated/Prolonged Grief and Stress-Related Symptoms

In a sample of 76 participants from the Pittsburgh area, most of whom were women, those with syndromal levels of traumatic grief, as assessed by the Inventory of Complicated Grief (Prigerson, Maciejewski, et al., 1995), were approximately five times more likely to report suicidal ideation than were participants with non-syndromal levels of traumatic grief (Prigerson, Bridge, et al., 1999). Latham and Prigerson (2004) used the Inventory of Complicated Grief-Revised (Prigerson, Shear, et al., 1999; Prigerson & Jacobs, 2001) to assess a sample of 309 bereaved adults at baseline (6.2 months post-loss) and again at follow up (10.8 months post-loss). Their results, after controlling for demographic factors, indicated that CG was associated with a 6.6 times greater likelihood of "high suicidality" at baseline, and an 11.3 times greater risk of high suicidality at follow-up. In a sample of 129 children and adolescents (age range 7–18 years) whose parents died of a sudden natural death, accident, or suicide, a modified version of the Inventory of Complicated

Grief-Revised (ICG-R), CG was related to functional impairment, including suicidal ideation, after controlling for MDD, PTSD, and anxiety (Melhem, Moritz, Walker, Shear, & Brent, 2007). In a studying assessing suicidal behavior, as compared to suicidal ideation, in a sample of 149 patients who met criteria for CG, 65% reported suicidal ideation following the death of a loved one, and more than half of this group (38% of the entire study sample) engaged in self-destructive behavior, including 9% who made a suicide attempt and 29% who engaged in indirect suicidal behavior (Szanto et al., 2006)

It was noted in the introduction to this chapter that loss of a spouse or significant other has long been considered among the most stressful of all life events (Holmes & Rahe, 1967; Prigerson et al., 1997; Zisook, Shuchter, & Lyons, 1987). The inherent stress associated with significant other loss is associated with compromised immune functioning (Irwin, Daniels, Smith, Bloom, & Weiner, 1987), more physician visits (Mor, McHorney, & Sherwood, 1986), and increased use of alcohol and cigarettes (Clayton, 1990; Lund, Dimond, & Caserta, 1985). In a sample of 150 widows and widowers who did and did not meet criteria for traumatic grief, those who met the criteria were significantly more likely to have heart trouble (19.2%) and cancer (15.4%) than those who did not meet the criteria (19.2% vs. 5.2%, and 15.4% vs. 0%, respectively) between 6 and 25 months after their loss (Prigerson et al., 1997). In a study comparing psychological, endocrine, and immune functioning over a 6-month period between 14 healthy participants who experienced *unpredictable* acute emotional stress, like the sudden death of a loved one, and 14 controls who did not experience loss, those who experienced the loss showed more stress as assessed by self-report (Hamilton Rating Scales), adrenocorticotropin and plasma concentrations, and nonsuppression in response to dexamethasone 10 days after the loss when compared to the controls (Gerra et al., 2003). Moreover, 40 days after bereavement, the unpredictable loss cohort showed decreased natural killer cell activity and other alterations in immune parameters not observed in the control group.

The development of neuroimaging techniques, such as functional magnetic resonance imaging scan (fMRI) and PET, has allowed researchers to investigate functional correlates of how bereavement affects task-related brain activity (Gündel, O'Connor, Littrell, Fort, & Lane, 2003); O'Connor, 2005; Ochsner & Lieberman, 2001). While many brain areas are noted to be activated during bereavement neuroimaging studies, a grief-eliciting paradigm (consisting of showing participants pictures or the deceased with a caption or words), a few of the most salient areas of the brain activated are the posterior cingulate cortex, which is activated during autobiographical memories and emotionally salient stimuli (Maddock, Buonocore, Kile, & Garrett, 2003), the medial/superior frontal cortex, and the cerebellum (Gündel, O'Connor, Littrell, Fort, & Lane, 2003; O'Connor). A more recent study by O'Connor and colleagues (2008) comparing event-related fMRI to idiopathic grief-related stimuli in 23 bereaved women (11 of whom had CG) showed that only those with CG evinced reward-related activity in the nucleus accumbens. This suggests that reminders of the deceased still activated reward activity, which may interfere with adapting to the loss.

Grief and Traumatic Events

Disasters, which by nature are sudden and unexpected, can result in multiple deaths (including children), mutilated bodies, devastated surroundings, and social disarray. Moreover, for survivors who may have witnessed horrific events, experienced the loss of loved ones and possibly blame themselves for what occurred, the process of grief and bereavement may be even more profound (Bonanno et al., 2007; Kaltman & Bonanno, 2003; Parkes, 2008). As noted by Parkes, the psychological interventions required of bereaved individuals following disasters are essentially the same as other bereavements, but high levels of anxiety and fear, along with anger, guilt, and aggression, may require anxiety-management programs or anger-management skills to mitigate severe or disabling symptoms that persist for more than 1 month.

Following the 1995 Oklahoma City bombing, Pfefferbaum and colleagues (2001) reported a positive relation between self-reported posttraumatic stress symptoms and grief. In a convenience sample, 704 bereaved adults surveyed 2.5–3.5 years after the September 11, 2001, terrorist attacks on the World Trade Center, 43% screened positive for CG reactions on a nine-item survey (Neria et al., 2007). Moreover, close to 65% of participants who lost a child screened positive for CG, 36% with CG had probable depression, and 43% had probable PTSD. Also of interest, and consistent with other data presented in this volume (see Chap. 19 on Sleep and Stress), nearly half (47%) of those who watched the attacks live on television screened positive for CG. In a sample of 262 (199 women and 63 men) bereaved inhabitants affected by the 2004 tsunami in Southeast Asia, 84% were identified as being severely emotionally distressed on the Hopkins Symptoms Checklist-25, and 77% were identified as being depressed 1 year after the tragedy (Souza, Bernatsky, Reyes, & de Jong, 2007). In a 2009 study (Johannesson et al. 2009) conducted 14 months after the tsunami that included 187 bereaved relatives of tsunami victims, 40% of the relatives reported CG and suicidal ideation. In addition, being chased by the tsunami waves was associated with more distress in the bereaved relatives.

Intervention

As noted previously, most normally grieving individuals will not require formal grief therapy (Jordan & Neimeyer, 2003). Usually with the passage of time, support from others, making sense of the loss through talking or writing about it, and integrating it into a new reality, productive resolution will typically occur in a relative timely fashion. In other words, part of the intervention task is to help the grieving individual reconfigure his or her sense of identity and create new meanings and new assumptions (Jeffreys, 2005). Jeffreys suggests various ways to facilitate this post-loss reality including: keeping a record of positive experiences that occur during the week, create a new hobby that is not dependent on another person, rehearse responses to people who are unaware of the loss, and utilize relaxation strategies. For caregivers, suggestions for dealing with grieving individuals include: don't be or look rushed, be comfortable with silence, remain nonjudgmental, be prepared to normalize the myriad emotions being displayed ranging from sadness, fear, confusion, helplessness, hopelessness, dread, anhedonia, and anger, help the person remain active, be sensitive to cultural norms, and be sensitive and aware of your own compassion fatigue when trying to assist others (Jeffreys; Love, 2007).

There are times, however, when grief does not remit and more formal therapeutic interventions are warranted for GC. Clearly the communication styles noted above will apply; however, there are also likely to be tailored procedures that incorporate more formal cognitive-behavioral techniques (e.g., counterfactual thinking, exposure techniques), family-focused therapy, and more evidence-based treatments (e.g., modified interpersonal therapy). From a constructionist therapy perspective, which is a postmodern approach that focuses on people's need to impose meaning on their life experiences or life stories (Neimeyer, 2009), resolution following death involves assimilating and accommodating the loss into a coherent and meaningful self-narrative and involves techniques such as narrative retelling (recounting the death under safe conditions), therapeutic writing, use of metaphor, evocative visualization (encouraging the person to "enter" and "experience" the scene at a visual and tactile level in order to foster meaning), and encountering the pro-symptom position (the proclivity to construct meaning that maintains the problem despite its distress) (Neimeyer, Burke, MacKay, & van Dyke Stringer, 2010; Neimeyer, van Dyke, & Pennebaker, 2008) .

Grief and Children: Developmental Stages and Intervention

Developmental Stages

Children of all ages grieve, but they are impacted by loss very differently than adults. It is relevant to note that while children are individually and uniquely impacted by the experience of death, they may react to death from a general developmental perspective. For example, children under the age of 5 years may view death as a "separation" that may be temporary and reversible and do not fathom that all functions of life have ceased (Dyregrov, 2008; Worden, 2008). Between the ages of 5–9 years, most children are gradually developing a sense of mortality. However, they may still not envision death as personal, meaning that they somehow believe they will be able to escape it (Worden). From the ages of around nine through adolescence, they begin to fully comprehend the finality of death, the existential aspects of death, including that they too will die someday.

Evidence of Grieving in Children and Adolescents

Fortunately, children tend to be highly resilient, but they may still experience signs and symptoms associated with death and the grieving process. The following are some of the common ways children may respond to a death (Dyer, 2002; Dyregrov, 2008):

- Sadness
- Shock, denial, and confusion
- Anger and fear
- Sleep difficulties
- School performance drop
- Physical complaints
- Guilt
- Regressed behavior (e.g., thumb-sucking, bedwetting)
- Anhedonia
- Repeated questions about the deceased
- Decreased appetite
- Vivid memories
- Acting out
- Isolation

Helping Children Understand Death

There are many ways to help children understand the impact of death, but one of the biggest challenges is communicating with a young child. First of all, recognize your own fear and discomfort in talking with children about death, spend time listening to them and giving them the opportunity to explore their curiosity. When talking with young children, they respond well to straightforward, brief, simple, and *concrete* explanations done in a timely manner (Dyregrov, 2008; Raveis, Siegel, & Karus; 1999; Worden, 2008). According to Grollman (1998), death may be made more understandable by explaining it in terms of the absence of normal life functions (e.g., when people die they do not think, breath, eat, or feel anymore; when dogs die they do not bark or dig anymore; dead flowers do not bloom anymore). Make sure a child not only listens but also hears what you say; therefore, repetition and having him or her paraphrase back what you say can be helpful. Some children, for example, confuse death with sleep, particularly when they may hear adults say things like "eternal rest" or "rest in peace." It is important, therefore, that they know that going to sleep does not mean that they may die. Additionally, religious statements, such as "this is God's will" or that the deceased is at peace because he or she "is with God now" may be unnerving to a young child. Young children may also be predisposed to feeling guilty and somehow believing that they caused the death of a loved one.

Even though for younger children the concept of death may not be fully developed, there is no reason to doubt that they may react strongly to loss. Therefore, depending on if the child is old enough to understand the concept of death, and more importantly if he or she wants to participate in the funeral, being included may help him or her accept the reality of the loss and say good-bye to the deceased. However, it is important that the child be prepared about what he or she will see and hear before, during, and after the service.

Overall, for children experiencing the various types of normal grief reactions associated with death, different approaches are likely to be helpful, and all are based on the premise of openness and honesty. For example, incorporating creative approaches, such as play, art, and dance may help to facilitate emotional expression.

Despite being highly resilient, there are instances, however, when a child may be particularly overwhelmed by a loss and may require more formal interventions. If, for example, the signs noted above show very little remittance after about three months, then it is an indication that the child is having problems that may respond to professional help (American Academy of Child and Adolescent Psychiatry, 2011; Dyer, 2002). Other possible warning signs that more professional help following a death may be warranted include (Dyer; Dyregrov, 2008; Worden, 2008):

- Repeated statements of wanting to join the deceased person
- Refusal to attend school
- Alcohol or drug use
- Recurrent, unexplainable temper tantrums
- Stealing, vandalism, or other illegal behavior
- Phobias or panic attacks
- Withdrawal from friends
- Excessive imitation of the deceased

Summary

Dealing with the grief and mourning associated with the death of a loved one is considered to be one of the most stressful situations we will encounter. Fortunately, the challenges of sadness and hurt usually remit within six months of the loss and we are able to return to our normal level of functioning. As this chapter noted, there are times, however, when the signs and symptoms of grief are more profound, do not remit, and may result in PGD. With approximately 2.4 million deaths per year in the USA in 2009 (Kochanek, Xu, Murphy, Mini o, & Kung, 2011), and with an estimated 4 survivors per death, and using the estimated 15–20% rate of PGD following deaths from natural causes (Bonanno, Wortman, & Neese, 2004), then there are more than one million cases of PGD in the USA alone.

This chapter has provided a general overview of the relation between grief, loss, and stress. Let us review the main points of the chapter.

1. We began with a diffe=rentiation between the terms bereavement, grief, and mourning.
2. The major theories of grief, including Lindemann's (1944), Kübler-Ross' (1969), Bowlby's (1980), and Worden's (2008) were reviewed.
3. The construct of complicated/prolonged grief was reviewed and the proposed criteria for a diagnosis were presented.
4. The general criteria for the proposed DSM V condition of persistent complex bereavement-related disorder were briefly reviewed.
5. Research results have shown how complicated/prolonged grief results in stress-related symptoms, including suicidal ideation and behavior (Melhem, Mortiz, Walker, Shear, & Brent, 2007), compromised immune function (Gerra et al., 2003), and alterations in brain activity (Gündel, O'Connor, Littrell, Fort, & Lane, 2003; O'Connor et al., 2008).
6. Data have also shown how traumatic events, including man-made and natural disasters, impact symptoms of CG reactions, such as increased symptoms of depression and probable PTSD (Neria et al., 2007; Souza, Benatsky, Reyes, & de Jong, 2007).
7. The chapter concluded with proposed intervention strategies for adults (Jeffreys, 2005; Love, 2007) and children (Dyer, 2002; Dyregrov, 2008) to mitigate the impact of loss.

References

American Academy of Child & Adolescent Psychiatry (2011). Facts for families: Children and Grief (No. 8). http://www.aacap.org/galleries/factsforfamilies/08_children_and_grief.pdf

American Psychiatric Association. (2000). *Diagnostic and statistical manual of mental disorders* (4th ed. Text revision). Washington, DC: Author

Barry, L. C., Kasl, S. V., & Prigerson, H. G. (2001). Psychiatric disorders among bereaved persons: The role of perceived circumstances of death and preparedness for death. *The American Journal of Geriatric Psychiatry, 10*, 447–457.

Boelen, P. A., van den Bout, J., & de Keijser, J. (2003). Traumatic grief as a disorder distinct from bereavement-related depression and anxiety: A replication study with bereaved mental health care patients. *The American Journal of Psychiatry, 160*, 1229–1241.

Bonanno, G. A. (2001). Grief and emotion: A social-functional perspective. In M. S. Stroebe, R. O. Hansson, W. Stroebe, & H. Schut (Eds.), *Handbook of bereavement research: Consequences, coping, and care* (pp. 493–516). Washington, DC: American Psychological Association.

Bonanno, G. A. (2004). Loss, trauma, and human resilience: Have we underestimated the human capacity to thrive after extremely aversive events? *The American Psychologist, 59*(1), 20–28.

Bonanno, G. A., Neria, Y., Mancini, A., Coifman, K. G., Litz, B., & Insel, B. (2007). Is there more to complicated grief than depression and posttraumatic stress disorder? A test of incremental validity. *Journal of Abnormal Psychology, 116*(2), 342–351.

Bonanno, G. A., Wortman, C. B., & Neese, R. M. (2004). Prospective patterns of resilience and maladjustment during widowhood. *Psychology and Aging, 19*, 260–271.

Bowlby, J. (1980). *Loss: Sadness and depression. Attachment and loss* (Vol. 3). New York, NY: Basic Books.

Clayton, P. J. (1990). Bereavement and depression. *The Journal of Clinical Psychiatry, 51*, 34–51.

DeSpelder, L. A., & Strickland, A. L. (2005). *The last dance: Encountering death and dying* (7th ed.). New York, NY: McGraw Hill.

Dillen, L., Fontaine, J. R. J., & Verhofstadt-Denève, L. (2008). Are normal and complicated grief different constructs? A confirmatory factor analytic test. *Clinical Psychology and Psychotherapy, 15*, 386–395.

Dyer, K. (2002). *Coping strategies for children*. http://www.journeyofhearts.org/jofh/grief/kids_cope

Dyregrov, A. (2008). *Grief in children: A handbook for adults* (2nd ed.). London: Jessica Kingsley Publishers.

Gerra, G., Monti, D., Panerai, A. E., Sacerdote, P., Anderlini, R., Avanzini, P., & Franceschi, C. (2003). Long-term immune-endocrine effects of bereavement: Relationships with anxiety levels and mood. *Psychiatry Research, 121*(2), 145–158.

Goodkin, K., Baldewicz, T. T., Blaney, N. T., Asthana, D., Kumar, M., Shapshak, P., & Zheng, W. L. B. (2001). Physiological effects of bereavement and bereavement support group interventions. In M. S. Stroebe, R. O. Hansson, W. Stroebe, & H. Schut (Eds.), *Handbook of bereavement research: Consequences, coping, and care* (pp. 671–703). Washington, DC: American Psychological Association.

Grollman, E. A. (1998). *Explaining death to children*. Cincinnati, OH: Forward Movement Publication.

Gündel, H., O'Connor, M. F., Littrell, L., Fort, C., & Lane, R. (2003). Functional neuroanatomy of grief: An fMRI study. *American Journal of Psychiatry, 160*, 1946–1953.

Holmes, T. H., & Rahe, R. (1967). The social readjustment rating scale. *Journal of Psychosomatic Research, 11*, 213–218.

Howarth, R. A. (2011). Concepts and controversies in grief and loss. *Journal of Mental Health Counseling, 33*(1), 4–10.

Irwin, M., Daniels, M., Smith, T. L., Bloom, E., & Weiner, H. (1987). Life events, depressive symptoms, and immune function. *American Journal of Psychiatry, 144*, 437–441.

Jeffreys, J. S. (2005). *Helping grieving people: When tears are not enough*. New York, NY: Brunner-Routledge.

Johannesson, K. B., Lundin, T., Hultman, C. M., Lindam, A., Dyster-Aas, J., Arnberg, F., & Per-Olof, M. (2009). The effect of traumatic bereavement on tsunami-exposed survivors. *Journal of Trauamtic Stress, 22*(6), 497–504.

Jordan, J., & Neimeyer, R. (2003). Does grief counseling work? *Death studies, 27*, 765–786.

Kaltman, S., & Bonanno, G. A. (2003). Trauma and bereavement: Examining the impact of sudden and violent deaths. *Journal of Anxiety Disorders, 17*(2), 131–147.

Kochanek, K. D., Xu, J., Murphy, S. L., Miniño, A. M., & Kung, H.-C. (2011). Deaths: Preliminary data for 2009. *National Vital Statistics Reports, 59*(4). Hyattsville, MD: National Center for Health Statistics.

Kübler-Ross, E. (1969). *On death and dying: What the dying have to teach doctors, nurses, clergy and their own families*. New York: Macmillian Publishing.

Kyrouz, E. M., Humphreys, K., & Loomis, C. (2002). A review of the research on the effectiveness of self-help mutual aid groups. In B. J. White & E. J. Madara (Eds.), *American Self-Help Group Clearinghouse self-help group sourcebook* (7th ed., pp. 71–86). Denville, NJ: American Self-Help Group Clearinghouse.

Latham, A. E., & Prigerson, H. G. (2004). Suicidality and bereavement: Complicated grief as psychiatric disorder presenting greatest risk for suicidality. *Suicide and Life Threatening Behavior, 34*, 350–362.

Lichtenthal, W. G., Cruess, D. G., & Prigerson, H. G. (2004). A case for establishing complicated grief as a distinct mental disorder in the *DSM-V*. *Clinical Psychology Review, 24*, 637–662.

Lindemann, E. (1944). Symptomatology and management of acute grief. *American Journal of Psychiatry, 101*, 141–148.

Love, A. W. (2007). Progress in understanding grief, complicated grief, and caring for the bereaved. *Contemporary Nurse, 27*, 73–83.

Lund, D., Dimond, M., & Caserta, M. S. (1985). Identifying elderly with coping difficulties two years after bereavement. *Omega: Journal of Death and Dying, 16*, 213–224.

Maddock, R. J., Buonocore, M. H., Kile, S. J., & Garrett, A. S. (2003). Brain regions showing increased activation by threat-related words in panic disorder. *Neuroreport, 14*, 325–328.

Malkinson, R., Rubin, S., & Witztum, E. (2005). Terror, trauma, and bereavement: Implications for theory and therapy. In Y. Danieli, D. Brom, & J. Stills (Eds.), *The trauma of terrorism: Shared knowledge and shared care, an international handbook* (pp. 467–477). New York: Haworth Press.

Melhem, N. M., Mortiz, G., Walker, M., Shear, M. K., & Brent, D. (2007). Phenomenology and correlates of complicated grief in children and adolescents. *Journal of the American Academy of Child & Adolescent Psychiatry, 46*(4), 493–499.

Mor, V., McHorney, C., & Sherwood, S. (1986). Secondary morbidity among the recently bereaved. *American Journal of Psychiatry, 143*, 158–163.

Neimeyer, R. A. (2009). *Constructivist psychotherapy*. New York: Routledge.

Neimeyer, R. A., Burke, L. A., Mackay, M. M., & van Dyke Stringer, J. G. (2010). Grief therapy and the reconstruction of meaning: From principles to practice. *Journal of Contemporary Psychotherapy, 40*, 73–83.

Neimeyer, R. A., van Dyke, J. G., & Pennebaker, J. W. (2008). Narrative medicine: Writing through bereavement. In H. Chochinov & W. Breitbart (Eds.), *Handbook of psychiatry in palliative medicine* (pp. 454–469). New York: Oxford.

Neria, Y., Gross, R., Litz, B., Maguen, S., Insel, B., Seirmarco, … Marshall, R. D. (2007). Prevalence and psychological correlates of complicated grief among bereaved adults 2.5 – 3.5 years after September 11th attacks. *Journal of Traumatic Stress, 20*(3), 251–262

O'Connor, M.-F. (2005). Bereavement and the brain: Invitation to a conversation between bereavement researchers and neuroscientist. *Death Studies, 29*, 905–922.

O'Connor, M.-F., Lasgaard, M., Shevlin, M., & Guldin, M. B. (2010). A confirmatory factor analysis of combined models of the Harvard Trauma Questionnaire and the Inventory of Complicated Grief-Revised: Are we measuring complicated grief or posttraumatic stress? *Journal of Anxiety Disorders, 24*, 672–679.

O'Connor, M.-F., Wellisch, D. K., Stanton, A. L., Eisenberger, N. I., Irwin, M. R., & Lieberman, M. D. (2008). Craving love? Enduring grief activates brain's reward center. *Neuroimage, 42*(2), 969–972.

Ochsner, K. N., & Lieberman, M. D. (2001). The emergence of social cognitive neuroscience. *American Psychologist, 56*, 717–734.

Parkes, C. M. (2008). Bereavement following disasters. In M. S. Stroebe, R. Hansson, H. Schut, & W. Stroebe (Eds.), *Handbook of bereavement research and practice* (pp. 463–484). Washington, D.C.: American Psychological Association.

Pfefferbaum, B., Call, J. A., Lensgraf, J., Miller, P.D., Flynn, B. W., Doughty, D. E., … Dickson, W. L. (2001). Traumatic grief in a convenience sample of victims seeking support services after a terrorist incident. *Annals of Clinical Psychiatry, 13*(1), 19–24

Prigerson, H. G. (2004). Complicated grief: When the path of adjustment leads to a dead-end. *Bereavement Care, 23*, 38–40.

Prigerson, H. G., Bierhals, A. J., Kasl, S. V., Reynolds, C. F., Shear, M. K., Day, N., … Jacobs, S. (1997). Traumatic grief as a risk factor for mental and physical morbidity. *American Journal of Psychiatry, 154*, 616–623.

Prigerson, H. G., Bierhals, A. J., Kasl, S. V., Reynolds, C. F., III, et al. (1996). Complication grief as a disorder distinct from bereavement-related depression and anxiety: A replication study. *The American Journal of Psychiatry, 153*(11), 1484–1486.

Prigerson, H. G., Bridge, J., Maciejewski, P. K., Berry, L. C., Rosenheck, R. A., Jacobs, S. C., … Brent, D. A. (1999a). Influence of traumatic grief on suicidal ideation among young adults. *American Journal of Psychiatry, 156*, 1994–1995.

Prigerson, H. G., Frank, E., Kasl, S. V., Reynolds, C. F., III, Anderson, B., Zubenko, G. S., et al. (1995). Complicated grief and bereavement-related depression as distinct disorders: Preliminary empirical validation in elderly bereaved spouses. *American Journal of Psychiatry, 152*, 22–30.

Prigerson, H. G., Horowitz, M. J., Jacobs, S. C., Parkes, C. M., Aslan, M., Goodkin, K., … Maciejewski, P. K. (2009). Prolonged Grief Disorder: Psychometric validation of criteria proposed for *DSM-V* and *ICD-11*. *PLoS Med 6*(8): e1000121.

Prigerson, H. G., & Jacobs, S. C. (2001). Perspectives on care at the close of life. Caring for bereaved patients: "All the doctors just suddenly go". *Journal of the American Medical Association, 286,* 1369–1376.

Prigerson, H. G., Maciejewski, P. K., Reynolds III, C. F., Bierhals, A. J., Newsom, J. T., Fasiczka, A., ... Miller, M. (1995). Inventory of complicated grief: A scale to measure maladaptive symptoms of loss. *Psychiatric Research, 59*(1–2), 65–79.

Prigerson, H. G., Shear, M. K., Jacobs, S. C., Kasl, S. V., Maciejewski, P. K., Silverman, G. K., ... Bremner, J. D. (2000). Grief and its relationship to PTSD. In D. Nutt & J. R. T. Davidson (Eds.), *Post traumatic stress disorders: Diagnosis, management and treatment* (pp. 163–186). New York: Martin Dunitz.

Prigerson, H. G., Shear, M. K., Jacobs, S. C., Reynolds III, C. F., Maciejewski, P. K., Davidson, J. R., ... Zisook, S. (1999b). Consensus criteria for traumatic grief: A preliminary empirical test. *British Journal of Psychiatry, 174,* 67–73.

Prigerson, H. G., Vanderwerker, L. C., & Maciejewski, P. K. (2008). Prolonged grief disorder: A case for inclusion in DSM-V. In M. S. Stroebe, H. Hansson, W. Schut, & W. Stroebe (Eds.), *Handbook of bereavement research and practice: 21st century perspectives* (pp. 165–186). Washington, D.C.: American Psychological Association Press.

Raveis, V. H., Siegel, K., & Karus, D. (1999). Children's psychological distress following the death of a parent. *Journal of Youth and Adolescence, 28*(2), 165–180.

Shear, M. K., & Mulhare, E. (2008). Complicated grief. *Psychiatric Annals, 38*(10), 662–670.

Shuchter, S., & Zisook, S. (1993). The course of normal grief. In M. S. Stroebe, W. Stroebe, & R. O. Hansson (Eds.), *Handbook of bereavement: Theory, research and intervention* (pp. 23–43). Cambridge, England: Cambridge University Press.

Simos, B. G. (1979). *A time to grieve: Loss as a universal human experience.* New York: Family Service Association of America.

Souza, R., Benatsky, S., Reyes, R., & de Jong, K. (2007). Mental health status of vulnerable tsunami-affected communities: A survey in Aceh Province, Indonesia. *Journal of Traumatic Stress, 20*(3), 263–269.

Stroebe, M. S., Hansson, R. O., Schut, H., & Stroebe, W. (2008). Bereavement research: Contemporary Perspectives. In M. S. Stroebe, H. Hansson, W. Schut, & W. Stroebe (Eds.), *Handbook of bereavement research and practice: 21st century perspectives* (pp. 3–25). Washington, D.C.: American Psychological Association Press.

Stroebe, M., S., Schut, H., & Stroebe, W. (2007). Health outcomes of bereavement. *Lancet, 370,* 1960–1973

Szanto, K., Shear, K., Houck, P. R., Reyonlds, C. F., III, Frank, E., Caroff, K., & Silowash, R. (2006). Indirect sself-destructive behavior and overt suicidality in patients with complicated grief. *Journal of Clinical Psychiatry, 67*(2), 233–239.

Walter, C. A., & McCoyd, J. L. M. (2009). *Grief and loss across the lifespan.* New York: Springer Publishing Company.

Worden, J. W. (2008). *Grief counseling and grief therapy* (4th ed.). New York: Springer Publishing Company.

Zisook, S., Shuchter, S., & Lyons, L. (1987). Predictors of psychological reactions during the early stages of widowhood. *Psychiatric Clinics of North America, 19,* 355–367.

Chapter 21
Posttraumatic Stress Disorder

The posttraumatic stress syndrome has been recognized for decades (Freud, 1921), and systematic empirical inquiry dates back to the 1940s (Kardiner, 1941). Yet, it was not until 1980 that the now highly recognizable posttraumatic stress syndrome was officially catalogued within the official nosological compendium of the American Psychiatric Association, the *Diagnostic and Statistical Manual of Mental Disorders,* third edition (DSM-III; American Psychiatric Association, 1980). With this recognition of the syndrome as an official mental disorder came a surge of research efforts designed to lead to better diagnostic refinement as well as improved treatment.

Whereas once the syndrome was viewed almost exclusively as a result of armed combat, now posttraumatic stress disorder (PTSD) has been found to result from not only war-related situations but also a host of non-combat-related experiences as well. In 1987, and again in 1994 and 2000, the American Psychiatric Association revised its official nosology (1987, 1994, 2000). Are we coming closer to a comprehensive understanding of PTSD, or are we just beginning to scratch the surface of what may be a uniquely complex interaction of pathophysiological and psychopathological constituents? The purpose of this chapter is to review current evidence on the nature of PTSD as well to as offer an integrating phenomenological hypothesis regarding this disorder, which appears to be playing more and more a role in Western society.

The Prevalence of Trauma as a Public Health Problem

What is the magnitude of risk for experiencing a significant psychological trauma that might yield a significantly adverse impact upon one's mental health? Is the risk minimal, or does it represent a significant public health issue? To review Chap. 1, the reader will recall:

- Recent evidence suggests that 82.8% of adults in the USA will be exposed to a traumatic event during their lifetime (Breslau, 2009).
- Suicide rates in the military seem to be increasing (Kang & Bullman, 2009).

G.S. Everly and J.M. Lating, *A Clinical Guide to the Treatment*
of the Human Stress Response, DOI 10.1007/978-1-4614-5538-7_21,
© Springer Science+Business Media New York 2013

- Twelve-month DSM-IV disorders are highly prevalent in the USA, with 14% experiencing moderate to severe cases (Kessler, Chiu, Demler, Merikangas, & Walters, 2005).
- Suicide was the tenth leading cause of death in the USA in 2007, and an estimated 11 attempted suicides occur per every suicide death.
- An elevated rate of major depression was equal to the rate of PTSD in New York City residents several months after the attacks on the World Trade Center of September 11, 2001 (Galea et al., 2002).
- Rates of trauma occurrence related to violence, injury/shock trauma, trauma to others, and unexpected death peaked sharply at age 16–20 years (Breslau, 2009).
- The lifetime prevalence of criminal victimization was assessed among female health management organization patients and found to be about 57%.
- In 2001, the terrorist attacks against the World Trade Center and the Pentagon focus terrorism against the USA.
- Of 2050 American Airlines (AA) flight attendants, 18.2% reported symptoms consistent with probable PTSD in the aftermath of the September 11 attacks (Lating, Sherman, Everly, Lowry, & Peragine, 2004).
- Clearly, trauma and stress are at epidemic proportions in the USA. It seems clear that such conditions represent a "clear and present danger" to the psychological health of American society.
- Perhaps of greatest concern, from a public health perspective is the realization that veterans returning from military service in Iraq and Afghanistan are returning home with a high prevalence of PTSD and PTSD-like syndromes. A recent review of 29 published studies revealed varying estimates of PTSD. "Among previously deployed personnel not seeking treatment, most prevalence estimates range from 5 to 20%. Prevalence estimates are generally higher among those seeking treatment: As many as 50% of veterans seeking treatment screen positive for PTSD...Combat exposure is the only correlate consistently associated with PTSD" (Ramchand et al., 2010, p. 59).
- The Veterans Affairs (VA) estimate that about 26% of veterans seeking treatment at VA facilities meet criteria for PTSD (U.S. Department of Veteran Affairs, Veterans Health Administration, Office of Public Health and Environmental Hazards, 2010).

Clearly, trauma has reached epidemic proportions in the USA! It seems clear that such crisis events represent a "clear and present danger" to the psychological health of Americans.

Diagnostic Symptomatology

In 1941, Kardiner (1941) described five consistent clinical features of the syndrome now referred to as PTSD:

1. Constriction of personality functioning
2. Exaggerated startle reflex and irritability

3. Psychic fixation upon the trauma
4. Atypical dream experiences
5. A propensity for explosive and aggressive reactions

In 1942, Gillespie described an acute "war neurosis" as having as an important clinical feature an increased startle reaction characterized by increased and generalized muscular tension, palpitations, and a "sinking feeling," thus emphasizing a distinct autonomic nervous system (ANS) component to this posttrauma syndrome.

In 1980, the American Psychiatric Association described PTSD as a form of anxiety disorder:

> The essential feature is the development of characteristic symptoms following a psychologically traumatic event that is generally outside the range of usual human experience. ...
> The characteristic symptoms involve re-experiencing the traumatic event; numbing of responsiveness to, or reduced involvement with, the external world; and a variety of autonomic, dysphoric, or cognitive symptoms. (p. 236)

The specific criteria are listed in Table 21.1. PTSD was described in subvariations as well:

1. "Acute," in which the onset of symptoms occurred within 6 months of the trauma and lasted less than 6 months.
2. "Chronic or delayed," in which either or both of the following applied: duration of the symptoms for 6 months or more (chronic) and/or the onset of symptoms at least 6 months after the trauma (delayed).

In 1987, the American Psychiatric Association revised its criteria for PTSD (American Psychiatric Association, 1987). In doing so, the traumata giving rise to PTSD were somewhat better defined. Once again, the notion of a psychologically distressing event outside the normal range of human experience was emphasized. Yet, specific instances were cited:

> a serious threat to one's life or physical integrity; a serious threat or harm to one's children, spouse, or other close relatives and friends; sudden destruction of one's home or community; or seeing another person who has recently been, or is being, seriously injured or killed as a result of an accident or physical violence. In some cases the trauma may be learning about a serious threat or harm to a close friend or relative. (pp. 247–248)

Table 21.2. describes the specific criteria requisite for the PTSD diagnosis.

In 1994, the American Psychiatric Association once again changed the diagnostic criteria for PTSD as contained within the revised nosological compendium (DSM-IV; American Psychiatric Association, 1994). The DSM-IV criteria (see Table 21.3) represented major alterations in the official criteria for PTSD, and even recognized a more acute variant of the posttraumatic syndrome, acute stress disorder (ASD; see Table 21.4).

The major changes in the DSM-IV formulation of PTSD reside in the definition of the traumatic event. While DSM-III and DSM-III-R defined the traumatic stressor as an unusually distressing event, the DSM-IV actually restricted the nature of the stressor by limiting it to events that involve actual or threatened death or serious injury to oneself or others. The DSM-IV-R stressor of the sudden destruction to one's home or community, in the absence of injury or death, was now omitted. This

Table 21.1 Diagnostic criteria for posttraumatic stress disorder, DSM-III

A. Existence of a recognizable stressor that would evoke significant symptoms of distress in almost everyone

B. Reexperiencing the trauma as evidenced by at least one of the following:
1. Recurrent and instrusive recollections of the event
2. Recurrent dreams of the event
3. Suddenly acting or feeling as if the traumatic event were reoccurring, because of an association with an environmental or ideational stimulus

C. Numbing of responsiveness to or reduced involvement with the external world, beginning some time after the trauma, as shown by at least one of the following:
1. Markedly diminished interest in one or more significant activities
2. Feeling of detachment or estrangement from others
3. Constricted affect

D. At least two of the following symptoms that were not present before the trauma:
1. Hyperalertness or exaggerated startle response
2. Sleep disturbance
3. Guilt about surviving when others have not, or about behavior required for survival
4. Memory impairment or trouble concentrating
5. Avoidance of activities that arouse recollection of the traumatic event
6. Intensification of symptoms by exposure to events that symbolize or resemble the traumatic event

Source: *Diagnostic and Statistical Manual of Mental Disorders, III.* Copyright 1980 American Psychiatric Association. Reprinted with permission.

restriction in the nature of the traumatic stressor was not well received by many individuals who work in mass disaster venues.

While restricting one aspect of the traumatic criterion (Criterion A), the DSM-IV actually broadened another aspect of the traumatic stressor by including a subjective distress criterion.

As this volume is being written, the American Psychiatric Association is in the process of revising the criteria for PTSD once again through the publication of the DSM-5. The changes in the diagnostic formulation are proposed at this point, but are nevertheless worth mentioning. Simply stated, the A-2 criterion (fear, helplessness, and horror) would be dropped and a fourth cluster of signs and symptoms would be added ("depression"). More specifically a "depression" cluster consisting of "negative alterations in cognition and mood that are associated with the traumatic event (s)" would be added to the existing three clusters of re-experiencing, avoidance, and numbing, as well as, increased stress arousal. The "depression" cluster consists of psychogenic amnesia, negative expectations about self and the world, self-blame, negative affect, diminished interest in important activities, interpersonal estrangement, and anhedonia.

Are these diagnostic criteria of equal phenomenological importance, or are certain elements more important than others? Let us take a closer look at the posttraumatic stress concept with an appreciation for reformulation. Figure 21.1 presents a phenomenological algorithm that provides a hierarchical structure to the constituent

Table 21.2 Diagnostic criteria for posttraumatic stress disorder, DSM-III-R

A. The person has experienced an event that is outside the range of usual human experience and that would be markedly distressing to almost anyone (e.g., serious threat to one's life or physical integrity; serious threat or harm to one's children, spouse, or other close relatives and friends; sudden destruction of one's home or community; or seeing another person who has recently been, or is being, seriously injured or killed as the result of an accident or physical violence)

B. The traumatic event is persistently reexperienced in at least one of the following ways:
    1. Recurrent and intrusive distressing recollections of the event (in young children, repetitive play in which themes or aspects of the trauma are expressed)
    2. Recurrent distressing dreams of the event
    3. Suddenly acting or feeling as if the traumatic event were recurring (includes a sense of reliving the experience, illusions, hallucinations, and dissociative [flashback] episodes, even those that occur upon awakening or when intoxicated)
    4. Intense psychological distress at exposure to events that symbolize or resemble an aspect of the traumatic event, including anniversaries of the trauma

C. Persistent avoidance of stimuli associated with the trauma or numbing of general responsiveness (not present before the trauma), as indicated by at least three of the following:
    1. Efforts to avoid thoughts or feelings associated with the trauma
    2. Efforts to avoid activities or situations that arouse recollections of the traumas
    3. Inability to recall an important aspect of the trauma (psychogenic amnesia)
    4. Markedly diminished interest in significant activities (in young children, loss of recently acquired development skills such as toilet training or language skills)
    5. Feeling of detachment or estrangement from others
    6. Restricted range of affect (e.g., unable to have loving feelings)
    7. Sense of a foreshortened future (e.g., does not expect to have a career, marriage, or children, or a long life)

D. Persistent symptoms of increased arousal (not present before the trauma), as indicated by at least two of the following:
    1. Difficulty in falling or staying asleep
    2. Irritability or outbursts of anger
    3. Difficulty in concentrating
    4. Hypervigilance
    5. Exaggerated startle response
    6. Physiological reactivity upon exposure to events that symbolize or resemble an aspect of the traumatic event (e.g., a woman who was raped in an elevator breaks out in a sweat when entering any elevator)

E. Duration of the disturbance (symptoms in B, C, and D) of at least 1 month

Source: *Diagnostic and Statistical Manual of Mental Disorders, III - R*. Copyright 1987 American Psychiatric Association. Reprinted with permission.

elements. We have combined the depression, avoidance, and withdrawal clusters as we believe they are consistent with a singular phenomenological syndrome.

As the algorithm indicates, posttraumatic stress represents a dynamic "process" rather than a monothetic formulation. Figure 21.1 emphasizes the etiological role that subjective interpretation of the traumatic stressor can play in the determination of the amplitude and chronicity of the posttraumatic stress response. This view is in concert with the model utilized throughout this text as the overarching framework for

Table 21.3 Diagnostic criteria for posttraumatic stress disorder, DSM-IV

A. The person has been exposed to a traumatic event in which both of the following were present:

1. Event or events that involved actual or threatened death or serious injury, or a threat to the physical integrity of self or others

2. The person's response involved intense fear, helplessness, or horror. *Note.* In children, this may be expressed instead by disorganized or agitated behavior

B. The traumatic event is persistency reexperienced in one (or more) of the following ways:

1. Recurrent and intrusive distressing recollections of the event, including images, thoughts, or perceptions. *Note.* In young children, repetitive play may occur in which themes or aspects of the trauma are expressed

2. Recurrent distressing dreams of the event. *Note.* In children, there may be frightening dreams without recognizable content

3. Acting or feeling as if the traumatic event were recurring (includes a sense of reliving the experience, illusions, hallucinations, and dissociative flashback episodes, including those that occur on awakening or when intoxicated). *Note.* In young children, trauma-specific reenactment may occur

4. Intense psychological distress at exposure to internal or external cues that symbolize or resemble an aspect of the traumatic event

5. Physiological reactivity on exposure to internal or external cues that symbolize or resemble an aspect of the traumatic event

C. Persistent avoidance of stimuli associated with the trauma and numbing of general responsiveness (not present before the trauma), as indicated by three (or more) of the following:

1. Efforts to avoid thoughts, feelings, or conversations associated with the trauma

2. Efforts to avoid activities, places, or people that arouse recollections of the trauma

3. Inability to recall an important aspect of the trauma

4. Markedly diminished interest or participation in significant activities

5. Feeling of detachment or estrangement from others

6. Restricted range of affect (e.g., unable to have loving feelings)

7. Sense of a foreshortened future (e.g., does not expect to have a career, marriage, children, or a normal life span)

D. Persistent symptoms of increased arousal (not present before the trauma), as indicated by two (or more) of the following:

1. Difficulty falling or staying asleep

2. Irritability or outbursts of anger

3. Difficulty concentrating

4. Hypervigilance

5. Exaggerated startle response

E. Duration of the disturbance (symptoms in Criteria B, C, and D) is more than 1 month

F. The disturbance causes clinically significant distress or impairment in social, occupational, or other important areas of functioning

Specify if:

Acute: if duration of symptoms is less than 3 months

Chronic: if duration of symptoms is 3 months or more

Specify if:

With Delayed Onset: if onset of symptoms is at least 6 months after the stressor

Source: Diagnostic and Statistical Manual of Mental Disorders, Fourth Edition. Copyright © 1994 American Psychiatric Association. Reprinted with permission.

Table 21.4 Diagnostic criteria for acute stress disorder, DSM-IV

A. The person has been exposed to a traumatic event in which both of the following were present:

1. The person experienced, witnessed, or was confronted with an event or events that involved actual or threatened death or serious injury, or a threat to the physical integrity of self or others

2. The person's response involved intense fear, helplessness, or horror

B. Either while experiencing or after experiencing the distressing event, the individual has three (or more) of the following dissociative symptoms:

1. A subjective sense of numbing, detachment, or absence of emotional responsiveness

2. A reduction in awareness of his or her surroundings (e.g., "being in a daze")

3. Derealization

4. Depersonalization

5. Dissociative amnesia (i.e., inability to recall an important aspect of the trauma)

C. The traumatic event is persistently reexperienced in at least one of the following ways: recurrent images, thoughts, dreams, illusions, flashback episodes, or a sense of reliving the experience; or distress on exposure to reminders of the traumatic event

D. Marked avoidance of stimuli that arouse recollections of the trauma (e.g., thoughts, feelings, conversations, activities, places, people)

E. Marked symptoms of anxiety or increased arousal (e.g., difficulty sleeping, irritability, poor concentration, hypervigilance, exaggerated startle response, motor restlessness)

F. The disturbance causes clinically significant distress or impairment in social, occupational, or other important areas of functioning or impairs the individual's ability to pursue some necessary task, such as obtaining necessary assistance or mobilizing personal resources by telling family members about the traumatic experience

G. The disturbance lasts for a minimum of 2 days and a maximum of 4 weeks and occurs within 4 weeks of the traumatic event

H. The disturbance is not due to the direct physiological effects of a substance (e.g., a drug of abuse, a medication) or a general medical condition, is not better accounted for by Brief Psychotic Disorder, and is not merely an exacerbation of a preexisting Axis I or Axis II disorder

Source: Diagnostic and Statistical Manual of Mental Disorders, Fourth Edition. Copyright © 1994, American Psychiatric Association. Reprinted with permission.

understanding the human stress response. At the same time, Fig. 21.1 argues that much of the depressive avoidance, numbing, and withdrawal that is replete in the posttraumatic stress constellation may, indeed, be but a second-order symptom manifestation.

While acknowledging the important role that subjective interpretation plays in the traumatic response, Fig. 21.2 is presented as a means of understanding the variable impact of subjective interpretation of the trauma spectrum.

Let us take a closer look at posttraumatic stress through the utilization of a factorial taxonomy (i.e., a two-factor model of posttraumatic stress), including the notion of subjective appraisal. The A (2) criterion of the DSM-IV notes that the individual's response to the traumatic event must involve "intense fear, helplessness, or horror." This alteration has engendered some concern from victims' advocacy groups in that acknowledgment of the subjective aspects of the traumatic stressor may lead to a "blame the victim" attitude. Yehuda (1998) raised this issue and stated, "The stipulation in DSM-IV that individuals must experience a subjective response to an event now makes the study of risk factors necessary rather than inappropriate" (p. 3).

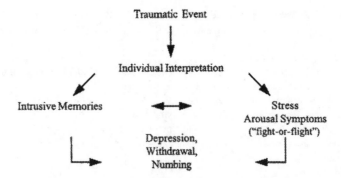

Fig. 21.1 As described by Everly and Lating (1995), the manifestation of the three symptom clusters consisting of intrusive memories, stress arousal symptoms, and withdrawal, depression, and numbing are predicated upon a complex interaction between the traumatic event and the individual experiencing the event

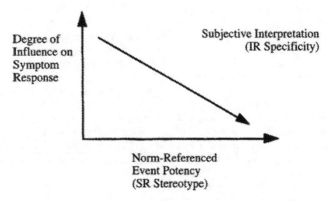

Fig. 21.2 As noted in Fig. 21.1, the nature and degree of manifest posttraumatic symptomatology is a function of the nature of the traumatic event and the individual experiencing the event. So as not to misinterpret this concept as reason to "blame the victim," the role of the victim's subjective interpretation is portrayed in overall event potency (severity). Traumatic events will vary in their normative severity, or potency. This is called stimulus–response (SR) stereotype and simply means that "mild" stressors usually engender "mild" responses, while "severe" stressors usually engender "severe" responses. Automobile accidents are less severe than torture. Thus, as the norm-referenced severity of the stressor event increases, the less a role-subjective interpretation, called individual response (IR) specificity, plays in determining the severity of the manifest symptom response. Thus, subjective interpretation plays less of a role in shaping the traumatic response to torture than it might to an automobile accident

The DSM-IV-TR also acknowledges the potential for PTSD to be associated with "… a change from the individual's previous personality characteristics" (American Psychiatric Association, 2000, p. 465). In recognizing that PTSD could alter something as concretized as personality, a new realm of psychological and biological phenomenological possibilities emerges.

A Two-Factor Theory of Posttraumatic Stress

Everly (1993; Everly & Lating, 1995, 2004) has analyzed the PTSD construct and found it to reveal two key factors, or constituents:

1. Neurological hypersensitivity
2. Psychological hypersensitivity (Everly, 1993; Everly & Lating, 1995, 2004)

Neurological Hypersensitivity

It is clear that the posttraumatic stress syndrome possesses a significant neurological constituency. Kolb (1987) has suggested that the PTSD symptoms fall within four categories (1) impaired perceptual, cognitive, and affective functions; (2) symptoms of released activation; (3) reactive affect and avoidance; and (4) restitutive symptoms and behaviors.

Yet, Kolb argues that the symptoms of released activation are the "constant" symptoms of the condition: the exaggerated startle reaction, irritability, hyperalertness, nightmares, and related psychophysiological expressions of ANS hyperfunction.

Similarly, (Foy, Sipprelle, Rueger, & Carroll 1984), in a comparison of methods for the concurrent discrimination of PTSD, found that self-report indices of anxiety and ANS arousal alone were capable of correctly identifying more than 90% of the study's participants. The investigation employed 21 Vietnam veteran PTSD patients and 22 Vietnam veterans with other psychiatric complaints.

In a review of three psychophysiological investigations into PTSD, Kolb (1984, 1987) concluded that indices of sympathetic nervous system (SNS) arousal were capable of differentiating PTSD from non-PTSD participants.

PTSD participants showed more autonomic arousal in response to trauma-related stimuli than did non-PTSD participants. Thus, Kolb (1987) concluded that "psychophysiological assessment offers strong potential not only for diagnostic identification … but also for assessment of severity of the disorder" (p. 991).

Finally, Horowitz, Wilner, Kaltreider, and Alvarez (1980) investigated the signs and symptoms of PTSD. Using a multi-inventory battery of self-report indices, they investigated the three major PTSD clusters: (1) intrusive re-experiencing of the trauma, (2) numbing/avoidance reactions, and (3) anxiety/stress reactions. The authors concluded that intrusive thinking and general symptoms of distress were of primary clinical prevalence and importance in the PTSD phenomenon. They added that the numbing and avoidance signs and symptoms are best understood as efforts of the PTSD patient to control the primary PTSD symptomatology.

From an anatomical perspective, in concert with the formulation of MacLean (1949), Gray (1982) has identified the septal–hippocampal complex as the neuroanatomical epicenter for the integration of exteroceptive as well as interoceptive, proprioceptive, and cognitive stimuli (Seifert, 1983; Van Hoesen, 1982). More specifically, Gray argues, as do Reiman et al. (1986), that the noradrenergic system within the septal–hippocampal nuclei bears primary responsibility for integrating and responding, via hypothalamic efferent mechanisms, to novel and unpleasant stimuli, and furthermore, that stimulation of these projections results in a heightened sensitivity and reactivity within all innervated regions, including neuroendocrine effector mechanisms, to environmental cues seen in any way as novel, threatening, or otherwise aversive. Similarly, Madison and Nicoll (1982) found that noradrenergic neurons from the locus ceruleus to the hippocampus serve to impair the ability of the septal–hippocampal region to accommodate to excitatory stimuli.

Reiman et al. (1986) have demonstrated through positron emission tomography that the septal–hippocampal complex plays a major role in panic attacks. They further conclude that via the septal–amygdalar complex, the septal–hippocampal nuclei can initiate a hypothalamically mediated stress response (see Aggleton, 1992; Cullinan, Herman, Helmreich, & Watson, 1995; LeDoux, 1995).

Gloor (1986) has reported that the hippocampus plays a major role in memory and fear reactions. Electrophysiological investigations of awake patients having surgery for epilepsy found that activation of the hippocampus was capable of engendering "flashbacks," affective lability, perceptual distortions, fear, worry, and even guilt reactions (see also Post, 1986; Seifert, 1983).

In summary, to this point, a wide range of evidence indicates that residing with the confines of the septal–hippocampal–amygdalar complex are nuclei responsible for engendering all of the major symptoms of PTSD, including intrusive recollections and flashbacks (Gloor, 1986), neurological hypersensitivity, hyperstartle reactions, and inhibited stimulus accommodation (Gray, 1982; Madison & Nicoll, 1982), panic-like responses (Reiman et al., 1986), fear, rumination, worry, guilt-like reactions (Gloor, 1986), and affective lability (Post, 1986). Cooper, Bloom, and Roth (1982) have suggested that the role of the locus ceruleus is to act as a general orienting system rather than as a specific organizing epicenter for panic and related dysfunction (see also Charney, Deutch, Southwick, Krystal, & Friedman, 1995).

The amygdala has been ascribed a preeminent role in the anatomical foundations of PTSD (Charney, Deutch, Krystal, Southwick, & Davis, 1993). Consistent with the survival orientation of the "fight-or-flight" response, the amygdala appears to possess a specialized mechanism for processing emotional, especially fear-related, memories (LeDoux, 1992). LeDoux has argued that the amygdala may process emotional memories in such a way that "memories established through the amygdala are indelible" (p. 342). This may help us understand the persistence of traumatic memories; that is, the maintenance of fear-related memories may serve as a means of assuring continued survival, especially if coupled with autonomic mobilization, hypervigilance, and explosive reactivity or withdrawal and avoidance behaviors (the fight-or-flight response). A more recent review has extended our initial understanding of the neuroanatomy of PTSD, however. Sripada, Gonzalez, Phan and Liberzon's (2011) analysis and Liberzon and Sripada's (2007) review correctly implicated the importance of contextualization and interpretation in generation of PTSD. Their work underscores the medial prefrontal cortex (mPFC) as an important structure in the psychological process of contextualization and thus as a critical anatomical foundation of PTSD.

If, indeed, the anatomical basis for PTSD is in the mPFC–septal–hippocampal–amygdalar system, what extraordinary physiology serves to sustain the phenomenon? The hypersensitivity formulations of van der Kolk, Greenberg, Boyd and Krystal (1985) and Kolb (1987) as generically extended within this text and elsewhere (Everly, 1985b, 1993; Everly & Benson, 1989) seem reasonable. Using the disorders of arousal model described earlier, it may be argued that PTSD represents a limbic-system-based condition of neurological hypersensitivity, where a pathognomic propensity for limbic hyperreactivity is related to intraneuronal alterations that result from and lead to further neural hypersensitivity/hyperexcitability.

The neurological hypersensitivity proposed as a factorial constituent of PTSD may possess several pathognomic and sustaining mechanisms (see Everly & Lating, 2004, for a review):

1. Increased excitatory neurotransmitter activity within the limbic circuitry (Black et al., 1987; Post, 1985; Post & Ballenger, 1981; Post, Weiss, & Smith, 1995; Post, Rubinow & Ballenger, 1986; Sorg & Kalivas, 1995).
2. Declination of inhibitory neurotransmitters and/or receptors (Cain, 1992; see Everly, 1993).
3. Augmentation of micromorphological structures (especially amygdaloidal and hippocampal dendritic branching) (Cain, 1992; Post et al., 1995; see Everly, 1993).
4. Changes in the biochemical bases of neuronal activation, for example, augmentation of phosphoproteins and/or changes on the transduction mechanism *c-fos* so as to change the genetic message within the neuron's nucleus (Cain, 1992; Horger & Roth, 1995; Sorg & Kalivas, 1995).
5. Increased arousal of neuromuscular efferents, with resultant increased proprioceptive bombardment of the limbic system (especially amygdaloidal and hippocampal nuclei) (Gellhorn, 1964b, 1968; Malmo, 1975; Weil, 1974).
6. Repetitive cognitive excitation (Gellhorn, 1964b, 1968; Gellhorn & Loofburrow, 1963; Post et al., 1986).

While examining the physiological bases of PTSD, a more specific look at the neurochemistry seems in order. It is clear that excitatory neurotransmitter activity is an essential component of the presentation of PTSD. Specifically, central amino acids such as glutamate and aspartate are implicated in hyperarousal as well as excitotoxic effects (Everly, 1995; Bermudo-Soriano, Perez-Rodriguez, Vaquero-Lorenzo, Baca-Garcia, 2012; Nair & Ajit, 2008). Corticotropin-releasing factor (CRF), endogenous opioids, vasopressin, and oxytocin are also implicated in extreme stress arousal (Selye, 1976; Rossier, Bloom, & Guillemin, 1980; Rochefort, Rosenberger, & Saffran, 1959; Nair & Ajit, 2008). Finally, there is evidence that serotonin, dopamine, and certainly norepinephrine play significant roles in extreme stress (Kolb, 1987; Sorg & Kalivas, 1995; van der Kolk et al., 1985; Charney, 2004).

The excitatory processes inherent in PTSD are not limited to the CNS. The mobilization of neuroendocrine and endocrine pathways carries the posttraumatic stress response throughout the human body. Especially implicated are the sympathoadrenomedullary (SAM) (Everly, 1990; Everly & Lating, 2004) and the hypothalamic–pituitary–adrenal

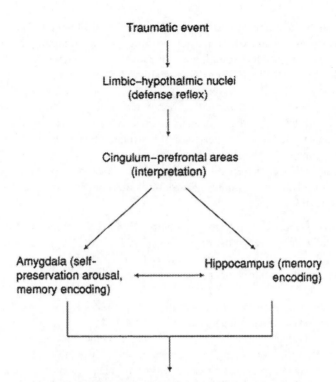

Fig. 21.3 Neurobiology of posttraumatic stress disorder

(HPA) systems (Yehuda, Giller, Levengood, Southwick, Siever, 1995; Everly & Lating). Figure 21.3 summarizes some of the key elements involved in the biology of PTSD.

Psychological Hypersensitivity

Psychological hypersensitivity is thought to arise from a violation of some deeply held belief, referred to as a worldview, or *Weltanschauung* (Everly, 1993, 1994, 1995; Everly & Lating, 2004). Thus, according to this perspective, a traumatic event is predicated upon some situation that violates a deeply held and important world-view. Most commonly, we think of the traumatic event as a life-threatening event—a violation of the assumption of safety discussed by writers such as Maslow (1970). But there appear to be at least five universally traumatogenetic themes:

1. Violation of the belief that the world is "just" or "fair." For example, why does an infant die in a motor vehicle accident?
2. Violation of a sense of who you are by having not done something you should, or by having done something you should not have done.
3. Abandonment, betrayal, and violation of trust.
4. Violation of a universal sense of safety.
5. Disruption of a religious or spiritually based belief.

Within his construct of "psychotraumatology," Everly (1993, 1994, 1995; Everly & Lating, 2004) discusses these issues in greater detail.

The Psychological Profile of Posttraumatic Stress Disorder

The work of Keane and his colleagues has been preeminent in the search for the psychological PTSD prototype. Using patients evaluated with the Minnesota Multiphasic Personality Inventory (MMPI) and 100 patients with other psychiatric diagnoses, Keane, Malloy, and Fairbank (1984) were able to identify an MMPI profile capable of correctly classifying 74% of all patients. The MMPI decision rule was $F \geq 66$, Depression (2)≥ 78, and Schizophrenia (8)≥ 79 (using T scores). Item analysis led to the creation of a 49-item MMPI PTSD subscale, the PTSD-Keane (PK) subscale (Keane et al.), that correctly identified 82% of the patients studied. On this MMPI subscale, patients who scored 35 out of 49 had an 87% chance of possessing a valid PTSD diagnosis, whereas patients who scored above 40 had a 90% chance of a true positive PTSD diagnosis. The MMPI-2 (Butcher et al., 1989, 2001) uses 46 items for PK subscale, and in a sample of veterans, a cut-off score of 28 correctly classified 76% of the overall sample, 67% of the PTSD group and 85% of the non-PTSD comparison group (Munley, Bains, Bloem, & Busby, 1995).

In a cross-validation of the aforementioned MMPI PTSD subscale, Fairbank, McCaffrey, and Keane (1985) found that patients with a T score above 88 on the F scale were most likely to possess a factitious disorder. Thus, the F decision rule became $66 \leq F \leq 88$ and correctly identified 93% of the sample studied when combined with the previous (2)≥ 78 and (8)≥ 79. On the MMPI-2, Tolin and associates (2004) reported that the Infrequency-Psychopathology $F(p)$scale, which consists of 27 items developed to distinguish between overreporting and accurate reporting of severe distress (Arbisi & Ben-Porath, 1995), is effective in determining over-reporting in Vietnam veterans being assessed for PTSD. In a study using the MMPI-2 to assess PTSD in a study of 90 trauma-exposed undergraduates, the MMPI-2 clinical scales of 7 (psychasthenia), 2 (depression), and 3 (hysteria), the content scales of Anxiety, Work Interference, and Low Self Esteem (LSE), and the two PTSD subscales (PK and PTSD-Schlenger (PS) subscale (Schlenger & Kulka, 1987)) discriminated between PTSD and a well-adjusted control group (McDevitt-Murphy, Weathers, Flood, Eakin, & Benson, 2007).

The work of McDermott (1987) sought to extend the psychometric diagnosis of PTSD beyond the MMPI. Using the Millon Clinical Multiaxial Inventory (MCMI), McDermott evaluated 22 Vietnam combat veterans, 11 of whom had been diagnosed with PTSD. The results of his study indicate that PTSD patients may present elevations on the MCMI schizoid and avoidant scales $(x>80)$, with a concomitant depression on the histrionic scale.

The MCMI-III contains a scale (R) that purports to assess PTSD with a 53% sensitivity and a positive predictive power of 73%. But the MCMI-III aggregate configural profile may take several forms:

1. Aggregate elevations on Schizoid, Avoidant, and Negativistic (passive–aggressive) scales are often viewed as the withdrawing "flight" variant of the MCMI posttraumatic stress profile.
2. Aggregate elevations on the Narcissistic, Aggressive, and Antisocial scales may be viewed as the aggressive "fight" variant of the MCMI posttraumatic stress profile.
3. Aggregate elevations on the Negativistic, Self-Defeating, Schizoid/Avoidant, Aggressive, and Borderline scales may be viewed as the affectively labile profile that is often characteristic of "complex PTSD" (i.e., indicative of early developmental trauma, abuse, and/or neglect).

Based on Kolb's (1987) hypothesis that PTSD represents a partial cognitive deficit, in combination with the belief that PTSD resides within the hippocampal complex, Everly and Horton hypothesized that there would be a short-term memory deficit among PTSD patients. Using 15- and 30-s trials of the Peterson Memory Paradigm, these authors found that 9 out of 14 (65%) non-combat-related PTSD patients failed to meet the 55% correct cutting-line criterion for the 15-s trials, and 11 out of 14 (79%) patients failed to meet the 45% correct cutting-line criterion for the 30-s trials. These data served to support the hypothesis that PTSD patients are likely to possess a cognitive deficit that manifests as an impairment to immediate and short-term memory function. Long-term memory was unimpaired in these participants. In one of the first controlled neuropsychological studies assessing active-duty Army soldiers, and after controlling for deployment-related heard injury, stress and depression, results revealed that Iraq deployment, when compared with non-deployment, was associated with reduced sustained attention, verbal learning, and visual-spatial memory, yet improved performance on a test of simple reaction time (Vasterling et al., 2006). Moreover, on self-report measures, deployment was associated with confusion and tension.

With the wars in Iraq and Afghanistan that have occurred in the last decade, there has been increased focus on the prevalence of PTSD in returning veterans. As noted earlier in this chapter, as many as 50% of Iraqi and Afghanistan veterans seeking treatment screen positive for PTSD. However, Ramchand and colleagues (2010) note in this same article that the prevalence rates in the studies they reported were as low as 4%. The authors attribute this variability to a number of factors, including the varied and multiple methods of assessment and diagnostic criteria used to determine a diagnosis of PTSD. Although there are inherent challenges in determining an accurate assessment of a PTSD psychological profile, the International Society for Traumatic Stress Studies (ITSS; Foa, Keane, Friedman, & Cohen, 2009) suggests using the following categories of evidence-based measures to complete a comprehensive PTSD assessment (1) structured diagnostic interviews, such as the Clinician-Administered PTSD Scale (CAPS) (Blake et al., 1990) or the Structured Clinical Interview for DSM-IV (SCID; First, Spitzer, Williams, & Gibbon, 2000), and (2) self-report measures, such as the MMPI-2, MCMI, or one of the many specific PTSD scales (e.g., PTSD Checklist; (PCL; Weathers, Litz, Herman, Huska, &, Keane, 1993)). According to Castro, Hayes, and Keane (2011), accurate assessment of PTSD within a military population is required to: (1) facilitate treatment planning, (2) allow for research progress, (3) provide valuable information used for policy making, and (4) to determine disability benefits.

Treatment of Posttraumatic Stress Disorder

This chapter has presented posttraumatic stress as a quintessential example of psychological and biological factors combining in an inextricable integration. Our two-factor model of PTSD implies that the recovery from posttraumatic stress is predicated upon improvement in both domains. This is not to say that every patient who suffers from PTSD requires medication, but it does suggest that the more severe the manifest symptomatology, the more psychotropic medications should be considered as an addition to the therapeutic mix. It is doubtful, however, that any PTSD patient has ever recovered on the basis of psychotropic medication alone. Because the "injury" is a psychological one, recovery will be based upon some alteration in the "psychological domain." That psychotherapeutic improvement may be greatly facilitated, indeed, by the addition of psychopharmacological agents. In instances when the amplitude of the neurological pathology has become self-sustaining, psychopharmacological agents will be mandatory. Let us take a look at current issues in the treatment of posttraumatic stress.

Psychopharmacotherapy

A wide variety of psychopharmacological agents have been used in the treatment of PTSD. As van der Kolk (1987) has stated, "Psychotherapy is rarely helpful as long as the patient continues to respond to contemporary events and situations with a continuation of physiological emergency reactions" (p. 75).

A review of the pharmacological treatment of PTSD has been offered by Platman (1999) and lists psychotropic agents for consideration by virtue of the symptoms they tend to target:

- *Learned helplessness*—clonidine, benzodiazepines, tricyclics (TCAs), and monoamine oxidase inhibitors (MAOI)
- *Hyperstartle response*—clonidine
- *Intrusive ideation*—selective serotonin reuptake inhibitors (SSRIs), TCAs, and MAOIs
- *Panic*—alprazolam and clonazepam
- *Depressed mood and avoidance*—SSRIs
- *Impulsive rage*—lithium and carbamazepine
- *Sleep disturbance*—trazodone

In 1999, the *Journal of Clinical Psychiatry* published findings from its Expert Consensus Panel for the Treatment of PTSD (Foa, Davidson, & Frances, 1999). The Panel recommended that psychopharmacological intervention either be followed or used in combination with psychotherapy for both acute and chronic PTSD. The medications of choice were the SSRIs. If no response was achieved, the Panel recommended that nefazodone or venlafaxine be initiated. If a partial positive response was achieved, it recommended a mood stabilizer in addition to the SSRI.

Given that some researchers consider severe posttraumatic stress a form of kindling, or subcortical ictus, the question of the utilization of mood stabilizers (carbamazepine and divalproex) as a primary medication becomes a relevant issue.

The UK's National Institute for Clinical Excellence (NICE, 2005) made the following recommendations: "Drug treatments for PTSD should not be used as a routine first-line treatment for adults (in general use or by specialist mental health professionals) in preference to a trauma-focused psychological therapy. Drug treatments (paroxetine or mirtazapine for general use, and amitriptyline or phenelzine for initiation only by mental health specialists) should be considered for the treatment of PTSD in adults who express a preference not to engage in trauma-focused psychological treatment" (NICE, p.5). In a review of consensus guidelines, such as NICE's, and several meta-analytic studies of pharmacotherapy in the treatment of PTSD, Stein, Ipser, & McAnda (2009) support that SSRIs, or some SSRIs and venlafaxine (a serotonin norepinephrine uptake inhibitor (SNRI)) are good first-line treatments.

Psychotherapy

The Expert Consensus Panel for the Treatment of PTSD (Foa et al., 1999) has recognized the superordinate role that psychotherapy initially plays in the therapeutic arsenal. The report notes that anxiety management, psycho-education, and cognitive therapy appear to be the safest and most acceptable psychotherapeutic interventions. This recommendation is echoed in part by NICE (2005). The NICE guidelines state:

"Trauma-focused cognitive behavioural therapy should be offered to those with severe post-traumatic symptoms or with severe PTSD in the first month after the traumatic event. These treatments should normally be provided on an individual outpatient basis. All people with PTSD should be offered a course of trauma-focused psychological treatment (trauma-focused cognitive behavioural therapy [CBT] or eye movement desensitisation and reprocessing [EMDR]). These treatments should normally be provided on an individual outpatient basis" (NICE, p. 4).

The work of Meichenbaum (1977, 1994) stands as a significant contribution in this regard. His treatise on the treatment of PTSD from a cognitive-behavioral perspective represents a powerful multidimensional approach to this complex and challenging disorder (Meichenbaum, 1994; also see Foy, 1992).

Other valuable resources in the area of treatment formulation for PTSD include the work of Foa, Keane, & Friedman (2000) and Flannery (1992). Wilson, Friedman, and Lindy (2001) offer an integrative perspective on PTSD treatment, and Wampold and colleagues (2010) provide a more recent review in determining what works in PTSD treatment.

Group therapy interventions have shown significant promise and have been summarized by van der Kolk (1987). The rationale for the use of group psychotherapy for PTSD includes the provision of peer support, a safe venue for therapeutic abreaction, consensual validation, and the minimization of regression and avoidance. A recent meta-analytic analysis of the efficacy of group treatment for PTSD (Sloan, Feinstein, Gallagher, & Beck, 2011) showed that while group treatment is better than no treatment for PTSD, it was not superior when compared to active treatment conditions that were used in the studies to control for nonspecific therapy effects (e.g., supportive therapy group). Moreover, the results indicate that group treatment might be less effective with men than women, and also in conditions where there is repeated trauma, such as child abuse and combat trauma, or more chronic PTSD.

Neurocognitive Strategic Therapy for Posttraumatic Stress

Everly (1993, 1994, 1995; Everly & Lating, 2004, 2005) has posited that posttraumatic stress represents a two-factor phenomenon (i.e., two inextricably intertwined factors that make up its core essence): (1) neurological hypersensitivity and (2) psychological hypersensitivity. We reviewed their respective constituencies earlier in this chapter, so we shall not reiterate them here. It may be argued that treatment should be the natural corollary of phenomenology. If so, then treatment formulations for posttraumatic stress reactions, including ASD and PTSD, should parallel, or match, their phenomenology. To put it another way, the treatment of posttraumatic stress reactions, including ASD and PTSD, should possess a two-factor constituency so as to match the two-factor phenomenology of the disorder.

Everly (1994, 1995) has proposed that a neurocognitive strategic treatment formulation for posttraumatic stress is likely to prove the most effective and is clearly the most theoretically sound. By way of explanation, it is clear that numerous therapies are effective for posttraumatic stress. In that it is unclear that any given "brand name" tactic is always superior to any other given tactic, Everly offers a strategic formulation for the treatment of posttraumatic stress rather than recommending a specific tactical approach. This strategic formulation recommends a phenomenologically driven *approach* to therapy rather than a specific *technique* for therapy. Thus, Everly suggests that *neurological desensitization* techniques should be used to address the neurological sensitivity of posttraumatic stress and be combined with techniques that address the *cognitive schemas* that have been threatened or destroyed by the traumatic event. Techniques for neurological desensitization might include meditation, Yoga, physical exercise, massage, neuromuscular relaxation techniques, hypnosis, psychotropic medications, imagery, and so on. Techniques to address the endangered cognitive schemas might include cognitive therapy, cognitive-behavioral therapy, dynamic therapies, group therapy, behavior therapy, and so on.

Eye Movement Desensitization and Reprocessing

Eye Movement Desensitization and Reprocessing (EMDR) may represent a unique example of an integrated neurocognitive therapy in that it may address both the neurological hypersensitivity and the cognitive schemas within the same therapeutic paradigm, virtually simultaneously. EMDR is a therapeutic method originated by Francine Shapiro in 1987, when she indiscriminately discovered that recurring, disturbing thoughts rapidly and permanently disappeared when she engaged in rapid, saccadic eye movements (Shapiro & Solomon, 1995). Shapiro first published her work in 1989 as EMD and reported on the successful controlled treatment of 22 rape/molestation victims and Vietnam veterans, using a one-session application that included as part of the protocol having the participant follow the repeated side-to-side movement of her fingers (Shapiro, 1989). The impressive treatment gains were maintained at a 3-month follow-up. The results of Shapiro's initial work generated tremendous excitement in area of PTSD treatment; however, it also raised considerable skepticism because of the lack of validated PTSD measures employed and the possibility of placebo effects, including demand characteristics (Feske, 1998).

The intense research scrutiny that resulted from the introduction of EMDR led in a relatively short period of time to numerous applied studies. However, the overall results of early studies of EMDR were largely equivocal due primarily to flawed methodology, poor experimental design, and inadequate treatment delivery (i.e., inexperienced or minimally trained therapists providing the treatment) (Shapiro, 1999). According to Shapiro (1999), it is important to acknowledge that EMDR is "an integrated form of therapy incorporating aspects of many traditional psychological orientations and one that makes use of a variety of bilateral stimuli besides eye movement" (p. 37). In fact, treatment effectiveness has been reported for bilateral auditory stimulation therapist (e.g., snaps fingers nearer one ear of the patient than the other) and bilateral tactile stimulation (e.g., participant rests palms on his or her knees and therapist alternatively taps the palms) (Lipke, 2000).

Therefore, the emphasis on eye movements is actually a misconception, but one that is certainly understandable given the name of the process. Shapiro is also quick to emphasize that other quite salient, nonspecific elements account for therapeutic success (Shapiro, 1995, 1999). She proposes that the general model of EMDR is predicated on the notion of accelerated information processing, which states that "there is an innate physiological system that is designed to transform disturbing input into an adaptive resolution and a psychologically healthy integration" (Shapiro, 1995, p. 53).

Within the past decade there have been numerous studies assessing the treatment efficacy of EMDR. Seidler and Wagner (2006) in a meta-analysis compared seven studies of "trauma-focused" cognitive behavioral therapy (CBT) to EMDR, and the results showed that both treatments were effective and that there were no differences between the two. A systematic review and meta-analysis of 38 randomized controlled trials of psychological treatments for chronic PTSD (participants need to have PTSD symptoms for at least 3 months) from search engine databases as well as the Cochrane Library, revealed that the treatments most supported were individually trauma-focused cognitive-behavioural therapy (TFCBT) and EMDR (Bisson et al., 2007). A meta-analysis of the efficacy of using EMDR in children with PTSD revealed an overall medium effect size ($d = 0.56$), suggesting that children benefited from EMDR treatment when compared to non-established trauma treatment or no-treatment control groups (Rodenburg, Benjamin, Roos, Meijer & Stams, 2009). Moreover, when compared to children receiving CBT, EMDR was shown to add small, but significant incremental efficacy. Overall, these results are supportive of EMDR as a treatment approach for PTSD, and also are clearly consistent with a neurocognitive treatment strategy for PTSD.

One of the most supported empirically based treatments for PTSD in the past two decades has been prolonged exposure (PE) therapy, a manualized 9–12 session treatment which emphasizes reduction of avoidance through repeated imaginal and in-vivo exposure (Foa, Rothbaum, Riggs, & Murdock, 1991; Foa et al., 1999; Nemeroff et al., 2006). The recent and impressive advances in virtual reality techniques have allowed exposure therapy to create much more realistic and somatosensory salient (i.e., sights, sounds, and smells) treatment environments, particularly when working with recent war veterans (Rizzo et al., 2011). We envision these virtual advances to continue and to expand PE to more diagnostic domains. In a study comparing the efficacy, speed, and adverse effects of exposure therapy, EMDR, and relaxation training in a sample of 60 participants (97% of whom were diagnosed with chronic PTSD), the results revealed that all three treatments were effective, but compared with EMDR and relaxation training, exposure therapy was the most efficacious in reducing experiencing and avoidance symptoms, more rapidly reduced avoidance, and resulted in the highest proportion of participants no longer meeting PTSD diagnostic criteria (Taylor et al., 2003). In a more recent meta-analytic review of PE for PTSD, Powers, Halpern, Ferenschak, Gillihan, and Foa (2010) reported on the treatment success of PE (86% of patients receiving PE fared better than control conditions), but noted as well that PE was no more effective than other active treatments, such as EMDR, stress inoculation training (SIT), or other cognitive therapies (see Chap. 8).

In the final analysis, and as suggested by Horowitz (1974) close to 40 years ago, psychotherapy should be directed toward cognitive control, improving self-image and interpersonal relationships, decreasing stress, and working through the "meaning" of the trauma. As noted by writers such as Janoff-Bulman (1992), addressing the "meaning" of the trauma becomes a pivotal aspect of the recovery process. This is clearly consistent with the two-factor model of PTSD introduced in this chapter, and also with the overarching formulation of the human stress response as used throughout this text, in that the "interpretation," or meaning, of the stressor event serves to contribute to the intensity and chronicity of the stress response itself.

Obviously, the treatment of PTSD needs to be tailored to the specific needs of the individual patient. Not only must the clinician consider the manifest symptomatology, but he or she must also strive to understand the "meaning" of the traumatic event. Once the symptoms have been stabilized and no longer represent a barrier to psychotherapy, the focus of the therapeutic process should most likely turn to the endangered or compromised belief about the world, or oneself, that lies at the foundation of the posttraumatic response (Everly, 1993, 1994, 1995).

Summary

This chapter addressed the subject of PTSD. Historically, in its more severe forms, PTSD has led to permanent partial disabilities. In some cases, permanent total disabilities have resulted. Because of the prevalence and propensity to remain undiagnosed for protracted periods of time, this stress-related disorder has been included in the present volume. Let us review the main points:

1. PTSD is generally thought to possess four key phenomenological constituents: (a) the presence of stressful experience generally acknowledged as being outside the usual realm of human experience; (b) intrusive, recollective experiences; (c) ANS hyperactivity; and (d) avoidance and numbing symptoms.
2. Within this chapter, we have argued that the "essence" of PTSD is the intrusive, recollective experience in combination with the ANS hyperfunction. The avoidant and numbing symptoms have been reformulated as attempts by the patient to control the pathological syndrome. Exposure to a stressor remains a necessary but insufficient diagnostic criterion.
3. Once viewed in the context of a combat-related syndrome, PTSD is now recognized as having the potential to arise out of virtually any life-threatening experience. Recent evidence has even suggested that PTSD can arise out of an accumulation of stressor experiences; exposure to certain solvents, toxins, and stimulants; and the experience or observation of traumatic, but not necessarily life-threatening, events such as the loss of personal property and/or physical injury.
4. Once suggested as residing within the hindbrain, PTSD has been reformulated from a physiological perspective as residing primarily as a condition of neurological hypersensitivity within the noradrenergic projections of the septal–

amygdalar–hippocampal complexes. Potential causes of the neuronal hypersensitivity include an augmentation of tyrosine hydroxylase, an increase in beta-1 postsynaptic excitatory receptors, a decrease in alpha-2 presynaptic inhibitory receptors, and an increase in postsynaptic dendritic spines.

5. Attempts to identify the psychological profile of the PTSD patient have focused upon the use of the MMPI. The $66 \leq F \leq 88$, $(2) \geq 78$, and $(8) \geq 79$ and decision rule for the MMPI seems a useful starting point. Other research utilizing the MCMI has found elevations on the Schizoid and Avoidant subscales, coupled with a diminution of the Histrionic subscale to be useful in identifying PTSD patients. Research has also found an impairment of short-term memory among PTSD patients. Finally, it should be noted that PTSD patients may frequently be misdiagnosed as sociopathic, hypochondriacal, and/or as substance abusers.

6. From a treatment perspective, PTSD, especially in its chronic forms, may require a combination of psychotherapeutic and pharmacological efforts to be truly effective. Antidepressants and anticonvulsants continue to be promising agents for the cases wherein psychotherapy alone seems insufficient.

7. Strategically, a two-factor neuro-cognitive strategic formulation for conceptualizing the treatment of posttraumatic stress, was offered.

References

Aggleton, J. P. (Ed.). (1992). *The amygdala*. New York, NY: Wiley-Liss.

American Psychiatric Association. (1980). *Diagnostic and statistical manual of mental disorders* (3rd ed.). Washington, DC: Author

American Psychiatric Association. (1987). *Diagnostic and statistical manual of mental disorders* (Rev. 3rd ed.). Washington, DC: American Psychiatric Association

American Psychiatric Association. (1994). *Diagnostic and statistical manual of mental disorders* (4th ed.). Washington, DC: Author

American Psychiatric Association. (2000). *Diagnostic and statistical manual of mental disorders* (4th ed. Text revision). Washington, DC: Author

Arbisi, P. A., & Ben-Porath, Y. S. (1995). An MMPI-2 infrequent response scale for use with psychopathological populations: The Infrequency-Psychopathology scale, $F(p)$. *Psychological Assessment, 7*, 424–431.

Bermudo-Soriano, C. R., Perez-Rodriguez, M. M., Vaquero-Lorenzo, C., & Baca-Garcia, E. (2012). New perspectives in glutamate and anxiety. *Pharmacology Biochemistry, and Behavior, 100*(4), 752–774.

Bisson, J. I., Ehlers, A., Matthews, R., Pilling, S., Richards, D., & Turner, S. (2007). Psychological treatments for chronic post-traumatic stress disorder: Systematic review and meta-analysis. *The British Journal of Psychiatry, 190*, 97–104.

Black, I., Adler, J., Dreyfus, C., Friedman, W., Laganuna, E., & Roach, A. (1987). Biochemistry of information storage in the nervous system. *Science, 236*, 1263–1268.

Blake, D. D., Weathers, F. W., Nagy, L. M., Kaloupek, D. G., Klauminzer, G., Charney, D., & Keane, T. M. (1990). A clinician rating scale for assessing current and lifetime PTSD: The CAPS-1. *Behavior Therapist, 18*, 187–188.

Breslau, N. (2009). The epidemiology of Trauma, PTSD, and other posttrauma disorders. *Trauma, Violence and Abuse: A Review Journal, 10*(3), 198–210.

Butcher, J. N., Dahlstrom, W. G., Graham, J. R., Tellegen, A., & Kaemmer, B. (1989). Manual for
    the restandardized Minnesota Multiphasic Personality Inventory: MMPI-2. An administrative
    and interpretative guideUniversity of Minnesota Press, Minneapolis, MN.
Butcher, J. N., Graham, J. R., Ben-Porath, Y. S., Tellegen, A., Dahlstrom,W. G., & Kaemmer, B.
    (2001). MMPI-2:Manual for administration, scoring and interpretation (Rev. ed.). Minneapolis:
    University of Minnesota Press.
Cain, D. P. (1992). Kindling and the amygdala. In J. P. Aggleton (Ed.), *The amygdala*
    (pp. 539–560). New York, NY: Wiley-Liss.
Castro, F., Hayes, J. P., & Keane, T. M. (2011). Issues in assessment of PTSD within the military
    culture. In B. A. Moore & W. E. Penk (Eds.), *Treating PTSD in military personnel. A clinical
    handbook* (pp. 23–41). New York, NY: Guilford.
Charney, D. S. (2004). Psychobiological mechanisms of reslience and vulnerability. Implications
    for successful adaptation to extreme stress. *Focus, 2*, 368–391.
Charney, D. S., Deutch, A., Krystal, J., Southwick, S., & Davis, M. (1993). Psychobiologic mecha-
    nisms of posttraumatic stress disorder. *Archives of General Psychiatry, 50*, 294–299.
Charney, D. S., Deutch, A. Y., Southwick, S. M., Krystal, J. H., & Friedman, M. J. (1995). Neural
    circuits and mechanisms of post-traumatic stress disorder. In D. S. Charney & A. Y. Deutsch
    (Eds.), *Neurobiological and clinical consequences of stress: From normal adaptation to post-
    traumatic stress disorder* (pp. 271–287). Philadelphia, PA: Lippincott Williams & Wilkins
    Publishers.
Cooper, J. R., Bloom, F., & Roth, R. (1982). *The biochemical basis of neuropharmacology.*
    New York, NY: Oxford University Press.
Cullinan, W., Herman, J. P., Helmreich, D., & Watson, S. (1995). A neuroanatomy of stress. In M.
    J. Friedman, D. Charney, & A. Deutch (Eds.), *Neurobiological and clinical consequences of
    stress* (pp. 3–26). Philadelphia, PA: Lippincott-Raven.
Everly, G. S., Jr. (1985b, November). *Biological foundations of psychiatric sequelae in trauma and
    stress-related "disorders of arousal."* Paper presented to the 8th National Trauma Symposium,
    Baltimore, MD.
Everly, G. S., Jr. (1990). Post-traumatic stress disorders as a "disorder of arousal. *Psychology and
    Health: An International Journal, 4*, 135–145.
Everly, G. S., Jr. (1993). Psychotraumatology: A two-factor formulation of posttraumatic stress
    disorder. *Integrative Physiology and Behavioral Science, 28*, 270–278.
Everly, G. S., Jr. (1994). Brief psychotherapy for posttraumatic stress disorder. *Stress Medicine,
    10*, 191–196.
Everly, G. S., Jr. (1995). An integrative model of posttraumatic stress. In G. S. Everly Jr. & J. M.
    Lating (Eds.), *Psychotraumatology* (pp. 27–48). New York, NY: Plenum.
Everly, G. S., Jr., & Benson, H. (1989). Disorders of arousal and the relaxation response.
    International Journal of Psychosomatics, 36, 15–21.
Everly, G. S., Jr., & Lating, J. (Eds.). (1995). *Psychotraumatology.* New York, NY: Plenum.
Everly, G. S., Jr., & Lating, J. M. (2004). *Personality guided therapy of posttraumatic stress disor-
    der.* Washington, DC: American Psychological Association.
Everly, G. S., Jr., & Lating, J. M. (2005). Integration of cognitive and personality-based conceptu-
    alization and treatment of psychological trauma. *International Journal of Emergency Mental
    Health, 7*, 263–276.
Fairbank, J., McCaffery, R., & Keane, T. (1985). Psychometric detection of fabrication symptoms
    of PTSD. *American Journal of Psychiatry, 142*, 501–503.
Feske, U. (1998). Eye movement desensitization and reprocessing treatment for posttraumatic
    stress disorder. *Clinical Psychology: Science and Practice, 5*(2), 171–181.
First, M., Spitzer, R., Williams, J., & Gibbon, M. (2000). Structured Clinical Interview for DSM-IV
    Axis I Disorders (SCID-I). In *American Psychiatric Association handbook of psychiatric mea-
    sures* (pp. 49–53). Washington, DC: American Psychiatric Association.
Flannery, R. B., Jr. (1992). *Posttraumatic stress disorder. The victim's guide to healing and
    recovery.* New York, NY: Continuum.
Foa, E., Davidson, J., & Frances, A. (1999). *Journal of Clinical Psychiatry,* Entire Supplement 16.

Foa, E. B., Hembree, E. A., Jaycox, L. H., Meadows, E. A., & Street, G. P. (1999). A comparison of exposure therapy, stress inoculation training, and their combination for reducing posttraumatic stress disorder in female assault victims. *Journal of Consulting and Clinical Psychology, 67*(2), 194–200.

Foa, E., Keane, T., & Friedman, M. (Eds.). (2000). *Effective treatments for PTSD*. New York, NY: Guilford.

Foa, E. B., Keane, T. M., Friedman, M. J., & Cohen, J. (Eds.). (2009). *Effective treatments for PTSD* (2nd ed.). New York, NY: Guilford Press.

Foa, E. B., Rothbaum, B. O., Riggs, D. S., & Murdock, T. B. (1991). Treatment of posttraumatic stress disorder in rape victims: A comparison between cognitive-behavioral procedures and counseling. *Journal of Consulting and Clinical Psychology, 59*(5), 715–723.

Foy, D. W. (1992). *Treating PTSD*. New York, NY: Guilford.

Foy, D., Sipprelle, R., Rueger, D., & Carroll, E. (1984). Etiology of PTSD in Vietnam veterans. *Journal of Consulting and Clinical Psychology, 52*, 79–87.

Freud, S. (1921). *Forward in psychoanalysis and the war neurosis*. New York, NY: International Psychoanalytic Press.

Galea, S., Ahern, J., Resnick, H., Kilpatrick, D., Bucuvalas, M., Gold, J., & Vlahov, D. (2002). Psychological sequelae of the September 11 terrorist attacks in New York City. *New England Journal of Medicine, 346*, 982–987.

Gellhorn, E. (1964b). Sympathetic reactivity in hypertension. *Acta Neurovegetative, 26*, 35–44.

Gellhorn, E. (1968). Central nervous system tuning and its implications for neuropsychiatry. *Journal of Nervous and Mental Disease, 147*, 148–162.

Gellhorn, E., & Loofburrow, G. (1963). *Emotions and emotional disorders*. New York, NY: Harper & Row.

Gillespie, R. D. (1942). *Psychological effects of war on citizen and soldier*. New York, NY: Norton.

Gloor, P. (1986). Role of the human limbic system in perception, memory, and affect. In B. Doane & K. Livingston (Eds.), *The limbic system* (pp. 159–169). New York, NY: Raven Press.

Gray, J. (1982). *The neuropsychology of anxiety*. New York, NY: Oxford University Press.

Horger, B. A. & Roth, R. H. (1996). The role of mesoprefrontal dopamine neurons in stress. *Critical Reviews in Neurobiology, 10(3–4)*, 395–418.

Horowitz, M. (1974). Stress response syndrome. *Archives of General Psychiatry, 31*, 768–781.

Horowitz, M., Wilner, N., Kaltreider, N., & Alvarez, W. (1980). Signs and symptoms to posttraumatic stress disorder. *Archives of General Psychiatry, 37*, 85–92.

Janoff-Bulman, R. (1992). *Shattered assumptions*. New York, NY: Free Press.

Kang, H. K., & Bullman, T. A. (2009). Is there an epidemic of suicides among current and former military personnel? *Annals of Epidemiology, 19*(10), 757–760.

Kardiner, A. (1941). *The traumatic neuroses of war*. New York: Hoeber.

Keane, T., Malloy, P., & Fairbank, J. (1984). Empirical development of an MMPI scale for combat related PTSD. *Journal of Consulting and Clinical Psychology, 52*, 888–891.

Kessler, R. C., Chiu, W. T., Demler, O., Merikangas, K. R., & Walters, E. E. (2005). Prevalence, severity, and comorbidity of 12-month DSM-IV disorders in the National Comorbidity Survey Replication. *Archives of General Psychiatry, 62*, 617–627.

Kolb, L. C. (1984). The post-traumatic stress disorders of combat: A subgroup with a conditioned emotional response. *Military Medicine, 149*(5), 237–243.

Kolb, L. C. (1987). A neuropsychological hypothesis explaining post traumatic stress disorders. *American Journal of Psychiatry, 144*, 989–995.

Lating, J. M., Sherman, M. F., Everly, G. S., Lowry, J. L., & Peragine, T. F. (2004). PTSD reactions and functioning of American airlines flight attendants in the wake of September 11. *Journal of Nervous and Mental Disease, 192*(6), 435–441.

LeDoux, J. E. (1992). Emotion and the amygdala. In J. P. Aggleton (Ed.), *The amygdala* (pp. 339–352). New York: Wiley-Liss.

LeDoux, J. E. (1995). Emotion: Clues from the brain. *Annual Review of Psychology, 46*, 209–235.

Liberzon, I., & Sripada, C. S. (2007). The functional neuroanatomy of PTSD: a critical review. *Progress in Brain Research, 167*, 151–69.

Lipke, H. (2000). *EMDR and psychotherapy integration: Theoretical and clinical suggestions with focus on traumatic stress.* Boca Raton, FL: CRC Press.

MacLean, P. D. (1949). Psychosomatic disease and the "visceral brain. *Psychosomatic Medicine, 11*, 338–353.

Madison, D., & Nicoll, R. (1982). Noradrenaline blocks accommodation of pyramidal cell discharge in the hippocampus. *Nature, 299*, 636–638.

Malmo, R. B. (1975). *On emotions, needs, and our archaic brain.* New York: Holt, Rinehart & Winston.

Maslow, A. H. (1970). *Motivation and personality.* New York: Harper & Row.

McDermott, W. (1987). The diagnosis of PTSD using the MCMI. In C. Green (Ed.), *Proceedings of the conference on the Millon inventories* (pp. 257–262). Minneapolis: National Computer Systems.

McDevitt-Murphy, M. E., Weathers, F. W., Flood, A. M., Eakin, D. E., & Benson, T. A. (2007). The utility of the PAI and the MMPI-2 for discriminating PTSD, depression, and social phobia in trauma-exposed college students. *Assessment, 14*, 181–195.

Meichenbaum, D. (1977). *Cognitive-behavior modification.* New York: Plenum Press.

Meichenbaum, D. (1994). *A clinical handbook/practical therapist manual for assessing and treating adults with posttraumatic stress disorder.* Waterloo: Institute.

Munley, P. H., Bains, D. S., Bloem, W. D., & Busby, R. M. (1995). Post-traumatic stress disorder and the MMPI-2. *Journal of Traumatic Stress, 8*(1), 171–178.

Nair, J., & Ajit, S. S. (2008). The role of the glutamtergic system in posttraumatic stress disorder. *CNS Spectrum, 13*(7), 585–591.

National Institute for Clinical Excellence. (2005). *Post-traumatic stress disorder.* London: National Collaborating Center for Mental Health.

Nemeroff, C. B., Bremner, J. D., Foa, E. B., Mayberg, H. S., North, C. S., & Stein, M. B. (2006). Posttraumatic stress disorder: A state-of-the-science review. *Journal of Psychiatric Research, 40*(1), 1–21.

Platman, S. R. (1999). Psychopharmacology and posttraumatic stress disorder. *International Journal of Emergency Mental Health, 3*, 195–199.

Post, R. (1985). Stress sensitization, kindling, and conditioning. *Behavioral and Brain Sciences, 8*, 372–373.

Post, R. (1986). Does limbic system dysfunction play a role in affective illness? In B. Doane & K. Livingston (Eds.), *The limbic system* (pp. 229–249). New York: Raven Press.

Post, R., & Ballenger, J. (1981). Kindling models for the progressive development of psychopathology. In H. van Pragg (Ed.), *Handbook of biological psychiatry* (pp. 609–651). New York: Marcel Dekker.

Post, R., Rubinow, D., & Ballenger, J. (1986). Conditioning and sensitisation in the longitudinal course of affective illness. *British Journal of Psychiatry, 149*, 191–201.

Post, R. M., Weiss, S., & Smith, M. (1995). Sensitization and kindling. In M. J. Friedmean, D. Charney, & A. Deutch (Eds.), *Neurobiological, and clinical consequences of stress* (pp. 203–224). Philadelphia: Lippincott-Raven.

Powers, M. B., Halpern, J. M., Ferenschak, M. P., Gillihan, S. J., & Foa, E. B. (2010). A meta-analytic review of prolonged exposure for posttraumatic stress disorder. *Clinical Psychology Review, 30*, 635–641.

Ramchand, R., Schell, T. L., Karney, B. R., Osilla, K. C., Burns, R. M., & Caldarone, L. B. (2010). Disparate prevalence estimates of PTSD among service members who served in Iraq and Afghanistan: Possible explanations. *Journal of Trauma and Stress, 23*(1), 59–68.

Reiman, E., Raichle, M. E., Robins, E., Butler, F. K., Herscovitch, P., Fox, P., & Perlmutter, J. (1986). The application of positron emission tomography to the study of panic disorder. *American Journal of Psychiatry, 143*, 469–477.

Rizzo, A., Parsons, T. D., Lange, B., Kenny, P., Buckwalter, J. G., Rothbaum, B., … Reger, G. (2011). Virtual reality goes to war: A brief review of the future of military behavioral healthcare. *Journal of Clinical Psychology in Medical Settings, 18*, 176–187

Rochefort, G. J., Rosenberger, J., & Saffran, M. (1959). Depletion of pituitary corticotropin by various stresses and by neurohypophyseal preparations. *Journal of Physiology, 146*, 105–116.

Rodenburg, R., Benjamin, A., de Roos, C., Meijer, A. M., & Stams, G. J. (2009). Efficacy of EMDR in children: A meta-analysis. *Clinical Psychology Review, 29*(7), 599–606.

Rossier, J., Bloom, F., & Guillemin, R. (1980). In H. Selye (Ed.), *Selye's guide to stress research* (pp. 187–207). New York: Van Nostrand Reinhold.

Schlenger, W. E., & Kulka, R. A. (1987, August). *Performance of the Keane-Fairbank MMPI Scale and other self-report measures in identifying posttraumatic stress disorder.* Paper presented at the meeting of the American Psychological Association, New York

Seidler, G. H., & Wagner, F. E. (2006). Comparing the efficacy of EMDR and trauma-focused cognitive-behavioral therapy in the treatment of PTSD: A meta-analytic study. *Psychological Medicine, 36*(11), 1515–1522.

Seifert, W. (Ed.). (1983). *Neurobiology of the hippocampus.* New York: Academic Press.

Selye, H. (1976). *Stress in health and disease.* Boston: Butterworth.

Shapiro, F. (1989). Efficacy of the eye movement desensitization procedure in the treatment of traumatic memories. *Journal of Traumatic Stress, 2*, 199–223.

Shapiro, F. (1995). *Eye movement desensitization and reprocessing: Basic principles, protocols, and procedures.* New York: Guilford.

Shapiro, F. (1999). Eye movement desensitization and reprocessing (EMDR) and the anxiety disorders: Clinical and research implications of an integrated psychotherapy treatment. *Journal of Anxiety Disorders, 13*(1–2), 35–67.

Shapiro, F., & Solomon, R. (1995). Eye movement desensitization and reprocessing: Neuro-cognitive information processing. In G. S. Everly Jr. (Ed.), *Innovations in disaster and trauma psychology* (Applications in emergency services and disaster response, Vol. 1, pp. 217–237). Ellicott City, MD: Chevron.

Sloan, D. M., Feinstein, B. A., Gallagher, M. W., & Beck, J. G. (2011). Efficacy of group treatment for posttraumatic stress disorder symptoms: A meta-analysis. *Psychological Trauma: Theory, Research, Practice, and Policy.* No pagination specified

Sorg, B. A., & Kalivas, P. (1995). Stress and neuronal sensitization. In M. J. Friedman, D. Charney, & A. Deutch (Eds.), *Neurobiological, and clinical consequences of stress* (pp. 83–102). Philadelphia: Lippincott-Raven.

Sripada, C. S., Gonzalez, R., Phan, K. L., & Liberzon, I. (2011). The neural correlates of intertemporal decision-making: contributions of subjective value, stimulus type, and trait impulsivity. *Human Brain Mapping, 32*(10), 1637–1648.

Stein, D. J., Ipser, J., & McAnda (2009). Pharmacotherapy of posttraumatic stress disorder: A review of meta-analyses and treatment guidelines. *CNS Spectrums, 14*(1) (Suppl 1), 25–31

Taylor, S., Thordarson, D. S., Maxfield, L., Fedoroff, I. C., Lovell, K., & Ogrodniczuk, J. (2003). Comparative efficacy, speed, and adverse effects of three PTSD treatments: Exposure therapy, EMDR, and relaxation training. *Journal of Consulting and Clinical Psychology, 71*(2), 330–338.

Tolin, D. F., Maltby, N., Weathers, F. W., Litz, B. T., Knight, J. A., & Keane, T. M. (2004). The use of the MMPI-2 Infrequency-Psychopathology Scale in the assessment of posttraumatic stress disorder in Vietnam veterans. *Journal of Psychopathology and Behavioral Assessment, 26*, 23–29.

U.S. Department of Veterans Affairs, Veterans Health Administration, Office of Public Health and Environmental Hazards. (2010). Analysis of VA health care utilization among U.S. Global War of Terrorism (GWOT) veterans. Unpublished quarterly report (cumulative through 4th quarter FY 2009). Washington, DC: Author.

van der Kolk, B. A. (1987). *Psychological trauma.* Washington, DC: American Psychiatric Press.

van der Kolk, B. A., Greenberg, M., Boyd, H., & Krystal, J. (1985). Inescapable shock, neurotransmitters, and addition to trauma. *Biological Psychiatry, 20*, 314–325.

Van Hoesen, G. W. (1982). The para-hippocampal gyrus. *Trends in Neuroscience, 5*, 345–350.

Vasterling, J. J., Proctor, S. P., Amoroso, P., Kane, R., Heeren, T., & White, R. F. (2006). Neuropsychological outcomes of Army personnel following deployment to the Iraq War. *Journal of the American Medical Association, 296*(5), 519–529.

Wampold, B. E., Imel, Z. E., Laska, K. M., Benish, S., Miller, S. D., Flückiger, C., … Budge, S. (2010). Determining what works in the treatment of PTSD. *Clinical Psychology Review, 30,* 923–933

Weathers, F. W., Litz, B. T., Herman, D. S., Huska, J. A., & Keane, T. M. (1993, October). *The PTSD Checklist (PCL): Reliability, validity, and diagnostic utility.* Poster session presented at the annual meeting of the International Society for Traumatic Stress Studies, San Antonio, TX

Weil, J. (1974). *A neurophysiological model of emotional and intentional behavior.* Springfield, IL: Charles C. Thomas.

Wilson, J., Friedman, M., & Lindy, J. (Eds.). (2001). *Treating psychological trauma & PTSD.* New York: Guilford.

Yehuda, R. (1998). Reslience and vulernability factors in the course of adaptation to trauma. *Clinical Quarterly, 8*(1), 1–5.

Yehuda, R., Giller, E., Levengood, R., Southwick, S., & Siever, L. (1995). Hypothalamic–pituitary–adrenal-functioning in post-traumatic stress disorder. In M. J. Friedman, D. Charney, & A. Deutch (Eds.), *Neurobiological, and clinical consequences of stress* (pp. 351–366). Philadelphia: Lippincott-Raven.

Chapter 22
Crisis Intervention and Psychological First Aid

Throughout this text, we have discussed the body and mind's continuing struggle to maintain homeostasis. As the body struggles to maintain a physical homeostasis (Cannon, 1932), or "steady state," the mind struggles to maintain a similar balance. As a medical crisis is a state wherein physiological homeostasis has been disrupted with resultant physical distress and dysfunction, we then see the possibility of a psychological analogue. A psychological crisis is a *response* to a critical incident or distressing event wherein the individual's psychological balance has been disrupted. There is, in effect, a psychological disequilibrium. This disequilibrium results because the individual's usual coping mechanisms have failed. The predictable result is the emergence of evidence of acute psychological or behavioral distress coupled with some degree of functional impairment.

More practically speaking, a crisis may be defined as a state of acute distress wherein one's usual coping mechanisms have failed in the face of a perceived challenge or threat and there results some degree of functional impairment (see Caplan, 1961, 1964). This description argues more for an acute stress management-based intervention platform rather than traditional psychotherapeutic engagements. In 1952, F. C. Thorne wrote

> "In our opinion, ... preoccupation with depth psychology [psychotherapy] has had a very detrimental effect in causing us to overlook presenting complaints which may be very distressing to the client and about which he urgently wishes us to do something ... Prophylactically, it is probable that many disorders could be nipped in the bud if prompt attention could be given to germinating seeds which may later grow into tall oaks ... Diagnostically, one of our problems is to identify these emergency situations so that we can discriminate what needs to be done immediately...Therapeutically, much will be gained if the client can be made more comfortable even though no deep cure can be effected by first aid methods" (Thorne, 1952, p. 210).

In this chapter, we shall examine crisis intervention and psychological first aid (PFA) as interventions that target acute distress seeking stabilization and acute mitigation rather than resolution and therapeutic growth.

G.S. Everly and J.M. Lating, *A Clinical Guide to the Treatment of the Human Stress Response*, DOI 10.1007/978-1-4614-5538-7_22,
© Springer Science+Business Media New York 2013

Crisis Intervention

The natural corollary of a psychological crisis is psychological crisis intervention (hereafter referred to as crisis intervention). The term crisis intervention may be thought of as urgent psychological/behavioral care designed to first stabilize, then reduce symptoms of distress/dysfunction so as to achieve a state of adaptive functioning; or, to facilitate access to continued care, when necessary.

Crisis intervention is sometimes confused with counseling and psychotherapy. The P-I-E principles, derived and currently adapted from military psychiatry (Salmon, 1919; Artiss, 1963), may assist in this differentiation. P-I-E represents the defining characteristics of crisis intervention:

P—proximity (the provision of services wherever needed),

I—immediacy (urgency; rapid intervention as close to the emergence of adverse reactions as possible),

E—expectancy (the view that the current state of disequilibrium is a result of a current perturbation; therefore, the goal of intervention is to address that current reaction, not cure any pre-existing psychiatric syndrome, even if it is present). Perhaps a useful way of conceptualizing crisis intervention is in the context of medical therapeutics. "As physical first aid is to surgery, crisis intervention is to psychotherapy."

Simply stated, the goals of crisis intervention should include (1) stabilization and mitigation of the individual's symptoms of acute distress, (2) restoration of a more "steady state" of psychological functioning (i.e., psychological homeostasis), and (3) reduction of the level of manifest functional impairment, that is, to assist the person in returning to an adaptive level of functioning (see Artiss, 1963; Neil, Oney, DiFonso, Thacker, & Reichart, 1974; Caplan, 1964). When the goal of restoration of adaptive independent functioning is not deemed to be obtainable, it becomes the responsibility of the crisis interventionist to move the individual in crisis to a more advanced level of psychological care. It should be remembered that the focus of the intervention is always the present crisis reaction. Pre-existing problems are attended to only as so far as they contribute to the current crisis.

In a 1982 study of Israeli soldiers, Solomon and Benbenishty (1986) investigated the core crisis intervention principles of proximity, immediacy, and expectancy. Their investigation revealed that all three were positively correlated with returning to the fighting unit. Further analyses revealed that immediacy and expectancy were correlated inversely with the development of posttraumatic stress disorder. "The effects of proximity, immediacy, and expectancy seem to be interrelated . . . the findings of this study clearly demonstrate the cumulative effect of implementing all three treatment principles" (Solomon and Benbenishty, 1986, p. 616). Most importantly, however, are the implications of the 20-year longitudinal follow-up by Solomon et al. (2005). The study evaluated the long-term effectiveness of the frontline interventions provided to combat stress reaction casualties. Using a longitudinal quasi-experimental design, the same combat stress reaction casualties of the 1982 Lebanon War who received frontline treatment ($N=79$) were compared to matched combat stress reaction casualties who did not receive frontline treatment ($N=156$), and other soldiers who did not experience combat stress reaction ($N=194$). Twenty years after the war, traumatized soldiers who received frontline crisis intervention, following the core principles of proximity, immediacy, expectancy, had lower rates of post-traumatic and psychiatric symptoms and reported better social functioning than similarly exposed soldiers who did not receive frontline intervention. The cumulative effect of the core crisis principles was documented in that the more principles applied, the stronger the effect. The authors conclude, "Frontline treatment is associated with improved outcomes even two decades after its application. This treatment may also be effective for nonmilitary precursors of posttraumatic stress disorder" (p. 2309).

In the wake of a terrorist mass casualty disaster, Boscarino, Adams, and Figley, (2005) conducted a random sample of 1,681 New York adults interviewed by telephone at 1 year and 2 years after 9/11. Results indicate that crisis interventions had a beneficial impact across a variety of outcomes, including reduced risks for binge drinking, alcohol dependence, PTSD symptoms, major depression, somatization, anxiety, and global impairment, compared with individuals who did not receive these interventions. A follow-up analysis (Boscarino et al.), found that 1–3 sessions of brief crisis intervention were useful at reducing various forms of distress from mass disasters.

Boscarino, Adams, Foa, and Landrigan (2006) utilized a propensity score analysis of brief worksite crisis interventions after the World Trade Center disaster. In a prospective cohort design of 1,121 employees, 150 received interventions. Interventions consisted of 1–3 brief interventions by a mental health clinician. Results indicated that the brief post-disaster interventions yielded positive outcome up to 2 years post-disaster in the forms of reduced depression, alcohol dependence, PTSD severity, and anxiety.

Boscarino, Adams, and Figley (2011) found that brief community-based crisis intervention was actually superior to traditional multi-session psychotherapeutic approached when applied after the World Trade Center disaster. Even more interestingly, the traditional multi-session cohort tended to get worse with time, not better. These findings raise serious doubts about the application of traditional multi-session therapeutics post-disaster.

Lastly, Stapleton, Lating, Kirkhart, & Everly (2006) in a meta-analytic review found brief crisis intervention effective in reducing stress, depression, and anxiety among medical patients. A meta-analysis of 11 studies ($N=2,124$) investigating the impact of individual crisis intervention with medical patients yielded a significant, overall moderate effect size, $d=0.44$. The strongest effect of individual crisis intervention was on posttraumatic stress symptoms ($d=0.57$) and anxiety symptoms ($d=0.52$). Specific moderating factors, such as single versus multiple sessions, single versus multiple components of intervention, and level of interventionists' training, were also analyzed. The results support the use of a brief multi-session approach to intervention. The interventionist having received specific training in crisis intervention almost doubled the effectiveness of the intervention. This latter finding suggests that crisis intervention and acute disaster mental health interventions should be applied only after receiving specialized training therein.

A Systems Approach

As defined by Everly and Mitchell (1999), Critical Incident Stress Management (CISM) represents an integrated and comprehensive multi-component approach to the provision of crisis intervention and disaster mental health services. More specifically, CISM is a framework by which the psychosocial aspects of crisis and disaster may be described, analyzed, and responded to. Operationally, CISM is an integrated multi-component continuum of crisis and disaster intervention services (Everly & Mitchell, 1999; Everly & Langlieb, 2003) consisting of a myriad of tactical elements including, but not restricted to, pre-disaster preparedness, acute assessment of need, individual crisis intervention, small group crisis intervention, psychological triage, large group crisis intervention, and follow-up assessment. In 1986, Australian psychiatrist Beverley Raphael wrote most cogently on the need for a multitude of psychosocial services, including PFA, in the wake of disaster (Raphael, 1986). In 1990, the British Psychological Society's Working Party wisely argued that psychosocial disaster services needed to be multi-component in nature, rather than a single one-off intervention applied without consideration for the situation or the recipient population (British Psychological Society's Working Party, 1990). Mitchell (1983), Mitchell and Everly (2000) argued for an even more highly integrated combinatorial program to insure the potency of the intervention. Bordow and Porritt (1979) were presumably the first to actually demonstrate, in a well-controlled investigation, the dose–response potency of combined crisis intervention technologies (also see Solomon & Benbenishty, 1986; Solomon, Shklar, & Mikulincer, 2005), such as we see in CISM. Thus, the natural corollary of the critical incident at the strategic level is an approach similar to CISM.

The CISM formulation is actually broader and more comprehensive in scope than the historical applications of crisis intervention and is more consistent with Caplan's comprehensive (1961, 1964) formulations of preventive psychiatry (Mitchell & Mitchell, 2006). Specifically, CISM embodies:

1. Primary prevention (i.e., the identification and mitigation of pathogenic stressors)
2. Secondary prevention (i.e., the identification and mitigation of acute distress and dysfunctional symptom patterns)
3. Tertiary prevention (i.e., follow-up mental health treatment and rehabilitation services)

The core tactical elements of the CISM model consist of:

1. Pre-incident strategic planning and preparedness as a form of psychological "inoculation" (to enhance "resistance")
2. Surveillance and field assessment/triage capabilities

3. Crisis intervention with individuals (face-to-face or telephonically), including PFA
4. Crisis intervention with small groups
5. Crisis intervention with large groups >20
6. Leadership and incident command consultation
7. Pastoral or spiritually based crisis intervention
8. Establishment of mechanisms for follow-up and referral for continued care

Unfortunately, CISM is commonly confused with terms and concepts such as "debriefing," Critical Incident Stress Debriefing (CISD), and "psychological debriefing" (see Hawker, Durkin, & Hawker, 2010, and Regel, 2007, for interesting reviews of the debate on CISD effectiveness) all of which represent various tactical interventions that may or may not be applied within a strategic continuum of care such as CISM (Tuckey, 2007; Robinson, 2008), but clearly are not synonyms for the CISM-like continua of care which reviews generally recommend (Jacobson, Paul, & Blum 2005; Regel, 2010).

Psychological First Aid

A brief review of current literature on crisis intervention and disaster mental health reveals differing points of view on the methods that should be employed, however (Raphael, 1986; NIMH, 2002). Nevertheless, there appears to be virtual universal endorsement, by relevant authorities, of the value of acute "psychological first aid" (American Psychiatric Association, 1954; DHHS, 2004; Raphael, 1986; NIMH, 2002; Institute of Medicine, 2003; WHO, 2003).

In 1944, a curriculum was developed to implement PFA in the US Merchant Marine (Blain, Hoch, & Ryan, 1944). This was the first known widely used curriculum in PFA. In 1954, the American Psychiatric Association published the monograph titled *Psychological First Aid in Community Disasters* (APA, 1954). That document therein defined and argued for the development of an acute mental health intervention in the "Cold War" era. This early exposition noted,

> "In all disasters, whether they result from the forces of nature or from enemy attack, the people involved are subjected to stresses of a severity and quality not generally encountered...It is vital for all disaster workers to have some familiarity with common patterns of reaction to unusual emotional stress and strain. These workers must also know the fundamental principles of coping most effectively with disturbed people. Although [these suggestions have] been stimulated by the current needs for civil defense against possible enemy action... These principles are essential for those who are to help the victims of floods, fires, tornadoes, and other natural catastrophes" (APA, 1954, p. 5).

This document delineated three important points:

1. The constituents of PFA consist of the ability to recognize common (and one might assume uncommon) reactions post-disaster.
2. The constituents of PFA further consist of the fundamentals of coping.

3. That ALL disaster workers should be trained, not just mental health clinicians.

More recently, the Institute of Medicine (2003) has written,

"In the past decade, there has been a growing movement in the world to develop a concept similar to physical first aid for coping with stressful and traumatic events in life. This strategy has been known by a number of names but is most commonly referred to as psychological first aid (PFA). Essentially, PFA provides individuals with skills they can use in responding to psychological consequences of [disasters] in their own lives, as well as in the lives of their family, friends, and neighbors. As a community program, it can provide a well-organized community task to increase skills, knowledge, and effectiveness in maximizing health and resiliency" (IOM, 2003, p. 4–5).

Raphael, in her seminal clinical treatise (1986) suggests that PFA consists of the following:

1. Comfort and consolation.
2. Physical protection.
3. Provision of physical necessities.
4. Channeling energy into constructive behaviors.
5. Reuniting victims with friends and family.
6. Provision of behavioral and/or emotional support, especially during emotionally taxing tasks.
7. Allowing emotional ventilation.
8. Re-establishing a sense of security.
9. Utilization of acute social and community support networks.
10. Triage and referral for those in acute need.
11. Referral to sub-acute and on-going support networks.

Everly and Flynn (2005) attempted to provide further guidance into the nature of PFA by defining PFA as a compassionate and supportive presence designed to stabilize and mitigate acute distress. They enumerated the core elements as:

1. Assessment of need for intervention (level one assessment) [Note that the present use of the term "assessment" is not intended to refer to formal mental health assessment per se, rather, it is designed to refer more to an appraisal of functional psychological and behavioral status.]
2. Stabilize—Subsequent to an initial assessment and determination that intervention of some form is warranted, act so as to prevent or reduce a worsening of the current psychological or behavioral status.
3. Assess and triage (level two assessment)—Once initial stabilization has been achieved, further assessment is indicated with triage as a viable option. Assessment of functionality is the most essential aspect of this phase.
4. Communicate—Communicate concern, reassurance, and information regarding stress management.
5. Connect—Connect the person in distress to informal and/or formal support systems, if indicated.

At the Johns Hopkins' Center for Public Health Preparedness (CPHP), the following set of guidelines for the practice of PFA was developed. The model is referred to as the RAPID PFA model. The RAPID PFA model was developed specifically for utilization by individuals with little or no formal mental health training to assist both primary and secondary survivors. The Hopkins RAPID PFA approach has shown initial content validation (Everly, Barnett, & Links, in press).

The RAPID PFA model, then, is designed to be taught to public health personnel as well as emergency services and disaster response personnel (educators, administrators, and first-line supervisors could also be trained in PFA). These individuals can then be the functional platform for surveillance, stabilization, and triage. More formal mental health services would be applied subsequent to the PFA as part of the over continuum of care. Such a framework will also serve to allow mental health clinicians to attend to those requiring more advanced clinical intervention. The elements of RAPID PFA are briefly outlined below:

1. *R*eflective listening of

   - The event or critical incident
   - Personal reactions sustained

2. *A*ssessment of need (Maslow's hierarchy)

   - Medical
   - Physical
   - Safety

     - Ability to function so as to discharge daily responsibilities

3. *P*rioritize—Triage benign distress vs. malignant dysfunctional reactions
4. *I*ntervention—Brief cognitive-behavioral interventions

   - Education: Explanatory (Use "Fight–Flight") and/or Anticipatory Guidance
   - Acute Cognitive/Behavioral Refocusing/Re-orienting
   - Deep Breathing/Relaxation
   - Cognitive Reframing

     - Correction of Errors in Fact
     - Disputing Illogical Thinking
     - Challenging Catastrophic Thinking
     - Instillation of a Future Orientation…Hope

   - Delay Making Any Life-altering Decisions/Changes
   - *Caution! Do* Not Interfere With Natural Recovery Processes

5. *D*isposition: Assess that person can adequately function. If person is unable to adequately function, the interventionist should serve as advocate/liaison for further support using friends, family, community, or workplace resources

   - Identify relevant resources
   - Make initial contacts, as appropriate

     - Follow-up, as indicated

Summary

In this chapter, we have reviewed the concepts of crisis intervention and the most recent variation thereof, "psychological first aid" (PFA). To summarize:

1. From both the acute clinical and public health preparedness perspectives, crisis intervention and its subset of acute PFA represent a potentially valuable skill set that is easily applied, not only in the wake of disasters but also on a daily basis responding to the crises of everyday living. Arguably, wherever there is a need for the application of physical first aid, there can be a need for the application of acute crisis intervention technologies.
2. "[A] acute distress following exposure to traumatic stressors is best managed following the principles of psychological first aid. This entails basic, non-intrusive pragmatic care with a focus on listening but not forcing talk; assessing needs and ensuring that basic needs are met; encouraging but not forcing company from significant others; and protecting from further harm. This type of aid can be taught quickly to both volunteers and professionals" (Sphere Project, 2004, p. 293).
3. Boscarino et al. (2011) found that brief community-based crisis intervention was actually superior to traditional multi-session psychotherapeutic approached when applied after the World Trade Center disaster.
4. At the Johns Hopkins' Center for Public Health Preparedness (CPHP), the following set of guidelines for the practice of PFA was developed. The model is referred to as the RAPID PFA model. The RAPID PFA model was developed specifically for utilization by individuals with little or no formal mental health training to assist both primary and secondary survivors. Thus it would seem to be almost "ideal" for training "peer support" personnel in high-risk occupations such as law enforcement, fire suppression, emergency medicine, disaster response, and the military.

The elements of RAPID PFA are briefly outlined below:

1. Reflective listening
2. Assessment of need

   - Medical
   - Physical
   - Safety

   Ability to function so as to discharge daily responsibilities

3. Prioritize—triage benign distress vs. malignant dysfunctional reactions
4. Intervention—brief cognitive-behavioral interventions
5. Disposition: Assess that person can adequately function

Follow-up, as indicated

References

American Psychiatric Association. (1954). *Psychological first aid in community disasters.* Washington, DC: Author

Artiss, K. (1963). Human behavior under stress: From combat to social psychiatry. *Military Medicine, 128*, 1011–1015.

Blain, D., Hoch, P., & Ryan, V. G. (1944). *A Course in Psychological First Aid and Prevention: A Preliminary Report.* Paper read at the Centenary Meeting of The American Psychiatric Association, Philadelphia, Pa., May 15–18

Bordow, S., & Porritt, D. (1979). An experimental evaluation of crisis intervention. *Social Science and Medicine, 13*, 251–256.

Boscarino, J. A., Adams, R. E., & Figley, C. R. (2005). A prospective cohort study of the effectiveness of employer-sponsored crisis interventions after a major disaster. *International Journal of Emergency Mental Health, 7*, 9–22.

Boscarino, J., Adams, R., & Figley, C. (2011). Mental health service use after the World Trade Center disaster: Utilization trends and comparative effectiveness. *The Journal of Nervous and Mental Disease, 199*, 91–99.

Boscarino, J. A., Adams, R. E., Foa, E. B., & Landrigan, P. J. (2006). A propensity score analysis of brief worksite crisis interventions after the World Trade Center disaster: Implications for intervention and research. *Medical Care, 44*(5), 454–462.

British Psychological Society. (1990). *Psychological aspects of disaster.* Leicester, UK: Author.

Cannon, W. (1932). *The wisdom of the body.* New York, NY: Horton.

Caplan, C. (1961). *An approach to community mental health.* New York, NY: Grune & Stratton.

Caplan, G. (1964). *Principles of preventive psychiatry.* New York, NY: Basic Books.

Everly, G. S., Jr., Barnett, D., & Links, J. (in press). The Johns Hopkins Model of Psychological First Aid (RAPID – PFA): Curriculum development and content validation. *International Journal of Emergency Mental Health*

Everly, G. S., Jr., & Flynn, B. W. (2005). Principles and practice of acute psychological first aid after disasters. In G. S. Everly Jr. & C. L. Parker (Eds.), *Mental health aspects of disasters: Public health preparedness and response, revised* (pp. 79–89). Baltimore, MD: Johns Hopkins Center for Public Health Preparedness.

Everly, G. S., Jr., & Langlieb, A. (2003). Evolving nature of disaster mental health. *International Journal of Emergency Mental Health, 5*, 113–119.

Everly, G. S., Jr., & Mitchell, J. T. (1999). *Critical Incident Stress Management: A new era and standard of care in crisis intervention* (2nd ed.). Ellicott City, MD: Chevron.

Hawker, D. M., Durkin, J., & Hawker, D. S. J. (2010). To debrief or not to debrief our heroes: That is the question. *Clinical Psychology and Psychotherapy,* Published online in Wiley Online Library (wileyonlinelibrary.com).

Institute of Medicine. (2003). *Preparing for the psychological consequences of terrorism: A public health strategy.* Washington, DC: The National Academy of Sciences.

Jacobson, J. M., Paul, J., & Blum, D. (2005). The EAP work-place critical incident continuum. *Journal of Employee Assistance, 32*, 28–30.

Mitchell, J. T. (1983). When disaster strikes… the Critical Incident Stress Debriefing process. *Journal of Emergency Medical Services, 8*, 36–39.

Mitchell, J. T, & Everly, G. S. (2000). The CISD and CISM: Evolution, effects and outcomes. In B. Raphael & J. Wilson (Eds.), *Psychological debriefing* (pp. 71–90). Cambridge: Cambridge University Press.

National Institute of Mental Health. (2002). Mental Health and Mass Violence: Evidence-Based Early Psychological Intervention for Victims/Survivors of Mass Violence: A Workshop to Reach Consensus on Best Practices. NIMH (NIH Publication No 02–5138). Washington, DC

Neil, T. C., Oney, J. E., DiFonso, L., Thacker, B., & Reichart, W. (1974). *Emotional First Aid.* Louisville, KY: Kemper-Behavioral Science Associates.

Raphael, B. (1986). *When disaster strikes.* NY: Basic Books.

Regel, S. (2007). Post-trauma support in the workplace: the current status and practice of critical incident stress management (CISM) and psychological debriefing (PD) within organizations in the UK. *Occupational Medicine, 57*, 411–416.

Regel, S. (2010). Does Psychological Debriefing work? *Healthcare Counselling and Psychotherapy Journal, 10*(2), 14–18.

Robinson, R. (2007). Commentary on "Issues in the debriefing debate for the emergency services: Moving research outcomes forward". *Clinical Psychology, 14*, 121–123.

Salmon, T. (1919). War neuroses and their lesson. *New York Medical Journal, 108*, 993–994.

Solomon, Z., & Benbenishty, R. (1986). The role of proximity, immediacy, and expectancy in frontline treatment of combat stress reaction among Israelis in the Lebanon War. *American Journal of Psychiatry, 143*, 613–617.

Solomon, Z., Shklar, R., & Mikulincer, M. (2005). Frontline treatment of combat stress reaction: A 20-year longitudinal evaluation study. *American Journal of Psychiatry, 162*, 2309–2314.

Sphere Project. (2004). *Sphere Project Handbook, Revised.* Geneva: Author

Stapleton, A. B., Lating, J., Kirkhart, M., & Everly, G. S., Jr. (2006). Effects of medical crisis intervention on anxiety, depression, and posttraumatic stress symptoms: A Meta-Analysis. *Psychiatric Quarterly, 77*(3), 231–238.

Thorne, F. C. (1952). Psychological first aid. *Journal of Clinical Psychology, 8*(2), 210–211.

Tuckey, M. (2007). Issues in the debriefing debate for the emergency services: Moving research outcomes forward. *Clinical Psychology, 14*, 106–116.

U.S. Department of Health and Human Services. (2004). *Mental health response to mass violence and terrorism: A training manual.* DHHS Pub. No. SMA 3959. Rockville, MD: Center for Mental Health Services, Substance Abuse and Mental Health Services Administration.

World Health Organization. (2003). *Mental health in emergencies.* Geneva: Author.

Chapter 23
Hans Selye and the Birth of the Stress Concept

Paul J. Rosch
President, The American Institute of Stress, Clinical Professor of Medicine
and Psychiatry, New York Medical College, American Institute of Stress,
Yonkers, NY 10703, USA

> *This chapter has been published in previous forms in Stress*
> *Medicine and the International Journal of Emergency Mental*
> *Health. Used with permission.*

This volume has been dedicated to assist the reader in developing greater proficiency in the treatment of the human stress response. Such a proficiency must be based upon a foundation of increased phenomenological understanding; more specifically, clinical proficiency is based upon an understanding of the phenomenology of the human stress response. Chapters 1–7 have provided the reader with a scientifically accurate yet clinically relevant introduction to the phenomenology of the stress response and its clinical implications and manifestations. But no review of phenomenology would be complete without a historical review. Virtually every chapter of this volume is replete with important historical references. Yet the authors decided to offer a final, rather unique contribution to this volume. Most of what we know about stress is attributable to one man—Hans Selye. While not always correct, Selye is nevertheless the father of the science of human stress. What drove the scientific investigations of human stress was not only the personality of the man but also his brilliance. We offer this chapter as a means of understanding the "background" of the nature and treatment of the human stress response.

For those who knew him intimately, Hans Selye would easily qualify for the *Reader's Digest*'s "Most Unforgettable Character I Ever Met" designation. However, few individuals, especially those in the scientific community, ever enjoyed that privilege because of his apparently aloof attitude. His father Hugo was a surgeon in the Imperial Austro-Hungarian Army, and it was possibly his early upbringing that resulted in his stiff, authoritarian, Prussian demeanor, which many interpreted as an air of arrogance. Born in 1907 in Komarom, a small town that at the time was in the Hungarian part of the Empire, midway between Vienna and Budapest, he attended school at a Benedictine monastery. Since his family had produced four generations of physicians, Selye entered the German Medical School in Prague at the age of 17 and later earned a doctorate in organic chemistry.

In medical school, Selye noted that patients suffering from very different diseases often exhibited identical signs and symptoms in the very early stages of their illness. All had low grade fevers, feelings of malaise, fatigue, generalized aching, and "they just looked sick." Excited about the possibility of studying the biochemical changes and mechanisms that might be responsible for these common findings and possibly lead to some treatment or form of relief,

Selye made an appointment to speak to the Chairman of the Department of Physiology to ask if he could study in the laboratory on weekends or in his free time after school. This individual's full name, including titles, was Hofrat Professor Doktor Armin Tschermak Edler (Nobleman) von Sysenegg. Since that was quite a mouthful, it was agreed that his highest title should be used; he, therefore expected to be addressed as "Herr Hofrat" (Counsel to the Imperial Court). Selye, who was 19 at the time and unaware of this, innocently called him "Herr Professor."

Apparently, that was the only part of his enthusiastic presentation that sank in, because when he had finished, the only response was "Well, if you are that chummy, why don't you just call me by my first name, Armin." Even after his profuse apologies, Selye's request was rejected as being so childish that it was not worth discussing. He was told that obviously, if a person is sick, he looks sick, just as if he is fat, he looks fat. He was warned not to bring the subject up again, and to concentrate on studying for his exams. Selye obeyed this edict and graduated first in his class.

Because of his obvious talent, Selye received a Rockefeller scholarship to study at Johns Hopkins University. He arrived in Baltimore in 1931, rented a cheap room with a kitchenette near the university, and learned how to cook for himself, so that he could save some of his $150 per month stipend. Selye subsisted on mostly canned foods and often referred to this as his "sardine period," since a large tin was a bargain at 10 cents, and he ate sardines daily for months. He was warmly accepted by the other postdoctoral students, and well-meaning faculty wives, who were sorry for "the poor lonely foreign students," constantly arranged parties and social events so that the students could meet people. Although he spoke English fairly well, Selye quickly realized that Americans had their own lingo. On one occasion at a party, when he met a very attractive daughter of a prominent professor, Selye asked if they could meet again to go to a movie or dinner, and he offered to walk her home. Her response was "Yes, but would you give me a ring first?" Selye was petrified, thinking that she meant an engagement ring; he had heard many stories of the strict enforcement of "breach of promise" laws in the USA. When he congratulated another girl on her beautiful complexion by saying that her "hide" was of the finest quality, she did not take the remark as a compliment. Unfortunately, there was no distinction between hide and skin in any of the several languages Selye spoke.

He also had difficulties adapting to faculty life at Johns Hopkins, having been reared in a formal, academic European environment, where the rigid class distinctions were much like the military. Full professors were respected and obeyed as if they were Generals in the Army, and Department Heads were demigods. Selye was appalled at the sight of such distinguished middle-aged and older individuals playing charades and acting in an undignified fashion at faculty parties to which underlings and even medical students were invited. Jackets and ties were discarded, and often everyone seemed to be on a first-name basis. Unable to conceive of Professor Hofrat or his other teachers acting in such a degrading way, Selye suffered from a severe case of culture shock. He was confused, and even considered returning home, but was told by friends that Canada was more European, traditional, and sedate. After making inquiries, Selye found that he could transfer the second half of his fellowship to McGill University in Montreal, to work under the renowned biochemist, J. B. Collip. Although fluent in Parisian French, Selye quickly found out that the language spoken by the Quebeçois was quite different. He quickly adapted and ultimately joined the McGill Faculty, became a Canadian citizen, and, in 1945, moved to his own Institute of Experimental Medicine and Surgery at the University of Montreal.

Selye once told me that he never felt he really had any nationality of his own. He spoke fluent German, Hungarian, Czech, Slovak, French, and English, since each had been his national language at one time or another. Based on the personal experience, I can confirm that he was also comfortably conversant in Russian, Spanish, Italian, and Portuguese, and could understand Swedish and a few other languages, if they were spoken slowly. Whereas his first name was Austrian, his surname was Hungarian. He was looked down on and considered an Austrian when he was in Hungary, and vice versa. When the Empire collapsed in 1918, Selye became Czechoslovakian without ever moving out of his house. The Czechs and the Slovaks had many disagreements with one another, but they both detested the Austrians and Hungarians. After Selye became an international celebrity, Czechoslovakia, Austria, and Canada, all wanted to claim him as their own. He readily accepted these accolades but confided in me that he was most proud of his Magyar Hungarian heritage. He was particularly fond of Hungarian Bull's Blood, and on several occasions when I visited his home, we consumed liberal amounts of this red wine, along with the superb Hungarian goulash he loved to make.

As instructed, he had not thought anymore about the "just being sick" syndrome that intrigued him in medical school, but by a strange twist of fate, the idea resurfaced a decade later at McGill. At the time, only two types of female hormones had been identified, but Professor Collip thought there was a third, and he assigned Selye to this research. Selye was sent to the slaughterhouses with a large bucket and told to retrieve as many cow ovaries as possible, which Collip then reduced to various extracts for Selye to inject into female rats for several days or weeks. The animals would later be autopsied to look for any changes in their sex organs or other tissues that could be attributed to this new ovarian hormone. However, no such effects could be demonstrated, and to add injury to insult, many of the rats became quite sick, and some died. Although there were no changes in the ovaries of breasts, all of the rats showed enlargement of the adrenals, shrinkage of the thymus and lymphoid tissues, and ulcerations in the stomach. This did not make any sense at all, and Selye searched for some explanation. One possibility was that the changes were due to some contaminant in his chemical concoction. One day, with a bottle of formaldehyde, a toxic substance used to fix tissues for microscopic study, right in front of him, he injected liberal amounts of formaldehyde into several rats on a whim, and was amazed to find that it produced identical results.

He began to wonder if other, or all, noxious substances or stimuli could also produce these same three effects, and what ensued is now history. He exposed rats not only to powerful chemicals but also to the frigid Canadian winter, by leaving them exposed on the windswept roof of the McGill medical building. He put others in a revolving, barrel-like treadmill contraption driven by an electric motor, so that they had to constantly run to stay upright. Sure enough, all who survived developed the same pathology in the adrenals, lymphoid tissues, and stomach. Selye viewed this syndrome as a nonspecific response to what he referred to as "biologic stress." He published these findings in the form of a 74-line letter to the editor of the British journal *Nature* in 1936, entitled "A Syndrome Produced by Diverse Nocuous Agents." He avoided using the word *stress* because of previous criticisms that, in everyday English, it implied nervous strain, and he did not want to create any confusion. However, Selye did suggest the term *alarm reaction* to describe this response, since he viewed it as a generalized mobilization of the body's defensive mechanisms.

In subsequent studies, he found that the same changes could be produced by other noxious challenges and stimuli. Animal activists were not as vocal at the time, and many of these experiments could never be performed today, including exposing rats to brilliant lights after their eyelids had been sewn back, bombarding them with constant deafening noise, making them continuously swim to the point of exhaustion to avoid drowning, and subjecting them to intense psychological frustration that bordered on torture. He also showed that the pathological changes characteristics of the "Alarm Reaction" occurred not only in rats but also in mice, rabbits, dogs, cats, and all other animals subjected to such acute insults.

Selye then studied the effects of animals' longer exposure to noxious but not lethal stimuli, noting that this resulted in a "Stage of Resistance" during which the body's defense mechanisms were maximized to adapt to these threatening challenges. However, if they persisted, a final "Stage of Exhaustion" ensued, with deterioration and death. He termed this three-stage response the "General Adaptation Syndrome." He performed numerous, detailed autopsies during the various stages of this syndrome, and observed, on gross and microscopic examination, changes identical to those seen in patients with arthritis, kidney disease, hypertension, coronary heart disease, and gastrointestinal ulcers. He suspected that perhaps "stress" might also cause these disorders in humans as well, and therefore considered them to be "Diseases of Adaptation." Actually, "Diseases of Maladaptation" would have been more appropriate. After thousands of additional experiments, Selye found that he could produce many of these disorders selectively, by sensitizing or conditioning the animals through certain dietary or hormonal manipulations, and subjecting them to different types of distressful insults.

He subsequently traced the pathways and mechanisms responsible for the changes seen in the "Alarm Reaction" and demonstrated that they were due to increased pituitary stimulation of the adrenal cortex to produce steroids that would reduce inflammation. This explained why the adrenals were enlarged. Similarly, the stomach ulcers and lymphoid tissue shrinkage were due to the increased amounts of cortisone-like hormones. If he removed the pituitary and repeated the experiments, these manifestations of damage in different organs and structures did not occur. He reasoned that if he could show how such injuries were caused, then perhaps he could also find a way to prevent them, or to treat the resultant diseases more effectively. These were entirely new and very radical concepts.

As a result of Pasteur's research and Koch's postulates, physicians had always been taught that each disease had its own, very specific cause. Tuberculosis was caused by the tubercle bacillus; pneumonia by the pneumococcus; rabies, anthrax, and cholera by other specific microorganisms, and so on. What Selye proposed was actually the complete reverse of this. He had demonstrated that very different, and even opposite physical challenges such as extremes of heat and cold, as well as severe emotional threats, could indeed produce identical pathological findings. While each of these might also have their own specific hallmarks, such as a burn, or frostbite, all nevertheless caused the same nonspecific changes in the adrenal, stomach, and lymphoid tissue he had first seen following the injection of his new ovarian hormone extract. Perhaps this also explained the curious and very common syndrome of "just being sick" that he had observed as a medical student, in the early stage of illness in patients who later went on to develop very different diseases.

He chose the word *stress* to describe this phenomenon, defining it as "the nonspecific response of the body to any demand for change." It turned out to be an unhappy decision that would haunt him the rest of his life. The term had evolved from the Latin *strictus* (tight, narrow) and *stringere* (to draw tight). This became *strece* (narrowness, oppression) in Old French, and *stresse* (hardship, oppression) in Middle English. In vernacular speech, and in Selye's opinion, stress represented a contraction or variant of distress, which would have been appropriate.

Unfortunately, he was not aware that the word *stress* had been used for centuries in physics to explain elasticity, the property of a material that allows it to resume its original size and shape after having been compressed or stretched by an external force. As expressed in Hooke's Law of 1658, the magnitude of an external force, or *stress,* produces a proportional amount of deformation, or *strain,* in a malleable metal. The maximum amount of stress a material can withstand before becoming permanently deformed is referred to as its elastic limit. This ratio of stress to strain, a characteristic property of each material, is called the modulus of elasticity. Its value is high for rigid materials, such as steel, and much lower for flexible metals, such as tin. Selye complained several times to me that had his knowledge of English been more precise, he would have gone down in history as the father of the "strain" concept.

This created considerable confusion when his research had to be translated into foreign languages. There was no suitable word or phrase that could convey what he meant, since he was really describing strain. In 1946, when he was asked to give an address at the prestigious College de France, the academicians responsible for maintaining the purity of the French language struggled with this problem for several days and subsequently decided that a new word would have to be created. Apparently, the male chauvinists prevailed, and *le stress* was born, quickly followed by *el stress, il stress, lo stress,* and *der stress* in other European languages, and similar neologisms in Russian, Japanese, Chinese and Arabic. Stress is one of the very few words you will see preserved in English form among these latter languages. Twenty-four centuries previously, Hippocrates had written that disease was not only *pathos* (suffering) but also *ponos* (toil) as the body fought to restore normalcy. While *ponos* might have sufficed, the Greeks also settled on stress. Selye's concept of stress and its relationship to illness quickly spread from the research laboratory to all branches of medicine, and *stress* ultimately became a "buzz" word in vernacular speech. However, the term was used interchangeably to describe both physical and emotional challenges, the body's response to such stimuli, as well as the ultimate result of this interaction. Thus, an unreasonable and over-demanding boss might give you heartburn or stomach pain, which eventually resulted in an ulcer. For some people, stress was the bad boss, while others used stress to describe either their "agita" or their ulcer.

Because it was clear that most people viewed stress as some unpleasant threat, Selye had to create a new word, *stressor,* in order to distinguish between stimulus and response. Even Selye had difficulties when he tried to extrapolate his laboratory research to apply to humans. In helping to prepare the *First Annual Report on Stress* in 1951, I included the comments of one critic, who, using verbatim citations from Selye's own writings, concluded that "stress, in addition to being itself, was also the cause of itself, and the result of itself."

I first met Selye in 1949, when he was writing his monumental tome, *Stress.* He was already regarded internationally as one of the world's leading authorities on endocrinology, steroid chemistry, experimental surgery, and pathology. He had singly authored one of the first textbooks of endocrinology, as well as a 27-volume *Encyclopedia of Endocrinology,* covering every aspect of this subject. Selye did everything on a grandiose scale. *Stress,* which was published in 1950, was a huge book of over 1,000 pages, containing more than 5,000 references. However, it paled in comparison to his *Encyclopedia of Endocrinology,* where each of the proposed 27 volumes was the size of a metropolitan telephone directory.

A voracious reader, he consumed everything from the most technical and esoteric journals, in eight languages, to popular magazines and pulp fiction, and he did this with lightning speed. He read as fast as most people could skim, and he could skim a book in almost the time it took to turn pages. However, he seemed to retain as much from skimming a page as most of us would from reading it, because of an amazing photographic memory. He could sometimes quote almost verbatim part of an article he had seemingly only glanced at months before. His favorite lay publications were *The New Yorker Magazine,* with its cartoons by Price and Arno, and some obscure Hungarian publication similar to *The Police Gazette,* the forerunner of *The National Enquirer.* He almost compulsively retained copies of every article in any scientific or lay publication remotely dealing with stress, but it did not stop there. He would write away for reprints of all the pertinent citations listed in an article, retrieve the relevant references from those articles when they were received, and then send away for these reprints, repeating this process over and over, which resulted in a never-ending chain of requests for reprints in different languages from all over the world.

The problem lay in deciding where and how to file this mountain of material. If it had to do with cold stress in hypophysectomized and adrenalectomized rats on a high sodium diet to determine the development of hypertension and/or cardiac enlargement, should he make seven copies to store separately under cold stress, hypophysectomy, adrenalectomy, combined hypophysectomy–adrenalectomy, high sodium diet, hypertension, and cardiac hypertrophy? To overcome this problem, he devised his own "Symbolic Shorthand System for Medicine and Physiology," using mnemonic symbols and arrows that transcended language barriers. It was generally acknowledged to be a vast improvement over the conventional Cutter and Dewey decimal systems, since it provided instant retrieval of pertinent information on any stress-related subject from any publications. Subsequently published for others to use, it went through several editions, until the advent of the computer made it obsolete. Selye eventually amassed a monstrous collection of reprints and books in a library that became world renowned. Unfortunately, it was virtually destroyed by a fire in 1962, but since his classification system allowed him to identify each item, Selye immediately set about completely restoring it by writing to everyone he knew, asking them to send copies of all the reprints on stress in their collections—many of which they had originally obtained from him during the course of their research!

Few people were aware of Selye's superb skills as an experimental surgeon. In order to trace the pathways of the response to stress, it was necessary to demonstrate the role of the pituitary and adrenal glands by studying the effects of removal of these organs. Taking out the adrenals required only an abdominal incision and a rudimentary knowledge of anatomy, but the pituitary posed a formidable problem. In humans, removal of pituitary tumors at the time required opening the skull at a very specific site, followed by 5 h of painstaking surgery to go deep into the brain without damaging other important structures. Outside of Harvey Cushing and a few others, few neurosurgeons were experienced in this trans-cranial operative procedure, and morbidity and mortality rates were high. Removing a rat's pituitary without harming the animal was not much easier, and to obtain the dozen or more hypophysectomized but otherwise healthy animals required for each experiment would have taken weeks. Selye found a way to remove the pituitary within 2 min, and it was so simple and safe that we all quickly learned to do it on an assembly-line basis. It consisted of a rectangular block of wood with a 1-in. staple partially embedded in it at the top, and a very heavy rubber band encircling the bottom. To the right, we had a beaker filled with ether-soaked balls of cotton, next to which was a cage of rats to be operated on. We would put a rat in the beaker, and after it was anesthetized, which took a minute or two, we placed its upper teeth under the staple and pulled down on the body until the mouth was fully open, maintaining this position by snapping the rubber band over the lower portion of the body or tail. We wore flashlights on our foreheads and used magnifying spectacles, which allowed us to see clearly into the open mouth. Once we had identified where the soft palate met the hard palate, we used a dentist's drill to make a small hole in the center of this junction, which clearly revealed the pituitary and its stalk, and much like a little cherry on a stem, it could easily be removed. The comatose rat was then put in an empty cage on the left to wake up, a new anesthetized rat was taken from the beaker and laid out the same way, then replaced by another to be anesthetized. We hardly ever lost an animal, and with a little practice, most of us could obtain two dozen specimens in a half hour. Selye told me he was visited by Harvey Cushing, who had heard about this remarkable achievement, and also taught him how to perform the procedure.

In later experiments, it was necessary to study the effects of removal of part of the liver on the metabolism of hormones and responses to stress, but this had to be done in some standardized fashion, and without damaging other structures. Selye discovered a way to also accomplish this in less than 2 min. Since the lobes of the liver are well differentiated and readily apparent on opening the abdomen, it was simply necessary to tie a suture completely around two of them, which allowed their bloodless removal, resulting in a two-thirds partial hepatectomy. Selye also devised a unique technique for studying the inflammatory response in order to prove that ACTH and glucocorticoids reduced inflammation, while STH (growth hormone) and mineralocorticoids promoted it. This was much more complicated, since it required the ability to quantify the irritant and the body's response to allow accurate measurements and to ensure consistency. There was also the need to separate the two major components of inflammation, the cellular reaction, with its resultant tissue proliferation, and the production of inflammatory fluid. He solved this in an ingenious fashion by shaving the skin on the back of a rat and then injecting air, so that a transparent sac resulted. Various irritants could then be injected and the amount of inflammatory fluid that was produced could be visualized and quantified on a daily basis by trans-illuminating the sac with a flashlight. The effects of stress or of injecting various steroids were easily demonstrated, and the tissue response could be measured by studying the thickness of the wall of the sac under the microscope. This granuloma pouch technique was so simple and useful that we could only wonder why no one had thought of it before.

When I was at the Institute, Selye's average work day was 10–14 h, including weekends and holidays. He habitually rose around 5:30 A.M., took a dip in the small pool in the basement of his house, which was across from the McGill campus, and then rode his bike several miles to work. He was usually the first to arrive and the last to leave. On sunny days, he often put aside an hour or so after lunch to "take a nap in Miami." This was not Florida, but rather a solarium on the roof, where he had had the glass ceiling replaced with quartz, so that he could work on his tan during the winter. As a result of his research on the experimental production of myocardial necrosis and the benefits achieved by Sodi Pallares's polarizing solution containing potassium in acute heart attacks, he filled all his salt shakers with potassium chloride. It tasted horrible, but he was convinced it would protect his heart and reduce risk for hypertension and stroke. Recent research findings have shown that he was absolutely correct. He regularly took garlic pills, he told me, not only because of their health benefits but also because his breath discouraged prolonged, close conversations, especially with strangers who frequently cornered him during his travels, and he used this effectively.

Selye's office was a real inner sanctum, guarded by an anteroom of protective secretaries and librarians. We had to make an appointment with these watchdogs if we wished to speak with him. There was a prominent green and a red light over both sides of his entry door. When the red light was on, which was not infrequently, he was absolutely not to be disturbed by anyone, including these wardens. A green light indicated that he could now be approached with messages that had accumulated, or important incoming telephone calls. For some reason, I enjoyed a somewhat special relationship with him right from the start, possibly because he knew that I had been an English teacher before entering medical school. Although his command of the language was superb, he was still struggling with the confusion surrounding what "stress" really signified, and was concerned about the possible connotations of other words or expressions that might have escaped him. Since most of his publications were now in English, he wanted to make absolutely certain that they were letter perfect, and that he had not overlooked anything.

He was extremely generous, inviting me to coauthor the lead Chapter "Integration of Endocrinology" for the American Medical Association's *Textbook of Glandular Physiology and Therapy,* which included contributions from 32 leading authorities on various hormonal disorders. He had given a presentation to the New York Academy of Medicine in 1951, which they wanted to publish. However, it had been an extemporaneous speech, so he asked me to write something up from his notes and to add anything that I deemed appropriate, or that he might have neglected. When a preprint was submitted for his approval, he again insisted that I be listed as a full coauthor, explaining to the Academy that a major portion of this final version had been my contribution.

Selye was not well received by his peers, who considered him arrogant and aloof. Many also resented that they could not evaluate much of his research without purchasing expensive publications from Acta Inc., which Selye owned completely. Selye explained to me that he had established this company in self-defense to speed up publication of *Stress* and subsequent works, rather than for any financial gain. Conventional medical publishing houses often took up to a year to get a book into circulation, and it was difficult to make any changes once the galleys had been set. However, since he had complete control of Acta, located a few miles away, he could readily insert any late-breaking research to ensure accuracy and timeliness. He had quarrels and feuds with prominent endocrinologists such as Dwight Ingle and George Engel, and although he was not liked, he was respected. Even many of his adversaries felt that he should have shared in the Nobel Prize given to Kendall and Hench. I had arranged for him to give a talk at Johns Hopkins when I was involved in the Endocrine Clinic with giants such as John Eager Howard, Lawson Wilkins, Harry Klinefelter, and Sam Asper. Although he was well received, I was surprised at the somewhat antagonistic attitude of these good friends, who also viewed him as somewhat pompous.

We continued to keep in close contact while I was at Johns Hopkins, and later, when I headed the Endocrine Section at Walter Reed Army Medical Center. He periodically commissioned me to write articles or review his own, even after I entered private practice. Over the next two decades, he became an international celebrity. Because of several books written for the public, which were high on the best-seller lists for months, he was in wide demand as a speaker all over the world, attracting large audiences and commanding huge fees. He had numerous requests for consultations but, to the best of my knowledge, never saw a patient. After I entered private practice, he regularly referred many patients to me, including several very famous individuals. He later developed a rare and usually fatal malignancy, and attributed his recovery to his strong desire to continue his research. He asked me to contribute a presentation on Stress and Cancer to a Symposium that his Institute conducted with Sloan-Kettering in 1978, which led to my present interest in this subject. He was adamant about my helping him establish the American Institute of Stress, and later assuming its Presidency, as well as serving on the Board of his International Institute of Stress.

In the final analysis, much of what he believed and proposed was not correct. However, his real legacy can be summed up by what he often reminded me, namely, that theories do not have to be correct—only facts do. He pointed out that many theories are of value simply because of their heuristic benefit, in that they encourage others to discover new facts that then lead to better theories. Hans Selye's propaedeutic contributions to our understanding of stress and its relationship to health and illness vividly illustrate this maxim.

Chapter 24
Summation and Conclusions

With all its sham, drudgery and broken dreams, it is still a
beautiful world. Be cheerful. Strive to be happy.

Max Ehrmann

"First study the science. Then practice the art which is born of that science." These words of Leonardo da Vinci have served as the guiding spirit of this volume. Perhaps more than any other pathological process, stress arousal represents the epitome of mind–body interaction. We suggested earlier in this volume that proper clinical understanding and treatment of such conditions that so intimately intertwine psychology and physiology demand that the clinician's attention be directed toward the "science" of physiology (and pathophysiology) as well as the art/science of behavior change. Thus, to be consistent with this stated bias, this volume has first introduced the reader to a rather detailed exploration of the physiological nature and foundations of the human stress response. This, as a preface to the subsequent chapters that directly addressed the treatment of excessive stress arousal and its pathological consequences.

A Treatment Model

In order to assist the reader in seeing the phenomenology of pathogenic stress arousal in its larger context, this volume has introduced an epiphenomenological model of the human stress response, from stressor to target-organ effect. This model

G.S. Everly and J.M. Lating, *A Clinical Guide to the Treatment*
of the Human Stress Response, DOI 10.1007/978-1-4614-5538-7_24,
© Springer Science+Business Media New York 2013

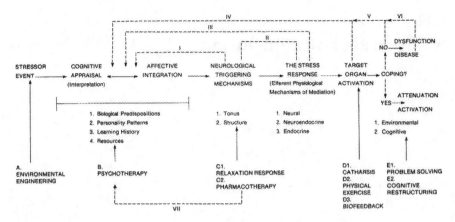

Fig. 24.1 A multidimensional treatment model for the human stress response

was first introduced in Chap. 2 as Fig. 2.6. It represents the larger "overview" of not just stress arousal but its antecedent and consequent constituents. This basic figure was employed again in Chap. 5 (Fig. 5.1) but this time with measurement technologies superimposed. The same basic model was again employed in the introduction to Part II, to demonstrate how treatment interventions might be conceptualized in a coherent and cogent manner via a unifying model. Finally, that same figure is replicated once again to assist in the summary of the text (see Fig. 24.1).

The stress response is predicated upon an event called a *stressor*. The stressor, which can be real or imagined, is typically then perceived and some *cognitive interpretation* is rendered by the individual. The obvious exception would be sympathomimetic and vasoactive stressors, which bypass interpretation. On the basis of the interpretation, the individual will experience some *affect* emerging from the limbic circuitry. Intimately intertwined with the creation of this affect is the activation of a *neurological triggering mechanism* that transduces psychological events into somatic realities, the most important of which is the initiation of the stress response itself: a psychophysiological mechanism of mediation characterized by arousal and possessing three basic efferent limbs: the neural, the neuroendocrine, and the endocrine. These stress arousal mechanisms then exert some *target-organ effect,* that is, signs and symptoms. If *coping* mechanisms employed by the person are not successful, continued arousal and a *psychosomatic disease* is the likely consequence (refer to Fig. 24.1).

Given an understanding of this oversimplified process, we can more appropriately select and implement treatment interventions. Listed in Table 24.1 are the major treatment interventions discussed within this volume and summarized in Fig. 24.1. Having used a treatment model to summarize this volume, let us turn to a clinical protocol to see how it all fits together.

Table 24.1 Treatment interventions

Treatment options	Chapter discussion	Purpose
Environmental engineering	Chapters 7, 8	To allow the patient to avoid or minimize exposure to stressors
Psychotherapy	Chapter 8	To avoid stressors; to reinterpret stressors; to increase perception of self-efficacy
Relaxation response	Chapters 9–15, Appendix B	To reduce pathogenic arousal; to increase perception of self-efficacy
Psychopharmacotherapy	Chapter 16	To reduce arousal
Reduction of target-organ arousal	Chapters 10–15	To ventilate the sress response in a health-promoting manner; to reduce target-organ arousal or dysfunction
Problem solving and cognitive restructuring	Chapters 8, 17, 20, 22	To attenuate excessive arousal

A Treatment Protocol

In Chap. 1, the reader may recall that on the basis of a review by Girdano, Dusek, and Everly (2009), we suggested that the treatment of excessive stress arousal may be categorized into three therapeutic genres, or "dimensions":

1. Strategies to avoid/minimize/modify stressors
2. Strategies to reduce excessive arousal and target-organ reactivity/dysfunction
3. Strategies to ventilate, or express, the stress response

The use of such a summative schema facilitates the creation of a generic, multi-dimensional treatment protocol. This protocol, compared with Fig. 24.1 and Table 24.1, more readily translates into a step-by-step guide for clinical practice and is summarized in Table 24.2.

Having the patient undergo a physical examination is desirable, especially if target-organ disease or dysfunction is manifest. The stress response is the epitome of mind-body interaction. For this reason, it is sometimes difficult to distinguish psychologically induced problems from those problems that possess little or no psychogenic etiology. In some cases, what appear to be stress-related signs and symptoms may in reality be indicative of some neurological pathology or neoplastic phenomenon.

As previously indicated, psychological assessment, especially personologic assessment, can play an important role in treatment planning. The concept of personologic diathesis, when operationalized, provides insight into not only diagnosis but also treatment (see Chap. 7). Broad-spectrum psychological assessments such as the Minnesota Multiphasic Personality Inventory (MMPI) or the Millon Clinical Multiaxial Inventory (MCMI) are useful and efficient assessment tools, especially the latter, which integrates personality assessment (refer also to Chap. 5).

Table 24.2 A general treatment protocol

Physical examination

Psychological assessment (especially personality assessment, see Chap. 5)

Intervention (three dimensions):

1. Helping the patient develop and implement strategies for the avoidance/minimization/modification of stressors
   (a) Patient education (see Chaps. 1, 2 for rationale)
   (b) Environmental engineering (see Chaps. 18, 19)
   (c) Psychotherapy (Chap. 8)
2. Helping the patient develop and implement skills that reduce excessive stress arousal and target-organ reactivity/dysfunction
   (a) Meditation (Chap. 10)
   (b) Neuromuscular relaxation (Chap. 12; Appendix B)
   (c) Respiratory control (Chap. 11)
   (d) Hypnosis (Chap. 13)
   (e) Biofeedback (Chap. 14)
   (f) Psychopharmacotherapy (Chap. 16)
3. Helping the patient develop and implement techniques for the healthful ventilation/expression of the stress response
   (a) Catharsis (Chap. 8)
   (b) Physical exercise (Chap. 15)
   (c) Religious belief (Chap. 17)

The general protocol described in Table 24.2 is not designed to be "blindly" adhered to by the practicing clinician; rather it is provided as a general guide to allow the clinician to formulate a multidimensional, individualized treatment protocol which is far superior to a unidimensional one. Furthermore, aided by the psychological assessment, the treatment plan can be tailored to the specific needs of the patient. Bhalla (1980) found that multidimensional, individualized treatment protocols were generally superior to unidimensional or otherwise "boilerplate" protocols (see also Millon, Crossman, Meagher, Millon, & Everly, 1999).

To reiterate the approach taken in this book, effective treatment emerges from accurate and specific diagnosis. To assess the notion of a personologic diathesis, to actively involve the patient in his or her own therapy, and to recognize the therapeutic value of patient education (see Chap. 8) seems a useful and humanistic approach to the treatment of the human stress response and its target-organ consequences.

A Word About Treatment Adherence

It would be naive to believe or expect that if all of the guidelines in this text are followed, treatment adherence would approach 100%. This is simply not the case. Patient adherence to lifestyle management programs designed to reduce health-related risk factors (e.g., stress management programs) reportedly ranges from a high of 80% to a low of 20%. It has been suggested that adherence to daily home relaxation sessions is as low as 40%. Even adherence to antihypertensive drug regimens may be as low as 60%. See Meichenbaum and Turk (1987) and Blackwell (1997) for a review of these and other treatment adherence issues.

Nevertheless, we hope that our review of the phenomenology and measurement of stress arousal will render clinical success superior to those treatment conditions where such has not been the case. We also highly recommended that the reader review a manual on facilitating treatment adherence before designing any treatment protocols (e.g., Blackwell, 1997; Meichenbaum & Turk, 1987; Millon et al., 1999).

Summary

In conclusion, within this chapter, we have seen two forms of summary: the first, a treatment model, provided a more conceptual summary; the second, a treatment protocol, provided a more clinically practical summary. We hope that, by providing both, we convey not only a sense of clinical practicality but also a conceptual understanding that will allow the reader to move beyond the limits of this volume.

References

Bhalla, V. (1980). Neuroendocrine, cardiovascular, and musculoskeletal analyses of a holistic approach to stress reduction. Unpublished doctoral dissertation, University of Maryland, College Park.

Blackwell, B. (Ed.). (1997). *Treatment compliance and the therapeutic alliance.* Australia: Harwood Academic Publishers.

Girdano, D., Dusek, D., & Everly, G. (2009). *Controlling stress and tension.* San Francisco, CA: Pearson Benjamin Cummings.

Meichenbaum, D., & Turk, D. (1987). *Facilitating treatment adherence.* New York: Plenum Press.

Millon, T., Crossman, S., Meagher, S., Millon, C., & Everly, G. S., Jr. (1999). *Personality-guided therapy.* New York: Wiley.

Appendices
Special Considerations in Clinical Practice

A. Self-Report Relaxation Training Form

When we teach the relaxation response, the typical protocol requires the patient to visit the office between one and three times per week. This limited frequency would make it difficult to realize the desired therapeutic effect of a cultivated lower arousal status. Therefore, patients commonly receive relaxation training "homework." This usually consists of asking the patient to employ the relaxation response once or twice a day. In order to provide a useful forum for communications and to improve compliance, it is highly desirable to have patients complete a relaxation training report from each time they practice the relaxation response. They are then asked to return the completed forms to the therapist at the beginning of each office session. The therapist then uses these forms as a means of reviewing patients' progress.

Following this introduction is a sample relaxation report form that may be used for reporting on the progress made in home relaxation training.

G.S. Everly and J.M. Lating, *A Clinical Guide to the Treatment of the Human Stress Response*, DOI 10.1007/978-1-4614-5538-7,
© Springer Science+Business Media New York 2013

Relaxation Report Form

Name: _____   Time Started _____

Date: _____   Time Finished _____

Beginning SURS* _____ (before the relaxation exercise begins)

Ending SURS   _____ (after the relaxation exercise has ended)

Were you able to relax?   YES   NO   (Circle one)
   If "No", why not? _____
_____

Did your mind wander?   YES   NO
   If "Yes", what were you distracted by? _____
_____

Did you experience anything unusual?   YES   NO
   If "Yes", what? _____
_____

Is there anything else you would like to report? _____
_____
_____
_____
_____
_____

   *The SURS (Subjective Units of Relaxation) indication is a method by which you may indicate your subjective levels of relaxation. A SURS of 10 will be indicative of a dreamlike state of profound relaxation; a SURS of 5 is indicative of how you believe the "average" person feels on an "average" day; and a SURS of 1 is indicative of a panic attack. Choose any number between 1 and 10, inclusive, to indicate your beginning and ending SURS levels.

B. Physically Passive Neuromuscular Relaxation

Earlier in this text, we stated that "neuromuscular relaxation" is the term usually reserved for isotonic and isometric contractions of the striated musculature designed to teach the client to relax. The entire discussion on neuromuscular relaxation has addressed that type of physically active procedure. By far the greater part of the literature has been generated on this active form of neuromuscular relaxation — hence our emphasis on reviewing that form. There does exist, however, what may be considered a physically passive form of neuromuscular relaxation. Here, we address that form of relaxation.

Physically passive neuromuscular relaxation fundamentally consists of having the patient focus sensory awareness on a series of individual striated muscle groups and then relax those muscles through a process of direct concentration. In the passive neuromuscular relaxation procedure described here, there is no actual muscular contraction initiated as part of the relaxation cycle — hence "passive" neuromuscular relaxation.

The physically passive neuromuscular relaxation procedure may be considered a form of mental imagery and directed sensory awareness. Mental imagery as a therapeutic intervention has a long and effective history for a wide range of clinical problems (see Leuner, 1969; Sheehan, 1972). When applied to the reduction of muscle tension, the basic mechanism involved in passive neuromuscular relaxation appears to be useful in tension reduction. In a review of investigations into the role of neuromuscular relaxation in general tension reduction, Borkovec et al. (1978) conclude: "Apparently, frequent attempts to relax while focusing on internal sensations are sufficient to promote tension reduction" (p. 527). In our own clinical experience, we have found passive neuromuscular relaxation to be quite effective in reducing subjective as well as electromyographically measured muscle tension.

There do appear to be several distinct advantages and disadvantages when comparing passive neuromuscular relaxation with a physically active form of neuromuscular relaxation. Passive neuromuscular relaxation has the advantage of having no potential limitations based on physical handicaps, as compared with neuromuscular relaxation that involves actual muscle tensing. Another advantage is the fact that the patient can execute a passive protocol without distracting others or drawing attention to him-or herself. Such is obviously not the case with a protocol that involves actual muscle contraction. A final advantage is that a passive protocol generally takes much less time to complete (usually half the time). The major disadvantage in using a passive form of neuromuscular relaxation is that, like meditation or other forms of mental images, it leaves the patient more vulnerable to distracting thoughts. This may be a significant drawback when using a passive protocol with obsessive-type patients or those who have a tendency to get bored easily.

Let us now examine one sample passive protocol (written as if being spoken directly to the patient). The "preparation for implementation" phase will be fundamentally the same as for the physically active form of neuromuscular relaxation, except for few alterations (refer to Chap. 12). In Step 1 of the preparation for implementation (precautions), the precautions are the same as those described for general relaxation. However, the special precautions for meditation prevail here, as opposed to those for the physically active neuromuscular relaxation. The physically passive component here dictates this alteration. Steps 2 through 4 may remain the same. Steps 5 through 8 may be omitted because of their reference to the actual tensing of muscles. The patient is instructed to breathe normally, in a relaxed manner.

Background Information

It has long been known that muscle tension can lead to stress and anxiety—thus, if you can learn to reduce excessive muscle tension, you will reduce excessive stress and anxiety.

What you are about to do is relax the major muscle groups in your body. You can do this by simply focusing your attention on each set of muscles that I describe. Research has shown that with *patience* and *practice*, you can learn to achieve a deeply relaxed state by simply concentrating on relaxing any of the various muscle groups in your body.

First, you should find a quiet place, without interruptions or glaring lights and a comfortable chair or bed to support your weight. Feel free to loosen restrictive clothing and remove glasses and contact lens if you desire.

Actual Instructions

OK, let's begin. I'd like you to close your eyes and get as comfortable as you can. Let the chair or bed support all your weight. Remember, your job is to concentrate on allowing the muscles that I describe to relax completely.

Chest and Stomach

I'd like you to begin by taking a deep breath. Ready? Begin... (*pause 3 s*) and now exhale as you feel the tension leave your chest and stomach. Let's do that one more time. Ready? Begin... (*pause 3 s*) and now relax and exhale as the tension continues to leave and your chest and stomach are relaxed.

Head

I'd like you to focus your attention on the muscles in your head. Now begin to feel those muscles relax as a warm wave of relaxation begins to descend from the top of your head. Concentrate on the muscles in your forehead. Now begin to allow those muscles to become heavy and relaxed. Concentrate as your forehead becomes heavy and relaxed (*pause 10 s*). Now switch your focus to the muscles in your eyes and cheeks and begin to allow them to become heavy and relaxed. Concentrate as your eyes and cheeks become heavy and relaxed (*pause 10 s*). Now switch your focus to the muscles in your mouth and jaw. Allow those muscles to become heavy and relaxed. Concentrate as your mouth and jaw become heavy and relaxed (*pause 10 s*).

Neck

Now you can begin to feel that wave of relaxation descend into the muscles of your neck. Your head will remain relaxed as you now shift your attention to your neck muscles. Allow your neck muscles to become heavy and relaxed. Concentrate as your neck becomes heavy and relaxed (*pause 10 s*).

Shoulders

Now you can begin to feel that wave of relaxation descend into your shoulder muscles. Your head and neck muscles will remain relaxed as you now shift your attention to your shoulder muscles. Allow your shoulder muscles to become heavy and relaxed. Concentrate as your shoulders become heavy and relaxed (*pause 10 s*).

Arms

Now you can begin to feel that wave of relaxation descend into your arms. Your head, your neck, and your shoulders will remain relaxed as you now shift your attention to the muscles in both your arms. Allow both your arms to become heavy and relaxed. Concentrate as your arms become heavy and relaxed (*pause 10 s*).

Hands

Now you can begin to feel that wave of relaxation descend into your hands. Your head, your neck, your shoulders, and your arms will remain relaxed as you now shift your attention to the muscles in both your hands. Allow both your hands to become heavy and relaxed. Concentrate as your hands become heavy and relaxed (*pause 10 s*).

Thighs

Now you can begin to feel that wave of relaxation descend into your thighs. Your head, your neck, your shoulders, your arms, and your hands will remain relaxed as you now shift your attention to the muscles in both your thighs. Allow both your thighs to become heavy and relaxed. Concentrate as your thighs become heavy and relaxed (*pause 10 s*).

Calves

Now you can begin to feel that wave of relaxation descend into your calves. Your head, your neck, your shoulders, your arms, your hands, and your thighs will remain relaxed as you now shift your attention to the muscles in both your calves. Allow both your calves to become heavy and relaxed. Concentrate as your calves become heavy and relaxed (*pause 10 s*).

Feet

Now you can begin to feel that wave of relaxation finally descend into your feet. The entire rest of your body will remain relaxed as you now shift your attention to the muscles in both your feet. Allow both your feet to become heavy and relaxed. Concentrate as your feet become heavy and relaxed (*pause 10 s*).

Closure

All the major muscles in your body are now relaxed. To help you remain relaxed, simply repeat to yourself each time you exhale, "I am relaxed." Take the next few minutes and continue to relax as you repeat to yourself, "I am relaxed"… "I am relaxed" (*pause about 5 min*).

Reawaken

Now I want to bring your attention back to yourself and the world around you. I shall count from 1 to 10. With each count, you will feel your mind become more and more awake, and your body become more and more responsive and refreshed. When I reach 10, open your eyes, and you will feel the *best* you've felt all day—you will feel alert, refreshed, full of energy, and eager to resume your activities. Let's begin: 1–2 You are beginning to feel more alert, 3–4–5 you are more and more awake, 6–7 now begin to stretch your hands and feet, 8– now begin to stretch your arms and legs, 9–10 open your eyes, *now*! You feel alert, awake, your mind is clear and your body refreshed.

On concluding the initial passive neuromuscular procedure, inform the patient that he or she can use this procedure to relax once or, preferably, twice a day—before lunch and before dinner. Other times can also be useful as well, particularly as an aid for sleeping.

In summary, Appendix B has presented the clinician with a physically passive alternative form of neuromuscular relaxation, not as a prescription, but as an example of how such a protocol might be created. This option is designed simply to expand the clinician's arsenal of stress-reduction interventions to meet the idiosyncratic needs of individual patients. The ultimate assessment of clinical suitability remains with the clinician and should be made on an individual, case-by-case basis.

C. Vascular Headaches and Vasoactive Substances

Many vascular headaches, including the classical migraine, can be induced by vaso-active stimuli. These stimuli interact with what may be a biogenic predisposition for vascular spasticity so as to set the stage for a vascular headache. More specifically, vasoactive stimuli are factors that have the ability to stimulate the sympathetic neural constituency of thusly innervated blood vessels. Through what may be either a vasospastic or a singular vascular rebound phenomenon, these stimuli are believed to have the capability to induce a vascular headache syndrome, including the classical migraine syndrome.

The primary vasoactive substances include the following:

1. Tyramine (a pressor amine)
2. Monosodium glutamate
3. Sodium nitrate
4. Histamine
5. Bright light that creates glare
6. Changes in barometric pressure, especially rapid declines
7. Strenuous physical exercise
8. Loud noise
9. Some sympathomimetics. (Despite the fact that sympathomimetic pharmaceuticals are prescribed to treat vascular headaches, the initial ingestion of some "hidden" or naturally occurring sympathomimetics may be sufficient to induce a vasospasm.)

Foods that are relatively high in vasopressor action include the following:

1. Liver
2. Most cheeses
3. Caviar
4. Sausages
5. Coffee (depending upon quantity)
6. Tea (depending upon quantity)
7. Chocolate (depending upon quantity)
8. Marinated herring
9. Hot dogs (if containing nitrates)
10. Chianti and other red wines
11. Many foods that contain brewer's yeast
12. Fava beans
13. Many fermented or overripened foods

These lists are provided as general information for the practicing clinician. They should not be used to prescribe medication or to alter the dietary regimen of patients. Rather, the information contained herein is designed to serve as a general guide to assist in formulating diagnostic and/or treatment impressions for appropriate medical and nutritional consultation.

D. The Etiology of Panic Attacks: Nonpsychological Factors

Panic attacks represent a very specific form of pathological stress response. Shader (1984) has suggested prevalence in the United States to be 2.0–4.7%. Any clinician who treats stress- and anxiety-related disorders will invariably be confronted with patients presenting some form of panic disorder and its predictable pattern of subsequent behavioral avoidance.

Panic attacks are characterized by paroxymal episodes of ANS hyperfunction usually combined with cognitive–affective symptoms that include dissociation, depersonalization, a generalized morbid fear, fear of dying, fear of losing control, and/or intense emotional manifestation. Proprioception is often interrupted, thus leaving the patient neuromuscularly unstable. Panic attacks typically may last but several minutes, although some attacks could last more than an hour, depending upon etiology.

Although it is widely known that panic attacks can be initiated by psychological factors, it is less widely known that panic attacks are sometimes secondary to variant medical/physiological conditions. Before treating a patient with panic-like symptomatology via psychotherapeutic or psychopharmacological interventions, the clinician should first attempt to determine to what degree medical or physiological factors serve as the etiological basis for the attacks.

Listed below are the most common primary medical/physiological factors that may give rise to secondary panic attacks; clinicians should be sensitive to these factors when constructing a medical history for the patient with some form of panic syndrome.

Acute hypoglycemia may serve as a panicogenic stimulus. It is well-established that the arcuate and ventromedial hypothalamic nuclei contain receptors responsible for the neurological monitoring of glucose. Buckley (1985) has argued that acute hypoglycemic inhibition of the hypothalamic glucoreceptor mechanisms prevents the release of the neurotransmitter beta endorphin and its inhibitory effect upon the panic-related neural networks of the locus ceruleus. When this inhibitory effect is removed, the locus ceruleus becomes far more likely to be massively depolarized. If such depolarization were to occur, a noradrenergically mediated panic attack would most likely result.

1. It has been suggested that some women will suffer panic-like symptoms at the point in their menstrual cycle when progesterone reaches its zenith. This point is usually within 7 days of the onset of menses. This conclusion is based upon the hypothesis that, for some, high levels of progesterone can act as a panicogenic substance (see Carr & Sheehan, 1984).
2. Vigorous anaerobic exercise is believed to be able to induce panic in those patients biologically inclined to suffer from panic disorders. One of the by-products of anaerobic exercise is lactic acid. Pitts and McClure (1967) found that some individuals manifest a biogenic hypersensitivity to lactate (a relative to

lactic acid) and this hypersensitivity is manifested in the form of panic attacks. Thus, factors that lead to a rise in lactic acid may be associated with panic.

3. According to Gorman, Liebowitz, and Klein (1984), there exist several medical disorders that either mimic or induce panic attacks. They include:

(a) Hyperthyroidism
(b) Hypothyroidism
(c) Mitral valve prolapse
(d) Cardiac arrhythmias
(e) Pheochromocytoma
(f) Drug or alcohol withdrawal
(g) Coronary insufficiency
(h) Amphetamine overdose
(i) Caffeine overdose

In summary, the assessment of any medical or physiological factors known to serve in the primary etiology of the panic syndrome seems a reasonable course of action prior to treating a patient with a history of panic-like symptoms.

E. How Do You Cope with Stress?

A Self-Report Checklist Designed for Health Education Purposes

DIRECTIONS: There are many ways to cope with the stress in your life. Some coping techniques are more effective than others. The purpose of this checklist is to help you, the reader, assess how effectively you cope with the stress in your life. Upon completing this checklist, you will have identified many of the ways you choose to cope with stress, while at the same time, through a point system, ascertaining the relative desirability of the coping techniques that you now employ. This is a health education survey, not a clinical assessment instrument. Its sole purpose is to inform you of how you cope with the stress in your life.

In order to complete the checklist, simply follow the instructions given for each of the items listed below. When you have completed all of the 14 items, place your total score in the space provided.

_____ 1. Give yourself 10 points if you feel that you have a supportive family.

_____ 2. Give yourself 10 points if you actively pursue a hobby.

_____ 3. Give yourself 10 points if you belong to some social or activity group that meets at least once a month (other than your family).

_____ 4. Give yourself 15points if you are within 5 pounds of your "ideal" body-weight, considering your height and bone structure.

_____ 5. Give yourself 15 points if you practice some form of "deep relaxation" at least three times a week. Deep relaxation exercises include meditation, imagery, yoga, etc.

_____ 6. Give yourself 5 points for each time you exercise 30 min or longer during the course of an average week.

_____ 7. Give yourself 5 points for each nutritionally balanced and wholesome meal you consume during the course of an average day.

_____ 8. Give yourself 5 points for each time you do something that you really enjoy, "just for yourself," during the course of an average week.

_____ 9. Give yourself 10 points if you have some place in your home that you can go to in order to relax and/or be by yourself.

_____ 10. Give yourself 10 points if you practice time-management techniques in your daily life.

_____ 11. Subtract 10 points for each pack of cigarettes you smoke during the course of an average day.

_____ 12. Subtract 5 points for each evening during the course of an average week that you take any form of medication or chemical substance (including alcohol) to help you sleep.

_____ 13. Subtract 10 points for each day during the course of an average week that you consume any form of medication or chemical substance (including alcohol) to reduce your anxiety or just calm you down.

_____ 14. Subtract 5 points for each evening during the course of an average week that you bring work home; work that was meant to be done at your place of employment.

_____ Total Score

Now that you've calculated your score, consider that the higher your score, the greater your health-promoting coping practices. A "perfect" score would be around 115. Scores in the 50–60 range are probably adequate to cope with most common sources of stress.

Also keep in mind that items 1–10 represent adaptive, health-promoting coping strategies, and items 11–14 represent maladaptive, health-eroding coping strategies. These maladaptive strategies are self-sustaining because they do provide at least some temporary relief from stress. In the long run, however, their utilization serves to erode one's health. Ideally, health-promoting coping strategies (items 1–10) are the best to integrate into your lifestyle and will ultimately prove to be an effective preventive program against excessive stress.

References

Borkovec, T., Grayson, J., & Cooper, K. (1978). Treatment of general tension: Subjective and physiological effects of progressive relaxation. *Journal of Consulting and Clinical Psychology, 46*, 518–526.

Buckley, R. (1985, November). *Post-prandial hypoglycemic anxiety.* Paper presented to the 32nd Annual Meeting of Psychosomatic Medicine, San Francisco, CA.

Carr, D., & Sheehan, D. (1984). Panic anxiety: A new biological model. *The Journal of Clinical Psychiatry, 45*, 323–330.

Gorman, J., Liebowitz, M., & Klein, D. (1984). *Panic disorder and agoraphobia.* Kalamazoo, MI: Upjohn.

Leuner, H. (1969). Guided affective imagery. *American Journal of Psychotherapy, 23*, 4–21.

Pitts, F., & McClure, J. (1967). Lactate metabolism in anxiety neurosis. *New England Journal of Medicine, 277*, 1329–1336.

Shader, R. (1984). Epidemiologic and family studies. *Psychosomatics, 25(Suppl.)*, 10–15.

Sheehan, P. (1972). *The function and nature of imagery.* New York: Academic Press.

Index

G.S. Everly and J.M. Lating, *A Clinical Guide to the Treatment of the Human Stress Response*, DOI 10.1007/978-1-4614-5538-7,
© Springer Science+Business Media New York 2013